REACTIVE
Oxygen Species
vs.
Antioxidants

$^{3}\Sigma_{g}O_{2}$ $O_{2}^{\cdot -}$ $^{1}\Delta_{g}O_{2}$ $H_{2}O_{2}$ $\cdot OH$ HOCl NO·

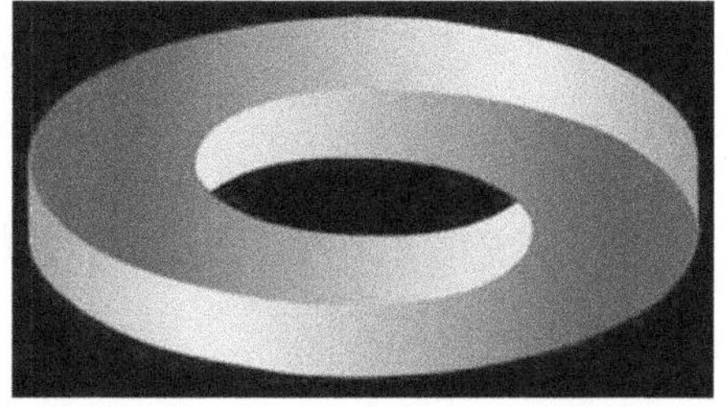

2

The Oxypocalypse or The War That Never Was

BY

PROF RANDOLPH M. HOWES MD, PhD

Surgeon, Scientist, Biochemist, Scholar and Author

Free Radical Publishing Co.
ISBN: 1-885458-08-8
Revised: 2014
ISBN-13: 9781497450417
ISBN-10: 1497450411

Address for communication: 27439 Highway 441, Kentwood, Louisiana 70444-8152, USA. Email: rhowesmd@hughes.net

REACTIVE

Oxygen Species

vs.

Antioxidants

$^{3}\Sigma_{g}O_2$ $O_2^{\cdot -}$ $^{1}\Delta_{g}O_2$ H_2O_2 $\cdot OH$ HOCl NO$\cdot$

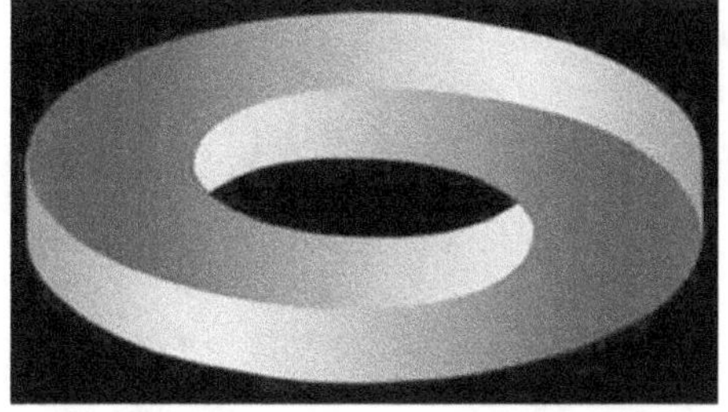

2

BY

PROF. HON. RANDOLPH M. HOWES, M.D., Ph.D.
Surgeon, Scientist, Biochemist, Scholar and Author

Adjunct Assistant Professor of Plastic Surgery (RET.),
The Johns Hopkins Hospital, Baltimore, MD USA

Espaldon Professor of Plastic and Reconstructive Surgery,
University of Santo Tomas, Manila, Philippines

Adjunct Professor of Biological Sciences,
Southeastern Louisiana University

Vice Chancellor/Dean, Louisiana University of Medical Sciences
(Also holds an Honorary Doctorate of Humanities, SLU)

DISCLOSURE AND DISCLAIMER

THE CONTENT OF THE MATERIAL PRESENTED HEREIN IS PROVIDED FOR INFORMATIONAL PURPOSES ONLY.

ANY DECISION BY THE READER TO ACT UPON THE MATERIAL PRESENTED HEREIN IS AT THE SOLE DISCRETION OF THE READER. NO ASSURANCE IS GRANTED OR IMPLIED AS TO THE ACCURACY OR COMPLETENESS OF THE MATERIAL HEREIN. ACTUAL PERFORMANCE, OR THE LACK THEREOF, MAY BE DIFFERENT THAN THE ESTIMATED PRESENTATIONS WITHIN THE MATERIAL. IN NO EVENT SHALL THE AUTHOR BE HELD LIABLE FOR DAMAGES, AND/OR ANY ALLEDGED HARM, INCURRED FROM THE USE OF, OR THE RELIANCE ON, THE CONTENT OF THE MATERIAL HEREIN CONTAINED.

ALL DECISIONS REGARDING PERSONAL HEALTH AND MEDICAL ISSUES SHOULD BE MADE IN CONSULTATION WITH A LICENSED MEDICAL PRACTIONER.

NOTE: This text is not presented as prescription, diagnosis nor treatment for any disease, illness, infirmity or physical condition. Any form of self-treatment or alternative health program necessarily must involve an individual's acceptance of some risk, and no one should assume otherwise. Persons needing medical care should obtain it from a qualified physician. Always consult your doctor before making any health decision.

It is understood that medicine is an ever-changing science. As new research and clinical experience broaden our knowledge, changes in treatment and drug therapy are required. The author and the publisher of this work have checked with sources believed to be reliable in their efforts to provide information that is complete and generally in accord with the standards accepted at the time of publication. However, in view of the possibility of human error or changes in the medical sciences, neither the authors nor the publisher nor any other party who has been involved in the preparation of publication of this work warrants that the information contained herein is in every respect accurate or complete, and they disclaim all responsibility to any errors or omissions or for the results obtained from use of the information contained in the work. Readers should confirm the information contained herein with other sources. For example and in particular, readers are advised to check the product information sheets (or labels) included in the package of each drug they plan to administer to be certain that the information contained in this work is accurate and that changes have not been made in the recommended dose or in the contraindications for administration. This recommendation is of particular importance in connection with new or infrequently used drugs, additives or supplements.

Disclaimers: Please note: only your personal physician or other health professional you consult can best advise you on matters of your health based on your medical history, your family medical history, your medication history, and how information from any of these databases may apply to you. Neither Dr. Howes nor any party involved in creating, producing or delivering this web site shall be liable for any damages arising out of access to or use of this material or web site, or any errors or omissions in the content thereof.

The information given herein is not intended as medical advice. Always consult with your doctor for underlying illness. Before beginning dietary investigation, consult a dietician or a physician with an interest in nutrition. Information is drawn from the scientific literature, web research, and personal enquiry; while all care is taken, information is not warranted as accurate and the author cannot be held liable for any errors and omissions.

Financial disclosure: Dr. Howes has no financial conflicts of interest and is not involved in the sale of dietary supplements or fitness equipment. The author holds no stocks or interests in companies in the food additive or antioxidant supplement business.

Companion Books:

Howes, R. M. *U.T.O.P.I.A. - Unified Theory of Oxygen Participation in Aerobiosis.* © 2004. Free Radical Publishing Co. Kentwood, LA, available at www.iwillfindthecure.org.

Howes R. M. *The Medical and Scientific Significance of Oxygen Free Radical Metabolism.* © 2005. Free Radical Publishing Co. Kentwood, LA. USA. available at www.iwillfindthecure.org.

Howes, R. M. *Hydrogen Peroxide Monograph 1: Scientific, Medical and Biochemical Overview.* © 2006; Free Radical Publishing Co. USA. 200 pages. available at www.iwillfindthecure.org.

Howes, R. M. Monograph 2: *Antioxidant vitamins A, C & E: Equivocal Scientific Studies*, © 2006; Free Radical Publishing Co. USA. 171 pages. available at www.iwillfindthecure.org.

Howes, R. M. *Cardiovascular Disease and Oxygen Free Radical Mythology*, © 2006; Free Radical Publishing Co. USA. 308 pages. available at www.iwillfindthecure.org.

Howes, R. M. *Diabetes and Oxygen Free Radical Sophistry*, © 2006;
Free Radical Publishing Co. USA. Free Radical Publishing Co. USA. 366 pages. available at www.iwillfindthecure.org.

Howes, R. M. *Reactive Oxygen Species Insufficiency (ROSI)*
as the Basis for Disease Allowance and Coexistence:
Extraordinary Support for an Extraordinary Theory
Vol I, II & III. © 2008; 1564 pages. available at www.iwillfindthecure.org.
Howes, R. M. Volume I 501 pages #7 © 2008. Free Radical Publishing Co. USA.
Howes, R. M. Volume II 505 pages #8 © 2008. Free Radical Publishing Co. USA.
Howes, R. M. Volume III 562 pages #9 © 2008. Free Radical Publishing Co. USA.

Howes, R. M. *THE HOWES PAPERS*
© 2009; Free Radical Publishing Co. USA. 211 pages

Howes R.M. *"COFFEE TABLE MUSINGS of the*
Da Vinci in COWBOY BOOTS"
Pithy Prose and Perspicacious Aphorisms. © 2009; 103 pages

Howes, R. M. Reactive Oxygen Species vs. Antioxidants:
"The Oxypocalypse" or
"The war that never was" © 2010; Free Radical Publishing Co. USA. 550 pages.
available at www.iwillfindthecure.org.

Howes R.M. *Death in Small Doses?:*
Antioxidant Vitamins A, C & E in the 21st Century
Book One: *A Health Impact Statement For The Layman*
© 2010; Trafford Publishing. Indianapolis, USA. 90 pages

Howes R.M. *Antioxidant Vitamins are Making A Killing;*
Antioxidant Vitamins A, C & E in the 21st Century
Book Two: *A Health Impact Statement For The Medical Scientist*
© 2010; 184 pages

Howes R.M. *Antioxidant Overkill:* An antioxidant guide for the educated consumer.
© 2011. CreateSpace and Free Radical Publishing Co. USA. 421 pages.

Howes R.M. *Dangers Of Excessive Antioxidants in Cancer Patients.* © 2011.
CreateSpace and Free Radical Publishing Co. 524 pages.

Companion Papers:

Dr. Howes has authored over 350 medical publications in health related editorials.

Citation: R. Howes: Mythology of Antioxidant Vitamins?. *The Journal of Evidence-Based Alternative and Complimentary Medicine.* April, 2011. 16(2): 149-189.

Citation: R. Howes: Cancer Therapy: A Review with Scientific Validation for the Role of Electronically Modified Oxygen Derivatives in Oncologic Treatment Modalities. *The Internet Journal of Alternative Medicine.* 2010 Volume 8 Number 1.

Citation: R. Howes: Hydrogen Peroxide: A review of a scientifically verifiable omnipresent ubiquitous essentiality of obligate, aerobic, carbon-based life forms. *The Internet Journal of Plastic Surgery.* 2010 Volume 7 Number 1.

Howes M.D., PhD., R. (2009). Dangers of Antioxidants in Cancer Patients: A Review. *PHILICA.COM Article number 153.* Published 7th February, 2009. (20 pages)

Howes M.D., PhD., R. (2008). Aging and anti-aging claims: a review on antioxidant vitamins A, C & E. *PHILICA.COM Article number 116*. Published on 12th January, 2008. (16 pages)

Howes M.D., PhD., R. (2007). Sleep: An original "radical" proposal. *PHILICA.COM Observation number 42*. Published on 5th October, 2007. (1 page)

Howes M.D., PhD., R. (2007). Antioxidant Vitamins A, C & E; Death in Small Doses and Legal Liability? *PHILICA.COM Article number 89*. Published on 5th April, 2007. (23 pages)

Howes M.D., PhD., R. (2007). Cancer, Apoptosis and Reactive Oxygen Species: A New Paradigm. *PHILICA.COM Article number 86*. Published on 26th February, 2007. (11 pages)

Howes M.D., PhD., R. (2007). Antioxidant Vitamins A, C and E: Assessing Potential for Harm. *PHILICA.COM Article number 83*. Published on 15th February, 2007. (14 pages)

Howes M.D., PhD., R. (2007). The Consequent Downfall of the Free Radical Theory. *PHILICA.COM Article number 75*. Published on 22nd January, 2007. (9 pages)

Howes, R.M.: "The Free Radical Fantasy," The Annals of New York Academy of Sciences, 2006, Vol. 1067, pp. 22-26.

(Howes, 2005) (Howes, R.M. Tumoricidal Activity of An Injectable Singlet Oxygen System Generated From Physiological Agents: The Howes Singlet Oxygen Cancer Therapy System). In The Medical and Scientific Significance of Oxygen Free Radical Metabolism. © 2005. Free Radical Publishing Co. Kentwood, LA. pp. 893-912).

(Howes, Farber, 2005) (Howes, R.M. and Farber, G. Tumoricidal Activity of the Howes Singlet Oxygen Delivery System in Human Basal Cell Carcinoma. In The Medical and Scientific Significance of Oxygen Free Radical Metabolism. © 2005. Free Radical Publishing Co. Kentwood, LA. pp. 883-892).

(Howes et al, 1977) (Howes, R.M., Steele, R.H. and Hoopes, J.E., The role of Electronic excitation states in collagen biosynthesis, Persp. In Biol. And Med., Summer 1977, 20; 4:539-544).

(Howes, Steele, 1976) (Howes, R.M., Steele, R.H. and Hoopes, J.E., Peroxide induced Chemiluminescence in an in vitro proline hydroxylation system, 1976, 8; 1:77-84).

(Howes et al, 1976) (Howes, R. M., Allen, R.C., Su, C.T. and Hoopes, J.E., Altered polymorphonuclear leukocyte bioenergetics in patients with thermal injury, the Surgical Forum, 1976, 27:558-560).

(Howes, Steele, 1972) (Howes, R.M. and Steele, R.H., Microsomal chemiluminescence induced by NADPH and its relation to aryl-hydroxylations, Res Commun. Chem. Path. Pharmacol., March 1972, 3; 2:349-357).

(Howes, Steele, 1971) (Howes, R. M. and Steele, R. H., Microsomal chemiluminescence induced by NADPH and its relation to lipid peroxidation, Res. Commun. Chem. Path. Pharmacol., July-Sept. 1971, 2; 4 & 5:619-626).

I despise precious time wasted,
for it alone, is the unfinished canvas
displaying the portrait of my life.
R. M. Howes, M.D., Ph.D.
9/7/09

"We are what we repeatedly do. Excellence then, is not an act, but a habit." ~Aristotle

OTHER BOOKS

PUBLISHED: Partial list.

The Fire Eaters, Molding your own destiny more easily, Carnivore Press, © 1982

Uplift, The Answer Book to your plastic and cosmetic surgery questions, Carnivore Press, © 1986

The Pundit Speaks, vol. I. An Anthology of Neoclassical Poetic Philosophy, Carnivore Press, © 1990

The Pundit Speaks, Volume II, An Anthology of Neoclassical Poetic Philosophy, Free Radical Press, © 1994

The Pundit Speaks, Volume III, An Anthology of Neoclassical Poetic Philosophy, Free Radical Press, © 1996

The Pundit Speaks, Volume IV, An Anthology of Neoclassical Poetic Philosophy, Free Radical Press, © 2000

The Fable of the Chocolate Covered Strawberry Coloring Book, Free Radical Press, © 2001

The Pundit Speaks, Volume IV, An Anthology of Neoclassical Poetic Philosophy, Free Radical Press, © 2003

The Pundit Speaks, Volume V, An Anthology of Neoclassical Poetic Philosophy, Trafford Publishing, © 2009

Coffee Table Musings of The DaVinci In Cowboy Boots, Trafford Publishing, © 2010

Death In Small Doses? Trafford Publishing, © 2010

Antioxidant Overkill, CreateSpace and Free Radical Publishing, © 2011

Dangers of Excessive Antioxidants in Cancer Patients, CreateSpace and Free Radical Publishing, © 2011

Heart Disease and Antioxidant Failures, CreateSpace and Free Radical Publishing, © 2011

Antioxidant Failures and Dangers, CreateSpace and Free Radical Publishing, © 2011

Anti-Aging Anti-oxidant Scams, CreateSpace and Free Radical Publishing, © 2011

Sports, Athletes, Exercise Facts and Antioxidant Myths, CreateSpace and Free Radical Publishing, © 2011

Alzheimer's Disease: Forget Antioxidants and Supplements, CreateSpace and Free Radical Publishing, © 2012

Antioxidants Linked To Deadly Unintended Consequences, CreateSpace and Free Radical Publishing, © 2012

Sex, Performance, Reproduction, Naked Radicals and Antioxidants, CreateSpace and Free Radical Publishing, © 2012
U.T.O.P.I.A.: Unified Theory of Oxygen Participation In Aerobiosis, CreateSpace and Free Radical Publishing, © 2013
Diabetes and Oxygen Free Radical Sophistry, CreateSpace and Free Radical Publishing, © 2014, revised

Available at: www.philica.com
www.medi.philica.com
www.iwillfindthecure.org
www.amazon.com

If you believe the implausible,
you will accept the indefensible and
not recognize the inexcusable.
R. M. Howes, M.D., Ph.D.
6/5/11

DOC
R_xANDOLPH
HOWES

RAD!CAL

ABOUT THE AUTHOR

Dr. Randolph M. Howes M.D., Ph.D.

Biographical sketch:

As a champion of the people, Dr. Howes anticipates and hopes for the active involvement of all connected parties (patients, caregivers, healthcare professionals, etc.) as an integral approach to educating consumers and the public about the potential dangers of excessive antioxidant-containing supplements and "antioxidant stacking."

Some people are born with a silver spoon in their mouth but Dr. Howes had to earn his. Even as a child, Dr. Howes could think with adult clarity. He could envision his future but it would require "decades of dedication" to make it a reality.

From childhood, Dr. Howes was motivated to become a medical doctor and scientist. Assuredly, having been born on a small strawberry farm in rural Louisiana, his journey to the top has proved to be arduous and demanding.

However, he was fortunate to acquire the confidence of Sister Elizabeth at St. Joseph's school and went on to gain the support of his high school speech teacher, Mrs. Iris Brann, who also had strong beliefs in his abilities and potential. Ultimately, with the help of his guitar and his singing ability, he defeated the star quarter back of the high school football team to become the president of the student body.

With the aid of a $25 dollar legislative scholarship, he went on to Southeastern Louisiana College (SLC). At SLC, he was selected for honors chemistry, made the Dean's list, worked at the Psychology Research Lab forty hours a week, maintained a premed study load, and was elected president of the Junior Class and the Interfraternity Council.

To earn badly needed funds, he played music on weekends in a small combo, The Three Blind Mice. Next, he matriculated to Tulane University School of Medicine.

His initial dream was to try to combine both medicine and science. In that regard, he began work as a technician with Dr. Andrew Schally at the Endocrine Polypeptide Lab in the isolation of thyrotropin releasing factor. This work led to a Nobel Prize for Dr. Schally.

Dr. Howes had been highly impressed with the enthusiasm of biochemist, Dr. Richard H. Steele, who accepted him as a doctoral candidate under his tutelage. Dr. Howes graduated in the top 10 of his class, won the Louisiana Pathology Association Award, was elected to the Sigma Xi honor fraternity and was the first in the history of Tulane to become a Doctor of Medicine and a Ph.D. in biochemistry concurrently.

Next, he was selected to pursue a career in surgery at the prestigious Johns Hopkins Hospital.

Unbelievably, at Dr. Howes' urging, he was allowed to operate his own research lab during his surgical internship and residency training while at Johns Hopkins Hospital. He worked hand in hand with the greats in American medicine and surgery.

Independently, he garnered grants, trained lab techs, wrote papers, slept on the cold floor, proudly served as a Captain in the U.S. Army Reserves Medical Corp and finished with board eligibility in both general and plastic surgery in an unheard of six year period.

In another first, he was appointed as an Adjunct Assistant Professor of Plastic Surgery at Johns Hopkins Hospital.

For decades, Dr. Howes gave unselfishly to pro bono medical missions in the Philippines and he holds the Ernesto Espaldon Chair as Professor of Plastic Surgery at the University of Santo Tomas.

Upon retirement from a career in cosmetic plastic surgery, he is living his dream of trying to revolutionize the treatment of cancer, heart disease, HIV/AIDS and malaria, with his in depth knowledge of the arcane biochemistry of oxygen metabolism. He is a work in progress! Dedicated and passionate, he is on a mission for mankind.

Dr. Howes invented the triple lumen venous catheter, which has been credited with helping save the lives of over 20 million critically ill patients worldwide. His catheter became the number one venous catheter in the world and his name is well recognized in over 100 countries. He has been recognized as a humanitarian, visionary, entrepreneur, singer, songwriter, inventor and author.

He received the Harper Award for innovative research from the American College for Advancement in Medicine, served as their keynote speaker and his peers refer to him as "a walking encyclopedia on oxygen metabolism."

He is a Dr. Norman Vincent Peale Unsung Hero award winner, which recognized his awesome versatility. Additionally, even though he is humble and does not like talking about it, he is a self made multi-millionaire.

He is currently doing extensive research on cures for cancer and heart disease and development of revolutionary treatment modalities. He has written 16 books over the past 8 years on the subject of oxygen metabolism, as it relates to protection from cancer, heart disease, diabetes, malaria, HIV/AIDS, Alzheimer's disease, aging and arthritis. He has written many scientific and medical papers and has lectured nationally and internationally.

His research has shown that currently common antioxidant vitamins, such as vitamins A & E, (and vitamin C to a lesser extent) can be harmful and that oxygen free radicals protect us from bacterial, fungal and viral infections and they help to control cancer growth.

He has developed an effective, inexpensive singlet oxygen generating system, from orthomolecular agents, for the treatment of cancer and heart disease. He is passionate about his research and hopes to have his discoveries at the patient's bedside in his lifetime. Admittedly, this is an extremely ambitious goal.

There are over 8,000 pages in his magnum opus and at the Howes World Selective Library on Oxygen Metabolism. **Over 3,000 pages of his opus are available online in a searchable format www.iwillfindthecure.org** © by R.M. Howes

NOTE: An avid researcher, Dr. Howes has authored more than 350 original publications, including over 30 medical and scientific books, such as Death In Small Doses (Antioxidant vitamins A, C & E in the 21st Century), Antioxidant Overkill and Dangers of Excessive Antioxidants In Cancer Patients. He has written numerous articles for medical and consumer publications, including The Journal of American Academy of Cosmetic Surgery, Annals of the New York Academy of Science, The Journal of Evidence Based Complementary And Alternative Medicine, The Baton Rouge Advocate, and The Houma Courier. He has a weekly science/

medicine column in the Hammond Daily Star and The Ponchatoula Times. His research interests include truthful reporting of antioxidant dangers, adverse effects of vitamins A, C & E, other antioxidant's deadly unintended consequences, free radicals, oxygen metabolism, and cancer and heart disease treatment and prevention, global health care policy, and oxidative means to revolutionize treating and preventing HIV/AIDS and malaria.

Dr. Howes is also an active and well-known speaker and media personality, having been featured on PBS's The American Health Journal, WWL-TV New Orleans and WDSU-TV New Orleans, Sirius/XM satellite radio, as well as many other national talk and news shows across America.

In 2013, he received from the American College for Advancement In Medicine the first Charles Farr Award for "excellence in oxidative medicine."

After reading Dr. Howes' book, *Dangers of Excessive Antioxidants In Cancer Patients,* Robert C. Allen, M.D., Ph.D., Chairman of the Department of Pathology at Creighton Medical School in Omaha, Nebraska, described Dr. Howes this way,

"During my forty-five-year association with Dr. Randolph M. Howes, I've been consistently impressed, and sometimes exhausted, by his brilliance, energy and intensity. Over the past several years his attention has been focused on debunking the meme that oxidants are "bad" and antioxidants are "good". We should all appreciate that oxidation provides the energy that drives all complex life forms. *Dangers of Excessive Antioxidants in Cancer Patients* presents convincing arguments with supporting evidence that simplistically assuming antioxidants are somehow "good" is not valid. Dr. Howes is *The Scientific Voyager* poetically described herein, and this book is the product of his voyage."

Dr. Allen answered the question, "If you or a loved one had cancer, would you now take or recommend antioxidants?" He answered, "If I had cancer and was undergoing chemotherapy, I certainly would not be taking BHT, vitamins A and E, or any "antioxidant" formulation, nor would I recommend antioxidants to my family, loved ones, or anyone else." His support of Dr. Howes' work is clear and undeniable.

Following the same scenario, Dr. Robert Muller, M.D. (Ob-Gyn) answered this way: "Dr Howes book shows the extensive research done on antioxidants, BUT the difficulty lies in overcoming the social norms established by the brainwashing of the public by the pharmaceutical industry. If common sense prevails, the choice becomes very clear—antioxidants are worthless in the prevention and treatment of cancer (and CVD)." Robert Muller, M.D. 5-12-11

These are just two examples of highly qualified, medically-involved, individuals who recognize the innovative brilliance of Dr. Howes' new approach to disease prevention, causation and coexistence.

Dr. Howes' origin from a small Louisiana farming community imbedded in him a unique level of morality, ethical behavior and common sense. He feels that common sense is "commonly missing" in the world of medical science today. True, one must be trained to deal with the arcane biological and physiological sciences but one must also be open-minded and willing to rely on common sense, especially when certain scientific theories go against or fly in the face of inductive/deductive reasoning and clear thinking.

If you can not see what is illogical,
you can not fix the irreconcilable.
If you can not sense flawed logic,
you will never taste truth.
R. M. Howes, M.D., Ph.D.
6/5/11

Dr. Howes spent over a quarter of a century in educational training to prepare himself for the challenging world of medical science. He is fulfilling his dreams of making significant contributions to the prevention and cure of some of mankind's most deadly diseases, such as cancer, heart disease, malaria and HIV/AIDS.

He feels strongly that he must place his innovative ideas onto the public forum, utilizing printed media and the world wide web. Thus, others can evaluate the validity of his contributions and continue in the pursuit of his dreams.

DEDICATION

To the country and educational system that has allowed me the opportunity to pursue the excitement of discovery

Note: == indicates an article related to EMOD induced apoptosis

TABLE OF CONTENTS:

The U.T.O.P.I.A. Institute and Free Radical Publishing Co.

DISCLOSURE AND DISCLAIMER 1
COMPANION BOOKS: 3
COMPANION PAPERS: 4
ABOUT THE AUTHOR 9
DEDICATION 15
"FINDING YOUR INNER RADICAL SELF" 33

1.0.0.0 INTRODUCTION 41
Nick Nolte
Angelina Jolie
Bruce Ames

- 1.0.0.1 Pall/Levine snake oil 43
- 1.0.0.2 Avoid prolix writing and overly wordy sophistry 46
- 1.0.0.3 Attempts to brain wash children on the dangers of EMODs 47
- 1.0.0.4 Skippy and Oaf: The Battle Against Oxygen Radicals 47
- 1.0.0.5 How some antioxidants can harm health 49
- 1.0.0.6 Calorie restriction and reduced oxidative stress 49
- 1.0.0.7 Exercise and antioxidants 50
- 1.0.0.8 Clinical trials of antioxidant supplements 52
- 1.0.0.9 Antioxidants used as food additives 53
- 1.0.1.0 Flavonoid polyphenolics (also known as bioflavonoids) 54
- 1.0.1.1 Other organic antioxidants 55
- 1.0.2.0 Speculation on anoxia and changes following death 55
- 1.0.2.1 Inflammation as the root of all evil 57
- 1.0.2.2 Hyperthermia speculation 58
- 1.0.3.0 Peroxidases 59
- 1.0.3.1 H_2O_2 60
- 1.0.3.2 Free Radical Shift: Antioxidants may not increase life span 62
- 1.0.3.3 Hekimi: C elegans and blocked SOD increases lifespan 62
- 1.0.3.4 Hekimi has problem with free radical theory 64
- 1.0.4.0 More Americans getting multiple chronic illnesses 65

- 1.0.4.1 Skin Cancer May Increase Risk of Other Cancers.......67
- 1.0.5.0 General discussion of cancer and oxygen.......69
- 1.0.5.1 The antioxidant, lactic acid == 71
- 1.0.6.0 Low O_2, cells mutate and high O_2, cells stop.......71
- 1.0.7.0 Tumor necrosis factor (TNF) and oxygen free radicals.......72
- 1.0.7.1 Tumor necrosis factor (TNF) and oxygen free radicals: potential effects for immunity.......72
- 1.0.7.2 Hydrogen Peroxide Enhances Tumor Necrosis Factor-Alpha Toxicity in Inducing Human Vascular Endothelial Cell Apoptosis: Reversal with Propofol == 73
- 1.0.7.3 TNF Blockers May Increase Cancer Risk in Kids == 75
- 1.0.8.0 Use of hydrogen peroxide in treating cancer.......76
- 1.0.8.1 High-Fat Diet Dramatically Increases Cancer Metastasis.......78
- 1.0.8.2 Dramatic Increase in Metastasis.......79
- 1.0.8.3 Increase in Circulating Tumor Cells.......80
- 1.0.8.4 Lack of Oxygen - the potential ability of Cancer survival and spread...81
- 1.0.8.5 Lack of oxygen and gangrene.......83
- *1.0.8.6 What are the causes of gangrene?*.......83
- *1.0.8.7 What are the risk factors for gangrene?*.......84
- *1.0.8.8 What are the symptoms of gangrene?*.......85
- 1.0.9.0 Methyglyoxal, Retine, Promine (Dr. Szent-Gyorgyi) 87
- 1.0.9.1 Chlorine.......89
- 1.0.9.2 A Doctor's Shocking Closed-Door Confession.......91
- 1.1.0.0 The Prime Cause and Prevention of Cancer: Dr. Otto Warburg.......93
- 1.1.0.1 The Prime Cause and Prevention of Cancer 97
- 1.1.0.2 The Fermentation of Morris Hepatomas.......99
- 1.1.0.3 Transformation of Embryonic Metabolism into Cancer Metabolism....100
- 1.1.0.4 Thermodynamics.......103
- 1.1.0.5 Chemistry of respiration.......104
- 1.1.0.6 A comment by Wilhelm H on the relationship of cancer researcher Dr. Johanna Budwig with Otto Warburg, Szent-Györgyi and other illustrious scientists:.......109
- 1.1.1.0 What Really Killed the Dinosaurs?.......110
- 1.1.1.1 Can glucose block oxygen transport 113
- 1.1.1.2 Diabetes, microvascular complications, and cardiovascular complications: what is it about glucose? 113
- 1.1.1.3 Organ Transplant Increases Risk of Skin Cancer 117
- 1.1.1.4 Why Organ Transplant Increases Risk.......117
- 1.1.1.5 Free radicals in the atmosphere.......118
- 1.1.1.6 The changing composition of the global atmosphere 119
- 1.1.1.7 Bistability of atmospheric oxygen and the Great Oxidation 122

- 1.1.2.0 Vitamin Mania: The Truth about Antioxidants 122
- 1.1.2.1 We love our vitamins 123
- 1.1.2.2 Rogue free radicals 123
- 1.1.2.3 Free to destroy 124
- 1.1.3.0 BHT and BHA 125
- 1.1.3.1 Antioxidants BHT and BHA can be carcinogenic and anti-carcinogenic 128
- 1.1.3.2 Are BHA and BHT safe? 130
- 1.1.3.3 BHA and BHT are tumor promoters 130
- 1.2.0.0 EMOD-induced apoptosis == 130
- 1.2.0.1 Oxygen Radicals Induce Poly(ADP-Ribose) Polymerase-Dependent Cell Death in Cytotoxic Lymphocytes 130
- 1.2.0.2 Methylglyoxal - methylglyoxal bis(guanylhydrazone) (mitoguazone) 133
- 1.2.0.3 Prooxidant thymoquinone induces apoptosis in colorectal cancer cells 133
- 1.2.0.4 Methylglyoxal-Induced Apoptosis in Human Prostate Carcinoma 134
- 1.2.0.5 Influence of methylglyoxal on antioxidant enzymes and oxidative damage 135
- 1.2.1.0 How I feel about antioxidants and the so-called experts 136
- 1.2.1.1 How I feel about redox induced apoptosis 136
- 1.2.1.2 EMOD-induced apoptosis in human leukemia cells 136
- 1.2.1.3 EMOD-induced apoptosis with radiation 137
- 1.2.1.4 Migraines associated with low EMOD levels and high antioxidants 138
- 1.2.1.5 EMODs, antioxidants and apoptosis: all antineoplastic drugs yield EMODs == 139
- 1.2.2.0 High Doses Of Antioxidants Taken By Many Breast Cancer Patients Despite Possible Consequences 140
- 1.2.2.1 Antioxidants must be good and EMODs bad 141
- 1.2.2.2 Free Radicals, Cancer Prevention, and Therapy (Ames) 141
- 1.2.2.3 Antioxidants Can Be Prooxidants When You Least Expect That to Be So 144
- 1.2.2.4 Signaling Pathways Activated by Oxidative Injury and Their Roles in Determining Cell Fate 146
- 1.2.2.5 Mechanisms of Pro- and Antioxidation 147
- 1.2.3.0 Iron, Free Radicals, and Oxidative Injury 149
- 1.2.3.1 Oxidative Stress and Human Genetic Variation 150
- 1.2.3.2 Session 2: Antioxidative effects—Pros and cons 152
- 1.2.3.3 Phytochemical Effects beyond Antioxidation 152
- 1.2.3.4 Tumor-Suppressing Effects of Antioxidants from Tea 153
- 1.2.3.5 Antioxidants Suppress Apoptosis: p53 increases EMOD-apoptosis 154

- 1.2.3.6 Green Tea Polyphenols, EGCG: Antioxidative and Prooxidative Effects.... 156
- 1.2.3.7 Rationale for Using High-Dose Multiple Antioxidants as an Adjunct to Radiation Therapy and Chemotherapy 158
- 1.2.5.0 Section 3: biomarkers 160
- 1.2.5.1 Biomarkers of Oxidative Stress: Fact or Artifact? 160
- 1.2.5.2 Plasma Antioxidant Measurements 161
- 1.2.5.3 DNA Oxidation Products, Antioxidant Status, and Cancer Prevention 163
- 1.2.5.4 Use of Biomarkers of Oxidative Stress in Research Studies 165
- 1.2.5.5 Manganese Superoxide Dismutase: Genetic Variation and Regulation 168
- 1.2.6.0 Session 4: Clinical aspects of antioxidant usage 169
- 1.2.7.0 Consumer Perspectives about Antioxidants 169
- 1.2.8.0 Antioxidant Supplement Use in Cancer Survivors and the General Population 170
- 1.2.9.0 Efficacy of Dietary Antioxidants to Prevent Oxidative Damage 171
- 1.3.0.0 Biomarkers for Assessing Antioxidant Nutrient Intakes and Status 174
- 1.3.1.0 Session 5a: Chemotherapy-antioxidant reactions 175
- 1.3.2.0 Chemotherapy and Antioxidants: An Overview 175
- 1.3.3.0 Redox and Vitamin C in Cell Signaling and Genomic Protection....... 177
- 1.3.4.0 Drugs, Glutathione, and ROS in Regulation of Proliferation 178
- 1.3.5.0 Session 5b: Radiation-antioxidant interactions 179
- 1.3.6.0 Novel Functional Imaging for Tissue Oxygen Concentration and Redox Status 181
- 1.3.7.0 Oxidative Genome Damage and the Pathogenesis of Prostate Cancer 182
- 1.3.8.0 Redox-Sensitive Signaling Factors and Antioxidants: How Tumor Cells Respond to Ionizing Radiation 183
- 1.3.9.0 Session 6: Wrap-up 186
- 1.4.0.0 Antioxidant (NAC) may stop pulling out of hair (trichotillomania)...... 189
- 1.4.1.0 Vitamins C and E and Beta Carotene Supplementation and Cancer Risk: A Randomized Controlled Trial 191
- 1.4.2.0 Nutritional Prevention of Cancer: basically a failure 192
- 1.4.3.0 Vitamin Supplements and Cancer Prevention: Where Do Randomized Controlled Trials Stand? 196
- 1.4.4.0 Failed studies and harmful endpoints 197
- 1.4.5.0 Low fat diets fail to prevent adenomas 198
- 1.4.6.0 Vitamins C and E fail to prevent cancer or heart disease 198
- 1.4.7.0 Vitamins C and E and B6 and B12 fail to prevent cardiovascular disease 198
- 1.4.8.0 Folic acid, B6 and B12 fail to prevent breast cancer 199

- 1.5.0.0 Selective Enhancement of Cellular Oxidative Stress by Chloroquine.....202
- 1.5.1.0 Summary.....202
- 1.5.2.0 Advances in Treatment of GBM, glioblastoma multiforme.....203
- 1.5.3.0 Importance of Oxidative Stress ==.....203
- 1.5.4.0 Chloroquine Enhances Oxidative Stress.....204
- 1.5.5.0 Therapeutic Benefit of Chloroquine: Potential Mechanisms.....206
- 1.5.6.0 The lamentable free radical story.....210
- 1.5.7.0 Vitamins C and E can undo health benefit of exercise.....212
- 1.5.8.0 Antioxidant stress (glutathione) leads to heart failure in mice.....214
- 1.5.9.0 Largest multivitamin study shows they do nothing.....216
- 1.6.0.0 Women's Health Initiative study 2-9-09 Multivitamins fail.....216
- 1.6.1.0 Group disputes cancer claims on One A Day vitamins.....218
- 1.6.2.0 The great vitamin debate.....219
- 1.6.3.0 Arthritis alternative treatments ineffective (also vitamins A, C & E).....222
- 1.6.4.0 Antler velvet.....223
- 1.6.5.0 Brain generates most EMODs.....224
- 1.6.6.0 Patients with major CNS disease showed a 50% reduction in cerebral oxygen utilization.....225
- 1.7.0.0 NAC.....225
- 1.7.1.0 NAC toxicity.....226
- 1.7.2.0 Chemo-brain/mental fog blocked by NAC.....227
- 1.7.3.0 Are Antioxidants Safe During Chemotherapy and Radiation Treatment?.....228
- 1.7.4.0 If you are having Chemotherapy or radiotherapy, should you take anti-oxidants like vitamin C?.....230
- 1.7.5.0 Chemotherapy and Radiation Therapy: antioxidants O.K......231
- 1.7.6.0 Cancer stem cell antioxidants protect cancers against oxidants and death.....232
- 1.7.7.0 Antioxidants May Affect Chemotherapy.....233
- 1.7.8.0 Vitamin C supplements reduce benefits of anticancer drugs.....233
- 1.8.0.0 Apoptosis controlled by p53 gene.....235
- 1.8.1.0 Cancer protection secret revealed.....235
- 1.8.2.0 Radiation doses.....236
- 1.8.3.0 Hepatitis C Virus: From Oxygen Free Radicals to Hepatocellular Carcinoma.....236
- 1.8.3.1 Hepatitis C Virus and Chronic Liver Damage.....237
- 1.8.3.2 Reactive Oxygen Species Production, DNA Oxidative Damage and Cancer.....238
- 1.8.3.3 Hepatitis C Virus, Reactive Oxygen Species and DNA Oxidative Damage.....239
- 1.8.3.4 Hepatitis C Virus, DNA Damage and Host Factors.....241

- 1.8.3.5 DNA Oxidative Damage, Cytokines and Molecular Targets 242
- 1.8.3.6 The Role of Sex Hormones 244
- 1.8.3.7 Conclusions 245
- 1.8.4.0 Hyperoxia causes cellular arrest and induces p53 246
- 1.8.5.0 Ozone/Oxygen Shot Helps Heal Herniated Disk 247
- 1.8.6.0 Mannitol is an antioxidant 249
- 1.8.7.0 Antioxidants increase mortality 249
- 1.8.8.0 Antioxidant vitamin recommendations, The Medical Letter, 2005 249
- 1.8.9.0 Current Patterns and Prevalence of the Public's Use of MVM Supplements 250
- 1.9.0.0 Data on Food Antioxidants Aid Research 250
- 1.9.1.0 Linnane argues against the free radical theory 251
- 1.9.2.0 Linnane argues of the essentiality of EMODs 252
- 1.9.3.0 CoQ is an essential prooxidant - Linnane 252
- 1.9.4.0 Denham Harmans' take on antioxidants and age, as of 2000 253
- 1.9.4.1 Origin and evolution of the free radical theory of aging: a brief personal history of Denham Harman, 1954–2009 254
- 1.9.5.0 Harman's logic proceeds from three observations: 254
- 1.9.6.0 Number of cancer deaths wrong 255
- 1.9.6.1 The Cancer Business 256
- 1.9.6.2 The Dark at the End of the Tunnel 256
- 1.9.6.3 The Solid Gold Source; cancer business is second only to petrochemicals 256
- 1.9.6.4 The Enemy Within 257
- 1.9.6.5 The Orthodox Cure Hoax 259
- 1.9.6.6 Early Detection 264
- 1.9.6.7 Breast Cancer 265
- 1.9.6.8 Bristol 266
- 1.9.6.9 Tamoxifen 268
- 1.9.6.10 Save the Children 270
- 1.9.7.0 The FRT and aging 271
- 1.9.7.1 Proponent/ Advocate Claims – Antioxidant Use in Treating Cancer 272
- 1.9.7.2 Professional Evaluation/ Critique - Antioxidant Use in Treating Cancer 273
- 1.9.8 0 Transmissible cancers (Tasmanian devils and Canine transmissible venereal tumor) 274
- 1.9.8.1 Evolution of a transmissible cancer 276
- 1.9.8.2 Is cancer a transmittable disease? 276
- 1.9.9.0 Prostate cancer not warded off by supplements, selenium and E 10/27/08. The SELECT study 277
- 1.9.9.1 The SELECT study (overall description) 278

- 1.9.9.2 Prostate Cancer Prevention: The Scoop on Supplements 1-30-09 288
- 1.9.9.3 What SELECT Revealed 289
- 1.9.9.4 What About Vitamin C? 289
- 1.9.9.5 Controlling Your Risk 289
- 1.9.9.6 Antioxidants fail again in cancer prevention study 290

2.0.0.0 DO THOSE ANTIOXIDANTS IN FOOD REALLY PREVENT CANCER? 293

- 2.0.0.1 Harmful effects of vitamins (references) 294
- 2.0.0.2 Antioxidants and Cancer: Researcher admits she got it wrong 296
- 2.0.0.3 Time for antioxidants v2.0 297
- 2.0.1.0 Antioxidants - Health Miracle or Profitable Hype? 297
- 2.0.1.1 Antioxidants quick True/False quiz 298
- 2.0.1.2 A little bit of history on vitamin C 299
- 2.0.1.3 What are polyphenols? 300
- 2.0.1.4 So what does all this have to do with collagen? 301
- 2.0.1.5 Can polyphenols recharge the iron-enzyme? 302
- 2.0.1.6 What do we know about polyphenols in the body? 303
- 2.0.1.7 The demise of vitamin P 307
- 2.0.1.8 A miracle drug is discovered - the anti-aging vitamin 308
- 2.0.2.0 Free radicals: general info 309
- 2.0.2.1 Elderly who exercise 1X/wk 30% more likely to maintain cognitive function 310
- 2.0.2.2 Oxidative stress and cancer: have we moved forward? 310
- 2.0.2.3 Soy sauce antioxidant gives unpredicted reaction in vivo 311
- 2.0.2.4 Ischemia decreases SOD 312
- 2.0.3.0 Vitamin C wards off gout in men 313
- 2.0.3.1 Vitamin E does not reduce AOM-induced cancer in mice 313
- 2.0.3.2 Vitamins E and C do not Prevent Cancer in Men 314
- 2.0.3.3 Vitamin E Supplements May Raise Lung Cancer Risk 317
- 2.0.3.4 Vitamin C May Interfere With Cancer Treatment 319
- 2.0.3.5 Antioxidants Vitamin C and Vitamin E for the Prevention and Treatment of Cancer 320
- 2.0.3.6 Vitamins E and C do not Prevent Cardiovascular Disease in Men 323
- 2.0.3.7 The Physicians' Health Study II Randomized Controlled Trial 11/09/08 323
- 2.0.3.8 US Vitamin supplement sales 325
- 2.0.4.0 One-third of US kids take vitamins 326
- 2.0.4.1 Vitamin and Mineral Supplement Use Among US Adults After Cancer Diagnosis 328
- 2.0.5.0 Avoid antioxidants in cancer patients 328

- 2.0.5.1 Can antioxidants block chemo or radiation therapy? 329
- 2.0.5.2 Do Antioxidants Interfere With Radiation Therapy for Cancer? 330
- 2.0.5.3 Should Supplemental Antioxidant Administration Be Avoided During Chemotherapy and Radiation Therapy? 331
- 2.0.5.4 Effects of Oncological Treatment and Mechanisms of Action of Antioxidants 333
- 2.0.5.5 Simone concludes that antioxidants increase cancer patient survival 339
- 2.0.5.6 Others caution antioxidant use in cancer patients 340
- 2.0.5.7 When a Potential for Harm Exists, Primum non nocere 341
- 2.0.5.8 Antioxidants Including Vitamin C Do Not Decrease the Efficacy of Chemotherapy 341
- 2.0.5.9 Should antioxidants be avoided during chemotherapy treatments? 346
- 2.0.6.0 Should patients undergoing chemotherapy and radiotherapy be prescribed antioxidants? 348
- 2.0.6.1 Selenium for alleviating the side effects of chemotherapy 349
- 2.0.7.0 LINUS PAULING INSTITUTE SPRING/SUMMER 2005 RESEARCH REPORT 351
- 2.0.7.1 Diabetes and supplemental vitamin C 351
- 2.0.7.2 Gastrointestinal cancers and antioxidants 352
- 2.0.7.3 Antioxidant vitamins and cancer chemotherapy 353
- 2.0.8.0 Vitamin C May Reduce Response to Chemotherapy 354
- 2.0.8.1 Reduction in Cytotoxic Effect == 355
- 2.0.8.2 Wide Variety of Chemotherapeutics Affected 355
- 2.0.8.3 Many Cancer Patients Take Vitamin C == 356
- 2.0.9.0 EMOD selective kill of cancer cells with beta-phenylethyl isothiocyanate (PEITC) == 357
- 2.0.9.1 Ascorbate generated H_2O_2 kills cancer cells (Human lymphoma cells) == 357
- 2.1.0.0 Failed antioxidant studies 359
- 2.1.0.1 Vitamin C and Major Cardiovascular Events 363
- 2.1.0.2 Randomized Trials of Vitamin E 364
- 2.1.0.3 Randomized Trials of Vitamin C 367
- 2.1.0.4 Potential Limitations 369
- 2.1.0.5 CONCLUSION 369
- 2.1.1.0 Effect of Combined Folic Acid, Vitamin B_6, and Vitamin B_{12} on Cancer Risk in Women. A Randomized Trial. Shumin M. Zhang, MD, ScD; Nancy R. Cook, ScD; Christine M. Albert, MD, MPH; J. Michael Gaziano, MD, MPH; Julie E. Buring, ScD; JoAnn E. Manson, MD, DrPH. JAMA. 2008;300(17):2012-2021. 370
- 2.1.1.1 Singlet oxygen 371
- 2.1.1.2 Singlet oxygen background 371

- 2.1.1.3 Viruses susceptible to EMODs (H_2O_2, singlet oxygen)........................372
- 2.1.1.4 Ascorbate reacts with singlet oxygen to produce hydrogen peroxide........................372
- 2.1.1.5 Singlet oxygen therapy........................373
- 2.1.1.6 Singlet oxygen toxicity is cell line-dependent........................374
- 2.1.2.0 Methylene blue to treat Alzheimer's and Parkinson's diseases........................374
- 2.1.2.1 Methylene blue produces hydrogen peroxide as a redox cycler (malaria)........................376
- 2.1.2.2 Malaria parasite has strong antioxidative defenses........................377
- 2.1.2.3 Methylene blue has syphilitic trypanocidal prooxidant activity........................378
- 2.1.2.4 Tropical diseases killed oxidatively........................378
- 2.1.3.0 SOD........................379
- 2.1.3.1 Faulty reasoning concerning oxygen and accelerated aging........................379
- 2.1.3.2 Oxygen and Accelerated Aging........................380
- 2.1.3.3 Low SOD associated with diseases........................381
- 2.1.3.4 SOD produces hydrogen peroxide........................382
- 2.1.3.5 SOD over expression increases peroxide levels and suppresses prostate cancer cells........................383
- 2.1.3.6 SOD is a virulence factor in bacteria........................383
- 2.1.3.7 SOD deficiency may cause AMD (adult-onset macular degeneration)........................385
- 2.1.3.8 SOD produced H2O2 and Gpx1 regulate cerebral vascular tone........................386
- 2.1.3.9 Life long SOD deficiency has negative effect on heart function........................387
- 2.1.3.10 SOD over expression protects cancer cell exposed to hyperthermia ==........................387
- 2.1.4.0 Hydrogen peroxide........................388
- 2.1.4.1 Hydrogen peroxide in the human body (Halliwell)........................388
- 2.1.4.2 Introduction........................388
- 2.1.4.3 Exposure of human tissues to H_2O_2........................389
- 2.1.4.4 The oral cavity, oesophagus and stomach........................390
- 2.1.4.5 The respiratory system........................390
- 2.1.4.6 The kidney, urinary tract and bladder........................390
- 2.1.4.7 Vascular endothelial and circulating blood cells........................391
- 2.1.4.8 Ocular tissues........................391
- 2.1.4.9 Conclusion........................391
- 2.1.5.0 T-cells contain 10-100 μM peroxide........................392
- 2.1.5.1 Hydrogen peroxide bactericidal activity is increased by blue light........................392
- 2.1.5.2 Hydrogen peroxide plus blue light kills germs in oral biofilms........................394
- 2.1.6.0 Myeloperoxidase is involved in H_2O_2-induced apoptosis of HL-60 human leukemia cells ==........................394
- 2.1.7.0 Hydrogen peroxide and melanogenesis........................395

- 2.1.7.1 The role of melanin in skin....396
- 2.1.7.2 Hydrogen peroxide & melanin....397
- 2.1.7.3 Dealing with the problem....397
- 2.1.8.0 Hydrogen peroxide and melanogenesis....398
- 2.1.8.1 Hydrogen peroxide & skin aging....398
- 2.1.8.2 How does hydrogen peroxide cause chronological ageing?....399
- 2.1.9.0 Hydrogen peroxide said to be causative of gray hair....401
- 2.2.0.0 Human body glows in the dark....402
- 2.2.1.0 Iron and ascorbate increase PDT effect....404
- 2.2.1.1 Ascorbate as a prooxidant....404
- 2.2.2.0 Effect of topically applied tocopherol on ultraviolet radiation-mediated free radical damage in skin....405
- 2.2.2.1 Vitamin E slows the rate of free radical-mediated lipid peroxidation in cells ==....405
- 2.2.3.0 EMODs and CVD....406
- 2.2.3.1 Multiple sclerosis not cured by antioxidants or vitamins B12 or D....407
- 2.2.4.0 Anthocyanins have unknown bioavailabity....407
- 2.2.4.1 Antioxidant and prooxidant activities of elderberry....408
- 2.2.4.2 Anthocyanin induces apoptosis in human leukemia cells via EMODs ==....409
- 2.2.4.3 Anthocyanins block colon cancer cells ==....410
- 2.2.4.4 Anthocyanins prevent cellular malignant transformation ==....410
- 2.2.5.0 Down Syndrome: The fallacy of the big vitamin deficiency....412
- 2.2.6.0 Pau d'Arco....412
- 2.2.7.0 EMOD generation in thyroid cells by naphthaquinone....416
- 2.2.8.0 Lapacho (naphthoquinone) generates tumoricidal EMODs ==....417
- 2.2.9.0 Oysters contain EMOD-apoptosis-inducing ceramides (blocked by antioxidants)....417
- 2.2.9.1 Onion oil EMOD-induced apoptosis blocked by NAC and glutathione ==....418
- 2.3.0.0 EMODs control apoptosis ==....419
- 2.3.1.0 EMODs cause spontaneous regression of cancer (melanoma)....420
- 2.3.1.1 Lipid coated viruses and bacteria....420
- 2.3.2.0 Spontaneous Cancer Regression in Melanoma Pigs....421
- 2.3.3.0 Hyperthermia inhibits tumor growth ==....422
- 2.3.4.0 Hyperoxia increases spontaneous regression....422
- 2.3.5.0 Spontaneous regression of cancer....422
- 2.3.5.1 Spontaneous regression of malignant breast cancer....424
- 2.3.5.2 Some breast cancers may resolve without treatment....424
- 2.3.6.0 Two paths for apoptosis death ==....429
- 2.3.7.0 Resveratrol....429

- 2.3.7.1 Resveratrol blocks EMOD-induced apoptosis == 429
- 2.3.7.2 Resveratrol prooxidant activity == 430
- 2.3.7.3 Resveratrol increases vascular oxidative stress resistance == 430
- 2.3.8.0 Catalase over-expression blocks apoptosis and increases tumor growth == 431
- 2.3.9.0 A Polyphenol antioxidant kills by increasing EMODs == 432
- 2.4.0.0 Lung cancer patients have higher GPx and lower SOD levels 433
- 2.4.1.0 Photodynamic therapy for Barrett's esophagus 434
- 2.4.2.0 Lung Cancer Chemoprevention: Evidence-Based Clinical Practice Guidelines (2nd Edition) 2007 434
- 2.4.3.0 No effect of vitamin C, E, or beta carotene on cardiovascular events among women at high risk for CVD 435
- 2.4.4.0 Supplemental vitamin E does not protect against prostate cancer 436
- 2.4.5.0 AHA Scientific Statement-2007. Do not recommend C or E 437
- 2.4.6.0 Thioredoxin blocks EMOD-induced apoptosis for human neuroblastoma == 438
- 2.4.7.0. Summary of American Heart Association Diet and Lifestyle Recommendations Revision 2006: supplements not recommended 438
- 2.4.8.0 American Cancer Society Guidelines on Nutrition and Physical Activity for Cancer Prevention 2006 439
- 2.4.9.0 AHA Scientific Statement. Diet and Lifestyle Recommendations Revision 2006: supplements not recommended for CVD 441
- 2.5.0.0 Vitamins C and E not recommended to treat or prevent cancer 442
- 2.5.1.0 How household bleach works to kill bacteria 443
- 2.5.2.0 Baths with Bleach Help Kids' Eczema 444
- 2.5.3.0 Lung airway cells activate vitamin D and increase immune response 446
- 2.5.4.0 HOCl vs H_2O_2 448
- 2.5.5.0 Oxidant stress and endothelial cell dysfunction 453
- 2.5.6.0 Exercise 454
- 2.5.6.1 Exercise and sleep drastically reduce cancer risk 454
- 2.5.6.2 Total antioxidant capacity tended to be lower in athletes 455
- 2.5.6.3 Antioxidants not recommended during strenuous exercise 455
- 2.5.6.4 "Exercise, Good; Antioxidants, Bad" 456
- 2.5.6.5 Habitual exercise and arterial aging 457
- 2.5.7.0 Oxidative stress in development of cardiovascular complications in diabetes mellitus 458
- 2.5.7.1 Endothelial dysfunction in diabetes mellitus 458
- 2.5.8.0 High Blood Glucose Levels in Early Pregnancy May Deprive Embryo of Oxygen and Lead to Birth Defects 459

- 2.5.8.1 Iron in Pregnancy: Free Radical Generation....462
- 2.5.8.2 Vitamin C, oxidative stress in pregnancy....463
- 2.5.9.0 Vitamin Deaths....467
- 2.5.9.1 Fifteen infant deaths in India may be due vitamin A....467
- 2.5.9.2 Vitamin death-link hard pill to swallow (*Bjelakovic*)....468
- 2.5.9.3 Orthomolecular News report *20th Apr 2008*....469
- 2.5.9.4 E-Ferol....469
- 2.5.9.5 Unusual Syndrome with Fatalities among Premature Infants: Association with a New Intravenous Vitamin E Product....470
- 2.5.9.6 Supplements have quality problems....471
- 2.6.0.0 Hyperuricemia Deaths....478
- 2.6.0.1 Antioxidant uric acid increases death risk....479
- 2.6.0.2 Hyperuricemia increases risk of death in all causes....480
- 2.6.0.3 Men with gout have increased all cause mortality....481
- 2.6.0.4 Framingham study: Uric acid not causal in deaths....482
- 2.6.0.5 Confusion: hyperuricemia induces oxidative stress....483
- 2.6.0.6 Hyperuricemic Syndromes in Cancer Patients....483
- 2.6.0 7 Hyperuricemia may cause chronic disease....484
- 2.6.1.0 Hyperbilirubinemia deaths....484
- 2.6.2.0 Earlier Jaundice Treatment Decreases Brain Injury In Preemies....486
- 2.6.3.0 Heart Disease Deaths Fall as Obesity and Diabetes Increase....486
- 2.6.4.0 Ginkgo Biloba and Cell Phone Free Radical Damage....488
- 2.6.5.0 Ginkgo Biloba Preserves Brain's Antioxidant Enzyme Activity, SOD & GPx....488
- 2.6.6.0 Cell phones can affect sperm quality....489
- 2.6.9 0 Metals, Fenton chemistry and antioxidants....498
- 2.7.0.0 Aging/anti-aging....499
- 2.7.1.0 Antioxidants can not extend normal life span....499
- 2.7.2.0 Support for antioxidants in aging is scarce and equivocal....500
- 2.7.3.0 Aging studies inconsistent on antioxidant defenses....501
- 2.7.4.0 Antioxidants 'cannot slow aging' (Nematode worms)....502
- 2.7.5.0 Aging Not Slowed By Antioxidants, Study Rejects 50 Year Old Theory....504
- 2.7.6.0 Survival Mode That Protects Cells When Oxygen Is Low (HIF) Also Slows Aging....506
- 2.7.7.0 Anti-aging creams don't work....508
- 2.7.8.0 Mice with increased catalase live longer....509
- 2.7.9.0 Superoxide is not a major determinant of aging in C. elegans: Against the oxidative damage theory of aging....512
- 2.8.0.0 Xanthine oxidase produces superoxide in route to making antioxidant, uric acid....512

- 2.8.1.0 A Fountain of Youth? 513
- 2.8.2.0 Hydrogen peroxide induces senescence in human fibrobsasts 513
- 2.8.3.0 Hydrogen peroxide increase senescence in Werner fibroblasts 513
- 2.8.4.0 Werner syndrome 514
- 2.8.6.0 Cytochrome produced EMODs do not contribute to aging 515
- 2.9.0.0 Hydrogen peroxide linked to longer life 515
- 2.9.1.0 Caloric restriction may raise ROS 517
- 2.9.1.1 Introduction 518
- 2.9.1.2 Hormesis and caloric restriction 519
- 2.9.2.0 Some pathogens have catalase to protect against peroxide 521
- 2.9.3.0 Hydrogen peroxide important signaling clue in cancer cells 521
- 2.9.4.0 Stem Cells 523
- 2.9.4.1 ROS required for signaling cascades initiating cardiovascular differentiation 523
- 2.9.5.0 Pro-vasculogenic stem cell effects are mediated by Ca^{2+}-induced ROS generation 524
- 2.9.6.0 Reactive Oxygen Species and Genomic Stability in Hematopoietic Stem Cells 525
- 2.9.7.0 ROS control hematolymphopoiesis 525

3.0.0.0 HYPOXIA 527

- 3.0.0.1 Intermittent Hypoxia: Cause of or Therapy for Systemic Hypertension? 527
- 3.0.1.0 Intermittent hypoxia has salutary effect 527
- 3.0.2.0 EMOD cardioprotection is blocked by NAC 528
- 3.0.3.0 Ischemic preconditioning 529
- 3.0.4.0 Controversial role of antioxidants 531
- 3.0.5.0 Antioxidant failures 536
- 3.0.6.0 British Nutrition Foundation says eat more fruits and vegetables (2001) 537
- 3.0.7.0 Fruits, veggies slash breast cancer risk: U.S. study 538
- 3.0.8.0 Hypertension 539
- 3.0.8.1 Antioxidants fail to stop hypertension 539
- 3.0.9.0 Antioxidants fail to reduce hypertension 544
- 3.1.0.0 EMODs in veins vs arteries 546
- 3.1.1.0 Producers and Destroyers of Reactive Oxygen Species 547
- 3.1.2.0 Mito-chondrial Respiratory Chain 548
- 3.1.3.0 Arteries and Veins: A Comparison of Structure and Function 550
- 3.1.4.0 Vascular EMOD production: veins have more EMODs 552
- 3.1.5.0 NADPH Oxidases: "the vascular oxidase" 553
- 3.1.6.0 Xanthine Oxidase 554

- 3.1.7.0 SODs 554
- 3.1.8.0 Atherosclerosis 554
- 3.1.9.0 Hypertension 555
- 3.2. 0.0 A comparison of EMODs in aorta vs vena cava 555
- 3.2.1.0 Obese children risk thyroid damage 556
- 3.2.2.0 American Heart Association Says Antioxidants do not decrease CVD 557
- 3.2.3.0 Vitamins C, E don't protect against cancer: studies 559
- 3.2.4.0 Supplementation with vitamin E or selenium does not reduce risk of prostate cancer 560
- 3.2.5.0 Editorial: Randomized Trials of Antioxidant Supplementation for Cancer Prevention-First Bias, Now Chance—Next, Cause 562
- 3.2.6.0 Nutritional Chemoprevention for Prostate Cancer Strikes Out Twice 563
- 3.2.7.0 Vitamins and antioxidants 'do not cut cancer risk' 566

4.0.0.0 IMPORTANCE OF OXYGEN LEVELS 569
- 4.0.1.0 The importance of adequate oxygen levels: altitude sickness 570
- 4.0.2.0 Low Brain Oxygen Ups Alzheimer's Risk 571
- 4.0.3.0 Anesthetic/Low Brain Oxygen Ups Alzheimer's Risk 572
- 4.0.4.0 Low Oxygen Accelerated the Great Dying (Permian-Triassic period) 572
- 4.0.5.0 Cell's Power Plants (mitochondria) Also Sense Low Oxygen 575
- 4.0.6.0 High altitude native Tibetans with high oxygen saturation survive better 577
- 4.0.7.0 High summits 'could harm brain' 578
- 4.0.8.0 'Earthly organisms developed in two sets' based on oxygen levels ... 579
- 4.0.9.0 High Tumor Oxygen Level essential for radiotherapy and chemotherapy 580
- 4.1.0.0 Breast cancer 582
- 4.1.1.0 Estrogen therapy increases breast cancer risk 582
- 4.1.2 0 Hormone Therapy-Breast Cancer Tie Grows 583
- 4.1.3.0 Hormone therapy may cut breast cancer risk in some 584
- 4.2.0 0 Quercetin 586
- 4.2.1.0 Quercetin blocks EMOD induced apoptosis == 586
- 4.2.2.0 Quercetin acts as a prooxidant == 586
- 4.2.3.0 Antioxidant and prooxidant effects of quercetin on GPDH 587
- 4.3.0.0 Vitamin D 587
- 4.3.1.0 What you need to know about vitamin D 587
- 4.3.2.0 Please remember that vitamin D is a prooxidant 589
- 4.3.3.0 Vitamin D often low in mothers and newborns 589

- 4.3.4.0 Vitamin D prevents cancer 590
- 4.4.0.0 Antioxidants and the free radical myth 591
- 4.4.1.0 Oxidative aging theories lack support 593
- 4.4.2.0 The free radical theory and aging 593
- 4.4.3.0 Mitohormesis: increased EMODs increased lifespan 596
- 4.4.4.0 Calorie restriction 597
- 4.4.5.0 EMODs may add to longevity and antioxidants may be harmful 597
- 4.4.6.0 EMODs challenge dogma: EMODs are anti-inflammatory 598
- 4.4.7.0 Inconsistencies of the free radical theory 599
- 4.5.0.0 Synta anticancer mechanism: STA-4783 causes EMOD apoptosis. NAC blocks apoptosis == 600
- 4.5.1.0 Brain plays key role in appetite by regulating free radicals: appetite controlled by EMODs 602
- 4.5.2.0 Exercise suppresses appetite by affecting appetite hormones 603
- 4.5.3.0 Treadmill versus weight lifting 604
- 4.5.4.0 Focus on active ghrelin 605
- 4.6.0 0 Asbestos increases antioxidant enzymes 605
- 4.6.1.0 Free oxygen radicals and kidney diseases--part I 605
- 4.7.0.0 The eye 607
- 4.7.1.0 Cataracts 608
- 4.7.2.0 Mechanisms of Light Damage to the Lens 609
- 4.7.3.0 Cataracts 610
- 4.7.4.0 Protection of the Lens Against Light Damage: antioxidants 610
- 4.7.5.0 Conclusion 611
- 4.8.0.0 Congenital cataracts 611
- 4.8.1.0 Causes 612
- 4.9.0.0 Sugar Cataracts 613
- 4.9.1.0 Vitamin D deficiency cataracts 614
- 4.9.2.0 Vitamins C and E do not prevent cataract development or progression 614
- 4.9.3.0 Vitamin E deficiency and long-term prednisolone treatment are subliminal cataractogenic risk factors 615

5.0.0.0 VITAMIN E DOES NOT PREVENT CVD 617

- 5.0.1.0 Failures of antioxidants to prevent cataract formation 617
- 5.0.2.0 Antioxidants not recommended 619
- 5.0.3.0 ATBC study fails to prevent cataracts 620
- 5.0.4.0 Antioxidants not recommended for Adult Macular Degeneration 621
- 5.0.5.0 Omega-3 Fatty Acids Appear To Impact AMD Progression 621
- 5.1.0.0 Hyperbaric Oxygen Therapy (HBOT) 623
- 5.1.1.0 Oxygen therapy benefit in autism 623

- 5.2.0.0 HBOT general information from emedicine....626
- 5.2.1.0 The Oxygen Revolution: Hyperbaric Oxygen Therapy....627
- 5.3.0.0 Exercise....628
- 5.4.0.0 Pills To Replace Exercising Could Soon Become Reality....628
- 5.5.0.0 A possible "exercise pill"....630
- 5.6.0.0 Disulfiram....631
- 5.6.1.0 General information from emedicine:....631
- 5.7.0.0 Disulfiram to treat cancer....634
- 5.7.1.0 Alcohol increases EMOD production....636
- 5.8.0.0 EMODs high in reproductive organs....637
- 5.9.0.0 WBCs....637
- 5.9.1.0 WBCs have an EMOD defect....637
- 5.9.2.0 WBC EMOD production inhibited by endothelial cells....638

6.0.0.0 STAUROSPORINE INDUCES APOPTOSIS VIA EMODs......641

- 6.0.1.0 Debunking The Detox Myth....641
- 6.0.2.0 Detox nonsense....644
- 6.1.0.0 Mangafodipir trisodium....644
- 6.1.1.0 Motexafin gadolinium....645
- 6.1.2.0 Metoxafin lutetium....645
- 6.2.0.0 Sonodynamic therapy....645
- 6.3.0.0 High-Intensity Focused Ultrasound Therapy: an Overview for Radiologists....646
- 6.3.1.0 Basic physics of sound and ultrasound....647
- 6.3.2.0 Biological interactions of US....648
- 6.3.3.0 Clinical Devices in use....649
- 6.3.4.0 Results of clinical studies....650
- 6.3.5.0 Limitations and Future Works....651
- 6.4.0.0 What is SPDT, PDT?....652
- 6.5.0.0 Light Therapy Spares the Scalpel and the Chemo....655
- 6.6.0.0 New light on medicine....657
- 6.6.1.0 Down's syndrome....659
- 6.6.2.0 Down's have lower risk of tumors, atherosclerosis and diabetic retinopathy....659
- 6.6.3.0 Free Radicals and Kundalini....660
- 6.6.4.0 TOP ANTIOXIDANT FOODS....665

"FINDING YOUR INNER RADICAL SELF"

As that famous "Okie" Will Rogers once said there are three ways to learn how to do something. Some people will learn by reading books, some will learn by watching what others do and there will be those who just have to piss on the electric fence to figure it out.

Howes Quotes

The magnanimous dance of the redox electron is the bona fide ballet of life.
R. M. Howes M.D., Ph.D.
11/18/08

Without educating the "radically" ignorant, convincing them of the dangers of antioxidant overuse is an impossibility.
R. M. Howes M.D., Ph.D.
11/18/08

Resolving redox confusion has proven fiendishly difficult.
R. M. Howes M.D., Ph.D.
11/21/08

The most important of all rules
is the rule that
no rule is immutable or
put another way,
the rule is that no rule remains the same rule....
forever.
Rules are progressive
and not everlasting.
R. M. Howes M.D., Ph.D.
11/22/08

When the expanding universe collapses,
we may experience
reverse evolution
or "devil-ution."
R. M. Howes M.D., Ph.D.
11/22/08

Two main quarries, oxidants and antioxidants,
supply the major building blocks
for electron and proton flow
in living entities.
Rock on!
R. M. Howes M.D., Ph.D.
11/23/08

Just about the time you begin to figure out life,
it's time to die
and you grasp just how little
you have figured out.
R. M. Howes M.D., Ph.D.
11/24/08

Just when you figure out that you can not
figure out life,
is when you realize that
we are all as dumb as a box of roxs....er, rocks.
R. M. Howes M.D., Ph.D.
11/28/08

"Antioxivores, gobble down
your synthetic supplements to
support billion dollar sales but
do so at your own peril.
R. M. Howes M.D., Ph.D.
12/18/08

Oxidants and antioxidants are like Wasabi or
a bass player---
i.e., they do not work well alone.
They are co-dependent in their life-sustaining quest
of promoting electron and proton flow.
R. M. Howes M.D., Ph.D.
1/8/09

The half century occurrence of the free radical theory
will merely represent a moment of confusion
in the overall history of redox thought,
aerobiosis and
oxygen appreciation.
R. M. Howes M.D., Ph.D.
1/19/09

Radicophobes can ignore the truth or
they can reject the truth but
they can not change the magnificent truths
regarding the crucial role
of EMODs in the life process
of all aerobes
or the inherent splendor of oxygen.
R. M. Howes M.D., Ph.D.
1/26/09

Under abnormal conditions,
electronically modified oxygen derivatives
may be toxic in excess but
the same can be said for water and food.
R. M. Howes M.D., Ph.D.
2/5/09

Friends do not let friends
injudiciously ingest antioxidants.
R. M. Howes M.D., Ph.D.
2/11/09

Amused and annoyed in equal measure,
I peruse the antioxidant vitamin ads.
Quotes are inspired by the marketing and business milieu,
which distort the facts to score a selling point....
so much for science.
Let's hear it for sales.
R. M. Howes M.D., Ph.D.
2/11/09

I toil to reveal the deceptive profit-driven agenda
of the
antioxivores and radicophobes.
R. M. Howes M.D., Ph.D.
2/11/09

The best thing about the free radical theory
is that you intuitively feel and
instinctively know that it is wrong,...
just plain old wrong.
R. M. Howes M.D., Ph.D.
2/11/09

Antioxidants: known harm for unknown benefit.
R. M. Howes M.D., Ph.D.
2/11/09

Comprehensive
Rejuvenating
Antioxidant
Program:
C.R.A.P.
Yes, this is their antiaging plan.
There are CRAP creams, CRAP pills, CRAP supplements,
CRAP shampoos, etc.
In short,
it's all a lot of CRAP.
R. M. Howes M.D., Ph.D.
2/22/09

**Hydrogen and oxygen are two of the
most flammable elements.
Yet, combine them into water and
they are a most effective extinguisher of their own fire.
The very essence of nature can be drastically altered
by associations and the company we keep.**

R. M. Howes M.D., Ph.D.
2/28/09

**Oxygen is the biomarker for life
on planet Earth and used as such
by those in the search
of life throughout the universe.
It is not the sentinel of death,
as espoused
by the ersatz free radi-crap theory.**

R. M. Howes M.D., Ph.D.
3/28/09

**Many faux theorist on aging
subscribe to the free radical theory,
which is like the theory of Bigfoot,
only with less credibility or substance.**

R. M. Howes M.D., Ph.D.
3/28/09

**Faith is the capacity of accepting, without question,
the incomprehensible as acknowledged
and simplified facts.**

R. M. Howes M.D., Ph.D.
5/9/09

**Theorists propose a multiplicity of parallel universes.
I have visited them many times.
I sleep
and enter via the dream-worm-hole portal.
It is as real as all of the other unprovable universes.
The dream dimension truly alters space and time
in a remarkable, mysterious
and inexplicable manner.**
R. M. Howes M.D., Ph.D.
5/19/09

**Humans are being rejected by the planet.
I feel it.**
R. M. Howes M.D., Ph.D.
6/8/09

**At 65, I have entered a strange place.
A place of looming questions and a
place where I realize that
I am nearer to death than I am
to life.
I am no longer all here,
parts of the whole have been lost
after passing my peak.
It is mucho unsettling.
Comprende?**
R. M. Howes M.D., Ph.D.
6/22/09

**Certain self evident truths
need not require additional evidence or proof,
such as the low toxicity of EMODs,
as evidenced by their omnipresent ubiquity.**
R. M. Howes M.D., Ph.D.
7/15/09

I believe that nature is composed of infinitely complex related factoids (convoluted factual cousins), each of which contains Byzantine elements beyond our realm of comprehension.

R. M. Howes M.D., Ph.D.
7/15/09

Based on the "design follows function" principle,
one should not be surprised
when a thing does what it was designed to do,
such as a radical seeking an electron or
a man seeking a woman or
of a woman satisfying a man.
One can not change the character of a thing
unless you permanently change
its basic nature,
human nature or
Mother Nature.

R. M. Howes M.D., Ph.D.
7/20/09

Please note: only your personal physician or other health professional you consult can best advise you on matters of your health based on your medical history, your family medical history, your medication history, and how information from any of these databases may apply to you. Neither Dr. Howes nor any party involved in creating, producing or delivering this web site shall be liable for any damages arising out of access to or use of this material or web site, or any errors or omissions in the content thereof.

1.0.0.0 INTRODUCTION

The Howes ratiocination of EMOD insufficiency and disease allowance.

EMODs do not cause wanton destruction to cells or within cells.

Epidemiology teaches that every statistical association has only 3 possible explanations: a) bias, b) chance, and c) cause. However, I impugn this statement and would add to this 1) partial fabrication of data, 2) unscrupulous manipulation of data and 3) completely made up data, i.e., bald-faced liars.

In actuality, free radicals perform many crucial roles in normal, healthy physiological processes like our immune system and promote beneficial oxidation. It is important to realize that many vitamins and supplements classified as antioxidants (or so-called antioxidants) are actually *redox agents*, meaning that they act as antioxidants in some instances and pro-oxidants in others. Both prooxidants and antioxidants are designed to exist in alternating redox states. This markedly increases the difficulty of intrepreting redox data and is seldom addressed in the literature or considered in arriving at so-called scientific conclusions.

Unfortunately, many believe that correlation equals causation.

The continued non-acceptance of the null findings of over 110 (over 500 as 2013) clinical trials on vitamin and antioxidant supplements has **no scientific basis or biochemical plausibility.** The underlying principles of the free radical theory have been proven to be unsound.

Radicophobes can ignore the truth or
they can reject the truth or
deny the truth but
they can not change the maginificent truths
regarding the crucial role
of EMODs in the life process
of all aerobes
or the inherent splendor of oxygen.

R. M. Howes M.D., Ph.D.
1/26/09

The researchers are using other technologies to determine how the loss of oxygen affects the functions of genes in the brain. Of the approximately 30,000 genes investigated to date, at least 6,000 are either inactivated or highly activated when a stroke reduces the oxygen in the brain. Their future work will explore the ramifications of those changed gene functions. I believe that this illustrates the crucial role of oxygen levels, EMOD levels and the redox status of the cell.

Normal redox homeostasis may be pathologically disturbed by overzealous use of antioxidants. My UTOPIA and ROS insufficiency theories present a new perspective more correctly informed by the most contemporaneous experimental findings and most reliable clinical studies.

The ideal drug to treat cancer would be not only potent and highly selective for tumors but also broken down quickly into harmless compounds and excreted from the body. This is exactly what my singlet oxygen delivery system does!

The average person breathes in about 6 pounds of oxygen a day, which is about the same amount by weight of food and water intake. Six has always been my lucky number. We breathe 21,600 times per day. To distribute oxygen throughout the body, the heart beats 100,000 times per day and pumps 5,000 gallons of blood. The free radical theory teaches the nonsense/nonscience approach that all of this effort is to bring a toxic agent into the body (i.e., oxygen) and distribute it to all aerobic cells on a continual basis. Thus, the free radical theory is not based on sound scientific reasoning and flies in the face of all teachings of evolution.

During a single hour of HBOT (hyperbaric oxygen therapy), a person will take in about 2.4 pounds of oxygen. This increases the oxygen content of the tissues by a factor of 10-15.

Half the protein produced in the body every day is enzymes and our endogenous antioxidant superoxide dismutase is the fifth most abundant protein in the body.

The brain must produce and use 20% of the body's total ATP production in order to maintain normal function

The radio airways are filled with nonscience/nonsense regarding antioxidants, energy production and oxidation. I was just listening to a station promoting antioxidant sales, with claims that antioxidants will cure damned near every disease out there. It claimed that CoQ 10 is like putting an internal ice pack on an inflamed joint. It claimed that one will get an incredible energy boost from antioxidants.

Please remember that it was the founder of the free radical theory, Denham Harman, who told Jack Chelam that taking too many antioxidants would cause fatigue, not an incredible energy boost.

NICK NOLTE'S RAVAGED FACE

Nick reportedly has a thousands-of-dollars-a-week vitamin habit.

He takes 60 supplements a day!

ANGELINA JOLIE'S SUPRAPUBIC TATTOO

"Quod me nutrit me destruit"
translates as "That which nourishes me, destroys me".
It bears a resemblance to some lines by Shakespeare (written a few years later): &lsquo:Consum'd with that which it was nourish&rlquo;d by' (Sonnet 73) and 'A burning torch that's turned upside down; / The word, *Qui me alit, me extinguit* [Who feeds me extinguishes me]' (Pericles, II.ii.33).

BRUCE AMES' QUOTE, "THE THING WE NEED MOST, OXYGEN, IS WHAT IS KILLING US."

1.0.0.1 Pall/Levine snake oil

I just received a small booklet from Stephen Levine's group pushing the sale of antioxidants to cure chronic fatigue syndrome (CFS).

To my knowledge, we do not know what CFS is, what causes it, if it is bonafide disease entity, or especially how to "cure" it. Here is the situation, CFS is an "unexplained illness" or a condition of fatigue. So, Levine and a character named Martin Pall, claim that by taking a fatigue inducing agent, i.e., an antioxidant, they can cure CFS. That makes no sense at all. They go into a conversation about high levels of peroxynitrite and superoxide and how it is the cause of CFS. But we have extreme difficulty measuring the more common so-called radicals, such as superoxide, peroxide, singlet oxygen, the hydroxyl radical or hypochlorous acid, let alone now trying to measure with accuracy peroxynitrite and then ascribing an accurate significance to it.

Their approach is: reducing NO-related free radical activity. Actually, these people rely on placebo to affect positive changes in the patients because the antioxidants ("free radical reducing supplements") that they use, would cause even greater fatigue. They evaluated 8 patients for 8 weeks. They were treating Chronic Fatigue Syndrome/Myalgic Encephalomyelitis (CFS/ME) and found that the most dramatic result was in the first four weeks, with a p value = .006 (p=.05 which is the minimum value required for stastical significance). **There were no significant results on mental symptom tests**.

Pall now talks about his so-called run away free radical damaging "NO/ONOO-" cycle mechanism, the No...oh no! syndrome and is allegedly found in patients with CFS, fibromyalgia, Gulf War syndrome, post-traumatic stress and multiple chemical sensitivity. These are the so-called five "mystery illnesses." They claim that these **five** illnesses are caused by the "NO/ONOO-" cycle and that **they can be completely ameliorated and completely reversed.** Wow, which means they can be CURED! (Nutricology Newsletter In Focus, July 2007).

Pall states that the initiator can be infection, toxic exposures, physical or mental trauma but they always cause the downstream effect of free radical damage medicated by raised levels of NO and ONOO. He says that the immune cells are particularly sensitive to oxidative stress. **Actually, I have found that immunocompetence depends upon maintaining adequate levels of EMODs**. Hulqvist has shown this with arthritis and it is also true in chronic granulomatous disease. Suppressing EMODs with antioxidants will theoretically suppress immunity. This is just the opposite of the Pall ascertions.

Pall claims to have a concoction of 16 nutrients that can improve these diseases: Trimethylglycine (betaine), Coenzyne Q10, Folic acid (folate), hydroxycobalamin (B12), Ecklonia cava extract, Acetyl-L-carnitine, Flavonoids, fish oil, magnesium, vitamin C, tocotrienols and carotenoids, multivitamins and minerals. His and Levine's group will sell you all of these so-called "cures." Please remember, as always to "follow the money."

Levine says this concerning Pall's results, "**These strong findings** on this small study present **compelling evidence** that Dr. Pall's hypothesis and suggested nutrients designed to reduce NO/ONOO and superoxide activity **are very useful in CFS/ME**."

Yet, on the last page of the IN FOCUS Nutricology Newsletter it states:

"In Focus publishes emerging nutritional science and scientific theories that **should not be construed to be conclusive scientific proof of any specific cause, effect or relationship.** The publication is for the educational use of healthcare practioners and physicians. The articles in the publication are the independent scientific views and theories of the authors. In Focus **takes no position on the views and theories** expressed but offers them for candid inquiry and debate. The articles are **not intended for use in support of the sale of any commercial product** and **should not be construed as indicative of the use or efficacy of any commercial product.** Emerging science and scientific theories do not constitute scientific proof of any specific cause, effect or relationship."

It seems to me that Levine is saying, contrary to his stated policy, that Pall has **"strong findings and compelling evidence that these products are very useful in treating CFS/ME."**

In my opinion, this whole scenario is a quintessential example of 21st century snake oil salesmanship!!! Snake oil now flows faster than Texas crude.

At worst, antioxidant supplements have dangerous consequences and at best, they are a waste of money. (RMH 1-5-09) In the absence of a proven vitamin deficiency, these supplement products are basically useless and do not have the same biochemical effect as the nutrients being obtained from a healthy diet.

With such a large portion of the population using antioxidant vitamins, even a small effect from antioxidant restriction could have a big public health impact. This should be combined with increasing overall oxidative capacity. RMH 1-26-10

Certainly, research findings have not been sufficiently compelling to convince most cellular biochemists that the free radical theory and overall disease causation are functionally linked. In fact, recent studies undermine this link.

A comprehensive literature review shows that antioxidant therapies have enjoyed unjustified support in preclinical studies across disparate animal models, but have shown little or no benefit in human intervention studies or clinical trials. A total reassessment of the role of antioxidant vitamins in human health is in order.

It has previously been believed that knockout of various antioxidant defense enzymes raises oxidative damage levels and promotes age-related cancer development in animals. In explaining this, most attention has been paid to direct oxidative damage to DNA by certain RS, such as hydroxyl radical (OH*). However, **increased levels of DNA base oxidation products such as 8OHdg (8-hydroxy-2'-deoxyguanosine) do not always lead to malignancy**, although malignant tumors often show increased levels of DNA base oxidation. Hence additional actions of RS must be important, possibly their effects on p53, cell proliferation, invasiveness and metastasis. Chronic inflammation predisposes to malignancy, but the role of RS in this is likely to be complex because **RS can sometimes act as anti-inflammatory agents** (Oxidative stress and cancer: have we moved forward? B. Halliwell. Biochem J (2007) 401: 1-11). **I believe that this discounts the suggestions that EMODs are both tumoricidal and inflammatory agents.**

1.0.0.2 Avoid prolix writing and overly wordy sophistry

I will attempt to avoid prolix writing and overly wordy sophistry (which is already overly wordy).

Paracelsus stated, "Practice should not be based on speculative theory; theory should be derived from practice. Experience is the judge; if a thing stands the test of experience, it should be accepted; if it does not stand this test, it should be rejected." **RMH Note: This could well refer to the situation with antioxidants. In theory, they should work but in practice, they do not. Ergo, they should be rejected.**

Antioxidants are (allegedly) especially important in the mitochondria of eukaryotic cells, since the use of oxygen as part of the process for generating energy produces reactive oxygen species. The process of aerobic metabolism requires oxygen because oxygen serves as the final resting place for electrons generated by the oxidation steps of the citric acid cycle (i.e. **oxygen is the final "electron acceptor"** of the redox reactions). However, the superoxide anion is produced as a by-product of this reduction of oxygen in the electron transport chain. Specifically, the reduction of coenzyme Q in complex III is currently believed to be the major source of superoxide anion, since a highly reactive free radical is formed as an intermediate (Q ·□). This unstable radical can lead to electron "leakage": instead of moving along the well-controlled reactions of the electron transport chain, the electrons jump directly to molecular oxygen, forming the superoxide anion (Finkel and Holbrook 2000). (http://articles.gourt.com/en/Antioxidant). **I interpret this to mean that oxygen is not ripping electrons away from reducing agents,**

but it is "accepting" electrons. Ripping is very aggressive process, whereas, accepting is passive. Please remember that oxygen is the "ultimate electron acceptor."

CONTRIVED SUPPORT FOR THE FREE RADICAL THEORY

1.0.0.3 Attempts to brain wash children on the dangers of EMODs

Skippy and Oaf is a blatant attempt to brainwash children against EMODs and to glorify antioxidants. This book is a prime example of nonsense/nonscience, written by a totally uninformed author for the purpose of making a buck.

1.0.0.4 Skippy and Oaf: The Battle Against Oxygen Radicals

(ISBN: 9781933255279), by Craig S. Cousineau, has just been released by DNA Press. **Heroic characters portray antioxidants battling evil oxygen radicals** in this lively, science-based story **(RMH Note: fairy tale.)**. Skippy and Oaf are rats living at a science and nutrition research laboratory. Skippy, a very intelligent rat, is concerned about his friend Oaf's terrible eating habits, and tries to get his friend to eat healthier food. Oaf is skeptical until Skippy explains, in his erroneous way, the science of nutrition at a molecular level, complete with descriptions of **battles between superheroes (antioxidants found in fruits and vegetables) and oxygen-radical villains**. Based on fascinating scientific information and including a lesson on genomes and DNA, the book is illustrated by playful drawings that clarify its key concepts.

This garbage is being used for propaganda and to endoctrinate the minds of children against the beneficence of oxygen.

(PRWEB) July 16, 2007 -- The DNA Press team is happy to announce the publication of "Skippy and Oaf: The Battle Against Oxygen Radicals", **a book that gives children the tools they need to make the right choices about the food they eat**. Craig Cousineau, a student at the University of Michigan, majoring in molecular biology, wrote the book while working as an intern at the Delta-Schoolcraft Intermediate School District.

"Skippy and Oaf" will help children and their parents understand the research behind nutrition and why fruits and vegetables are good for them," says the young author. "Oftentimes when a child is told what they should eat without being told why, they won't eat the right foods willingly or may completely refuse. This book not only explains to children what they should eat, but it also tells them why. It uses information about genetics and microbiology that they might not otherwise start learning about until they are in high school."

It inspires children to start eating more fruits and vegetables. The Center for Disease Control and Prevention reports that the number of overweight children in the United States has tripled over the past 30 years, with one in five children now being overweight.

"Parents and teachers are looking for books that deal with this topic and can help educate children," says Kristine Paulsen, General Education Director at the Delta-Schoolcraft Intermediate School District. "This book teaches children and their parents about health and nutrition in an entertaining way. Reading "Skippy and Oaf" inspires children to start eating more fruits and vegetables."

Delta-Schoolcraft ISD used "Skippy and Oaf" as the centerpiece in two pilot projects aimed at introducing elementary students to healthy eating and nutrition. 75% of participating students increased the number of healthy foods they were eating, 90% of the students talked about the book at home, and **76% of the parents believe this experience will impact the food choices their children will make in the future**.

Following is a sample of the many enthusiastic parent responses:

* "Skippy and Oaf made my son more aware of why fruits and vegetables are good for him and opened him to eating things he might avoid."

* "This book made my daughter aware that veggies are a good snack. It's not just Mom saying it."

* "My daughter tried new foods and I didn't have to 'make' her."

"Schools in Michigan, California and South Carolina have begun using this book and the feedback from teachers has been great," says Ms. Paulsen.

Joanne Woodard, a teacher in Poway, California, wrote, "My **first-grade children** loved the book. Every day they wanted to know when we were going to read the 'Skippy and Oaf' book and what the 'Skippy' snack was going to be that day. I can't believe how much the children understood and were fascinated by the information about DNA, oxygen radicals and antioxidants."

"Skippy and Oaf: The Battle Against Oxygen Radicals" can help children and their families improve their nutrition and become excited about the science behind good eating.

http://neutral-izer.blogspot.com/2007/07/skippy-and-oaf-battle-against-oxygen.html

1.0.0.5 How some antioxidants can harm health

Some of the plant based reducing acids, most notably oxalic and phytic, bind to needed dietary minerals, rendering them unabsorbable in the gastrointestinal tract. Some of the tannins also have this negative characteristic. Calcium and iron deficiencies are not uncommon in mideastern diets where there is high consumption of phytic acid present in beans and unleavened whole grain bread. Such antinutrients can sometimes result in deceptively high Oxygen Radical Absorbance Capacity (ORAC) ratings given to various "healthy" beverages and foods, particularly:

- cocoa/chocolate, spinach, and berries - oxalic acid
- whole grains, maize - phytic acid
- tea - tannins

Other extremely powerful nonpolar antioxidants such as eugenol also happen to have toxicity limits that can easily be exceeded with the misuse of essential oils.

High levels of antioxidants can be powerful agents against tumors, but in some scenarios can interfere with the effects of other cancer treatments.

Recent laboratory studies suggest that at levels much higher than occur through normal diets, antioxidant vitamins such as A, E and C can have pro-oxidant effects, increasing the formation of free radicals. Natural antioxidants are always ingested together with a wide variety of flavonoids and other phytochemicals are also likely to play a part. Many supplement manufacturers supply products containing antioxidants in combination with these other natural chemicals. Another significant factor is that the mechanisms by which different antioxidants regenerate each other require balanced levels to work optimally. Newer liquid nutritional supplements using plant ionic compounds are believed to be more readily absorbed in the human body. (http://articles.gourt.com/en/Antioxidant).

1.0.0.6 Calorie restriction and reduced oxidative stress

Virtually all studies of mammals have concluded that a restricted calorie diet (CR) extends median and maximum lifespan (CR is almost the only protocol to have achieved this). **This benefit appears to be at least partly due to substantially reduced oxidative stress.** Very large increases in lifespan (up to around 100%) have only been observed in short lived species and the effect in humans is expected to be far less dramatic. The best evidence from animal studies is likely to come from ongoing studies in primates where median life spans have already been shown to be increased and biomarkers of health significantly improved. Due to the long life span of primates, confirmation of maximum lifespan increase will not be available until around 2014. The striking results from animal experiments provide strong evidence that an excess of food reduces life expectancy, although the relationship is not a simple one. **Other research suggests that being a little overweight is actually a healthier option in humans (**New Scientist 26 November 2005), and a recent major study concluded that mortality rates were positively correlated with waist size, but for a fixed waist size mortality rates were negatively correlated with body mass index (particularly for underweight subjects). As **food produces free radicals (oxidants) when metabolized**, antioxidant-rich diets are thought to stave off the effects of aging significantly better than diets lacking in antioxidants. **(RMH Note: Research has not confirmed this.)** http://articles.gourt.com/en/Antioxidant).

1.0.0.7 Exercise and antioxidants

During exercise, oxygen consumption can temporarily increase by a factor of more than 10-15X. This leads to a temporary large increase in the production of oxygen free radicals, allegedly resulting in increased cell damage contributing to muscular fatigue during and after exercise. The body uses antioxidants to reduce the amount of such damage. The inflammatory response that occurs after strenuous exercise is also associated with increased occurrence of free radicals, especially during the 24 hours after an exercise session. In this phase too, antioxidants in the body reduce the damage. The immune system response to damage done by exercise peaks 2 to 7 days after exercise, the period during which adaptation resulting in greater fitness is greatest. During this process, free radicals are used by neutrophils in the immune system to identify damaged tissue. As a result, **excessive antioxidant levels have the potential to inhibit recovery and adaptation mechanisms.** [http://www.ncbi.nlm.nih.gov/entrez/query.fcgi?cmd=Retrieve&db=PubMed&list_uids=9839079&dopt=Abstract.]

There is a popular view that those who undertake vigorous exercise can benefit from increased consumption of antioxidants, but an examination of the literature finds support that this is the case only for certain antioxidants at certain levels, and **some evidence that very large intake of some antioxidants may be**

detrimental to recovery from exercise. There is strong evidence that one of the adaptations that result from exercise is a strengthening of the body's anti-oxidant defenses, particularly the glutathione system, to deal with the increased oxidative stress. It is possible that this effect may be to some extent protective against diseases which are associated with oxidative stress, which would provide a partial explanation for the lower incidence of major diseases and better health of those who undertake regular exercise.

The antioxidant system that protects lipid membranes from free radicals includes vitamin E, beta-carotene, vitamin A, and coenzyme Q10. The system that scavenges free radicals in the water based cytoplasm includes vitamin C, glutathione peroxidase, superoxide dismutase, and catalase. The effect of each of the exogenous antioxidants needs to be examined separately, although they work in a co-operative manner.

The body of research suggests no benefits from supplementing with vitamin A above normally recommended levels. Recent well-designed studies suggest **there are no ergogenic benefits from vitamin E** (except for those who do exercise at high altitude), (Mehdani et al, 1997), despite its key role in preventing lipid membrane peroxidation. For example, 6 weeks of vitamin E supplementation had no effect on muscle damage indicators in ultramarathon runners RDA is of any ergogenic benefit. However, for vitamin C there is considerable evidence that vitamin C requirements are greater in those who do vigorous exercise, with plasma levels falling with intake of 100mg (well over the accepted RDA) and around 300mg per day being required to maintain blood plasma levels (Keith, 1997). There is some evidence that supplementation with vitamin C increased the amount of intense exercise that can be done, and lowered the heart rate while doing it (which is indicative of greater efficiency) and that vitamin C supplementation before strenuous exercise reduces the amount of muscle damage, although the very short pre-exercise supplementation period in this study may have influenced the results. There is strong evidence that **vitamin C supplementation reduces upper respiratory tract infections in ultra-endurance athletes** [http://www.ncbi.nlm.nih.gov/entrez/query.fcgi?cmd=Retrieve&db=PubMed&list_uids=8185726&dopt=Abstract.

In summary, **a diet with at least 300mg of vitamin C is of benefit to those who undertake high intensity or high volume exercise**, but it is not clear that normal requirements for vitamin A, vitamin E or selenium are increased. (http://articles.gourt.com/en/Antioxidant).

1.0.0.8 Clinical trials of antioxidant supplements

Although some levels of antioxidant vitamins and minerals in the diet are required for good health, **there is considerable doubt as to whether antioxidant supplementation is beneficial,** and if so, which and what amount of antioxidant(s) are optimal.

One study of lung cancer patients found that those given beta-carotene supplements had worse prognoses. Two 1994 studies found an increased rate of lung cancer in smokers supplementing with beta carotene. This is believed to be due to antioxidant interference with the body's normal use of localised free radicals e.g. nitric oxide for cell signalling. Due to the complex nature of the interactions of antioxidants with the body, it is difficult to interpret the results of many experiments. In vitro testing (outside the body) has shown many natural antioxidants, in specific concentration, can halt the growth of or even kill cancerous cells.

In the early 1990s, it was hypothesized that oxidation of LDL cholesterol contributes to heart disease, and several observational studies found that people taking Vitamin E supplements had a lower risk of developing heart disease (Rimm 1993). Taken together, **this led researchers to conduct at least seven large clinical trials testing the effects of antioxidant supplement with Vitamin E, in doses ranging from 50 to 600 mg per day.** However, **none of these trials found a statistically significant effect of Vitamin E on overall number of deaths or on deaths due to heart disease** (Vivekananthan 2003).

While several trials have investigated supplements with high doses of antioxidants, the "Supplementation en Vitamines et Mineraux Antioxydants" (SU.VI.MAX) study tested the effect of supplementation with doses comparable to those in a healthy diet (Hercberg 2003). Over 12,500 French men and women took either low-dose antioxidants (120 mg of ascorbic acid, 30 mg of vitamin E, 6 mg of beta carotene, 100 \mug of selenium, and 20 mg of zinc) or placebo pills for an average of 7.5 years. The investigators found **there was no statistically significant effect of the antioxidants on overall survival, cancer, or heart disease.** However, **a subgroup analysis showed a 31% reduction in the risk of cancer in men, but not women.** The authors interpreted these results as suggesting that "an adequate and well-balanced supplementation of antioxidant nutrients, at doses that might be reached with a healthy diet that includes a high consumption of fruits and vegetables, had protective effects against cancer in men."

The significant effect of supplementary selenium in reducing incidence of prostate cancer was strongly supported by the Nutrition for the Prevention of Cancer (NPC) trial (designed primarily to determine the effect of selenium supplementation on skin cancers) and found **significant effects for subjects whose plasma selenium levels were in the middle and lower thirds, but not for those in the top third.** The **SELECT project** further investigating the effects of selenium supplementation (in combination with vitamin E) on prostate cancer incidence, but **final results will not be available until 2013** [http://www.ncbi.nlm.nih.gov/entrez/query.fcgi?cmd=Retrieve&db=pubmed&dopt=Abstract&list_uids=15753149&query_hl=5&itool=pubmed_docsum. (http://articles.gourt.com/en/Antioxidant).

1.0.0.9 Antioxidants used as food additives

Antioxidants used as food additives to help guard against food deterioration include:

- Ascorbic acid (vitamin C)
- Tocopherol-derived compounds
- BHA, BHT, EDTA
- Citric acid
- Acetic acid - found in vinegar; used for pickling
- Pectin
- Rosmarinic acid - in the form of the herb rosemary and Italian seasoning mixtures in naturally or minimally processed foods, and pet foods

Since the discovery of vitamins, it has been recognized that **antioxidants from the diet are essential for healthful lives in humans and many other mammals**. More recently, a large body of evidence has accumulated that suggests supplementation of the diet with various kinds of antioxidants can arguably improve health and extend life. Many nutraceutical and health food companies now sell formulations of antioxidants as dietary supplement.These supplements may include specific antioxidant chemicals, like resveratrol (from grape seeds), combinations of antioxidants, like the "ACES" products that contain beta carotene (provitamin **A**), vitamin **C**, vitamin **E** and **S**elenium, or specialty herbs that are known to contain antioxidants such as green tea and jiaogulan. (http://articles.gourt.com/en/Antioxidant).

There are hundreds of different types of antioxidants.

Melatonin is a natural hormone, occurring in every organism, which has many biological roles. Melatonin acts as an antioxidant and promoter of antioxidants in several different ways Recent research supports a specific role as an antioxidant in mitochondria, which have an high level of reactive oxygen species produced during aerobic metabolism, but lack some of the protective mechanisms of cell nuclei. **Melatonin has also been shown to have significant prooxidant activity.**

1.0.1.0 Flavonoid polyphenolics (also known as bioflavonoids)

Bioflavonoids, a subset of polyphenol antioxidants, are present in many dark berries such as pomegranate, seabuckthorn, noni, blueberries, and blackberries, as well as in certain types of coffee and tea, especially green tea.

Flavonols:

- Resveratrol - found in the skins of dark-colored grapes, and concentrated in red wine.
- Pterostilbene - methoxylated analogue of resveratrol, abundant in Vaccinium berries
- Kaempferol
- Myricetin - walnuts are a rich source
- Isorhamnetin
- Proanthocyanidins, or condensed tannins

Flavones:

- Quercetin and related, such as rutin
- Luteolin
- Apigenin
- Tangeritin

Flavanones:

- Hesperetin (metabolizes to hesperidin)
- Naringenin (metabolized from naringin)
- Eriodictyol

Flavan-3-ols (anthocyanidins):

- Catechin
- Gallocatechin
- Epicatechin and its gallate forms
- Epigallocatechin and its gallate forms
- Theaflavin and its gallate forms
- Thearubigins

Isoflavone phytoestrogens - found primarily in soy, peanuts, and other members of the Fabaceae family. Besides having antioxidant characteristics, isoflavones also protect and maintain the skeletal system.

- Genistein
- Daidzein
- Glycitein

Anthocyanins protect plants from UV damage:

- Cyanidin
- Delphinidin
- Malvidin
- Pelargonidin
- Peonidin
- Petunidin

1.0.1.1 Other organic antioxidants

- Citric acid
- Lignan - antioxidant and phytoestrogen found in oats, flax seeds, pumpkin seeds, sesame seeds, rye, soybeans, broccoli, beans, and some berries.
- **Antinutrients** - strong antioxidants that readily bind to needed dietary minerals, rendering them unabsorbable in the gastrointestinal tract. Examples: **oxalic acid** and **phytic acid**.
- Bilirubin, a breakdown product of blood, has been identified as a possibly significant antioxidant.
- Uric acid
- R-α-lipoic acid - fat and water soluble
- Silymarin - fat soluble; also available in water soluble form
- N-acetylcysteine - water soluble

(http://articles.gourt.com/en/Antioxidant).

1.0.2.0 Speculation on anoxia and changes following death

Previously, I have discussed the changes following anoxia and death and how rapidly the bacteria in the body replicated and decompose the body. Also, it is well known that a body can be kept alive on heart lung machine indefinitely. Then, what happens when the oxygen is turned off? Does this further illustrate my point that oxygen holds these bacteria in abeyance and can anything be learned by either nitrogen perfusion (oxygen displacement) or by studying in utero deaths, whereby the fetus is in a sense on a heart and lung machine?

In multicellular organisms, the total number of cells is a balance between the cell-generating effects of mitosis and cell death that is induced through apoptosis. A disruption of this delicate balance can lead to the development of cancer. (Apoptosis and cancer: the genesis of a research field. TG Cotter. Nat Rev Cancer (2009) 9: 501-7).

This has led to my theory of carcinogenesis, in which EMOD-induced apoptosis is the primary means of producing neoplastic cellular death. Thus, EMOD insufficiency allows for the development of malignancy.

When cellular superoxide dismutase comes into contact with superoxide, the SOD reaction takes place, which results in the production of hydrogen peroxide. For each two superoxides that are encountered by the SOD, one hydrogen peroxide (H_2O_2) is created. Hydrogen peroxide may however pose a great danger to the cell as it transforms easily into the highly reactive hydroxyl radical. **I believe that according to the predictions of the free radical theory, that patients without catalase (acatalasemia) would have disastrous consequences as the result of a fatal genetic flaw. However, acatalasemic patients live basically normal lives, troubled only by gum infections. This fact, alone, discounts the doom and gloom predictions of the free radi-crap theory.**

There does exist an efficient mechanism for dealing with the hydrogen peroxide. The enzyme catalase is produced by the rough endoplasmic reticulum and is concentrated in peroxisomes surrounding the mitochondria (as well as being present in lower concentrations throughout the cell). The catalase reacts with the hydrogen peroxide to produce water and oxygen. As stated before, **acatalasemics live basically normal lives and have a normal life span.**

Over 90% of the dioxygen used by an organism is processed in the mitochondria (B Chance, H Sies and A Boveris, Physiol Rev, 59, 527-605(1979).

If oxygen and its stochastic products are the cause of aging, then infinitely dividing cells, such as neoplasia, should also age and die, even though most cancer cells are relatively hypoxic. This alone discounts the free radical theory of aging. Even though these cancer cells use oxygen, they are immortal. Additionally, hypoxia is usually associated with

increased ROS production, which should rapidly end the life of cancerous cells, but it does not.

1.0.2.1 Inflammation as the root of all evil

Speculation points to **chronic inflammation** as not only being the problem of well recognized inflammatory diseases such as tuberculosis, rheumatoid arthritis or inflammatory bowel disease (Hensley et al., 2000) (Hensley K, Robinson KA, Prasad Gabbita S, Salsman S, Floyd RA. Reactive oxygen species, cell signaling and cell injury. Free Rad Biol Med 28(10):1456-1462, 2000), but also as a contributor to a growing number of mechanistically unconnected illnesses such as atherosclerosis, Alzheimer disease, and some cancers (Forrester, 2004) (Forrester JS. Common ancestors: Chronic progressive diseases have the same pathogenesis. Clin Cardiol 27:186-190, 2004).

The **allegation** that inflammation is involved in one way or another in almost all known diseases has led to the hypothesis that **"inflammation may be the root of all evil"** (Kreeger, 2003) (Kreeger K. Inflammation's inflamy. The Scientist 17(14):28-30, 2003). Please remember that inflammation is consistent with hypoxia.

RMH Note: To me, it makes sense that inflammation is going to be at disease sites and associated with disease. That is because inflammation is there to fight the disease and not to cause it. If the inflammatory response was great enough, it would likely reverse or cure the respective disease.

At sites of inflammation, H_2O_2 generated by activated phagocytes appears to modulate the inflammatory process, e.g. by up-regulating expression of adhesion molecules, controlling cell proliferation or apoptosis and modulating platelet aggregation.

It has been said that, "The essence of cell aging may be demonstrated with the example of high-specialized cells found in peripheral blood systems, which are either unable to divide or divide relatively seldom. Human blood cell life spans vary widely, from several hours to several years. There is the evidence that the level of specific activity of superoxide dismutase in different blood corpuscles also varies considerably. **Superoxide dismutase concentrations have been reported to be lowest in granulocytes;** at the same time, these cells aggressively generate exogenous superoxide radicals used in bactericidal activity. That is what the majority of oxygen consumed by granulocytes is used for; thus, the lifespan of these cells are, not surprisingly, short." (Doctor's Corner Newsletter Archive. Superoxide dismutase and aging. By Leonid Magidenko, MD. *Sunday, July 15, 2007*). **However, I believe that the WBCs are sacrificial. The true low toxicity of EMODs is demonstrated by post mitotic cells, such as brain and heart, which generate huge quantities of EMODs and they can exist for a century and still function well! This obviously indicates low toxicity, even in the presence of renewal and corrective enzymatic systems.**

Magidenko also states that, "phagocytosis accompanied by a surge in respiratory metabolism and **rocketing superoxide radical** generation accelerates the death of phagocytes, while **exogenous superoxide dismutase increases the survival rate for phagocytes to that of resting cells. (RMH Note: Increases in SOD directly increases the levels of peroxide.).** Although phagocytes have the highest superoxide dismutase levels, they generate exogenous superoxide radicals, which affect their lifespan substantially.

Red blood cells are also characterized by high level of superoxide dismutase; despite their low ability to generate superoxide radicals **(RMH Note: This makes no sense according to the free radical theorists.)**, red blood cells contain a high quantity of **hemoglobin which continuously interacts with oxygen to generate superoxide radicals.** They have a longer lifespan than platelets, but not much longer. Lymphocytes do not generate exogenous superoxide radicals; their lifespan is relatively long, apparently due to the high level of superoxide dismutase."

1.0.2.2 Hyperthermia speculation

A similar correlation has been reported between the speed of aging and body temperature. It is most apparent in cold-blooded organisms, which change their metabolic rate in accordance with their body temperature. **When earthworms adapt to a temperature rise from 15 to 30°C, its tissues undergo a 28% increase in the level of superoxide dismutase and its oxygen consumption rises by 135%.** Since this level of increased oxygen consumption cannot be accounted for by the rise in superoxide dismutase activity, it has been proposed to be the reason for the considerably higher lifespan of the earthworm at 15°C. **I believe that this may relate to our febrile response to infections and pathogen protection. This may also be the beneficial basis of hyperthermia therapy. Simply put, the higher the temp, the faster are the involved chemical reactions.**

Non-protein anti-oxidants may increase lifespan in short-living strains of mice by 30 to 33%. Experiments on transgenic animals are very promising but inconsistent. In a very early study of superoxide dismutase, the DNA of copper-bearing superoxide dismutase was implanted in drosophila by genetic engineering methods. This genetic modification resulted in its **increased activity and modest, but significant, lifespan increase.** Drosophila with complementary copies of genes of superoxide dismutase and catalase lived longer than control animals by 20 to 37%. Additionally, transgenic drosophila demonstrated signs of improved age-related characteristics; decreased accumulation of carbonyl proteins; decreased oxygen-sensitive enzyme inactivation as well as decreased accumulation of oxygen damaged DNA products; and reduced generation rate of oxidants in mitochondria. Recent studies have shown **lifespan increases of 40% in drosophila with abundant human superoxide dismutase gene expressions in motorneurons. I believe that this is directly due to the increased peroxide generation by SOD, which maintains an EMOD sufficiency.**

(Accessed 7-19-09 http://www.abcvitaminslife.com/HealthFacts/Article428.aspx)

It has occurred to me that conditions such as hypothyroidism could be because of a peroxide deficiency (EMOD insufficiency). Since peroxide serves as a substrate for thyroxine synthesis, a low level of peroxide would result in low levels of thyroxine synthesis. This could be extrapolated to other peroxidases, in that deficiencies in peroxide would result in low levels of their respective reaction products and with the consequent manifestation of the associated symptoms.

It appears to me that chronic disease syndrome is intimately related to energy metabolism, which is closely related to the electron transport chain and oxidative phosphorylation. This focuses attention to the EMODs being in a deficiency state.

1.0.3.0 Peroxidases

Peroxidases: Thyroperoxidase, Cytochrome c peroxidase, Eosinophil peroxidase, Myeloperoxidase, Thylperoxidase, Glutathione peroxidase, Prostaglandin synthase, Human salivary peroxidase, Chloroperoxidase.

If only researchers had stopped and wondered why neutrophils have a green hue! It is due to the content of myeloperoxidase.

When Weiss showed **that 25% of extracellular hydrogen peroxide was converted to HOCl it became clear that chlorine bleach is a major oxidant generated by neutrophils.** Subsequently, Hurst showed that **at least 10% of the oxygen consumed by neutrophils was converted to HOCl that reacted inside phagosomes.** These two results clearly confirmed **Klebanoff's earlier assertion that myeloperoxidase plays a central part in neutrophil oxidant production.**

1.0.3.1 H_2O_2

Peroxide plays an important role as a beneficial signaling molecule. In addition to the unwanted production of H_2O_2 in the body, ROS are also intentionally produced in the body and used for synthesis and detoxification processes as well as for immune defense. **H_2O_2 is produced** in the **thyroid gland** as a substrate for thyroperoxidase, which catalyzes the attachment of iodine to thryoglobulin, an important protein for the synthesis of thyroid hormone. **H_2O_2 is generously produced in peroxisomes to aid in the degradation of fatty acids** and other molecules, and **H2O2 is used for detoxification reactions involving the liver cytochrome P-450 system. Thus, how toxic can these EMODs be?**

True or not, it is now certain that just as **ROS and H_2O_2 can be considered "death molecules", they also can be called "molecules of life"** (Droege, W. Free radicals in the physiological control of cell function. Physiol Rev 82:47-95, 2001) (Rhee SG, Chang TS, Bae YS, Lee SR, Kang SW. Cellular regulation by hydrogen peroxide. J Am Soc. Nephrol 14:S211-S215, 2003).

H_2O_2 is well suited to act as cellular messenger since it does not randomly react with all molecules, as most other EMODs do, but instead primarily targets cysteine residues. It oxidizes the -SH group of cysteine to –·OH which is then reduced by cellular reducing agents such as glutathione and thioredoxin. However, these reactions are only possible when the cysteine is deprotonated (-S-), which is not often the case at physiological pH. Only a positively charged amino acid in the vicinity of the cysteine can keep it in an oxidizable form, which means that **only selected proteins are targets for H_2O_2.** (Reth M. Hydrogen peroxide as second messenger in lymphocyte activation. Nature Immunol 3(12):1129-1134, 2002).

The stability of H_2O_2 further depends on the cell's redox state. H_2O_2 is more stable in an oxidizing environment, such as the extracellular

space, than in a reducing environment like the cell interior. Therefore, H2O2 has also been proposed to act as an inter-cellular messenger (Reth M. Hydrogen peroxide as second messenger in lymphocyte activation. Nature Immunol 3(12):1129-1134, 2002).

The net H_2O_2 concentration depends on the site and source of H_2O_2 production, the numerous H_2O_2 activities within the cell, the spontaneous and enzymatic dismutation of H_2O_2, as well as the concentration of protective agents. In other words, it depends on the redox milieu. **Catalase does not appear to be nearly so important as SOD, judging from the weak phenotypes of cells that lack it (**Imlay, J. A., and Linn, S. (1988) *Science* 240, 1302-1309**) and persons with acatalasemia** (Eaton, J. W., and Ma, M. (1995) in *The Metabolic and Molecular Bases of Inherited Disease* (Scriver, C. R., Beaudet, A. L., Sly, W. S., and Valle, D., eds), 7th Ed., pp. 2371-2383, McGraw-Hill, Inc., New York).

Denham Harman told Jack Cheatam that taking excessive antioxidants would result in fatigue. Is it possible that conditions of chronic fatigue syndrome are due to "antioxidant stress" or an EMOD insufficiency? I suggest that is the case.

Oxygen is fundamentally essential for life and adequate concentrations are an important signal for virtually all cellular processes. Oxygen is an integral signal in all major aspects of stem cell biology including proliferation and tumorigenesis (EMOD insufficiency), cell death and differentiation, self-renewal, and migration. (Oxygen in the Cultivation of Stem Cells. Marie Csete. *Ann. N.Y. Acad. Sci.* 1049: 1–8 (2005).

The researchers are using other technologies to determine how the loss of oxygen affects the functions of genes in the brain. Of the approximately 30,000 genes investigated to date, at least 6,000 are either inactivated or highly activated when a stroke reduces the oxygen in the brain. Their future work will explore the ramifications of those changed gene functions. I believe that this illustrates the crucial role of oxygen levels, EMOD levels and the redox status of the cell.

The most important underlying cause of most ill health can be traced to inadequate production of cellular energy and **faulty oxygen metabolism. I am proposing the correction of an EMOD insufficiency state as the means of countering the development and progression of a wide variety of**

disease conditions and aging. Just as EMODs kill pathogens and nullify toxins on the outside of the body, they do likewise internally.

1.0.3.2 Free Radical Shift: Antioxidants may not increase life span

Scientific American Magazine - May 7, 2009 By Kate Wilcox

Antioxidants, abundant in pomegranates, counter free radical damage but may not delay aging. Companies have started putting antioxidants in goods as different as face creams and sodas, claiming that they clean out cells, prevent cancer and even stave off death. The idea is to prevent unstable oxygen molecules, which are normal by-products of metabolism, from damaging cells. But **a recent study suggests that when it comes to living longer, those antioxidants may not be the answer**.

The antioxidant theory of aging states that some of the oxygen molecules used by the body become negatively charged, making them reactive. As a result, they compromise health and age the body by damaging cell structures, proteins and DNA. Cells have a natural defense—superoxide dismutase (SOD), a special class of antioxidant that neutralizes the chemicals and prevents them from harming cells. According to the theory, proposed in 1956 by Denham Harman, now emeritus professor of medicine at the University of Nebraska, when the body gets older, SODs become less efficient at preventing oxidative stress. Over the past 50 years this widely accepted theory has held up in studies: when the SOD gene is knocked out in mice, flies or yeast, the organisms develop cancers and have shorter life spans.

RMH Note: SOD is in actuality a prooxidant. It converts superoxide to hydrogen peroxide (-330 eV to +320 eV). In other words, it converts a weaker oxidant into a stronger oxidant. Thus, the lack of SOD causes problems because of the lack of peroxide, which is part of an overall EMOD insufficiency and allows for disease manifestation.

1.0.3.3 Hekimi: C elegans and blocked SOD increases lifespan

But in the February 2009 PLoS Genetics, Siegfried Hekimi and Jeremy M. Van Raamsdonk, both at McGill University, report that **removing SODs from tiny Caenorhabditis elegans soil worms has the exact opposite effect—they live longer**. In the experiment, each of the worms' five SOD genes, which primarily work in the mitochondria (the cells' energy-producing organelles), was disabled in different combinations, hampering the worms' ability to make the antioxidant. **When the researchers turned off one SOD gene (namely, sod-2), the nematodes actually lived 30 percent longer. When four were disabled in follow-up work, the worms still had a normal life span.**

I believe that superoxide is still being formed and is spontaneously being converted to hydrogen peroxide. Thus, the impact of blocked SOD is nullified.

Hekimi believes that the findings throw a wrench in the entire free radical theory of aging. Instead he claims that cell damage is a product of aging, not the actual cause. "It's like the sun coming up every morning—they can't prove that it will," he says in reference to free radical proponents. "But I have to prove that it won't."

These modified worms are not healthy, though; they show evidence of oxidative stress. Without the antioxidants, their cells are left unprotected, and outside the lab the worms would have died from disease or cancer. But Hekimi separates such a condition from having a normal life span. The organism may be sicker, he observes, but it is living longer. **I believe that the sickly condition of these worms is due to the fact that SOD has been knocked out and superoxide is not rapidly converted to hydrogen peroxide.**

Other scientists doubt that the findings discredit free radicals entirely. "You can't take a single paper studying a single gene in a single organism and make sweeping conclusions about a theory," remarks John Phillips of the University of Guelph in Ontario, who has examined SODs in the fruit fly Drosophila melanogaster. Moreover, **C. elegans has five SOD genes, whereas humans have two.** "I think we need to know where the extra SODs are operating, like in tissues or muscles, and in which cellular compartments" to fully understand oxygen metabolism in C. elegans, Phillips says. Knowing the biological idiosyncrasies in the worm would elucidate how SODs work in general.

Hekimi proposes that his findings could bolster an alternative aging theory—specifically, the idea that a slower metabolism or lower temperatures decelerate the body and allow an organism to live longer. **Several studies have challenged the rate of living theory of aging,** but Hekimi thinks that "you have to take a broader version of the theory, that the rate at which things happen affects life span." As he sees it, in SOD-deficient worms, free radicals damage the mitochondria, which produce less energy and thereby slow the organism down.

Hekimi's idea stands in contrast with that of **Bart Braeckman of Ghent University in Belgium**, whose own 2007 experiments with C. elegans led him to rule out the metabolic theory of aging. But **Braeckman also does not think that the free radical theory is the only answer.** He notes that Hekimi's work joins **other recent studies that challenge the simplistic version of the theory. "The final conclusion was similar in all these papers: there is a problem with the free radical theory,"** he states.

1.0.3.4 Hekimi has problem with free radical theory

So what does this mean for the antioxidants everyone clamors for? **Synthetic antioxidants have failed to show any clear longevity benefit to humans, and that has been a problem for Harman ever since he conceived his theory.** Although antioxidants definitely prevent damage, there is still no consensus on how much they forestall aging. **"I'm glad there are challenges to the theory," Harman says. "It's the only way we get anything done."**

(http://www.scientificamerican.com/article.cfm?id=free-radical-shift&page=2#comments)

Dr. Siegfried Hekimi of McGill's Department of Biology, said most of the evidence for the oxidative stress theory is circumstantial, meaning oxidative stress could just as easily be a result of aging as its cause.

"The problem with the theory is that it's been based purely on correlative data, on the weight of evidence," explained Hekimi, McGill's Strathcona Chair of Zoology and Robert Archibald & Catherine Louise Campbell Chair in Developmental Biology. "It is true that the more an organism appears aged, whether in terms of disease, or appearance or anything you care to measure, the more it seems to be suffering from oxidative stress".

"This has really entrenched the theory," he continued, "because people think correlation is causation. But now this theory really is in the way of progress."

Hekimi and postdoctoral fellow Jeremy Van Raamsdonk studied mutant Caenorhabditis elegans worms. They progressively disabled five genes responsible for producing a group of proteins called superoxide dismutases (SODs), which detoxify one of the main ROS. Earlier studies seemed to show that decreased SOD production shortened an organism's lifespan, but Hekimi and Van Raamsdonk did not observe this. In fact**, they found quite the opposite.**

None of their mutant worms showed decreased lifespan compared to wild-type worms, even though oxidative stress was clearly raised. In fact, one variety actually displayed increased lifespan, the researchers said.

"The mutation that increases longevity affects the main SOD found in mitochondria inside the animals' cells," said Hekimi. "This is consistent with earlier findings that mitochondria are crucial to the aging process. It seems that reducing mitochondrial activity by damaging it with ROS will actually make worms live longer."

The researchers hasten to point out that they are not suggesting that oxidative stress is good for you. However, I am pointing out that adequate EMOD levels are good for you.

"ROS undoubtedly cause damage to the body," Hekimi said. "However, they do not appear to be responsible for aging.

1.0.4.0 More Americans getting multiple chronic illnesses

1-6-09 **More Americans are burdened by chronic illnesses such as diabetes and high blood pressure, often having more than three at a time**, and this has helped fuel a big rise in out-of-pocket medical expenses, a study released on 1-6-09 showed. **Coexistence of diseases argues for a systemic EMOD insufficiency, which allows them to manifest themselves.**

With prescription drugs playing a key role, average annual out-of-pocket medical costs -- those not covered by health insurance -- rose from $427 per American in 1996 to $741 in 2005, researchers wrote in the journal Health Affairs.

Adjusting for inflation, that translated to 39 percent more in out-of-pocket spending per person over that time, according to Kathryn Paez of Maryland-based health research organization Social & Scientific Systems Inc. and colleagues.

The figures were much higher among the elderly. For example, a person insured through the Medicare program for those 65 and older **who had three or more chronic conditions paid an average of $2,588 of out-of-pocket medical expenses.**

A separate report published in the journal on Tuesday showed U.S. health care spending rose to $2.2 trillion in 2007, or $7,421 per person.

Based on government survey data, **44 percent of Americans in 2005 had at least one chronic medical condition, which could include diabetes, high**

blood pressure, high cholesterol levels, cancer, arthritis, heart failure and others. That compares to 41 percent in 1996.

The study did not look directly at **the causes of the increases, but there appear to be several factors. I believe that the primary cause is EMOD insufficiency.**

The rise in Americans with multiple chronic illnesses comes as obesity and sedentary lifestyles have grown more common. Obesity contributes to many chronic ailments including diabetes. U.S. health officials say the rate of new cases of diabetes soared by about 90 percent in the past decade.

TRIPLE BURDEN

But **the percentage of Americans with three or more chronic illnesses rose even more sharply**.

It jumped from 13 percent in 1996 to 22 percent in 2005 for ages 45 to 64, to 45 percent for ages 65 to 79, and rose from 38 percent to 54 percent for those 80 and older. Among all ages, it went from 7 percent in 1996 to 13 percent in 2005.

"The burden of chronic conditions is becoming heavier. **People who already have chronic conditions no longer just have one. Now they might have three**," Paez said in a telephone interview.

Chronic disease accounts for three-fourths of the more than $2 trillion spent on health care yearly in the United States.

The chronic disease increase was seen not just among the very oldest age groups but also in middle age and early old age -- regardless of sex, race, ethnicity and income level.

President-elect Barack Obama takes office on January 20 with plans to try to tackle the rising costs of **the U.S. health care system, the world's most expensive.** This study suggests that growing amounts of chronic illness may complicate his efforts.

The increase in out-of-pocket medical expenses reflects not only more chronic illness, but likely other factors as well, including worrisome levels of people with no medical insurance as well as reduced coverage from some employers, Paez said.

The higher costs may make it harder for some people to pay for needed medications -- and they may not stay on them or skip doses, worsening their medical problems, Paez added.

The findings were based on nationally representative surveys of about **32,000 people in 2005 and 22,000 people in 1996.**

1.0.4.1 Skin Cancer May Increase Risk of Other Cancers

1-7-09 A new study from the US suggests that **people who have had nonmelanoma skin cancer (NMSC) may be at increased risk of developing** other cancers, including those that affect other parts of the body. **People with a history of non-melanoma skin cancer were found to face a two-fold increase in the risk of subsequent cancers.** Previous research has suggested that non-melanoma skin cancer survivors are at increased risk of developing melanoma in the future, but the researchers found that the disease also increases the risk of other forms of cancer.

The study is the work of Dr Jiping Chen of the National Cancer Institute in Bethesda, Maryland, and Dr Anthony Alberg of the Medical University of South Carolina, and colleagues, and is published on August 26 in the online issue of the *Journal of the National Cancer Institute.*

Previous research has already shown a link between a history of NMSC and increased risk of developing melanoma, a rarer but more malignant form of skin cancer that causes most deaths from skin cancer, but it is not clear whether NSMC is also a risk factor for cancers that affect other parts of the body.

Chen and Alberg and colleagues analyzed data from a prospective cohort study known as **CLUE II,** which is based in Washington County, also in Maryland. They found **769** people in the cohort had been diagnosed with NMSC during a 16 year follow up period since the study started in 1989, and 18,405 people had no history of the disease over the same period. They then compared the risk of developing other types of cancer in the two groups.

The results showed that:

- **The overall rate of cancer diagnosis was 293.5 cases per 10,000 person-years in the NMSC group and 77.9 per 10,000 in the non-NMSC group.**
- After adjusting for other known cancer risk factors such as age, sex, body mass index (BMI), smoking status, and educational level, **people with a history of NMSC were twice as likely to develop other cancers as people with no such history.**
- The increased risk was unaffected by the removal of melanoma from the list of other cancers.
- **The figures were the same for both types of NMSC, basal cell and squamous cell carcinoma.**
- The strongest links between a history of NMSC and the risk of developing other cancers was in participants aged 25 to 44.

The authors concluded that:

"This community-based, prospective cohort study provides evidence for an association between an NMSC diagnosis and an increased risk of subsequent cancer, even after adjusting for individual-level risk factors."

Speculating on the finding that the younger participants with a history of NMSC were the ones most likely to develop other cancers, the authors **suggested it could be because of an inherited predisposition to cancer.**

Discussing the limitations of the study, the editors suggested that people with a history of NMSC might be more likely to receive a diagnosis for another cancer because they are more closely monitored. Also, the people studied in this cohort were all from one county in Maryland and may not be representative of the population as a whole. And finally, the adjustments that were made to eliminate factors such as skin type and sunburn history had to include assumptions because a lot of the data was missing for those factors.

"Nonmelanoma Skin Cancer and Risk for Subsequent Malignancy."

Jiping Chen, Ingo Ruczinski, Timothy J. Jorgensen, Gayane Yenokyan, Yin Yao, Rhoda Alani, Nanette J. Liégeois, Sandra C. Hoffman, Judith Hoffman-Bolton, Paul T. Strickland, Kathy J. Helzlsouer, and Anthony J. Alberg.

Journal of the National Cancer Institute Advance Access published on August 26, 2008.

DOI 10.1093/jnci/djn260).

1.0.5.0 General discussion of cancer and oxygen

Cancerous cells are always being created in the body. It's an ongoing process that has gone on for eons. Specific parts of your immune system are designed to seek out and destroy cancer cells.

Poor oxygenation comes from a buildup of carcinogens and other toxins within and around cells, which blocks and then damages the cellular oxygen respiration mechanism. Clumping up of red blood cells slows down the bloodstream, and restricts flow into capillaries. This also causes poor oxygenation. Even lack of the proper building blocks for cell walls, essential fatty acids, restricts oxygen exchange.

(This is why the flax oil in cottage cheese treatment popular in Europe - 2 tablespoons of organic, refrigerated flax oil or freshly ground flax seed mixed in some cottage cheese - has become a well known cancer treatment. It provides essential fatty acids needed by cell walls so that oxygen can enter the cells.)

Decades ago, two researchers at the National Cancer Institute, Dean Burn and Mark Woods, (Dean translated some of Warburg's speeches) conducted a series of experiments where they measured the fermentation rate of cancers that grew at different speeds. What they found **supported Dr. Warburg's theory. <u>The cancers with the highest growth rates had the highest fermentation rates</u>. The slower a cancer grew, the less it used fermentation to produce energy**.

Naturally Warburg's contention was challenged and tested by other scientists.

Some researchers claimed his theory was not valid after they had measured a particularly slow growing cancer, and found no fermentation at all. And if cancer could grow with no fermentation, then fermentation, or lack of oxygen respiration, was not the cause of cancer. Dean Burn and Mark Woods checked those results.

Using more sophisticated equipment, they determined that the equipment these researchers used to measure fermentation levels was not accurate enough to detect fermentation at low levels. Their testing, using newer and more accurate equipment, showed that **even in those very slow growing cancer cells, fermentation was still taking place, at very low levels.**

Pietro Gullino, also at the National Cancer Institute, devised a test which showed **that this slow growing cancer always produced fermentation lactic**

acid. Silvio Fiala, a biochemist from the University of Southern California, also confirmed that this slow growing cancer produced lactic acid, and that its oxygen respiration was reduced.

Further research into Warburg's theory showed that when oxygen levels were turned down, cells began to produce energy anaerobically. *They ultimately became cancerous when levels went low enough. It took a reduction of 35% in oxygen levels for this to happen.* **NOTE: RMH this is the point I believe that low oxygen levels lead to low or insufficient EMOD levels, which allows neoplasia to manifest itself.**

J. B. Kizer, a biochemist and physicist at Gungnir Research in Portsmith, Ohio explains, "Since Warburg's discovery, this difference in respiration has remained the most fundamental (and some say, only) physiological difference consistently found between normal and cancer cells. Using cell culture studies, I decided to examine the differential responses of normal and cancer cells to changes in the oxygen environment.

"The results that I found were rather remarkable. I found that... **"High O_2 tensions were lethal to cancer tissue, 95 percent being very toxic**, whereas in general, **normal tissues were not harmed by high oxygen tensions**. Indeed, some normal tissues were found to require high O_2 tensions. It does seem to demonstrate the possibility that if the **0_2** tensions in cancer tissues can be elevated, then the cancer tissue may be able to be killed selectively, as it seems that the cancer cells are incapable of handling the **0_2** in a high **0_2** environment." **RMH Note: the high oxygen levels results in higher EMOD levels, which induce apoptosis in the cancer cells and are handled readily by normal cells.**

RMH NOTE: This, I believe, is EMOD-induced apoptosis.

Low oxygen levels in cells may be a fundamental cause of cancer. **RMH Note: I do not look at it as a cause of cancer but rather as a condition which allows for the development of cancer.** There are several reasons cells become poorly oxygenated. An overload of toxins clogging up the cells, poor quality cell walls that don't allow nutrients into the cells, the lack of nutrients needed for respiration, poor circulation and perhaps even low levels of oxygen in the air we breathe. **RMH NOTE: Any factor which produces an EMOD insufficiency will allow for cancer formation.**

Cancer cells produce *excess lactic acid* as they ferment energy. Lactic acid is toxic, and tends to prevent the transport of oxygen into neighboring normal cells. Over time as these cells replicate, the cancer may spread if not destroyed by the immune system. **I believe that the antioxidant lactic acid provides for an EMOD insufficiency, which is needed to sustain the cancer cells and avoid EMOD-induced apoptosis.**

1.0.5.1 The antioxidant, lactic acid ==

1.0.6.0 Low O_2, cells mutate and high O_2, cells stop

RMH Note: Lactic acid is an antioxidant and it is in this capacity that it is advantageous for cancer cells to produce it, such that EMODs can be kept at sub-apoptotic levels. In short, cancer cells produce high levels of antioxidants to protect themselves. Salts of lactic acid are used in foods as a humecticant and an antioxidant which can increase the effect of other antioxidants.

Chemotherapy and radiation are used because cancer cells are **weaker** than normal cells and therefore may die first.

However, chemo and radiation **damage respiratory enzymes** in healthy cells, and overload them with toxins, so they become more likely to develop into cancer. The underlying cancer causing conditions are worsened, not improved. And the cancer usually returns quickly a second time unless you make changes to support the health of your body.

The implication of this research is that an effective way to support the body's fight against cancer would be to **get as much oxygen as you can** into healthy cells, and improving their ability to utilize oxygen. Raising the oxygen levels of normal cells would help prevent them from becoming cancerous.

And increasing oxygen levels in cancer cells to high levels could help kill those cancer cells.

A nurse who works in medical research said, *"It's so simple. I don't know why I never thought of it before. When we're working with cell cultures in the lab, if we want the cells to mutate, we turn down the oxygen. To stop them, we turn the oxygen back up."*

Ma Lan, MD and Joel Wallach DVD, point out that one type of white blood cells kills cancer cells by injecting oxygen creating hydrogen peroxide into the cells.

It is not easy to get **additional oxygen** into cells. Most approaches don't work well. **Breathing oxygen is still limited by the amount of hemoglobin available, and pH levels.** Dr. Whittaker points out, quite rightly, that liquid oxygen supplements that release oxygen into the blood, which most of them only do, *can't* get oxygen into the cells.

He explains that a delivery mechanism is needed to transport oxygen into cells. And though the typical oxygen supplement gets oxygen into the blood, that doesn't mean it gets into the cells.

So what can you do to increase oxygen levels in your cells? The 11 Natural Therapies To Conquer Cancer e-book gives you not one, but two supplements that have the ability to get more oxygen into your cells.

There is a bit more to this oxygenation story.

1.0.7.0 Tumor necrosis factor (TNF) and oxygen free radicals

1.0.7.1 Tumor necrosis factor (TNF) and oxygen free radicals: potential effects for immunity

During various biological processes as inflammation or septic shock, free radical damages are produced by a direct production of oxygen radicals by phagocytes, but also by a TNF-mediated generation in target cells. **Antioxidants have been demonstrated as protective against TNF cytotoxicity.** We try to measure directly the free radical produced by murine recombinant TNF on L929 cells, by detecting the direct light produced by decomposition of superoxide using an adapted chemiluminometer. We measure also the chemiluminescence after addition of luminol. These techniques demonstrate the effective production of oxygen radicals. Unfortunately they have a rather poor specificity and sensitivity. So we use the protective effect of antioxidants on cytotoxicity to investigate the origin of the productive mechanism. We evaluate cytotoxicity of 1 U/ml TNF on L929 murine fibroblasts after 24 hours incubation with actinomycin D by the MTT and Cr51 release. Using the MTT test we observe that **addition of thiourea or catalase has the better protecting effect when Cu-Zn SOD had few effect**. Reversely using the Cr51 release we observe a good protective effect of Cu-Zn SOD simultaneously with a good protective effect of catalase. So the difference in the effect of various antioxidant agent do not permit to identify the species generated, but depend more on the ability of the antioxidant to reach the cell compartment tested by the method (membrane, or mitochondria). **The oxidative effect ofTNF is beneficial in physiological condition to destroy cancerous or virus infested cells infested by virus inside the body.** But this effect can be deleterious in situation of deficiency in some antioxidant.TNF-induced free radicals can increase the replication of virus as HIV-1 and destroy immunocompetent cells as T cells.This last action explains the defect in cellular immunity observed in oxidative stress and the immunostimulatory effect of many antioxidants (Tumor necrosis factor (TNF) and oxygen free radicals: potential effects for immunity. Ferlat S; Favier A. C R Seances Soc Biol Fil. 1993;187(3):296-307).

1.0.7.2 Hydrogen Peroxide Enhances Tumor Necrosis Factor-Alpha Toxicity in Inducing Human Vascular Endothelial Cell Apoptosis: Reversal with Propofol ==

TNF is a cytokine.

Investigators designed the present study to test the hypothesis that oxygen free radicals can enhance tumor necrosis factor (TNF)-α cellular toxicity, which might be reversed by **propofol, an anesthetic with antioxidant properties**, in human vascular endothelial cell line ECV304. Cultured ECV304 were either not treated, treated with 10 μM of hydrogen peroxide (H_2O_2), treated with TNF-α (40 ng/mL) alone, TNF-α in the presence of 10 μM of H_2O_2 (H+T), or propofol plus H_2O_2 for 24 h. Cell viability was measured by lactate dehydrogenate (LDH) assay. Cell apoptosis was assessed by flow cytometry and terminal deoxynucleotidyl transferase (TdT)-mediated deoxyuridine triphosphate (dUTP) nick end-labeling. The **antiapoptotic Bcl-2 and pro-apoptotic Bax protein** expressions were measured by immunocytochemical analysis. **Increases in apoptosis, Bax, lipid peroxidation product malondialdehyde, LDH, and decreases in Bcl-2, superoxide dismutase, and glutathione peroxidase were observed in TNF-α–treated cells. H_2O_2 10 μM did not cause significant lipid peroxidation** (0.75 ± 0.03 nmol/mg of malondialdehyde protein) as compared with control (0.70 ± 0.04 nmol/mg of malondialdehyde protein) ($P > 0.05$) but further enhanced TNF-α–induced lipid peroxidation, upregulated Bax, and down-regulated Bcl-2 expression and enhanced TNF-α–induced cell apoptosis ($P < 0.05$). **Propofol 50 μM attenuated TNF-α and H_2O_2-induced cell apoptosis,** accompanied by decreases in malondialdehyde and LDH production and restoration of Bcl-2 expression. Propofol exerts protective effects against H_2O_2-enhanced TNF-α cell toxicity by reducing oxidative injury.

The vascular endothelium plays an important role in maintaining cardiovascular homeostasis, including important functions such as the regulation of vascular tone and tissue perfusion, vascular permeability, myocardial function, blood fluidity, anticoagulant activity, and inflammatory responses. Various forms of endothelial cell injury occur in patients with shock, sepsis, and, in particular, during myocardial ischemia reperfusion injury, such as in patients undergoing cardiac surgery using cardiopulmonary bypass (Verrier ED, Boyle EM Jr. Endothelial cell injury in cardiovascular surgery. Ann Thorac Surg 1996;62:915–22).

One study suggests that circulatory pro-apoptotic inflammatory cytokines (such as tumor necrosis factor [TNF]-α) and reactive oxygen species (ROS), which are increased during myocardial ischemia reperfusion injury and atherosclerosis, promote cardiomyocyte apoptosis subsequent to the induction of endothelial cells apoptosis (Scarabelli T, Stephanou A, Rayment N, et al. Apoptosis of endothelial cells precedes myocyte cell apoptosis in ischemia/reperfusion injury. Circulation 2001;104:253–6).

Thus, inhibition of TNF-α– and ROS-induced endothelial cells apoptosis may represent an effective therapy for myocardial ischemia reperfusion injury.

Propofol, an IV anesthetic with potential antioxidant property, has a chemical structure similar to that of phenol-based free-radical scavengers, such as vitamin E, and reduces free radicals (Murphy PG, Myers DS, Davies MJ, et al. The antioxidant potential of propofol (2,6-diisopropylphenol). Br J Anaesth 1992;68:613–8).

Propofol has been shown to attenuate hydrogen peroxide (H_2O_2)-induced mechanical and metabolic derangements in the isolated rat heart. Our study showed that propofol can dose-dependently reduce TNF-α–induced human umbilical vein endothelial cells (HUVECs) apoptosis *in vitro*, and the effect was more profound at concentrations ≥50 μM. **TNF-α and ROS may work synergistically in inducing endothelial cell apoptosis**. It is unknown, however, whether ROS enhancements of TNF-α cellular toxicity was mediated through enhanced lipid peroxidation or primarily through the modulation of pro- and antiapoptotic proteins. **Apoptosis caused by TNF-α and H_2O_2 were reduced significantly by the addition of propofol.**

ROS, which could be generated by TNF-α in many tissue and cell types, plays an important role in inducing cell apoptosis. Studies have shown that both the application of exogenous antioxidants such as vitamin E and the overexpression of endogenous antioxidant proteins such as Bcl-2, SOD, catalase, GSH, or GSH-Px can attenuate apoptosis induced by lipopolysaccharide and cytokines such as TNF in different cell types.

H_2O_2 10 μM induced only a small amount of cell apoptosis. **The H_2O_2 concentration (10 μM) used in this study is in the smallest range that induces minimal endothelial cell apoptosis but not necrosis** (Burlacu A, Jinga V, Gafencu AV, et al. Severity of oxidative stress generates different mechanisms of endothelial cell death. Cell Tissue Res 2001;306:409–16).

Interestingly, H_2O_2, when used at such a small concentration (i.e., 10 μM), profoundly augmented TNF-α–induced vascular endothelial cell apoptosis. The possible mechanism for this phenomenon is likely that application of H_2O_2 could result in increased intracellular Bax and decreased Bcl-2 levels, which may make the cells more vulnerable to TNF-α.

A novel finding of the current study is that **H_2O_2, at a trace concentration (10 μM), did not cause significantly enhanced lipid peroxidation in ECV304 cells** and markedly exacerbated TNF-α–induced increases in ECV304 cell lipid peroxidation and pro-apoptotic Bax protein, leading to enhanced cell apoptosis. **Propofol attenuated H_2O_2-mediated exacerbation of TNF-α effects.**

In summary, results from the current study indicate that **H_2O_2 could enhance TNF-α–induced vascular endothelial cell apoptosis. Propofol can attenuate TNF-α and H_2O_2 cellular toxicity. I believe that this indicates the dangers of propofol in patients with precancerous or cancerous growths. It would block the killing of cancer cells.**

1.0.7.3 TNF Blockers May Increase Cancer Risk in Kids ==

8-5-09 Kids and teens treated with drugs called tumor necrosis factor (TNF) blockers may be at an increased risk for lymphoma and other cancers, according to the US Food and Drug Administration (FDA), which is updating black box warnings for the drugs.

The FDA's decision is based on a yearlong review of the childhood cancer risk associated with **TNF blocker drugs, which are used to treat rheumatoid arthritis, Crohn's disease, and other inflammatory diseases.**

These drugs -- which include adalimumab (Humira), etanercept (Enbrel), certolizumab pegol (Cimzia), golimumab (Simponi), and

infliximab (Remicade) -- work by blocking tumor necrosis factor, a protein that's overproduced in some immune system diseases. The FDA started investigating the drugs in 2008 after evidence suggested that **interfering with TNF may also increase the risk of some life-threatening infections and certain cancers. I believe that this is due to the blocking of TNF, which generates EMODs, and the creation of an EMOD insufficiency state, and the patient is unable to fight infections and allows cancer development.**

This analysis found **children and teens taking these drugs had an increased risk of cancer, with cases occurring on average after 30 months of treatment. About half were lymphomas, and some were fatal.** The FDA said it was working with TNF drug manufacturers, including Johnson & Johnson, Abbott, and Wyeth, to better understand the childhood cancer risk associated with these drugs.

Cancers in children often are hard to recognize. Parents should be sure that their children have regular medical check-ups and watch for any unusual signs or symptoms that do not go away. These may include:

- an unusual lump or swelling
- unexplained paleness and loss of energy easy bruising
- an ongoing pain in one area of the body
- limping
- unexplained fever or illness that doesn't go away
- frequent headaches, often with vomiting
- sudden eye or vision changes
- sudden unexplained weight loss

These symptoms are more likely to be caused by something other than cancer, but they should be checked out by your child's doctor. For more specific information on possible symptoms, see "What are the types of childhood cancers?"

(American cancer news center: http://www.cancer.org/docroot/NWS/content/NWS_1_1x_TNF_Blockers_May_Increase_Cancer_Risk_in_Kids.asp. Accessed 8-6-09)

1.0.8.0 Use of hydrogen peroxide in treating cancer

The following were part of a review of "Can Oxygen Cure Cancer?" http://www.amazon.com/dp/1594771774/ref=pe_606_12214760_pe_ar_t1 Accessed 8-07-09.

In 2001, a group of **researchers from the Department of Life Sciences at Nottingham Trent University injected hydrogen peroxide solutions in solid tumors in mice and found the solutions had the potential to cause tumor cell death without generating dangerous by-products.** They were impressed concluding that hydrogen peroxide was a potential cytotoxic agent. Hydrogen peroxide used as an anti-cancer drug benefits are that it is cheap and cost effective.

In 2003, Jackson State University in Mississippi explored the combined effect of oxidative stress with hydrogen peroxide, Nigella sativa, a medicinal herb from the Middle East, on breast cancer. **The combination of hydrogen peroxide, ethanol, and Nigella sativa could inactivate MCF-7 cancer cells.**

Carolinas Medical Center in Charlotte, NC, investigated the efficiency of using hydrogen peroxide as an adjuvant therapy after extended local curettage (scaping away lesions) for benign cell tumors of the bone. Cell cultures taken from the tumor tissue of six patients was cultured and treated with hydrogen peroxide for 2 minutes. **Hydrogen peroxide was very effective in killing giant tumors of bone.**

Researchers in 1989, found that peroxidase in Hodgkin's disease sensitizes the tumor cells to killing by low levels of hydrogen peroxide. The idea was to deliver cytotoxic quantities of hydrogen peroxide to Hodgkin's disease.

Dr. Carl F Nathan and Dr. Zanvil A Cohn wrote, "**Hydrogen peroxide contributes to the lysis [destruction] of tumor cells by macrophages [immune cells] and granulocytes [white blood cells] in vitro." They found that 8 milligrams of hydrogen peroxide was able to kill more than 90 percent of P338 lymphoma cells.**

http://www.med.cornell.edu/research/cnathan/

Tottori University School of Medicine **in Japan in 1966, fifteen patients suffering from maxilliary cancer (cancer of the nasal cavity) were given intra-arterial infusions of hydrogen peroxide daily for ten days** followed by daily injections of mitomycin C, an antibiotic showing anti-tumor activity. Of the fifteen cases treated with hydrogen peroxide and Mutamycin, **eight show almost a complete disappearance of the tumor, while six experienced a partial reduction.** One had little change. The changes involve either an actual shrinking of the tumor or a softening of a hard tumor.

During a Baylor University cancer study of inoperable abdominal tumors, **intra-arterial hydrogen peroxide and irradiation was administered.** The researchers wanted to see if hydrogen peroxide could shrink the tumors and make them amenable to surgery. Two of the three experience shrinkage of the tumor and underwent successful operations to remove the tumors. One of the patients experience not shrinkage and was sent home. He began to improve over the next several months and the tumor began shrinking considerably. The doctors removed the shrunken tumor.

Dr J.W Finney, in 1962 stated, **"The use of Hydrogen Peroxide as a source of oxygen in a Regional Intra-arterial Infusion System revealed that cancer cells become more sensitive to irradiation in the presence of increased oxygen tension produced by hydrogen peroxide."** The researchers noted increased regional oxygenation, which led them to believe that there is an increased therapeutic ratio in malignant tumors receiving radiation when oxygen levels of the affected area are increased with hydrogen peroxide.

Oxidative therapies increase the activity of immunocompetent cells, stimulate the release of cytokines, upregulate the body's antioxidant system and induce mild activation of the immune system. Activating the patient's neuroendocrine system causes the patient to experience less pain and greater sense of well-being.

1.0.8.1 High-Fat Diet Dramatically Increases Cancer Metastasis

March 5, 2009 — Although **the link between obesity and cancer is well established**, exactly why there is a link remains **unclear**. Now, an animal study shows that **a high-fat diet dramatically increases cancer metastasis**, and offers a mechanistic explanation for what has been, up to now, anecdotal evidence.

The study was published online January 30, 2009 in *BMC Cancer.*

"These findings demonstrate that **an increase in lipids leads directly to a rise in cancer metastasis**", said senior author Ji-Xin Cheng, PhD, assistant professor at the Weldon School of Biomedical Engineering, Purdue University, in West Lafayette, Indiana.

The study was conducted in mice implanted with a tumor that metastasized, but **there was a 300% increase in metastases in mice fed a high-fat diet**,

compared with those fed a lean diet. In addition, the researchers showed that the high-fat diet had a direct effect on cancer-cell membranes, which increased their aggressiveness.

The implication from this study is that **patients who already have cancer could be increasing the risk of it spreading if they eat a high-fat diet**, comments lead author Thuc Le, PhD, also from Weldon School of Biomedical Engineering.

However, when asked whether physicians should advise their patients about this, Dr. Le told *Medscape Oncology* that there are "many caveats."

"Firstly, our study was performed in laboratory animals," he noted. "It's unclear whether our observations hold true in humans."

"But, when our study is viewed in the context of many other clinical studies of human patients and the strong correlation between lipid-rich breast cancer and aggressive clinical behavior, including early death, then a link (albeit indirect) between high-fat diet and cancer aggressiveness should emerge," he added.

1.0.8.2 Dramatic Increase in Metastasis

The study was carried out in 32 mice implanted with a lung cancer cell line, injected subcutaneously into a hind leg. One group of animals was fed a lean diet (4.2% fat and 3.82 kcal/g) and the other was fed a high-fat diet (34.9% fat and 5.24 kcal/g).

The mice on the high-fat diet became "very sick" after 4 weeks, Dr. Le explained; this was "clearly due to a very high number of tumor colonies and very large tumor colonies in the lungs." These animals also "lost tremendous body weight and mobility. To minimize their suffering, they were euthanized on week 4."

In contrast, the mice fed a lean diet survived with normal weight and mobility until week 6, he added. **At 4 weeks after tumor implantation, there was a 3-fold increase in lung metastasis in mice on the high-fat diet,** compared with mice on the lean diet.

There was a strong correlation between the high-fat diet and increased cancer metastasis, Dr. Le noted.

However, there may also be a more general conclusion. **The mice on the high-fat diet had elevated visceral adipose tissue weight (belly-fat weight)**

and elevated levels of free fatty acids, and "these conditions are normally observed in obesity," Dr. Le pointed out. This suggests that obesity or a high-fat diet might accelerate cancer spread, he commented. **Adipose tissue produces the antioxidant, estrogen.**

1.0.8.3 Increase in Circulating Tumor Cells

In addition, **mice on the high-fat diet also showed an early increase in circulating tumor cells, with levels 3-fold higher than those seen in the lean-diet mice 2 weeks after tumor implantation**. However, **this difference gradually declined and became indistinguishable by week 4,** the researchers note.

"We don't know the exact reason because we don't have direct evidence showing the whereabouts of the circulating cancer cells at all times," Dr. Le explained. However, one speculative explanation is that, in the mice fed the high-fat diet, the cancer cells escaped from the primary tumor and into the bloodstream (intravasion) at a faster rate than in mice fed the lean diet.

A more detailed study of the cancer cells themselves revealed a direct effect of the diet on the cancer-cell membrane. The researchers studied this using an imaging method known as coherent anti-Stokes Raman scattering, and they found "physical perturbations" in the cancer-cell membrane, which contributed to increased cancer aggressiveness.

In mice fed a high-fat diet, the increased lipid levels resulted in increased membrane phase separation and membrane rounding in cancer cells, which enhanced their ability to separate and spread through the body. The more rounded shape leads to reduced cell–cell adhesion and increased tissue invasion, the authors explain.

"If the cancer cells don't have excess lipids, they stick together and form very tight junctions in tumors, but increasing lipids causes them to take on a rounded shape and separate from each other," Dr. Le explained.

The team further demonstrated that **linoleic acid, which is predominant in polyunsaturated fats, causes increasing membrane phase separation**, whereas oleic acid, found in monounsaturated fats, does not. (Coherent anti-Stokes Raman scattering imaging of lipids in cancer metastasis. Le TT, Huff TB, Cheng JX. BMC Cancer. 2009 Jan 30;9:42).

1.0.8.4 Lack of Oxygen - the potential ability of Cancer survival and spread

Sept. 18 (HealthDayNews) -- A sad fact of cancer is that some tumor cells spread, signaling a worse prognosis for the patient, while others don't. An enduring question in cancer research has been, "Why?"

"If you look at the public health problem of cancer, it's mostly due to cancer that has spread," says Dr. Max Sung, medical director of the Ruttenberg Cancer Treatment Center at the Mount Sinai Medical Center in New York City. "If there's a mechanism by which these cancer cells that have spread can be destroyed, that would be wonderful. The next best thing is to see if we could prevent the primary tumor from spreading in the first place."

An article appearing in the Sept. 18, 2009 issue of *Nature* looks into just this issue: why tumor cells spread and how that deadly process can be prevented. **Scientists already knew tumor cells that don't have enough oxygen, a condition known as hypoxia, have a greater tendency to spread than those with a regular supply of oxygen**. Now scientists have shown that **tumor cells that are deprived of oxygen also seem to have the ability to zoom in on certain organs, which explains why certain types of cancer tend to spread to certain parts of the body**.

Breast cancer, for instance, has a preference for bone marrow, lungs and the liver.

"This adds a novel dimension to our insight. It has shown that, not only do tumor cells acquire the ability to spread, but they also acquire the ability to home in on certain organs," says Rene Bernards, author of an accompanying article in the journal and a professor of molecular carcinogenesis at The Netherlands Cancer Institute in Amsterdam.

When faced with hypoxia, tumor cells respond by increasing production of a protein called hypoxia-inducible factor (HIF), which in turn binds to and activates different genes. The von Hippel-Lindau (VHL) tumor suppressor gene produces proteins that prevent cells from becoming malignant. It is also part of the oxygen-sensing machinery of the cell that controls the levels of the HIF.

"The question is 'What is the relationship of this gene to the tumor cells spreading?'" Sung says. In this study, the researchers introduced VHL into kidney cancer cells (which normally lack a copy of this gene) and then looked for changes in the activity of thousands of other genes under conditions of adequate oxygen. To their surprise, they found that VHL reduced the production of a receptor protein called CXCR4, which is known to be over-expressed in those breast cancer cells that spread to the bone. The CXCR4 acts as a sort of homing system. "**Now it turns out that if tumor cells become starved of oxygen, that they begin to express CXCR4, which allows tumor cells to migrate specifically to other organs,**" Bernards explains.

The findings do open up the possibility of gene therapy to correct the situation sometime in the future. At the same time, the results cast doubt on the concept of angiogenesis, which posits that cutting off blood supply to a tumor will shrink or kill it. **Oxygen is carried via the bloodstream.** "Although the concept that oxygen deprivation promotes tumor metastasis is not altogether novel, this is still an interesting and important study," says Charles Graham, assistant professor of anatomy and cell biology at Queen's University in Ontario. "The idea of using angiogenesis inhibitors to deprive tumors of their blood [and hence oxygen] supply as a therapeutic approach has been around for quite a while. However, this and **other studies... indicate that reducing the blood supply to a tumor may have unintended consequences, as it may promote the spread of malignant cells."**

There are other unresolved issues. "A key question that follows is whether these changes have already taken place in the primary tumor, allowing it to spread to a specific secondary site, or whether primary tumor cells that are carried to secondary organs undergo these changes after they have been exposed to the new environment," Bernards writes in his commentary.

The current results seem to suggest the changes leading to this deadly cascade happen early on. This supports research that Bernards and his colleagues previously conducted that was also published in *Nature*. "We showed that breast cancer comes in two flavors even if they are small primary tumors, either of good prognosis or bad prognosis. Even if the primary tumor is still small, it has either already decided very early in its life that it will become malignant and aggressive and metastatic or has started out on a relatively benign path," he says.

"In a way, that is good news for cancer patients because you can determine up front whether a cancer is likely to metastasize to other parts of the body or not, and we can adjust the chemotherapy requirements to this insight."

(Rene Bernards, Ph.D., professor, molecular carcinogenesis, The Netherlands Cancer Institute, Amsterdam; Max Sung, M.D., assistant professor, hematology/oncology, and medical director, Ruttenberg Cancer Treatment Center, Mount Sinai Medical Center, New York City; Charles Graham, Ph.D., assistant professor, anatomy and cell biology, Queen's University, Ontario; Sept. 18, 2003, *Nature.*).

1.0.8.5 Lack of oxygen and gangrene

7-24-09 **Gangrene** occurs when tissue dies (necrosis) because its blood supply is interrupted. Gangrene may be caused by an infection, injury, or a complication of a long-term condition that restricts blood circulation. It most commonly occurs in the extremities - the toes, fingers, arms and legs - but internal organs and muscles may also become gangrenous. There are five main types of gangrene: 1. Dry gangrene. 2. Wet gangrene. 3. Gas gangrene. 4. Internal gangrene. 5. Fournier's gangrene. **I believe that all forms of gangrene are due to an EMOD insufficiency, which allows the development of infection and tissue death.**

The word gangrene comes from the Latin word *gangreana* and the Greek word *gangraina*, which both mean "purification of tissues". There is no link to the English word "green".

The number of Americans hospitalized for the treatment of gangrene has been steadily growing over the last couple of decades. Experts believe this is partly because the number of Americans with diabetes has increased. According to the U.S. Agency for Healthcare Research and Quality, 45,400 Americans were hospitalized for gangrene in 2003, compared to 21,000 in 1991.

1.0.8.6 What are the causes of gangrene?

Our cells require nutrients and oxygen to survive and they get this from our blood. If their blood supply goes down below a certain level, the cells will become damaged and will eventually die. This illustrates the significance of an adequate oxygen supply, which is necessary to generate adequate levels of EMODs.

Tissues and cells are also attacked by organisms such as bacteria, viruses, parasites and fungi. Our white blood cells and the Thymus cells (T-cells) form part of our immune system and fight germs. **If the blood supply is cut there will be no white cells or T-cells to stop the organisms from multiplying and causing an infection. I believe that this blocks our continally operative**

protective system of oxygenation and EMOD production and thus the anoxic cell is vulnerable to infection and death.

1.0.8.7 What are the risk factors for gangrene?

- **Age** - gangrene is much more common in older people.
- **Diabetes** - the high blood sugar levels, which are common in diabetes, may eventually damage the nerves, especially in the feet. When the nerves are damaged the patient does not feel pain and will not know if he/she has an injury. The patient may continue walking without protecting the wound. The wound may get worse and develop into a foot ulcer. High blood sugar levels may also damage blood vessels, resulting in poor blood supply to the area. Less blood means less nutrients and oxygen for the tissue cells, and fewer white blood cells and T-cells to fight off infection. The ulcer becomes infected; the infection grows rapidly and gangrene develops. The oxygen/nutrient deprived cells are weak and rapidly die.
- **Vascular diseases** - diseases of the blood vessels, such as atherosclerosis (narrowed arteries) and blood clots can result in poor blood flow to various parts of the body.
- **Injury or surgery** - anything which wounds the skin and tissues below it will raise the risk of gangrene. People with underlying conditions which may affect blood flow who also wound their skin run an even higher risk. Approximately 40% of wet gangrenes are caused by infections that occur during surgery and about 50% are caused by serious traumatic injuries. Gangrene from frostbite and gunshot wounds are less common than from automobile accidents, crush injuries, burns and industrial accidents.
- **Weakened immune system** - people with weakened immune systems, such as those with AIDS/HIV, patients receiving chemotherapy or radiotherapy, as well as organ transplant recipients who are on immunosuppressants, are more susceptible to the complications of infection, which include gangrene.
- **Smoking** - smoking causes the blood vessels to narrow, resulting in less blood flow.

1.0.8.8 What are the symptoms of gangrene?

Symptoms of dry gangrene

Generally, dry gangrene develops slowly. It is the most common gangrene for patients with atherosclerosis and other vascular diseases.

- A red line appears on the skin which surrounds the affected tissue.
- The area will gradually become numb and cold.
- When necrosis (tissue death) occurs there may be some pain.
- Some patients, especially older ones, may feel nothing at all.
- The area will change from red, to brown, to black.
- The necrotized tissue then shrivels up and eventually falls off.

Symptoms of wet gangrene

Wet gangrene is much more painful than dry gangrene. The term 'wet' is used to refer to a bacterial infection in the affected tissue. It can develop as a result of an injury, a severe burn, or frostbite. This type of gangrene is common with diabetes patients who unwittingly injure a toe or foot. As it spreads rapidly and can be fatal it needs to be treated urgently.

- The affected area swells before any tissue dies.
- The skin will change color from red, to brown, to black.
- There will be pus and a foul smell.
- Fever (temperature).

Gas gangrene

Usually deep muscle tissue is affected. The surface of the skin may appear normal, but as the condition advances the skin may become pale, and then turn grey or purplish-red. Gas gangrene is usually caused by *Clostridium perfringens* bacteria. The bacteria multiply when the blood supply is depleted. The bacterial infection produces toxins that release a gas. Gas gangrene can become life-threatening. **I believe that the Baylor group was able to cure gas gangrene with simple hydrogen peroxide injections and by increasing EMODs.**

- The affected area feels heavy and painful. The pain is caused by the infection which produces a gas.

- The skin may appear to bubble.
- A crackling sound when area is pressed. This sound is caused by the gas.
- Sometimes there may be a watery discharge which does not usually have a foul smell.

Internal gangrene

The most common organs to be affected are the intestines, gallbladder, or the appendix. An infected person may have more than one affected organ. Gangrene in the intestine may be the result of a hernia; when a part of the intestine bulges through a weakened area of muscle and becomes twisted.

Patients will experience fever and pain in the affected area. Internal gangrene can be fatal if left untreated.

Fournier's gangrene

This type is very uncommon. It affects the male genital organs. It is usually the result of a urinary tract infection or an infection in the genital area. The patient will feel pain, tenderness, and swelling in the affected area. Women can also develop Fournier's gangrene, but much less so than men. Approximately half of all people who develop this type of gangrene have diabetes.

What is the treatment for gangrene?

Necrotized (dead) tissue cannot be saved, but a lot can be done to stop the gangrene from spreading.

- **Surgery** (Debridement)

The surgical removal of dead tissue (debridement) helps prevent the gangrene from spreading, and allows healthy tissue to recover.

Damaged or diseased blood vessels might also be repaired during surgery so that blood flow is restored to the affected area.

Skin graft - if damage is extensive the surgeon may remove some healthy skin from one part of the patient's body and spread it over the affected area. Sacrificed skin is usually taken from a part of the body that is hidden by clothing. **Skin grafts are only possible if the blood supply to the affected area is adequate.**

Amputation - if the gangrene is severe it is sometimes necessary to amputate the affected body part, for example a finger, toe, or limb.

- **Antibiotics**

  Antibiotics are administered to fight infection - these will usually be given intravenously.

- **Hyperbaric oxygen therapy**

- The patient will be placed on a padded table which slides into a special chamber. The chamber is pressurized with oxygen to about 2.5 times normal sea level atmospheric pressure. If the air pressure is high and oxygen rich more oxygen can be carried in the blood to the affected area. **Bacteria require environments that lack oxygen to thrive.** The oxygen chamber helps fight the bacteria and heal the wounds.

- These may help reduce the infection and speed up the healing process.

Written by Christian Nordqvist

Copyright: Medical News Today http://www.medicalnewstoday.com/articles/158770.php

Accessed 7-28-09

1.0.9.0 Methyglyoxal, Retine, Promine (Dr. Szent-Gyorgyi)

If you remember, according to Warburg, it is increased amounts of carcinogens, toxicity and pollution that cause cells to be unable to uptake oxygen efficiently. This is connected with over-acidity.

Cancer Strategy #4: Lack Of Methylglyoxal Causes Cancer...

Getting Methylglyoxal Into Cells Puts The Brakes On Cancer

Dr. Albert Szent-Gyorgyi was the Nobel Laureate in Medicine in 1937 for the isolation and discovery of Vitamin C. Known as the "Father of Nutritional Science", **he**

also discovered iso-flavones and vitamin P. In his last 40 years, he researched the regulatory processes of cell growth, and thereby the regulation of cancer itself.

He made a rather amazing breakthrough about cancer. In 1963 the prestigious magazine "Science" published a remarkable article about his research. In it Dr. Szent-Gyorgyi identified two substances, one called **Retine, which inhibited cancer growth, and the other called Promine, which promoted cell growth and made cancerous cells grow faster.**

He explained that these were very small molecules that were highly potent in controlling cell division. His research using mice achieved shrinkage of tumors by increasing the ratio of Retine to Promine with daily injections of Retine. Other researchers obtained similar results.

There were no harmful or toxic side effects.

In another "Science" article in 1967 he announced that his laboratory had isolated and manufactured Retine, which retards cell growth, in the form of a Carbonyl compound called **Methylglyoxal**.

Again, in animal studies he showed that injecting Methylglyoxal daily into mice with cancer was highly effective. The study was divided up into 5 groups of 20 mice each. Every mouse in the control group died in the first 26 - 34 days. All mice were observed for 300 days. The first group began treatment 1 hour after inoculation with cancer. 15 survived.

In the second group, beginning treatment 4 hours after inoculation, 13 animals survived. The third group began treatment 24 hours afterwards and 7 survived. The fourth group waited 48 hours and 4 survived.

In an interview in Prevention magazine in 1972 conducted by Jane Kinderlehrer, he explained that he and "Dr. Egyud have found that **retine (methylglyoxal) stops the growth of cancer cells without poisoning other cells.** When retine is present in sufficient concentration, no cell division can occur while vital cellular processes go on unhindered."

The article goes on, "And what is a good bit of luck, and not my cleverness, the white-haired scientist pointed out, "is that if a cancer cell cannot grow, it dies by itself.' According to the researchers, **retine is normally produced by the body** and, when it is, it prevents the growth of existing cancer cells. But the body can lose its ability to produce this substance...

"Putting the retine back in the body, just as we put insulin back into a diabetic's body, can stop the growth of cancer...The scientists at Woods Hole found that **cancer cells are much more sensitive to retine than normal ones, and so cancer cells may be inhibited specifically**."

To sum it up, **the Carbonyl group - Glyoxal & Methylglyoxal, are retine**. They arrest cell division and make cells return to a resting state. If Carbonyl is missing, uncontrolled proliferation goes on, and cells grow wildly and uncontrollably which leads to cancer. Glyoxal & Methylglyoxal are a non-toxic substance that is supposed to be in your cells. Putting them back in your cells has significant anti-cancer activity.

Another well known Nobel Prize winner of that period, Dr. William Koch, worked on this same issue with a different approach. Dr. Szent-Gyorgyi acknowledged his work saying, "**A decade ago, a very intuitive researcher, Dr. William F. Koch, came to the same conclusion about the possible importance of Carbonyls in regulation of cell division and carcinostasis.**"

While both work best when used together, one of these two supplements is a much stronger cancer killer than the other.

1.0.9.1 Chlorine

The French **do not** drink chlorinated water. They ozonate their water to purify it.

Does this make a difference? Absolutely.

"We are quite convinced... that there is an association between cancer and chlorinated water."

Medical College Of Wisconsin research team

We don't use chlorine because it's safe, we use it because it is *cheap*. We essentially still pour bleach in our water before we drink it. The long-term effects of chlorinated drinking water are disastrous.

According to the U.S. Council Of Environmental Quality, "Cancer risk among people drinking chlorinated water is 93% higher than among those whose water does not contain chlorine."

It may cause much heart disease too. Dr. Joseph Price wrote a highly controversial book in the late sixties titled Coronaries/Cholesterol/Chlorine, and concluded that nothing can negate the incontrovertible fact, that **the basic cause of arteriosclerosis, heart attacks and stroke, is chlorine.**

Dr. Price later headed up a study using chickens as test subjects, where two groups of several hundred birds were observed throughout their span to maturity.

One group was given water with chlorine and the other without. The group raised *with* chlorine, when autopsied, showed some level of heart or circulatory disease in every specimen, the group *without* had **no incidence of disease.** The group without chlorine grew faster, larger and displayed vigorous health.

This study was well received in the poultry industry, and is still used as a reference today. As a result, most large poultry producers use dechlorinated water.

When chlorine is added to our water, it combines with other natural compounds to form Trihalomethanes (chlorination byproducts), or THMs. These chlorine byproducts trigger the production of **free radicals** in the body, causing cell damage, and are highly **carcinogenic**.

"Although concentrations of these carcinogens (THMs) are low, it is precisely these low levels that cancer scientists believe are responsible for the *majority* of human cancers in the United States". *The Environmental Defense Fund*

Dr. Robert Carlson, a highly respected University of Minnesota researcher, sums it up by claiming, **"Chlorine is the greatest crippler and killer of modern times!"**

Breast cancer, which now affects one in every eight women in North America, has recently been linked to the **accumulation of chlorine compounds in the breast tissue.** A study carried out in Hartford Connecticut, the first of it's kind in North America, found that:

"Women with breast cancer have **50% to 60% higher levels** of organochlorines (chlorination byproducts) in their breast tissue than women without breast cancer."

It is not just *drinking* chlorinated water that is the problem.

Up to <u>two thirds</u> of our exposure to chlorine is due to **inhalation of steam and skin absorption while showering.** A warm shower opens up the pores of the skin and allows for accelerated absorption of chlorine and other chemicals in water.

The steam we inhale while showering can contain up to 50 times the level of chemicals than tap water due to the fact that chlorine and most other contaminants vaporize much faster and at a lower temperature than water. Inhalation is a much more harmful means of exposure since the chlorine gas (chloroform) we inhale goes directly into our blood stream.

"Showering is suspected as the primary cause of elevated levels of chloroform in nearly every home because of chlorine in the water."

Dr Lance Wallace, *U.S. Environmental Protection Agency.*

If you take showers using chlorinated water and are dealing with cancer, clearly installing a **shower filter** to dechlorinate your shower water makes good sense.

Another reason we have too much free radical damage and too much cancer is that processed foods generate more free radicals than whole foods, and have fewer nutrients to act as free radical scavengers to help protect you from those free radicals. On top of this, you are **exposed to 70,000 chemicals** -- 20,000 of which are **known cancer-causing** agents. These all cause free radical damage.

For this strategy, the e-book focuses on a **unique free radical scavenger** that has the ability to **kill cancer cells** by increasing the amount of energy the mitochondria on the cancer cell is producing. The cancer cell's energy pathways are shut down because normally they produce very little energy. The extra energy this one of a kind supplement causes the cancer cell's mitochondria to produce cannot be handled by the cancer cell. And causes it to die. *It is one of the strongest cancer killers we have seen.*

1.0.9.2 A Doctor's Shocking Closed-Door Confession

In a survey of 79 oncologists from McGill University Cancer Center in Canada, 64 said they would not consent to treatment with Cisplatin, a common chemotherapy drug, while **58 oncologists** said they would reject <u>**all**</u> the current trials being carried out by their establishment. Why? "The ineffectiveness of chemotherapy and its unacceptable degree of toxicity." Philip Day, *Cancer: Why We're Still Dying to Know the Truth*

In 2004, the Journal of Clinical Oncology published a study about chemotherapy's success rates when looking at how many cancer patients were still alive after 5 years. It states:

RESULTS: The overall contribution of curative and adjuvant cytotoxic chemotherapy to 5-year survival in adults was estimated to be 2.3% in Australia and 2.1% in the USA.

CONCLUSION: As the 5-year relative survival rate for cancer in Australia is now over 60%, it is clear that cytotoxic chemotherapy only makes a minor contribution to cancer survival. To justify the continued funding and availability of drugs used in cytotoxic chemotherapy, a rigorous evaluation of the cost-effectiveness and impact on quality of life is urgently required.

You'd be hard pressed to find anything still being touted as your best shot at a cure with an average success rate of just over 2 percent, which chemotherapy has, if it wasn't for the fact that big profits were driving the recommendation. For stage 4 cancers the rate is less than half of one percent.

Fundamentally, chemotherapy rarely works. Worse, some drug treatments also promote the spread of cancer. But somehow the rationale to avoid these agents because they might promote cancer does not apply when it comes to drugs.

– A Cancer Journal for the Clinician article concludes by stating:

"Pending the publication of suitable trials, clinicians must be guided by existing data in the context of a fundamental principle of medicine, "Primum non nocere." (First do no harm.)

And yet, conventional cancer treatments can in no way, shape or form ever be considered harmless.

"...as a chemist trained to interpret data, it is incomprehensible to me that physicians can ignore the clear evidence that chemotherapy does much, much more harm than good."

Alan C Nixon, PhD, former president of the American Chemical Society

http://www.cancerfightingstrategies.com/?engine=adwords!800&keyword=%2Acancer%2A&match_type=&gclid=CJ-Z096Vo5gCFQpuGgodkDTGmA

1.1.0.0 The Prime Cause and Prevention of Cancer: Dr. Otto Warburg

Lecture delivered to Nobel Laureates on June 30, 1966

at Lindau, Lake Constance, Germany

There are prime and secondary causes of diseases. For example, the prime cause of the plague is the plague bacillus, but secondary causes of the plague are filth, rats, and the fleas that transfer the plague bacillus from rats to man. By the prime cause of a disease, I mean one that is found in every case of the disease.

Cancer, above all other diseases, has countless secondary causes. Almost anything can cause cancer. But, even for cancer, there is only one prime cause. **The prime cause of cancer is the replacement of the respiration of oxygen (oxidation of sugar) in normal body cells by fermentation of sugar.**

All normal body cells meet their energy needs by respiration of oxygen, whereas cancer cells meet their energy needs in great part by fermentation. All normal body cells are thus obligate aerobes, whereas **all cancer cells are partial anaerobes.** From the standpoint of the physics and chemistry of life this difference between normal and cancer cells is so great that one can scarcely picture a greater difference. Oxygen gas, the donor of energy in plants and animals, is dethroned in the cancer cells and replaced by the energy yielding reaction of the lowest living forms, namely the fermentation of sugar.

In every case, during the cancer development, the oxygen respiration always falls, fermentation appears, and the highly differentiated cells are transformed into fermenting anaerobes, which have lost all their body functions and retain only the now useless property of growth and replication. Thus, when respiration disappears, life does not disappear, but the meaning of life disappears, and what remains are growing machines that destroy the body in which they grow.

All carcinogens impair respiration directly or indirectly by deranging capillary circulation, a statement that is proven by the fact that **no cancer cell exists without exhibiting impaired respiration.** Of course, respiration cannot be repaired if it is impaired at the same time by a carcinogen.

To prevent cancer it is therefore proposed first to keep the speed of the blood stream so high that the venous blood still contains sufficient

oxygen; second, to keep high the concentration of hemoglobin in the blood; third, to add always to the food, even of healthy people, the active groups of the respiratory enzymes; and to increase the doses of these groups, if a precancerous state has already developed. If at the same time exogenous carcinogens are excluded rigorously, then much of the endogenous cancer may be prevented today.

These proposals are in no way utopian. On the contrary, they may be realized by everybody, everywhere, at any hour. Unlike the prevention of many other diseases, the prevention of cancer requires no government help, and not much money.

Many experts agree that one could prevent about 80% of all cancers in man, if one could keep away the known carcinogens from the normal body cells. But how can the remaining 20%, the so-called spontaneous cancers, be prevented? It is indisputable that all cancer could be prevented if the respiration of body cells were kept intact.

Nobody today can say that one does not know what the prime cause of cancer is. On the contrary, there is no disease whose prime cause is better known, so that today ignorance is no longer an excuse for avoiding measures for prevention. That the prevention of cancer will come there is no doubt. But how long prevention will be avoided depends on how long the prophets of agnosticism will succeed in inhibiting the application of scientific knowledge in the cancer field. **In the meantime, millions of men and women must die of cancer unnecessarily.**

Otto Warburg

1883-1970

Preface to the Second Revised German Edition of the Lindau Lecture

(The way to prevention of cancer)

Since the Lindau lecture of June 1966 many physicians have examined - not unsuccessfully - the practical consequences of the anaerobiosis of cancer cells. The more who participate in these examinations, the sooner will we know what can be achieved. It is a unique aspect of these examinations that they can be carried out on human patients, on the largest scale, without risk; whereas **experiments on animals have been misleading many times. The cure of human**

cancer will be the resultant of biochemistry of cancer and of biochemistry of man.

A list of selected active groups of respiratory enzymes will soon be published, to which we recently added **cytohemin and d-amino-Levulinic acid, the precursor of oxygen-transferring hemins.** In the meantime commercial vitamin preparations may be used that contain, besides other substances, many active groups of the respiratory enzymes. Most of these may be added to the food. Cytohemin and vitamin B 12 may be given subcutaneously. (A synonym of "active group" is "prosthetic" group of an enzyme.)

There exists no alternative today to the prevention of cancer as proposed at Lindau. It is the way that attacks the prime cause of cancer most directly and that is experimentally most developed. Indeed millions of experiments in man, through the effectiveness of some vitamins, have shown, that cell respiration is impaired if the active groups of the respiratory enzymes are removed from the food; and that cell respiration is repaired at once, if these groups are added again to the food. No way can be imagined that is scientifically better founded to prevent and cure a disease, the prime cause of which is an impaired respiration. Neither genetic codes of anaerobiosis nor cancer viruses are alternatives today, because no such codes and no such viruses in man have been discovered so far; but anaerobiosis has been discovered.[8]

What can be achieved by the active groups, when tumors have already developed? The answer is doubtful, because **tumors live in the body almost anaerobically**, that is under conditions that the active groups cannot act.

On the other hand, because young metastases live in the body almost aerobically, inhibition by the active groups should be possible. Therefore we propose first to remove all compact tumors, which are the anaerobic foci of the metastasis. Then the active group should be added to the food, in the greatest possible amount, for many years, even for ever. This is a promising task. If it succeeds, then cancer will be a harmless disease.

Moreover, we discovered recently[a)] in experiments with growing cancer cells in vitro that very low concentrations of some selected active groups inhibit fermentation and the growth of cancer cells completely, in the course of a few days. From these experiments it may be concluded that **de-differentiated cells die if one tries to normalize their metabolism.** It is a result that is unexpected and that encourages the task of inhibiting the growth of metastases with active enzyme groups.

As emphasized, **it is the first precondition of the proposed treatment that all growing body cells be saturated with oxygen**. It is a second precondition that exogenous carcinogens be kept away, at least during the treatment. All carcinogens impair respiration directly or indirectly by deranging capillary circulation, a statement that is proved by the fact that **no cancer cell exists, the respiration of which is not impaired.** Of course, respiration cannot be repaired if it is impaired at the same time by carcinogens.

It has been asked after the Lindau lecture why the repair of respiration by the active groups of the enzymes was proposed as late as 1966, although the fermentation of the cancer cell was discovered as early as 1923. Why was so much time lost?

He who asked this questions ignored that in 1923 the chemical mechanism of enzyme action was still a secret of living nature alone.[1] The first active group of an enzyme, "Iron, the Oxygen-Transferring Part of the Respiratory Enzyme" was discovered in 1924[2]. There followed in two decades the discoveries of the O2-transferring metalloproteins, the flavoproteins and the pyridinproteins, a period that was concluded by the "Heavy Metals as Prosthetic Groups of Enzymes"[3] and by the "Hydrogen Transferring Enzymes"[4] in 1947 to 1949.

Moreover, during the first decades after 1923 glycolysis and anaerobiosis were constantly confused, so that nobody knew what was specific for tumors. **The three famous and decisive discoveries of DEAN BURK and colleagues[5] of the National Cancer Institute at Bethesda were of the years 1941, 1956 and 1964: first, that the metabolism of the regenerating liver, which grows more rapidly than most tumors, is not cancer metabolism, but perfect aerobic embryonic metabolism; second, that cancer cells, descended in vitro from one single normal cell, were in vivo the more malignant, the higher the fermentation rate; third, that in vivo growing hepatomas, produced in vivo by different carcinogens, were in vivo the more malignant, the higher the fermentation rate.** Furthermore, the very unexpected and fundamental fact, that tissue culture is carcinogenic and that **a too low oxygen pressure is the intrinsic cause** were discovered[6-8] in the years 1927 to 1966. Anaerobiosis of cancer cells was an established fact only since 1960 when methods were developed[7] to measure the oxygen pressure inside of tumors in the living body.

This abridged history shows that even the greatest genius would not have been able to propose in 1923, what was proposed at Lindau in 1966. As unknown as the prime cause of cancer was in 1923 was the possibility to prevent it.

Life without oxygen in a living world that has been created by oxygen[9] was so unexpected that it would have been too much to ask that anaerobiosis of cancer cells should be accepted at once by all scientists. But most of the resistance disappeared when at Lindau it was explained that on the basis of anaerobiosis there is now a real chance to get rid of this terrible disease, if man is willing to submit to experiments and facts. It is true that more than 40 years were necessary to learn how to do it. But 40 years is a short time in the history of science.[10]

Wiesenhof über Idar-Oberstein, August 1967

OTTO WARBURG

a) In press in Hoppe-Seylers Zeitschrift für Physiologische Chemie 1967. 10 g riboflavin per ccm or 10 g d-Aminolevulinic acid inhibit in vitro growth and fermentation completely but inhibit respiration less. As expected, ascites cancer in vivo is not cured.

Two years after the Lindau lecture LINUS PAULING (Science Vol. 160, Page 265, 1968) proposed to control mental diseases by adding to the food the active groups of respiratory enzymes. But here the experimental basis was lacking. No mental disease is known so far, the prime cause of which is an impairment of the respiration of brain cells

1.1.0.1 The Prime Cause and Prevention of Cancer

(Revised Lindau Lecture)

By OTTO WARBURG

(Director, Max Planck Institute for Cell Physiology, Berlin-Dahlem, Germany) English Edition by DEAN BURK*), National Cancer Institute, Bethesda, Maryland*)

Note by DEAN BURK: Adapted from a lecture originally delivered by O. Warburg at the 1966 annual meeting of Nobelists at Lindau, Germany. **O. Warburg won the Nobel Prize in Medicine in 1931 for his discovery of the oxygen-transferring enzyme of cell respiration, and was voted a second Nobel Prize in 1944 for his discovery of the active groups of the hydrogen transferring enzymes.** Many universities, like Harvard, Oxford, Heidelberg have offered him honorary degrees. He is a Foreign member of the Royal Society of London, a Knight of the Order of Merit founded by Frederick the

Great, and was awarded the Great Cross with Star and Shoulder ribbon of the Bundesrepublik. His main interests are Chemistry and Physics of Life. In both fields no scientist has been more successful.

There are prime and secondary causes of diseases. For example, the prime cause of the plague is the plague bacillus, but secondary causes of the plague are filth, rats, and the fleas that transfer the plague bacillus from rats to man. By a prime cause of a disease I mean one that is found in every case of the disease.

Cancer, above all other diseases, has countless secondary causes. But, even **for cancer, there is only one prime cause. Summarized in a few words, the prime cause of cancer is the replacement of the respiration of oxygen in normal body cells by a fermentation of sugar. All normal body cells meet their energy needs by respiration of oxygen, whereas cancer cells meet their energy needs in great part by fermentation.** All normal body cells are thus obligate aerobes, whereas all cancer cells are partial anaerobes. From the standpoint of the physics and chemistry of life this difference between normal and cancer cells is so great that one can scarcely picture a greater difference. Oxygen gas, the donor of energy in plants and animals is dethroned in the cancer cells and replaced by an energy yielding reaction of the lowest living forms, namely, a fermentation of glucose.

The key to the cancer problem is accordingly the energetics of life, which has been the field of work of the Dahlem institute since its initiation by the Rockefeller Foundation about 1930. In Dahlem the oxygen transferring and hydrogen transferring enzymes were discovered and chemically isolated. In Dahlem the fermentation of cancer cells was discovered decades ago; but only in recent years has it been demonstrated that cancer cells can actually grow in the body almost with only the energy of fermentation. Only today can one submit, with respect to cancer, all the experiments demanded by PASTEUR and KOCH as proof of the prime causes of a disease. If it is true that the replacement of oxygen-respiration by fermentation is the prime cause of cancer, then all cancer cells without exception must ferment, and no normal growing cell ought to exist that ferments in the body.

An especially simple and convincing experiment performed by the [US] Americans MALMGREN and FLANEGAN confirms the view. **If one injects tetanus spores, which can germinate only at very low oxygen pressures, into the blood of healthy mice, the mice do not sicken with tetanus, because the spores find no place in the normal body where the oxygen pressure is sufficiently low. Likewise, pregnant mice do not sicken when**

injected with the tetanus spores, because also in the growing embryo no region exists where the oxygen pressure is sufficiently low to permit spore germination. However, if one injects tetanus spores into the blood of tumor-bearing mice, the mice sicken with tetanus, because the oxygen pressure in the tumors can be so low that the spores can germinate. These experiments demonstrate in a unique way the anaerobiosis of cancer cells and the non-anaerobiosis of normal cells, in particular the non-anaerobiosis of growing embryos.

1.1.0.2 The Fermentation of Morris Hepatomas

A second type of experimentation demonstrates a quantitative connection between fermentation of tumors and growth rate of tumors.

If one injects rats with cancer-inducing substances of different activities, one can create, as HAROLD MORRIS of the National Cancer Institute in Bethesda has found, liver cancers (hepatomas) of very different degrees of malignancy. Thus, one strain of tumor may double its mass in three days, another strain may require 30 days. Recently DEAN BURK and MARK WOODS 3), also of the National Cancer Institute, measured the in vitro rates of anaerobic fermentation in different lines of these hepatomas, and obtained a curve (Fig. 1) that shows a quantitative relationship between fermentation and growth rate, and therefore between fermentation and malignancy, in these various tumor strains. The fermentation increases with the malignancy, and indeed the fermentation increases even faster than the malignancy.

Special interest attaches to the fermentation of the most slowly growing hepatomas, because several investigators in the United States believed that they had found *) that such tumors had no fermentation; that is that anaerobiosis cannot be the prime cause of cancer.

*) For example see C. H. BÖHRINGER SON, Ingelheim am Rhein, the factory Work-Journal "Das Medizinische Prisma", Vol. 13, 1963. Here a lecture of VAN POTTER (Madison, Wisconsin) is reprinted where owing to the slow-growing Morris-tumors anaerobiosis as prime cause of cancer is rejected and the lack of "intracellular feeding back" is claimed to be the real cause of cancer.

Fig. 1. Velocity of growth and fermentation of the Morris-Hepatomas, according to DEAN BURK and MARK WOODS

DEAN BURK and MARK WOODS saw immediately from their curves that in the region of the zero point the rate of fermentation was so small that it could no longer be measured by the usual gross methodology employed by the aforementioned workers, whereas in the same region the smallest growth rate was always easily measurable. BURK and WOODS saw, in other words, that in the region of the zero point of their curves the growth test was more sensitive than the usual fermentation test. With refined and adequate methods for measuring fermentation of sugar (glucose) they found, what any physical chemist after a glance at the curve would realize, that even the most slow-growing Morris hepatomas fermented sugar.

The results of DEAN BURK and MARK WOODS were confirmed and extended by other workers with independent methods. PIETRO GULLINO, also in Bethesda, developed a perfusion method whereby a Morris hepatoma growing in the living animal could be perfused for long periods of time, even weeks, by means of a single artery and single vein, and the blood entering and leaving any given tumor could be analyzed. **GULLINO found with this method that the slow-growing Morris hepatomas always produced fermentation lactic acid during their growth. This was in contrast to liver, where, as known since the days of CLAUDE BERNARD, lactic acid is not produced but consumed by liver**; the difference between liver and Morris tumors in vivo is thus infinite (+ vs. -). GULLINO further found that tumors grow in vivo with diminished oxygen consumption. In summary, GULLINO's findings indicate that the slow-growing Morris hepatomas are partial anaerobes. SILVIO FIALA, a biochemist at the University of Southern California, found that **not only did the slow-growing hepatomas produce lactic acid, but also that the number of their oxygen-respiring grana was reduced.**

The slow-growing Morris hepatomas are therefore far removed from having refuted the anaerobiosis of tumors. On the contrary, they are the best proof of this distinctive characteristic. For forty years cancer investigators have searched for a cancer that did not ferment. When finally a non-fermenting tumor appeared to have been found in the slow-growing Morris tumors, it was shown to be a methodological error.

1.1.0.3 Transformation of Embryonic Metabolism into Cancer Metabolism

A third type of experiment, from the institute in Dahlem with coworkers GAWEHN, GEISSLER and LORENZ, is likewise highly pertinent. Having established that anaerobiosis is that property of cancer cells that distinguishes them from all normal body cells, we attacked the question, namely, how normal body cells may become transformed into anaerobes 6)7)8).

If one puts embryonic mouse cells into a suitable culture medium saturated with physiological oxygen pressures, they will grow outside the mouse body, in vitro, and indeed as pure aerobes, with a pure oxygen respiration, without a trace of fermentation. However, if during the growth one provides and oxygen pressure so reduced that the oxygen respiration is partially inhibited, the purely aerobic metabolism of the mouse embryonic cells is quantitatively altered within 48 hours, in the course of two cell divisions, into the metabolism characteristic of fermenting cancer cells. Fig. 2 illustrates the very simple experimental procedure involved.

If one then brings such cells, in which during their growth under reduced oxygen pressure a cancer cell metabolism has been produced, back under the original high oxygen pressure, and allows the cell to grow further, the cancer metabolism remains. **The transformation of embryonic cell metabolism into cancer cell metabolism can thus be irreversible, and important result, since the origin of cancer cells from normal body cells is an irreversible process.** It is equally important that these body cells whose metabolism has thus been transformed into cancer metabolism now continue to grow in vitro as facultative anaerobes. The duration of our experiments is still too limited to have yielded results of tests of inoculation of such cells back into mice, but according to all previous indications such cells will later grow as anaerobes upon transplantation into animals.

In any case, these experiments belong to the most important experiments in the field of cancer investigation since the discovery of the fermentation of tumors. For cancer metabolism, heretofore, measured so many thousand of times, has now been induced artificially in body cells by the simplest conceivable experimental procedure, and with this artificially induced cancer metabolism the body cells divide and grow as anaerobes in vitro*).

*) The experiments were at once repeated, when they were published, of course without acknowledgment. See for example Th. Goodfriend, D. M. Sokol and N. O. Kaplan, J. molecular Biol. 15, 18, 1966.

In recent months we have further developed our experimental arrangements so that we can measure manometrically the oxygen respiration and fermentation of the growing mouse embryonic cells during the metabolic transformation. Fig.

3 shows the experimental arrangement. We find by such experiments that 35 percent inhibition of oxygen respiration already suffices to bring about such a transformation during cell growth**). Oxygen pressures that inhibit respiration 35 percent can occur at the end of blood capillaries in living animals, so that the possibility arises that **cancer may result when too low oxygen pressures occur during cell growth in animal bodies.**

**) These experiments show, like the curve of Dean Burk and Mark Woods in Fig. 1, that it is more correct to designate tumor cells as "partial anaerobes" rather than "facultative anaerobes". A body cell is transformed into a tumor cell if only a part of the respiration is replaced by fermentation.

Fig. 2. Method to transform embryonic metabolism into cancer metabolism by decreasing the oxygen pressure

(Weniger O_2 = Less O_2 Viel O_2 = Much O_2)

The induction of cancers by solid materials injected into animals is a further experimental indication of this possibility. If one implants discs of solid substances under the skin of rats, the discs will soon be surrounded by capsules of living tissue that will be nourished with blood vessels from the hypodermis. Sarcomas very frequently develop in these capsules. **It is immaterial whether the solid discs are chemically plastics, gold, or ivory, etc. What produces the cancer is not the chemical nature of the solid discs, but the special kind of blood nourishment supplied to the tissue encapsulating the discs. This blood provision varies with the site and in adequacy within a given animal, and induces cancer from the low oxygen pressure in the encapsulating disc.**

Fig. 3. Method to measure manometrically respiration and fermentation during the transformation of embryonic into cancer metabolism*)

(Luft = Air)

*) The vessels are not shaken, because shaking inhibits growth. Therefore, the oxygen pressure in the liquid phase at the bottom of the vessels is much lower than in the gasphase. For example, when the oxygen pressure in the gas phase was 2000 mm H2O it was at the bottom of the vessels 130 mm H2O. (O. Warburg, A. Geissler and S. Lorenz, Zeitschr. für Naturforschung 20b, 1070, 1965.)

1.1.0.4 Thermodynamics

If a lowered oxygen pressure during cell growth may cause cancer, or, more generally, if any inhibition of respiration during growth may cause cancer, then a next problem is to show why reduced respiration induces cancer. Since we already know that with a lowering of respiration fermentation results, we can re-express our question: Why does cancer result if oxygen-respiration is replaced by fermentation?

I believe that fermentation generates the antioxidant, lactic acid, which in turn causes an EMOD insufficiency and "allows" for cancer development and metastasis. the EMOD insufficiency effectively blocks EMOD induced apoptosis of the neoplastic cells.

The early history of life on our planet indicates that life existed on earth before the earth's atmosphere contained free oxygen gas. The living cells must therefore have been fermenting cells then, and, as fossils show, they were undifferentiated single cells. Only when free oxygen appeared in the atmosphere - some billion years ago - did the higher development of life set in, to produce the plant and animal kingdoms from the fermenting, undifferentiated single cells. **What the philosophers of life have called "Evolution créatrice" has been and is therefore the work of oxygen.**

The reverse process, the dedifferentiation of life, takes place today in greatest amount before our eyes in cancer development, which is another expression for dedifferentiation. To be sure, cancer development takes place even in the presence of free oxygen gas in the atmosphere, but this oxygen may not penetrate in sufficient quantity into the growing body cells, or the respiratory apo-enzymes of the growing body cells may not be saturated with the active groups. In any case, **during the cancer development the oxygen-respiration always falls,** fermentation appears, and the highly differentiated cells are transformed to fermenting anaerobes, which have lost all their body functions and retain only the now useless property of growth. Thus, when respiration disappears, life does not disappear, but the meaning of life disappears, and what remains are growing machines that destroy the body in which they grow.

But why oxygen differentiates and why lack of oxygen dedifferentiates? Nobody would dispute that the development of plants and animals and man from unicellular anaerobes is the most improbable process of all processes in the world. Thus

there is no doubt, that EINSTEIN descended from a unicellular fermenting organism - to illustrate the miracle, molecular O2 achieved. But according to the thermodynamics of Boltzmann, improbable processes require work to take place.

It requires work to produce temperature differences in a uniformly temperatured gas; whereas the equalization of such temperature differences is a spontaneous process that does not require work. It is the oxygen-respiration that provides in life this work, and dedifferentiation begins at once when respiration is inhibited in any way. **In the language of thermodynamics, differentiation represents a forced steady state, whereas dedifferentiation - that is, cancer - is the true equilibrium state**. Or, illustrated by a picture: the differentiated body cell is like a ball on an inclined plane, which, would roll down except for the work of oxygen-respiration always preventing this. If oxygen respiration is inhibited, the ball rolls down the plane to the level of dedifferentiation.

But why respiratory energy and not fermentation energy can differentiate, whereas in general, for example in growth, respiratory energy and fermentation energy are equivalent? Obviously, there would be no cancer if there were not this discrimination of fermentation energy, that is, if fermentation like respiration could differentiate. Then, when respiration is replaced by fermentation, fermentation would take over differentiation, and a high state of differentiation would be maintained even in the fermenting body cells.

1.1.0.5 Chemistry of respiration

Physics cannot explain why the two kinds of energy are not equivalent in differentiation; but chemistry may explain it. Biochemists know that both respiration energy and fermentation energy do their work as phosphate energy, but the ways of phosphorylation are different. If one applies this knowledge to carcinogenesis, it seems that only oxidative phosphorylation but not fermentative phosphorylation can differentiate, a result, that may in future explain the mechanism of differentiation.

Yet Biochemistry can explain already today why fermentation arises, when respiration decreases. Figure 4 shows that the pathways of respiration and fermentation are common as far as pyruvic acid. Then the pathways diverge. The endproducts of fermentation is reached by one single reaction, the reduction of pyruvic acid by dihydro-nicotinamide to lactic acid. On the other hand, the endproducts of the oxidation of pyruvic acid, H_2O and CO_2, are only reached after many additional reactions. Therefore, when cells are harmed, it is probable that first respiration is harmed.

In this way the frequency of cancer is explained by reasons of probability.

To sum up:

1. Impairment of respiration is [more] frequent than impairment of fermentation because respiration is more complicated than fermentation.
2. The impaired respiration can be easily replaced by fermentation, because both processes have a common catalyst, the nicotinamide.
3. The consequence of the replacement of respiration by fermentation is mostly glycolysis, with death of the cells by lack of energy. Only if the energy of fermentation is equivalent to the lost energy of respiration, is the consequence anaerobiosis. Glycolysis means death by fermentation, anaerobiosis means life by fermentation.
4. Cancer arises, because respiration, but not fermentation, can maintain and create the high differentiation of body cells.

To conclude the discussion on the prime cause of cancer, the virus-theory of cancer may be mentioned. It is the most cherished topic of the philosophers of cancer. If it were true, it would be possible to prevent and cure cancer by the methods of virology; and all carcinogens could be eaten or smoked freely without any danger, if only contact with the cancer virus would be avoided.

It is true that some virus-caused cancer[b)] occur in animals, but no one sure human virus-cancer has been observed so far, whereas innumerable substances cause cancer without viruses in animals and man. Thus viruses do not **meet the demands of Pasteur, that is must be possible to trace the prime cause in every case of the disease.** Therefore science classifies viruses as remote causes of cancer, leading to anaerobiosis, the prime cause that meets the demands of Pasteur.

b) The chicken Rous sarcoma, which is labeled today as a virus tumor, ferments glucose and lives as a partial anaerobe like all tumors. O. WARBURG, Bioch. Zeitschrift 160, 307, 1925; F. WIND, Klinische Wochenschrift, Nr. 30, 1926.

Many may remember how anaerobiosis as prime cause of cancer was recently disputed emphatically, when one single cancer - the slow Morris hepatomas - was believed (wrongly) to lack in fermentation. In contrast the virus theory is adhered to although all cancers of man are lacking in virus-origin. This means the surrender of the principles of Pasteur and the relapse into bygone times of medicine

Applications

Of what use is it to know the prime cause of cancer? Here is an example. In Scandinavian countries there occurs a cancer of throat and esophagus whose precursor is the so-called Plummer-Vinson syndrome. This syndrome can be healed when one adds to the diet the active groups of respiratory enzymes, for example: iron salts, riboflavin, nicotinamide, and pantothenic acid. When one can heal the precursor of a cancer, one can prevent this cancer. According to ERNEST WYNDER 3) of the Sloan-Kettering Institute for Cancer Research in New York, the time has come when one can exterminate this kind of cancer with the help of the active groups of the respiratory enzymes.

It is of interest in this connection that with the help of one of these active groups of the respiratory enzymes, namely nicotinamide, tuberculosis can be healed quite as well as with streptomycin, but without the side effects of the latter [c)]. Since the sulfonamides and antibiotics, this discovery made in 1945 is the most important event in the field of chemotherapy generally, and encourages, in association with the experiences in Scandinavia, efforts to prevent cancer by dietary addition of large amounts of the active groups of the respiratory enzymes. Since there can scarcely be overdosage, such experiments can do no harm.

c) V. CHORINE: C. R. sci. Paris, 220, 150 (1945). – H. FUST and A. STUDER, Schweizerische Z. für allgemeine Pathologie, Band 14; Fasc 5 (1951).

I would like to go further and propose always making dietary additions of large amounts of the active groups of the respiratory enzymes after successful operations when there is danger from metastatic growths. One could indeed never succeed in redifferentiating the dedifferentiated cancer cells, since during the short duration of human life the probability of such a back-differentiation is zero. But one might increase the respiration of growing metastases, and thereby inhibit their fermentation, and - on the basis of the curve of DEAN BURK and MARK WOODS obtained with the Morris hepatomas - thereby inhibit the growth of metastases to such an extent that they might become as harmless as the so-called **"sleeping" cancer cells in the prostates of elderly men.**

A Second Example of Application

The physicist MANFRED VON ARDENNE has recently attacked the problem of the therapy of cancer. ARDENNE discovered **that cancer cells owing to their fermentation, are more acid – inside and on their surface – than normal cells and hence are more sensitive to high temperatures**. On this basis, he and his medical colleagues have treated cancer patients, after surgical removal of the primary tumors, by raising the body temperature of the patients to about **109° Fahrenheit for an hour**, in the hope that the metastases will then be killed or their growth so slowed up as to become harmless. It is not yet decided whether this idea can be described as a practical success. But the provisional work of ARDENNE is already of great significance in a field where hopes of conventional chemotherapy have been dimmed but might be brightened by combination with extreme or moderate hyperthermy.

A third application. According to an estimate by K. H. Bauer of the Cancer Institute in Heidelberg, at least one million of the now living twenty five million male inhabitants of West Germany will die of cancer of the respiratory tract; still more will die from other cancer. When one considers that cancer is a permanent menace, one realizes that cancer has become one of the most dangerous menaces in the history of medicine.

Many experts agree that one could prevent about 80% of all cancers in man, if one could keep away the known carcinogens from the normal body cells. This prevention of cancer might involve no expenses, and especially would require little further research to bring about cancer prevention in up to 80 percent *).

*) Since this estimate was published, some thought 80% even too low. Yet prevention remained taboo and early diagnosis was the only consolation that was offered.

Why then does it happen that in spite of all this so little is done towards the prevention of cancer? The answer has always been that one does not know what cancer or the prime cause of cancer [might] be, and that one cannot prevent something that is not known.

But nobody today can say that one does not know what cancer and its prime cause [may] be. On the contrary, **there is no disease whose prime cause is better known**, so that today ignorance is no longer an excuse that one cannot do more about prevention. That prevention of cancer will come there is no doubt, for man wishes to survive. But how long prevention will be avoided depends on how long the **prophets of agnosticism** will succeed in inhibiting the application of scientific knowledge in the cancer field. In the meantime, millions of men must die of cancer unnecessarily.

Literature to Preface of Second Edition:

1. WILLSTAETTER, WIELAND and EULER, Lectures on enzymes at the centenary of the Gesellschaft Deutscher Naturforscher. Berichte der Deutschen

Chemischen Gesellschaft, 55, 3583, 1922. The 3 lectures of the 3 chemists show that in the year 1922 the action of all enzymes was still a mystery. No active group of any enzyme was known.

2. OTTO WARBURG, Biochem. Zeitschrift, 152, 479, 1924.

3. OTTO WARBURG, Heavy Metals as prosthetic groups of enzymes, Clarendon Press, Oxford, 1949.

4. OTTO WARBURG, Wasserstoffübertragende Fermente, Verlag Werner Sänger, Berlin, 1948.

5. DEAN BURK, 1941. On the specificity of glycolysis in malignant liver tumors as compared with homologous adult or growing liver tissues. In Symposium of Respiratory Enzymes, Univ. of Wisconsin Press. pp. 235-245, 1942. DEAN BURK, Science 123,314, 1956. Woods, M.W., Sandford, K. K., Burk, D., and Earle, W. R. J. National Cancer Institute 23, 1079-1088, 1959. DEAN BURK, Burk, D., Woods, M. and Hunter, J. On the Significance of Glucolysis for Cancer Growth, with Special Reference to Morris Rat Hepatomas. Journ. National Cancer Institute 38, 839-863, 1967.

6. O. WARBURG und F. KUBOWITZ, Bioch. Z. 189, 242, 1927; H. GOLDBLATT und G. CAMERON, J. Exper. Med. 97, 525, 1953.

7. O. WARBURG, 17. Mosbacher Kolloquium, April 1966. Verlag Springer, Heidelberg, 1966.

8. O. WARBURG, K. GAWEHN, A. W. GEISSLER, D. KAYSER and S. LORENZ, Klinische Wochenschrift 43, 289, 1965.

9. O. WARBURG, Oxygen, The Creator of Differentiation, Biochemical Energetics, Academic Press, New York, 1966.

10. O. WARBURG, New Methods of Cell Physiology, Georg Thieme, Stuttgart, and Interscience Publishers, New York, 1962.

Literature to Preface of First Edition:

1. OTTO WARBURG, A. W. GEISSLER, and S. LORENZ: Über die letzte Ursache und die entfernten Ursachen des Krebses. 17. Mosbacher Kolloquium, April 1966. Verlag Springer, Heidelberg 1966.

2. Any book on vitamins, such as Th. Bersin. Biochemie der Vitamine. Akad. Verlags.-Ges. Frankfurt 1966.

3. ERNEST L. WYNDER, SVEN HULTBERG, FOLKE JACOBSSON, and IRWIN J. BROSS, Environmental Factors in Cancer. Cancer, Vol. 10, 470, 2057.

1.1.0.6 A comment by Wilhelm H on the relationship of cancer researcher Dr. Johanna Budwig with Otto Warburg, Szent-Györgyi and other illustrious scientists:

The lecture of Warburg is very interesting. It is obviously very good since he was the discoverer of the importance of oxygen in cell respiration. Yet it was also a sad witness of **his closed mind** towards Dr. Budwig's discovery. He gave the lecture some 15 years after Dr. Budwig had found the missing link which he had unsuccessfully searched for. Dr. Budwig was by this time in full swing of healing cancer patients with her Oil-Protein Diet. Here is what Dr. Budwig said:

"I assumed that Professor Warburg would recognize the significance of my discovery regarding the essential fatty acids and their role in the electro-kinetic power of the cell. In 1952 I repeatedly sent him my works and wrote to him. He refused to meet with me to discuss it."

Official history unscrupulously omits Dr. Budwig's contribution, and telling the truth tarnishes some shining names. Warburg was not the only Nobel winner to ignore Dr. Budwig's vital discovery. **Other giants of scientific history missed the significance of "fat."**

Dr. Budwig is quoted in an interview in the following manner: "Szent-Gyorgyi dealt with my published works, but he never acknowledged me," she said bitterly. "For example, he ignored me in his book Electronic Biology and Cancer, even though he was fully aware of my discovery."

More on Budwig's relationships to other scientists at Linseed and Fatty Acids: Johanna Budwig. For a thorough introduction to the subject of Johanna Budwig's natural healing protocol for cancer and other degenerative disease, see Dr. Budwig's Healing Diet & Protocol, including the complete list of Healing Cancer Naturally articles on Dr. Budwig's protocol. Unsolicited visitor's comment: "I have been educating myself on the Budwig protocol and your site is by far the most informative."

While the animal research (vivisection results) quoted by Dr. Warburg may indeed be transferrable to humans in that in the cited cases humans react similarly as did the animals, in the great majority of cases the opposite is true, see Animal Experimentation Unscientific: Physicians Convincingly Argue That Animal Testing Seriously Impedes Progress in Human Medicine While Vivisection Industry Profits

1.1.1.0 What Really Killed the Dinosaurs?

December 13, 2007 http://www.newmediaexplorer.org/sepp/2007/12/13/what_really_killed_the_dinosaurs.htm

Today, oxygen makes up about 21 percent of the atmospheric gases. But, historically that level seems to have fluctuated a lot. Much higher and much lower levels are thought to have occurred in geological times linked to the development of our current biodiversity of life on the planet:

According to recently developed geochemical models, ***oxygen levels are believed to have climbed to a maximum of 35 percent and then dropped to a low of 15 percent during a 120-million-year period that ended in a mass extinction at the end of the Permian****.*

Such a jump in oxygen would have had dramatic biological consequences by enhancing diffusion-dependent processes such as respiration, allowing insects such as dragonflies, centipedes, scorpions and spiders to grow to very large sizes. ***Fossil records indicate, for example, that one species of dragonfly had a wing span of 2 1/2 feet****.* From: Evolution of the Atmosphere

While oxygen is essential to human life, the flip side of the coin is of course the *oxygen radical,* formed during metabolic processes, which has destructive and disruptive properties. **(RMH Note: here we go again, with the same old "redox ignorant" party line).** We counteract **these naturally occurring "terrorist" molecules** by the use of anti-oxidants, vitamins, minerals and similar biological substances formed in plants that defuse and largely prevent the destructive effects of oxygen radicals. Much of our health revolves around a balance between supplying enough oxygen to tissues for normal function and blocking the destructive effects of too much oxygen by the use of anti-oxidant mechanisms.

Beldeu Singh has written several articles on the importance of anti-oxidants for the prevention and cure of cancer and the lowered immunity we call Aids. And here is Beldeu's view on how **oxygen likely was involved in the extinction of the dinosaurs**...

The change in oxygen content began to favor the emergence and selection of warm blooded animals and comparatively smaller reptiles in contrast to the huge dinosaurs. The key factor **may have been** the availablity of the oxygen molecule for metabolism rather than any disaster event.

What is apparent is that **after the mass extinction of the large-bodied dinosaurs due to the rapid decline of oxygen in the atmosphere**, the lower oxygen levels could only support the tiny foraminifera species that were only 1/20th the size following the mass extinction of the large-bodied dinosaurs.

It appears that since life first appeared on earth about a billion years ago, its evolution has been directed by many factors including biochemistry that requires sunlight in electron transfer as in photosynthesis which saw a major change to another form of L-form molecules called antioxidants being involved in electron transfer bio-reactions to sustain life without photosynthesis but in which system, the antioxidant molecules produced by photosynthesis (from plant cells) could be incorporated into animal cell biochemistry. **In both biological systems, the availability of oxygen is of critical importance.**

There is one special point to note in the role of the availibity of oxygen in evolution. When the oxygen content increases over time, say from 11% to 22%, there is too much oxygen in metabolic reactions that leads to excess oxygen free radicals and the small-bodied animal cannot consume enough antioxidants to scavenge it. **(RMH Note: This is another SWAG (scientific wild a$$ed guess).).** That environment favors larger-bodied dinosaurs with larger hearts that beat more slowly, in the region of 20-22 beats per minute. The heart of an elephant beats at around 28 beats per minute. On the other hand, as oxygen content declines significantly, say from 40% to 24%, **the slow beating heart cannot deliver enough oxygen to all parts of the huge animals and the cell function suffers from low oxygen**.

Birds are more suited to oxygen levels below 24% and their bio-engineering shows the adaptation of a relatively large heart to body-size ratio that beats around 300-1000 beats per minute during flight depending on the size of the bird. A bird's heart rate can increase rapidly when it takes off for flight and the heart rates of **small birds can easily rise above 1000 beats per minute during flight.** Their alimentary system is different and can digest the same amount of food at about four times faster than mammals to provide the additional energy and nutrients.

Bird lungs are smaller than those of mammals. They are part of the most efficient respiratory machinery known in vertebrates and even with this efficient respiratory system, **birds breathe rapidly during flight - up to 450 breaths per minute for a pigeon.** A bird's heart is much like the four chambered mammalian heart whereas reptiles have a three chambered heart but a bird's heart weighs up to twice as much as that of a mammal of equal size because **flying requires more energy and more oxygen**. Natural selection favoured the bioengineering of a bigger, faster beating heart to supply plenty of oxygen derived from faster breathing and nutrients derived from a faster digestive system. **RMH Note: yet, birds live very long lives, compared to mammalian species. This discounts the free radical theory. I believe that a bird would have been better designed if it possessed a central, oxygen-absorbing, conduit for flying (like a gill tube), instead of having to breathe in and back out so rapidly.**

Smaller birds and mammals lead fast-paced lifestyles and generally have faster heart rates than large ones. The heart of a hummingbird has about 600 beats per minute at rest. The heart of pigeon has 200 beats per minute at rest while the heart of an ostrich has 65 beats per minute at rest. **Domestic chicken heart beats are around 240 per minute. The human heart beats at 70-72 beats per minute at rest.** Elephants have a much lower heart beat at around 28 beats per minute. If dinosaur hearts beat hard and fast like those of birds, it would damage the lung and brain tissue and result in death.

Bird blood is similar to mammalian blood in that it contains both red cells (erythrocytes) and white blood cells called leucocytes. The red blood cells are iron-based proteins as in the mammalian system and do the work of transporting oxygen around the system and taking the waste carbon dioxide away from the muscles and organs. However, **unlike ours, a bird's red blood cells are nucleated, meaning they have a nucleus, where our red corpuscles have no nucleus.** So, the four chambered heart and blood quite similar to mammalian blood had already appeared before the mass extinction of the large-bodied dinosaurs but more evolutionary niches opened up due to the declining oxygen levels that meant lower photosynthetic output that would yield lower amounts of natural antioxidants for the same volume of leaves and fruits which said antioxidants are required in the metabolic activity of cells.

Natural selection favored the warm blooded mammalian physiology that could make do with lower oxygen levels in the atmosphere, a lower metabolic rate and a slower beating heart, smaller reproductive cells and a relatively longer gestation, all of which could be supported by the lower photosynthetic output.

In summary, it seems that evolutionary changes were related to the oxygen molecule levels in the atmosphere and to oxygen's role in metabolic activity which gives life but at the same time also yields the oxygen *free radical* that is toxic to life. That is what may have shaped the biodiversity we see today and ended the dominance of the large-bodied dinosaurs rather than any disaster events or any single disaster event in one part of the world.

1.1.1.1 Can glucose block oxygen transport

Glucose can attach to the hemoglobin molecule and does so in diabetes. Hemoglobin is a substance found inside red blood cells. It carries oxygen for transport to all the cells in the body. Hemoglobin can also attach itself to glucose.

When too much glucose stays in the bloodstream for an extended period of time, the glucose will attach itself to the hemoglobin inside the red blood cells. **The more glucose there is in the blood stream, the more glucose will be attached to the hemoglobin.** A hemoglobin A1c blood test will be able to determine the average glucose level over a period of two to three months. Elevated hemoglobin A1c levels are associated with increased risk for cardiovascular disease.

Approximately 65 to 75 percent of persons with diabetes die from some form of heart or vascular disease. Diabetes alone, without the other risk factors, accelerates the rate of atherosclerosis formation.

Elevated blood glucose levels are associated with increased risk for heart disease and stroke. **I believe that the reduced ability for oxygen transport is responsible for the coexistence of these diseases.**

1.1.1.2 Diabetes, microvascular complications, and cardiovascular complications: what is it about glucose?

Glycemic control is the primary mediator of diabetic microvascular complications and also contributes to macrovascular complications. A new study reveals a previously unrecognized association between oxidant activation of poly(ADP ribose) polymerase (PARP) and upregulation of known mediators of glycemic injury. Inhibitors of PARP may have potential therapeutic roles in the prevention of diabetic complications.

The prevalence of obesity, diabetes, and the metabolic syndrome is increasing in the US and worldwide at astonishing rates. Diabetes is the leading cause of blindness, renal failure, and amputation in the United States. These conditions can be slowed or prevented with optimal glycemic control. Accompanying the diabetes epidemic is a concomitant two- to four-fold excess risk for cardiovascular disease (Hanson RL, Imperatore G, Bennett PH, Knowler WC. Components of the "metabolic syndrome" and incidence of type 2 diabetes. *Diabetes*. 2002;**51**:3120–3127) (Abbasi F, Brown BW, Jr, Lamendola C, McLaughlin T, Reaven GM. Relationship between obesity, insulin resistance, and coronary heart disease risk. *J. Am. Coll. Cardiol.* 2002;**40**:937–943).

Modification of traditional cardiovascular risk factors has an impressive impact on morbidity and mortality in subjects with diabetes and insulin resistance as reported in various studies, including the Scandinavian Simvastatin Survival Study, the Cholesterol and Recurrent Events (CARE) study, the MRC/BHF Heart Protection Study, the Steno-2 study, the Losartan Intervention For Endpoint reduction in hypertension study (known as LIFE), and the Heart Outcomes Prevention Evaluation study (known as HOPE).

Even with these effective interventions, people with diabetes still have increased morbidity and mortality when compared to the nondiabetic population. The question remains, **what is it about diabetes (defined by high blood glucose levels) that leads to excess vascular risk?** In this issue of the *JCI*, Du and colleagues present a new molecular target — poly(ADP ribose) polymerase (PARP) — dysregulated by hyperglycemic injury, which may have implications for prevention of both microvascular disease and macrovascular disease because this enzyme affects critical targets in the endothelial cell.

Glucose is the driving force in microvascular complications of diabetes, yet **the action of glucose alone seems inadequate and unable to account for the excess atherosclerosis observed in subjects with diabetes.** In type 2 diabetes, insulin resistance, and the metabolic syndrome, the vasculature is exposed to a frontal assault by hypertension, dyslipidemia (increased triglycerides, low HDL and high LDL cholesterol), inflammation, and impaired fibrinolysis. This toxic metabolic environment increases atherosclerotic risk in persons with the metabolic syndrome.

The heightened risk observed in the metabolic syndrome inevitably sets the stage for increased vascular disease in type 2 diabetics, but hyperglycemia adds additional risk.

Strong epidemiological evidence suggests a correlation among glucose, atherosclerotic plaque burden, cardiovascular events, and increased morbidity and mortality (Tominaga M, et al. Impaired glucose tolerance is a risk factor for cardiovascular disease, but not impaired fasting glucose. The Funagata Diabetes Study. *Diabetes Care*. 1999;**22**:920–924) (Ledru F, et al. New diagnostic criteria for diabetes and coronary artery disease: insights from an angiographic study. *J. Am. Coll. Cardiol.* 2001;**37**:1543–1550).

In an autopsy study of 18- to 34–year-olds there was an increase in atherosclerotic plaque burden in subjects with elevated hemoglobin A1C (Ledru F, et al. New diagnostic criteria for diabetes and coronary artery disease: insights from an angiographic study. *J. Am. Coll. Cardiol.* 2001;**37**:1543–1550).

The Honolulu Heart Program demonstrated a predictive correlation between fasting plasma glucose levels (nondiabetic, impaired glucose tolerance, and diabetic ranges) and cardiovascular events and mortality. Large population studies from Northern Europe indicate a direct correlation between glycemic control (as measured by glycohemoglobin) and cardiovascular morbidity and mortality. As will be discussed later, **hyperglycemia has specific deleterious effects upon vascular endothelial function that could account for these epidemiological correlations between hyperglycemia and poor vascular outcomes**.

One would predict, based upon epidemiological data, that interventional studies targeting hyperglycemia would show improved cardiovascular outcomes. To date, no such compelling evidence has emerged. In fact, in the largest prospective glucose-lowering trial in type 2 diabetes patients, the United Kingdom Prospective Diabetes Study, **there were no statistical improvements in cardiovascular outcomes when glucose was lowered using insulin or sulfonylureas**. Only in the small metformin cohort (n = 342) were cardiovascular outcomes improved by optimal glycemic control. A few small studies have suggested a positive impact of glycemic control on cardiovascular events, but this point remains highly debated. The conclusions of a recent panel convened by the American Heart Association suggest that **while glycemia contributes to cardiovascular risk, treatment of glycemia, exclusive of other potent cardiovascular risk factor intervention, is inadequate to reverse or reduce the complex atherosclerotic process**.

The negative impact of hyperglycemia on endothelial function and pathological changes observed in diabetes is supported in the literature. **Endothelial cells in vitro are exquisitely sensitive to high glucose (25mM).** Nishikawa et al. and others have carefully characterized four major molecular signaling mechanisms activated by hyperglycemia in endothelial cells and other cell types **vulnerable to hyperglycemic injury**. These include activation of PKC (via diacylglycerol), increased hexosamine pathway flux, increased advanced glycation end product (AGE) formation, and increased polyol pathway flux.

Nishikawa et al. recently proposed the existence of a unifying mechanism that integrates the above pathways: **increased production of reactive oxygen species (ROS) (specifically superoxide) by the mitochondrial electron transport chain** (Nishikawa T, et al. Normalizing mitochondrial superoxide production blocks three pathways of hyperglycaemic damage. *Nature.* 2000;**404**:787–790).

In their original report, numerous theoretical constructs were outlined for the impact of altered redox state upon formation of polyols, AGEs, and PKC. What remained unclear were the downstream targets of oxidant stress. In the paper by Du et al. in this issue of the *JCI,* this group takes their seminal observation one step further and defines one consequence of increased ROS, namely activation of PARP. PARP activation leads to ribosylation and inactivation of GAPDH. Inhibition of GAPDH increases delivery of glycolytic intermediates to the mitochondria. **This change in turn would be expected to increase mitochondrial superoxide production** and also to increase flux through the AGE and PKC glucotoxic pathways.

It has been well established that diabetes leads to microvascular complications, and it has also been suggested that hyperglycemia plays an accelerating role in macrovascular disease. This excess disease burden is driven by glucose-related activation of PKC, accumulation of AGEs, excess polyol flux, and accumulation of glucosamine. Interventions for each of these mechanisms have had great efficacy in animal models but **disappointing outcomes in clinical trials** (Brownlee M. Biochemistry and molecular cell biology of diabetic complications. *Nature.* 2001;**414**:813–820).

It was concluded that a cocktail of inhibitors might be necessary to effectively block these deleterious cellular responses in a complex human model of fluctuating hyperglycemia.

The observation that these pathways reflect a single hyperglycemia-induced process, namely oxidative stress, suggested that antioxidants could serve as a single agent in the prevention of diabetes complications. To date, human studies with α lipoic acid suggest a therapeutic benefit, but **the use of conventional antioxidants has been disappointing in larger trials** (Heart Outcomes Prevention Evaluation Study Investigators. Effects of ramipril on cardiovascular and microvascular outcomes in people with diabetes mellitus: results of the HOPE study and MICRO-HOPE substudy. *Lancet.* 2000;**355**:253–259).

Thus, I conclude that EMODs are not causative of diabetes.

Conventional antioxidants scavenge free radicals in an inefficient stoichiometric manner so that one molecule of the antioxidant would be needed to neutralize each free radical generated. Novel small molecular weight compounds that function as superoxide dismutase mimetics may offer more reliable benefits due to the catalytic properties that could permit enzymatic detoxification. The observation that PARP drives glucotoxicity through inhibition of GAPDH suggests PARP inhibitors as another therapeutic tool for complication prevention. In theory, these agents could have an effect equivalent to combination inhibitor therapy due to positive effects on AGE, PKC, and NF-κB. Indeed, the few reports employing PARP inhibitors in animal models of diabetes support the therapeutic potential of these agents. With the incidence of diabetes and its complications on the rise, these results offer hope for new treatments in the foreseeable future. (**Diabetes, microvascular complications, and cardiovascular complications: what is it about glucose?** Jane E.B. Reusch. J Clin Invest. 2003 October 1; 112(7): 986–988).

1.1.1.3 Organ Transplant Increases Risk of Skin Cancer

In study after study, the finding is the same. **Organ-transplant recipients have an increased risk of developing skin cancer, and with each passing year, this risk grows.** Some dermatologists report that **these patients tend to develop their first skin cancer 2 to 4 years after the transplant operation.** http://www.skincarephysicians.com/skincancernet/organ_transplant.html Accessed 1-07-09.

1.1.1.4 Why Organ Transplant Increases Risk

The medication taken to prevent organ rejection plays a key role, but it is not the only reason for this increased risk. **Unprotected sun exposure, which allows ultraviolet (UV) rays to harm the skin, also affects a person's risk. The more life time sun exposure, the greater the risk. Research shows that 20 years after receiving an organ, recipients who live in a temperate climate have a 40% overall increased risk of developing skin cancer. This risk exceeds 80% in sun-intense areas such as Australia.**

Having naturally pale to olive skin and contracting an infection caused by a human papillomavirus (HPV) also seem to increase the risk of an organ-transplant recipient developing skin cancer. I believe that this means that if one is susceptible to a viral infection, they are also susceptible to development of cancer, since the same EMOD protective system is involved in both. Further, because of organ transplantation, immunosuppression causes an EMOD insufficiency, which "allows" for cancer formation and progression.

I believe that the skin, which has the lowest levels of oxygen, is a setup for cancer and infections, due to low EMOD levels.

When skin cancer develops in an organ-transplant recipient, multiple skin cancers may appear and the cancer can be more aggressive. An aggressive cancer has greater potential to recur (return after treatment) and to metastasize (spread). Being aware of this and learning what can reduce the risk are likely to improve one's quality of life (Berg D, Otley CC. Skin cancer in organ transplant recipients: Epidemiology, pathogenesis, and management. *Journal of the American Academy of Dermatology* 2002; 47: 1-17; quiz 8-20) (Carucci, JA. Update on Transplant Related Skin Cancer. Presented during a surgical symposium (SYM 308) at the Summer Academy Meeting of the American Academy of Dermatology, August 2007; New York City) (Euvrard S, Kanitakis J, Claudy A. Skin cancers after organ transplantation. *The New England Journal of Medicine* 2003; 348: 1681-91) (Harwood CA, Leedham-Green M, Leigh IM *et al.* Low-dose retinoids in the prevention of cutaneous squamous cell carcinomas in organ transplant recipients: a 16-year retrospective study. *Archives of Dermatology* 2005; 141: 456-64) (Harwood CA, Proby CM, McGregor JM *et al.* Clinicopathologic features of skin cancer in organ transplant recipients: a retrospective case-control series. *Journal of the American Academy of Dermatology* 2006; 54: 290-300) (Martinez JC, Otley CC, Stasko T *et al.* Defining the clinical course of metastatic skin cancer in organ transplant recipients: a multicenter collaborative study. *Archives of Dermatology* 2003; 139: 301-6) (Ong CS, Keogh AM, Kossard S et al. Skin cancer in Australian heart transplant recipients. *Journal of the American Academy of Dermatology* 1999; 40: 27-34).

1.1.1.5 Free radicals in the atmosphere

Dry air contains roughly (by molar content – equivalent to volume, for gases) 78.08% nitrogen, 20.95% oxygen, 0.93% argon, 0.038% carbon dioxide, and trace amounts of other gases; but air also contains a variable amount of water vapor, on average around 1%. This mixture of gases is commonly known as **air**. The atmosphere protects life on Earth by absorbing ultraviolet solar radiation. **This means that 21% of the atmosphere is made up of the diradical, oxygen. In space, hydrogen is the most common element and since it has only one outer unpaired electron, it is a free radical. Consequently, I believe that we basically live on a "radical planet and in a radical universe."**

Atmospheric gases scatter blue light more than other wavelengths, giving the Earth a blue halo when seen from space.

Actually, the sun is composed mainly of the radical, hydrogen. This radical star emits photons, which are collected by plant life on earth and converted into oxygen and carbohydrates. We utilize the oxygen to produce energy and regenerate carbon dioxide for the plants' survival. Plants use excited states and photosynthesis to produce the oxygen, which we convert to EMODs, for pathogen and cancer protection and healing.

Thus, we have a "radical star" as our source of solar energy.

1.1.1.6 The changing composition of the global atmosphere

by David Etheridge

david.etheridge@dar.csiro.au

The levels of many trace gases and aerosol particles are changing in the atmosphere, largely as a result of human activities. Although totalling less than 0.1 per cent of the mass of the atmosphere, these constituents determine much of its chemical and physical state. Changes in atmospheric composition have significant impacts, often a long way from the origins of the emissions (for example, stratospheric ozone depletion, volcanic aerosols, global warming). As a result, the issues are broadening from urban or regional concerns to being at the centre of global environmental protocols.

Precise measurements of oxygen concentration provide another powerful tracer. **The concentration of oxygen in the atmosphere is decreasing**, because oxygen is being combined stoichiometrically with carbon from fossil fuels and from forest burning to form carbon dioxide. The increase in carbon dioxide is well known, but the related decrease in oxygen is very small compared to its approximately 20 per cent atmospheric abundance. Measurement of the oxygen change has presented a major measurement challenge. Although oxygen's decrease could be viewed with concern, it will not have a noticeable effect for thousands of years. **Previously, I have postulated that the decrease in atmospheric oxygen is related to EMOD insufficiency and that it is directly related to the increase in global diseases, such as cancer, atherosclerosis, diabetes, arthritis, etc.**

The global oxygen trend measured over the last 20 years or so in air archived at Cape Grim, could be explained quantitatively by the amount of fossil fuel carbon known to have been burnt over this period. However, we know that large areas of forests have also been cleared and combusted, so the oxygen decrease from this cause must have been approximately balanced by the release of oxygen from a greater rate of photosynthesis of the remaining terrestrial biosphere. This is possibly a result of higher plant growth rates caused by higher CO_2 levels, or climate change. The biosphere over this period is said to be in mass balance.

The most common atmospheric gas, nitrogen (chemical symbol N_2) accounts for about 78% of the atmosphere. Nitrogen gas is largely inert, meaning that it does not readily react with other substances to form new chemical compounds. The next most common gas, oxygen (O_2), makes up about 21% of the atmosphere. Oxygen is required for the **respiration** (breathing) of all animal life on **Earth**, from humans to **bacteria**. In contrast to nitrogen, oxygen is extremely reactive. It participates in **oxidation, a type of chemical reaction that can be observed everywhere.** Some common examples of oxidation are apples turning from white to brown after being sliced, the rusting of **iron**, and the very rapid oxidation reaction we call fire. Just under 1% of the atmosphere is made up of argon (Ar), which is a very inert noble gas, meaning that it does not take part in any **chemical reactions** under normal circumstances.

Together, these three gases account for 99.96% of the atmosphere. The remaining 0.04% contains a wide variety of trace gases, several of which are crucial to life on Earth, such as CO2. Despite its relative scarcity**, atmospheric water probably has more of an impact on the earth than any of the major gases, aside from oxygen**.

Ozone (O_3) is almost all found in a layer about 9–36 mi (15–60 km) in attitude. Ozone gas is irritating to peoples' eyes and skin, and chemically attacks rubber and plant **tissue**. Nevertheless, it is vital to life on Earth because it absorbs most of the high energy radiation from the sun that is harmful to plants and animals. A portion of the energy radiated by the sun lies in the ultraviolet (UV) region. This shorter wavelength radiation is responsible for suntans, and is sufficiently powerful to harm cells, cause skin **cancer**, and burn tissue, as anyone who has had a painful sunburn knows. The ozone molecules, along with molecules of O_2, absorb nearly all the high energy UV rays, protecting the earth's surface from the most damaging radiation. The first step in this process occurs high in the atmosphere, where O_2 molecules absorb very high energy UV radiation. Upon doing so, each absorbing **molecule** breaks up into two oxygen atoms. The oxygen atoms eventually collide with another O_2molecule, forming a molecule of ozone, O_3 (a third molecule is required in the collision to carry away excess energy). Ozone in turn may absorb UV of slightly longer wavelength, which knocks off one of its oxygen atoms and leaves O_2. The free oxygen atom, being very reactive, will almost immediately recombine with another O_2, forming more ozone. The last two steps of this cycle keep repeating but do not create any new chemical compounds; they only act to absorb ultraviolet radiation. The amount of ozone in the stratosphere is minute. If it were all transported to the surface, the ozone gas would form a layer about 0.1–0.16 in (2.5–4.0 mm) thick. This layer, as thin as it is, is sufficient to shield the earth's occupants from harmful solar radiation.

The upper mesosphere and the lower thermosphere contain charged atoms and molecules (ions in a region known as the ionosphere. The atmospheric constituents at this level include nitrogen gas, atomic oxygen and nitrogen (O and N), and nitric oxide (NO). All of these are exposed to strong solar **emission** of ultraviolet and x ray radiation, which can result in ionization, knocking off an **electron** to form an atom or molecule with a positive charge. The ionosphere is a region enriched in free electrons and positive ions. This charged particle region affects the propagation of radio waves, reflecting them as a mirror reflects light. The ionosphere makes it possible to tune in radio stations very far from the transmitter; even if the radio waves coming directly from the transmitter are blocked by **mountains** or the curvature of the earth, one can still receive the waves bounced off the ionosphere. After the sun sets, the numbers of electrons and ions in the lower layers drop drastically, since the sun's radiation is no longer available to keep them ionized. Even at night, however, the higher layers retain some ions. The result is that the ionosphere is higher at night, which allows radio waves to bounce for longer distances. This is the reason that one can frequently tune in more distant radio stations at night than during the day.

The upper thermosphere is also where the bright nighttime displays of colors and flashes known as the aurora occur. The aurora are caused by energetic particles emitted by the sun. These particles become trapped by **Earth's magnetic field** and collide with the relatively few gas atoms present above about 60 mi (100 km), mostly atomic oxygen (O) and nitrogen gas (N_2). These collisions cause the atoms and molecules to emit light, resulting in spectacular displays.

http://science.jrank.org/pages/590/Atmosphere-Composition-Structure.html. Accessed 1-07-09.

1.1.1.7 Bistability of atmospheric oxygen and the Great Oxidation

The history of the Earth has been characterized by a series of major transitions separated by long periods of relative stability. **The largest chemical transition was the 'Great Oxidation', approximately 2.4 billion years ago**, when atmospheric oxygen concentrations rose from less than 10^{-5} of the present atmospheric level (PAL) to more than 0.01 PAL, and possibly to more than 0.1 PAL. This transition took place long after oxygenic photosynthesis is thought to have evolved, but the causes of this delay and of the Great Oxidation itself remain uncertain. Here we show that **the origin of oxygenic photosynthesis gave rise to two simultaneously stable steady states for atmospheric oxygen.** The existence of a low-oxygen (less than 10^{-5} PAL) steady state explains how a **reducing atmosphere** persisted for at least 300 million years after the onset of oxygenic photosynthesis. **The Great Oxidation can be understood as a switch to the high-oxygen (more than 5×10^{-3} PAL) steady state.** The bistability arises because ultraviolet shielding of the troposphere by ozone becomes effective once oxygen levels exceed 10^{-5} PAL, causing a nonlinear increase in the lifetime of atmospheric oxygen. Our results indicate that the existence of oxygenic photosynthesis is not a sufficient condition for either an oxygen-rich atmosphere or the presence of an ozone layer, which has implications for detecting life on other planets using atmospheric analysis and for the evolution of multicellular life (Bistability of atmospheric oxygen and the Great Oxidation. Colin Goldblatt et al. *Nature* 443, 683-686 (12 October 2006).

1.1.2.0 Vitamin Mania: The Truth about Antioxidants

By Christopher Wanjek, LiveScience's Bad Medicine Columnist

posted: 02 May 2006

Studies showing the negative or null effects of vitamins supplements are so common, it is nonsensical that many doctors still find these negative studies to be surprising or disappointing. Vitamins are not as simple as A-B-C.

The latest bit of confusion appears in the April 27, 2006 issue of the *New England Journal of Medicine*. **Doctors in Australia provided nearly 1,900 pregnant women with either supplements of vitamins C and E or a placebo**

to see whether the vitamins would lower the risk of developing high blood pressure during pregnancy. It didn't work.

Surprisingly, the doctors said, **the vitamin C and E group had a slightly higher rate of high blood pressure compared to the placebo group**.

1.1.2.1 We love our vitamins

The levels of vitamins C and E were greater than those found in an ordinary multivitamin tablet—1,000 milligrams of C and 400 IU of E, or roughly 10 and 20 times the recommended daily allowance. In an editorial accompanying the study, doctors said that supplements at these levels should not be prescribed routinely.

But we *love* our vitamins.

Americans spend about $2 billion a year on vitamins C and E, along with beta carotene (a precursor of vitamin A) and selenium, according to *Nutrition Business Journal*. These are the most popular antioxidants, a class of chemicals said to cure just about everything.

The trouble is, science can't seem to support the bad movie script created by the vitamin supplement industry.

No simple movie plot...

1.1.2.2 Rogue free radicals

Here's the plot, a battle between good and evil: **Rogue chemicals called free radicals** roam about the body like brazen street punks, smashing cellular walls and roughing up innocent DNA molecules, causing cancers and the diseases of middle- and old-age. Their flagrant disregard for the law would continue unchecked if it weren't for **swashbuckling antioxidants** swooping in on the wings of vitamin supplements, disarming the free radicals of their menacing electrons and converting them into respectable molecular citizens.

But the body, it seems, is not governed by a Hollywood "B" script. **Free radicals are as good as they are bad, and too many antioxidants may do the body harm**.

It is true that antioxidants serve as sort of a rust protector for the body, stopping a process called oxidation. Important molecules in the body, such as those that form artery walls, become oxidized when they lose an electron. Once oxidized, they become unstable and easily break apart.

The culprit, without a doubt, is the free radical. **NOT! This is unproved.**

1.1.2.3 Free to destroy

Free radicals are highly reactive molecules or single atoms with unpaired electrons looking for a mate. So they steal an electron from the first thing they encounter, perhaps a cell wall or DNA. As free-radical damage mounts, cells can no longer perform properly. Disease sets in. **An excess of free radicals has been cited in cardiovascular disease, Alzheimer's disease, Parkinson's disease and cancer. (But not proven)**

Aging itself has been defined as a gradual accumulation of free-radical damage.

Yet **free radicals are necessary for life. The body's ability to turn air and food into chemical energy depends on a chain reaction of free radicals. Free radicals are also a crucial part of the immune system, floating through the veins and attacking foreign invaders.**

Hydrogen peroxide is a prime example of a free radical. **(RMH Note: peroxide is not a free radical). Your blood actually contains trace amounts of hydrogen peroxide,** an internal germ fighter. In fact, **you could not fight bacteria without free radicals.**

How antioxidants work is an utter mystery, which explains the contradicting results of very large and well-conducted studies in the past decade showing, for example, that **vitamin E slowed the progress of coronary artery disease but increased the risk of a heart attack. I believe that it is obviously because the free radi-crap theory is wrong.**

One thing that studies do reveal is that **a diet rich in antioxidants, as opposed to supplements, is associated with lower rates of cancer and circulatory disease**. Richard Veech of the National Institute on Alcohol Abuse and Alcoholism, whom I interviewed a few years ago, sums it up best, I think:

"People don't want to exercise," he said. "They don't want to eat healthy food. They don't want to stop drinking; they don't want to stop smoking; they don't want to stop having dangerous sex. They want to take a pill. Well, good luck."

1.1.3.0 BHT and BHA

Butylated Hydroxytoluene- BHT, and Butylated Hydroxyanisole- BHA are preservatives (antioxidants) for oil containing products due to their antioxidant properties. BHA is generally used to keep fats from becoming rancid and BHT is used to prevent oxidative rancidity of fats. BHT has been used since 1949 and despite it being a known carcinogen, it is still used today.

These two closely related chemicals can still be found in many foods and personal care products like, cosmetics, pharmaceuticals, personal ointments, meat, beer, butter, meats, cereals, chewing gum, baked goods, snack foods, dehydrated potatoes, rice products, dried soup, food packaging, animal feed and rubber and petroleum products.

Based on animal tests, a chemical that causes cancer in at least one organ in three different species indicates that it might be carcinogenic in humans. BHT has caused various disorders in animals such as cancer, reduced body weight, increased blood cholesterol levels, and it has been linked to birth defects in rats. That is why the **U.S. Department of Health and Human Services considers BHA to be "reasonably anticipated to be a human carcinogen"**. Nevertheless, the Food and Drug Administration still permits **BHA to be used in foods. Japan has banned the use of BHT and BHA and the U.K. and several European countries have severely restricted it's use all citing considerable safety risks**.

Serious concerns have been raised about the use of BHT in food products. BHT is a suspected mutagen and carcinogen. There have been cases in which some individuals have had difficulty metabolizing BHT, resulting in health and behavior changes.

BHT has been banned for use in food in Japan (1958), Romania, Sweden, and Australia. The US has barred it from being used in infant foods. However some food industries have eliminated it from their products including McDonald's as of 1986.

Some foods in which BHA is used include: butter, meats, cereals, chewing gum, baked goods, snack foods, dehydrated potatoes, and beer.

Butylated hydroxytoluene (BHT) is a fat-soluble organic compound primarily used as an antioxidant food additive (E number E321). It also used as an antioxidant in cosmetics, pharmaceutical drugs, jet fuels, rubber and petroleum products, and embalming fluid.

BHT is produced by the reaction of *p*-cresol with isobutylene. It was patented in 1947 and received approval of the Food and Drug Administration for use as a food additive and preservative in 1954. BHT reacts with free radicals, slowing the rate of autoxidation in food, preventing changes in the food's color, odor, and taste.

Listed in reverse date order, linked to extracts below and abstracts in MedLine:

Klein 2003 — Effects of dietary butylated hydroxytoluene on aflatoxin B(1)-relevant metabolic enzymes in turkeys.

Umemura 2002 — The mouse rasH2/BHT model as an in vivo rapid assay for lung carcinogens.

Sarafian 2002 — Synergistic cytotoxicity of Delta(9)-tetrahydrocannabinol *(THC in marijuana smoke)* and butylated hydroxyanisole. *(BHA)*

Yu 2000 — Molecular mechanisms of butylated hydroxylanisole-induced toxicity: induction of apoptosis through direct release of cytochrome c.

Patrick 1999 — Depigmentation with tert-butyl hydroquinone using black guinea pigs.

Malkinson 1999 — Lung tumor promotion by BHT.

Chung 1999 — Effects of butylated hydroxyanisole (BHA) and butylated hydroxytoluene (BHT) on the acetylation of 2-aminofluorene and DNA-2-aminofluorene adducts in the rat.

Tryphonas 1999 — The effect of butylated hydroxytoluene on selected immune surveillance parameters in rats bearing enzyme-altered hepatic preneoplastic lesions.

Takami 1999 — Antioxidants reversibly inhibit the spontaneous resumption of meiosis.

Stolze 1999 — Free radical formation and erythrocyte membrane alterations during MetHb formation induced by the BHA metabolite, tert-butylhydroquinone *(TBHQ)*.

Safer 1999 — Hepatotoxicity induced by the anti-oxidant food additive, butylated hydroxytoluene (BHT), in rats: an electron microscopical study.

McFarlane 1997 — Hepatic and associated response of rats to pregnancy, lactation and simultaneous treatment with butylated hydroxytoluene.

Gudz 1997 — Effect of butylhydroxytoluene and related compounds on permeability of the inner mitochondrial membrane.

Peters 1996 — Glutathione conjugates of tert-butyl-hydroquinone, a metabolite of the urinary tract tumor promoter 3-tert-butyl-hydroxyanisole, are toxic to kidney and bladder.

Siman 1996 — Effect of butylated hydroxytoluene on alpha-tocopherol content in liver and adipose tissue of rats.

Jobling 1995 — A variety of environmentally persistent chemicals, including some phthalate plasticizers, are weakly estrogenic.

Kahl 1993 — Toxicology of the synthetic antioxidants BHA and BHT in comparison with the natural antioxidant vitamin E.

Tanaka 1993 — Three generation toxicity study of butylated hydroxytoluene administered to mice.

Parke 1992 — Safety aspects of food preservatives.

Briggs 1989 — hort-term effects of butylated hydroxytoluene on the Wistar rat liver, urinary bladder and thyroid gland.

Thompson 1988 — Cytotoxicity of butylated hydroxyanisole and butylated hydroxytoluene in isolated rat hepatocytes.

Zoccarato 1987 — Inhibition by some phenolic antioxidants of Ca2+ uptake and neurotransmitter release from brain synaptosomes.

Kahl 1984	Synthetic antioxidants: biochemical actions and interference with radiation, toxic compounds, chemical mutagens and chemical carcinogens.
Ohno 1984	Differentiation induction of murine erythroleukemia cells by butylated hydroxytoluene.
Kovaleva 1983	Effect of antioxidants on the release of 3H-serotonin by rat brain synaptosomes.
Gould 1982	Inhibition of norepinephrine uptake into synaptic vesicles by butylated hydroxytoluene.
Juhlin 1981	Recurrent urticaria: clinical investigation of 330 patients.
Vorhees 1981	Developmental neurobehavioral toxicity of butylated hydroxyanisole (BHA) in rats.
Osmundsen 1980	Contact urticaria from nickel and plastic additives (butylhydroxytoluene, oleylamide).
Kawano 1980	Species and strain differences in the butylated hydroxytoluene (BHT)-producing induction of hepatic drug oxidation enzymes.
Meyer 1980	Behavioural and developmental effects of butylated hydroxytoluene dosed to rats in utero and in the lactation period.
Stokes 1974	The effect of butylated hydroxyanisole and butylated hydroxytoluene on behavioral development of mice

1.1.3.1 Antioxidants BHT and BHA can be carcinogenic and anti-carcinogenic

When administered prior to or at the time of carcinogen exposure, the phenolic antioxidants butylated hydroxyanisole (BHA) and butylated hydroxytoluene (BHT) are effective inhibitors of carcinogenesis in several target organs.

However, **chronic, postcarcinogen administration of BHT apparently enhances tumorigenesis in certain animal models for liver and lung cancer**. The present study was performed to determine the effects of BHA and BHT on mammary carcinogenesis when antioxidant exposure is limited to defined periods encompassing or following carcinogen availability. At 50 days of age (Time 0), virgin female Sprague-Dawley rats (25/group) were given a single intragastric dose of 8 mg of 7,12-dimethylbenz(*a*)athracene. Basal diet (Wayne Lab Meal) was supplemented with 5000 or 2500 mg of BHA or BHT/kg by the following protocol: 2 weeks before until 1 week after carcinogen administration; 1 week after carcinogen administration until the end of the study; or none. The experiment was terminated 210 days after 7,12-dimethylbenz(*a*)anthracene administration, and all mammary tumors were confirmed histologically. When administered by the 2 weeks before to 1 week after schedule, both BHA and BHT were effective inhibitors of mammary carcinogenesis. However, the compounds also were active in chemoprevention when administered by the 1 week after to end protocol. These data indicate that the anticarcinogenic activity of antioxidants is not limited to influences on carcinogen metabolism, since both BHA and BHT inhibited mammary tumor induction when their administration was begun following clearance of the carcinogen from the mammary gland. **The anticarcinogenic activity of postcarcinogen administration of BHA and BHT in the mammary gland is in contrast to the apparent tumor-enhancing activity of BHT in the liver and lung** (Inhibition of 7,12-Dimethylbenz(*a*)anthracene-induced Rat Mammary Carcinogenesis by Concomitant or Postcarcinogen Antioxidant Exposure. David L. McCormick, Nancy Major and Richard C. Moon. Cancer Research *44, 2858-2863, July 1, 1984*).

Yet, BHT has been tested extensively for toxicity and used widely for many years. It does not contain any ingredient designated as a known, probable, or suspected human carcinogen by IARC, NTP, ACGIH, or OSHA.

And still others claim: **BHA & BHT** are widely used as preservatives, stabilizers and antioxidants. **BHA is known to cause cancer in humans. Both BHA and BHT are toxic to the liver and kidneys.** BHT may react with other ingested substances to cause the formation of carcinogens. BHT is banned in England. http://www.healthyeatingadvisor.com/9cancer-causingchemicals.html accessed 8-9-09.

BHA has at least epigenetic carcinogenic activity and BHT causes hemorrhagic complications and alters offspring fed BHT. http://www.mindfully.org/Plastic/Antioxidants/BHA-BHT.htm

(Madhavi et al, 1996) (Butylated hydroxyanisole (BHA; *tert*-butyl-4-hydroxyanisole) and Butylated hydroxytoluene (BHT; 2,6-di-*tert*-butyl-p-cresol) in *Food Antioxidants: Technological, Toxicological, and Health Perspectives*. Edited by DL Madhavi, SS Deshpande, and DK Salunkhe / Dekker 1996).

1.1.3.2 Are BHA and BHT safe?

Both BHA and BHT have undergone the additive application and review process required by the US Food and Drug Administration. However, the same chemical properties which make BHA and BHT excellent preservatives may also be implicated in health effects. The oxidative characteristics and/or metabolites of BHA and BHT may contribute to carcinogenicity or tumorigenicity; however the same reactions may combat oxidative stress. There is evidence that certain persons may have difficulty metabolizing BHA and BHT, resulting in health and behavior changes.

http://chemistry.about.com/od/foodcookingchemistry/a/bha-bht-preservatives.htm

1.1.3.3 BHA and BHT are tumor promoters

"...Specific toxic effects to the lung have only been observed with BHT. The other described toxic effects of BHA and BHT are less characteristic and often occur only after high dosage and long-term treatment. However, BHA induces in animals tumours of the forestomach, which are dose dependent, whereas BHT induces liver tumours in long-term experiments. ... all published findings agree with the fact that **BHA and BHT are tumour promoters.** In contrast to BHA and BHT, vitamin E is not carcinogenic." (Toxicology of the synthetic antioxidants BHA and BHT in comparison with the natural antioxidant vitamin E. Kahl R, Kappus H, *Z Lebensm Unters Forsch* 1993 Apr;196(4):329-38).

The American Academy of Pediatrics (AAP) had real concerns about major drug additives: -- **Sulfites, antioxidants** found in many anti-asthma drugs, have been known to induce "serious reactions" such as wheezing, breathing difficulties and chest tightening in asthmatic children. Sulfites are also found in some anti-inflammatories, antibiotics, and the anti-allergy drug epinephrine.

1.2.0.0 EMOD-induced apoptosis ==

1.2.0.1 Oxygen Radicals Induce Poly(ADP-Ribose) Polymerase-Dependent Cell Death in Cytotoxic Lymphocytes

The PARP/apoptosis-inducing factor axis is critically involved in oxygen radical-induced apoptosis in cytotoxic lymphocytes.

Oxygen radicals are produced by phagocytes as part of a defense strategy against intra- and extracellular pathogens. The radicals are formed by the assembly and activation of a membrane enzyme complex, the NADPH oxidase, which transforms molecular oxygen into superoxide anion, which in turn is converted to hydrogen peroxide, toxic halids, and other radical species. **Extracellularly released oxygen radicals are toxic to a variety of cells and tissues** ("oxidative stress") (Hellstrand, K.. 2003. Melanoma immunotherapy: a battle against radicals?. *Trends Immunol.* 24: 232-233) (Klebanoff, S. J.. 1980. Oxygen metabolism and the toxic properties of phagocytes. *Ann. Intern. Med.* 93: 480-489).

During the past decade, much attention has been directed toward the ability of mononuclear phagocytes to adversely affect cytotoxic lymphocyte function (Elgert, K. D., D. G. Alleva, D. W. Mullins. 1998. Tumor-induced immune dysfunction: the macrophage connection. *J. Leukocyte Biol.* 64: 275-290), with a focus on the **immunosuppressive role of phagocyte-derived oxygen radicals** (Hansson, M., A. Asea, U. Ersson, S. Hermodsson, K. Hellstrand. 1996. Induction of apoptosis in NK cells by monocyte-derived reactive oxygen metabolites. *J. Immunol.* 156: 42-47) (Kono, K., F. Salazar-Onfray, M. Petersson, J. Hansson, G. Masucci, K. Wasserman, T. Nakazawa, P. Anderson, R. Kiessling. 1996. Hydrogen peroxide secreted by tumor-derived macrophages down-modulates signal-transducing zeta molecules and inhibits tumor-specific T cell-and natural killer cell-mediated cytotoxicity. *Eur. J. Immunol.* 26: 1308-1313) (Schmielau, J., O. J. Finn. 2001. Activated granulocytes and granulocyte-derived hydrogen peroxide are the underlying mechanism of suppression of t-cell function in advanced cancer patients. *Cancer Res.* 61: 4756-4760) (Samlowski, W. E., R. Petersen, S. Cuzzocrea, H. Macarthur, D. Burton, J. R. McGregor, D. Salvemini. 2003. A nonpeptidyl mimic of superoxide dismutase, M40403, inhibits dose-limiting hypotension associated with interleukin-2 and increases its antitumor effects. *Nat. Med.* 9: 750-755). **I believe that the paper by Samlowski argues for EMOD-induced apoptosis.**

Thus, several investigators have demonstrated that **phagocyte-derived oxygen radicals strongly inhibit the antitumor cytotoxicity and other functions of T cells and NK cells.** Typically, these tumor-killing lymphocyte cells are functionally suppressed by relatively low concentrations of exogenous oxygen radicals and are equally strongly inhibited by oxygen radicals produced by adjacent phagocytes.

The action of oxygen radicals on T and NK cells has been shown not only to comprise inhibition of tumor-killing activity, but **oxygen radicals have also been found to trigger cell death by apoptosis in several phenotypes of tumor-killing lymphocytes** (Hansson, M., A. Asea, U. Ersson, S. Hermodsson, K.

Hellstrand. 1996. Induction of apoptosis in NK cells by monocyte-derived reactive oxygen metabolites. *J. Immunol.* 156: 42-47) (Hansson, M., S. Hermodsson, M. Brune, U. H. Mellqvist, P. Naredi, A. Betten, K. R. Gehlsen, K. Hellstrand. 1999. Histamine protects T cells and natural killer cells against oxidative stress. *J. Interferon Cytokine Res.* 19: 1135-1144) (Betten, A., J. Bylund, T. Cristophe, F. Boulay, A. Romero, K. Hellstrand, C. Dahlgren. 2001. A proinflammatory peptide from *Helicobacter pylori* activates monocytes to induce lymphocyte dysfunction and apoptosis. *J. Clin. Invest.* 108: 1221-1228), **in addition to inducing the disappearance of critical signal transduction structures on remaining viable cells** (Betten, A., J. Bylund, T. Cristophe, F. Boulay, A. Romero, K. Hellstrand, C. Dahlgren. 2001. A proinflammatory peptide from *Helicobacter pylori* activates monocytes to induce lymphocyte dysfunction and apoptosis. *J. Clin. Invest.* 108: 1221-1228) (Aoe, T., Y. Okamoto, T. Saito. 1995. Activated macrophages induce structural abnormalities of the T cell receptor-CD3 complex. *J. Exp. Med.* 181: 1881-1886) (Otsuji, M., Y. Kimura, T. Aoe, Y. Okamoto, T. Saito. 1996. Oxidative stress by tumor-derived macrophages suppresses the expression of CD3 zeta chain of T-cell receptor complex and antigen-specific T-cell responses. *Proc. Natl. Acad. Sci. USA* 93: 13119-13124).

Importantly, in vitro studies demonstrate that T cells and NK cells are refractory to activating stimuli, including the prototypic T and NK cell activator IL-2, in the presence of phagocytes, and that the lack of response to IL-2 is, at least in part, explained by the release of oxygen radicals from phagocytes.

Oxygen radicals have been proposed to significantly contribute to cytotoxic lymphocyte dysfunction in several forms of human cancer, including solid cancers such as melanoma, colorectal cancer, renal cell cancer, and prostate cancer (Kono, K., F. Salazar-Onfray, M. Petersson, J. Hansson, G. Masucci, K. Wasserman, T. Nakazawa, P. Anderson, R. Kiessling. 1996. Hydrogen peroxide secreted by tumor-derived macrophages down-modulates signal-transducing zeta molecules and inhibits tumor-specific T cell-and natural killer cell-mediated cytotoxicity. *Eur. J. Immunol.* 26: 1308-1313) (Rabinowich, H., M. Banks, T. E. Reichert, T. F. Logan, J. M. Kirkwood, T. L. Whiteside. 1996. Expression and activity of signaling molecules in T lymphocytes obtained from patients with metastatic melanoma before and after interleukin 2 therapy. *Clin. Cancer Res.* 2: 1263-1274) (Healy, C. G., J. W. Simons, M. A. Carducci, T. L. DeWeese, M. Bartkowski, K. P. Tong, W. E. Bolton. 1998. Impaired expression and function of signal-transducing ζ chains in peripheral T cells and natural killer cells in patients with prostate cancer. *Cytometry* 32: 109-119), **as well as in hematological malignancies such as acute and chronic myelogenous leukemias**. Therefore, understanding the molecular events underlying radical-induced lymphocyte inactivation could be useful in identifying therapeutic strategies to alleviate cancer-related immunosuppression. **I believe that these results have been misinterpreted in view of the crucial role of EMODs in apoptosis induction.**

It is concluded that **caspase activation is a late event during oxygen radical-induced lymphocyte apoptosis and that the role of caspases is rather in the execution phase than in the induction phase of apoptosis**. In contrast, PARP/AIF axis may be critically involved in initiating phagocyte-mediated, oxygen radical-induced lymphocyte apoptosis. (Oxygen Radicals Induce Poly(ADP-Ribose) Polymerase-Dependent Cell Death in Cytotoxic Lymphocytes. Fredrik B. Thorén, Ana I. Romero and Kristoffer Hellstrand. The Journal of Immunology, 2006, 176: 7301-7307).

1.2.0.2 Methylglyoxal - methylglyoxal bis(guanylhydrazone) (mitoguazone)

The "secret" of the "miracle" lies in the anti-tumor effect of Methylglyoxal - a property shared by hundreds of toxic chemicals. Methylglyoxal, it is claimed, inhibits electron flows in cancerous cells and blocks a crucial step necessary for the production of ATP, the cellular energy "currency".

1.2.0.3 Prooxidant thymoquinone induces apoptosis in colorectal cancer cells

Thymoquinone Triggers Inactivation of the Stress Response Pathway Sensor *CHEK1* and Contributes to Apoptosis in Colorectal Cancer Cells

There are few reports describing the role of p53-dependent gene repression in apoptotic cell death. To identify such apoptosis-associated p53 target genes, we used **the pro-oxidant plant-derived drug thymoquinone** and compared p53+/+ and p53–/– colon cancer cells HCT116. The p53 wild-type (wt) status correlated with more pronounced DNA damage and higher apoptosis after thymoquinone treatment. A significant up-regulation of the survival gene *CHEK1* was observed in p53–/– cells in response to thymoquinone due to the lack of transcriptional repression of p53. In p53–/– cells, transfection with p53-wt vector and CHEK1 small interfering RNA treatment decreased CHEK1 mRNA and protein levels and restored apoptosis to the levels of the p53+/+ cells. p53–/– cells transplanted to nude mice treated with thymoquinone up-regulated CHEK1 expression and did not undergo apoptosis unlike p53+/+ cells. Immunofluorescence analysis revealed that the apoptosis resistance in p53–/– cells after thymoquinone treatment might be conveyed by shuttling of CHEK1 into the nucleus. We confirmed the *in vivo* existence of this CHEK1/p53 link in human colorectal cancer, showing that tumors lacking p53 had higher levels of CHEK1, which was accompanied by poorer apoptosis. CHEK1 overexpression was correlated with advanced tumor stages (P = 0.03), proximal tumor localization (P = 0.02), and worse prognosis (1.9-fold risk, univariate Cox regression; Kaplan-Meier, P = 0.04). We suggest that the inhibition of the stress response sensor CHEK1 might contribute to the antineoplastic activity of specific DNA-damaging drugs. [Thymoquinone Triggers Inactivation of the Stress Response Pathway Sensor *CHEK1* and Contributes to Apoptosis in Colorectal Cancer Cells. **Hala Gali-Muhtasib** et al. Cancer Res 2008;68(14):5609–18]

1.2.0.4 Methylglyoxal-Induced Apoptosis in Human Prostate Carcinoma

Investigators examined the cellular effects of methylglyoxal (MG), a toxic physiological metabolite, on human prostatic cancer PC-3 cells.

Methods: The effects of MG on cell growth and viability were evaluated first, and then its effects on the cell cycle and the glycolytic process were analyzed by Western blots and specific assays. Possible MG-induced apoptosis was also assessed by DNA analysis using agarose gel electrophoresis.

Results: MG ≥3 m*M* caused severe growth inhibition, resulting in nearly 100% cell death by 24h. The time course study revealed that expression of cyclin D_1, cdk2, and cdk4 was significantly (>50%) downregulated in 3 h of MG (3 m*M*) exposure, followed by the dephosphorylation of retinoblastoma protein by 6 h. Both the glyceraldehyde 3phosphate dehydrogenase activity and the cellular lactate level were also reduced by ~50 and 80%, respectively, following 6-hour MG exposure. Induction of apoptosis by MG was indicated by partial degradation of poly(ADP-ribose) polymerase and further confirmed by discrete DNA fragmentation detected on an agarose gel.

Conclusion: MG is capable of inducing apoptosis in prostatic cancer PC-3 cells, due primarily to a blocking of the cell cycle progression (G_1 arrest) and glycolytic pathway. Therefore, **MG could be a potent apoptosis inducer**, which may have a potential for prostate cancer treatment. (**Methylglyoxal-Induced Apoptosis in Human Prostate Carcinoma: Potential Modality for Prostate Cancer Treatment.** Dan M. Milanesa, Muhammad S. Choudhury, Camille Mallouh, Hiroshi Tazaki, Sensuke Konno. *Eur Urol* 2000;37:728-734).

1.2.0.5 Influence of methylglyoxal on antioxidant enzymes and oxidative damage

The effect of different doses of methylglyoxal (50–400 mg/kg body wt.) were examined using enzymes involved in the antioxidant function, glutathione (GSH) content and lipid peroxidation in the liver and spleen of Swiss albino mice (7–8 week old) after 6, 12 and 24 h. Significant changes were observed predominantly in the liver. The specific activities of superoxide dismutase (SOD), glutathione-*S*-transferase (GST), catalase, glyoxalase I (gly I) and glyoxalase II (gly II) were found to decrease in the liver. The mode and magnitude of change in the specific activities was seen to depend on the dose of methylglyoxal and the time after its administration. Methylglyoxal also decreased the GSH content and enhanced the lipid peroxidation in the liver. These findings are suggestive of the adverse effect of methylglyoxal on the antioxidant defence system. It is likely that **methylglyoxal undergoes a redox cycle and generates the free radicals** which in turn lower the antioxidant status in animals. The increased levels of lipid peroxidation provide support for the involvement of free radical processes in the detrimental effects of methylglyoxal. The response of DT-diaphorase (DTD) seems to be adaptive (Influence of methylglyoxal on antioxidant enzymes and oxidative damage. Dharamainder Choudhary, Dhyan Chandra and Raosaheb K. Kale. Toxicology Letters. Volume 93, Issues 2-3, 1 December 1997, Pages 141-152).

In 1963 the prestigious magazine "Science" published a remarkable article about his research. In it Dr. Szent-Gyorgyi identified two substances, one called Retine, which inhibited cancer growth, and the other called Promine, which promoted cell growth and made cancerous cells grow faster. These compounds are Ketoaldehydes and are found in the body naturally as a byproduct of the Krebs Cycle and the Glyoxylase System. His research using mice achieved shrinkage of tumors by increasing the ratio of Retine to Promine with daily injections of Retine. There were no harmful or toxic side effects.

Dr.Szent-Gyorgyi explained that he and "Dr. Egyud have found that retine (methylglyoxal) stops the growth of cancer cells without poisoning other cells. When retine is present in sufficient concentration, no cell division can occur while vital cellular processes go on unhindered." The article goes on, "And what is a good bit of luck, and not my cleverness, the white-haired scientist pointed out, "is that if a cancer cell cannot grow, it dies by itself.' According to the researchers, Retine is normally produced by the body and, when it is, it prevents the growth of existing cancer cells. But the body can lose its ability to produce this substance..." Putting the retine back in the body, just as we put insulin back into a diabetic's body, can stop the growth of cancer...The scientists at Woods Hole found that cancer cells are much more sensitive to retine than normal ones, and so cancer cells may be inhibited specifically."

Before the AAAS (American Academy of Science), April 24, 1967 he announced his work results with Methylglyoxal. He stated "We along with Dr.L. Egyud, synthesized a number of methylglyoxal derivatives...The cardinal question thus was: do tissues contain glyoxal derivatives? ...The answer was YES. "To sum up, our experiments indicate that ketone aldehydes are normal constituents of tissues and have a high biological activity. THE CHEMICAL SIGNAL WHICH REGULATES CELL DIVISION MAY THUS BE A KETONE ALDEHYDE (Methylglyoxal). These glyoxal derivates, together with the enzymes responsible for their formation and deletion, form a complex system with complex equilibria, the disturbance of which may be connected with cancer. http://www.arrowheadhealthworks.com/Retine_C.htm

It is amazing to me that I have found this work by Szent-Gyorgi, my mentor's mentor, and that it is actually based on my UTOPIA theory.

1.2.1.0 How I feel about antioxidants and the so-called experts

The case for direct intervention does not arise from a narrow, professional, "expert" consideration, but a simple human one. Decent science cannot tolerate lack of transparency, abuse of human rights, and disrespect for safety. To condone such abuses in the name of science is to degrade and berate it, and to vulgarise a rational pursuit - thereby demeaning rationality itself as something whimsical and indifferent to human dignity. It is also to legitimise hierarchy, the rule of the powerful, and the tyranny of "experts". Nothing could be worse for democracy. http://www.hinduonnet.com/fline/fl1817/18170960.htm. Accessed 2-4-09.

1.2.1.1 How I feel about redox induced apoptosis

The precise mechanisms critical for cellular suicide are still unknown. Apoptosis is a combination of several complex interconnected actions, especially redox involvement. Arguing which mechanism is more critical may not be important, and these clarified mechanisms should be connected and utilized in homeostatic maintenance and pathogen and neoplasia protection.

1.2.1.2 EMOD-induced apoptosis in human leukemia cells

Investigators used a human leukemia cell line that, after homologous recombination knockout of the gp91-phox subunit of the phagocyte respiratory-burst oxidase cytochrome b-558, **mimics chronic granulomatous disease** (X-CGD) to study the role of oxygen radicals in apoptosis. **Camptothecin (CPT),** a topoisomerase I inhibitor, induced significantly more apoptosis in PLB-985 cells than in X-CGD cells. Sensitivity to CPT was enhanced after neutrophilic differentiation, but was lost after monocytic differentiation. No difference between the two cell lines was observed after **treatment with other apoptosis inducers, including etoposide, ultraviolet radiation, ionizing radiation, hydrogen peroxide, or 7-hydroxystaurosporine.** After granulocytic differentiation of both cell lines, CPT still induced apoptosis, suggesting independence from replication in fully differentiated and growth-arrested cells. **Pyrrolidine dithiocarbamate (an antioxidant inhibitor of NF-kappaB) and catalase partially inhibited CPT-induced DNA fragmentation in granulocytic-differentiated PLB-985 cells,** but had no effect in X-CGD cells. Flow cytometry analysis revealed that reactive oxygen intermediates were generated in CPT-treated PLB-985 cells. These data indicate that **oxygen radicals generated by NADPH oxidase may contribute directly or indirectly to CPT-induced apoptosis in human leukemia and in neutrophilic-differentiated cells** (Role of oxygen radicals generated by NADPH oxidase in apoptosis induced in human leukemia cells. W Hiraoka, N Vazquez, W Nieves-Neira, S J Chanock and Y Pommier. *J. Clin. Invest.* 102(11): 1961-1968 (1998). **I believe that these same EMOD producers could be used clinically to prevent or treat various malignancies. This study supports the role for EMOD induced apoptosis.**

I would hypothesize that chemotherapy and irradiation decrease EMOD levels, which is responsible for the second primary cancers in survivors of chemo and radiation.

1.2.1.3 EMOD-induced apoptosis with radiation

Oxidative damage is an important mechanism in X-ray-induced cell death. Radiolysis of water molecules is a source of reactive oxygen species (ROS) that contribute to X-ray-induced cell death. In this study, we showed by ROS detection and a cell survival assay that **NADPH oxidase has a very important role in X-ray-induced cell death. Under X-ray irradiation, the upregulation of the expression of NADPH oxidase membrane subunit gp91^{phox} was dose-dependent**. Meanwhile, the cytoplasmic subunit p47^{phox} was translocated to the cell membrane and localized with p22^{phox} and gp91^{phox} to form reactive NADPH oxidase. Our data suggest, for the first time, that **NADPH oxidase-mediated generation of ROS is an important contributor to X-ray-induced cell death.** This suggests a new target for combined gene transfer and radiotherapy (NADPH oxidase-mediated generation of reactive oxygen species: A new mechanism for X-ray-induced HeLa cell death. Qing Liu et al. Biochemical and Biophysical Research Communications

Volume 377, Issue 3, 19 December 2008, Pages 775-779).

Major further improvement can be expected from the design and exploration of drugs that influence the pathways leading to cell death after irradiation. Examples include topoisomerase I (topo I) inhibitors, alkyl-lysophospholipids, epidermal growth factor receptor (EGFR) receptor inhibitors.

1.2.1.4 Migraines associated with low EMOD levels and high antioxidants

The oxidant-antioxidant balance disorders underlie a number of acute and chronic diseases of the central nervous system (CNS). It is **believed that oxidative stress plays a role in the pathogenesis of migraine.** The study objective was to assess the processes of lipid peroxidation with malondialdehyde (MDA) as its major indicator and to determine the activities of **antioxidant enzymes: superoxide dismutase (SOD), glutathione peroxidase (GSH-Px) and glutathione reductase (GSSG-R)** in the serum and erythrocytes of patients at developmental age with migraine with and without aura. The study group consisted of **34 patients at the age of 10-18 years** (mean +/- standard deviation: 14.04 +/- 2.29 years), **suffering from migraine.** The **control group included 38 patients**, aged 4-17 years (mean age 12.11 +/- 3.46). MDA concentration and activities of SOD, GSH-Px and GSSG-R were determined in serum and erythrocytes of all the patients. **In the migraine group, the MDA levels in serum and erythrocytes were statistically significantly lower** than in control subjects ($p < 0.001$). **In the migraine group, serum GSH-Px activity was significantly higher** ($p < 0.05$). **The GSSG-R activity in the erythrocytes of migraine children was significantly higher compared** to controls ($p < 0.001$). **SOD activity was decreased** and GSH-Px was increased (non-significantly) in erythrocytes of migraineurs. Our results confirm the disturbances of lipid peroxidation processes in migraine and suggest the activation of antioxidant mechanisms. Its important indicator seems to be the increase in the GSSG-R activity in the erythrocytes and the GSH-Px activity in serum between migraine attacks. (Serum and intraerythrocyte antioxidant enzymes and lipid peroxides in children with migraine. Boćkowski L, Sobaniec W, Kułak W, Smigielska-Kuzia J. Pharmacol Rep. 2008 Jul-Aug;60(4):542-8). **I interpret this data to indicate that migraneurs have low EMOD levels and high antioxidant levels, which is contrary to the predictions of oxidative stress.**

Cluster headaches are said to be relieved by breathing pure oxygen for 15 minutes.

1.2.1.5 EMODs, antioxidants and apoptosis: all antineoplastic drugs yield EMODs ==

The drugs of many classes of antineoplastic agents are known to generate a high level of oxidative stress in biological systems. These classes of drugs include the anthracyclines, most alkylating agents, platinum-coordination complexes, epipodophyllotoxins, and camptothecins. For these drugs, the hepatic microsomal monooxygenase system is a primary site where ROS are generated, although other enzymatic (e.g., xanthine oxidase) and nonenzymatic (Fenton and Haber-Weiss reactions) mechanisms also play a role. The electron transport system of cardiac mitochondria is another site where significant levels of ROS are generated by anthracyclines.

Although some classes of antineoplastic agents generate high levels of oxidative stress, others, including the taxanes, vinca alkaloids, antifolates, and nucleoside and nucleotide analogues, generate only low levels. Nevertheless, all drugs generate some free radicals as they induce apoptosis in cancer cells.

Although superoxide is not highly toxic, mitochondrial superoxide dismutase generates hydrogen peroxide from superoxide and, in the presence of reduced iron that is abundant in mitochondria, highly toxic hydroxyl radicals are formed via Fenton and Haber-Weiss reactions. Thus, all drugs that induce apoptosis by this mechanism generate some degree of oxidative stress, although this does not imply that free radical generation is necessary for a drug to exert its cytotoxic effect on neoplastic cells, because the apoptotic process is initiated by cytochrome c release and superoxide generation may occur secondarily. (Supplement: Free Radicals: The Pros and Cons of Antioxidants. Cancer Chemotherapy and Antioxidants. Kenneth A. Conklin. The American Society for Nutritional Sciences J. Nutr. 134:3201S-3204S, November 2004). **This view is contrary to mine.**

1.2.2.0 High Doses Of Antioxidants Taken By Many Breast Cancer Patients Despite Possible Consequences

A new study finds that many women with breast cancer take antioxidant supplements while undergoing cancer treatment, even though **the consequences of doing so are unknown**. Published in the July 15, 2009 issue of *CANCER*, a peer-reviewed journal of the American Cancer Society, the study indicates that **additional research should be undertaken to determine the effects of antioxidant supplementation on the health and survival of breast cancer patients.**

Antioxidant supplements include vitamin C, vitamin E, beta-carotene, and selenium. They are found in individual supplements as well as in many multivitamins. **Many breast cancer patients believe that antioxidant supplements will protect them from the side effects of breast cancer treatment, help prevent breast cancer recurrence, and improve their overall health.**

However, the actual effects of taking antioxidants during cancer treatment are poorly understood and the **findings to date are mixed.**, which often **Some physicians believe antioxidants may in fact interfere with radiation and some types of chemotherapy** attacks tumor cells by generating reactive oxygen species (ROS), very small molecules that play a role in cell development.

Researchers led by Heather Greenlee, ND, PhD, Assistant Professor of Epidemiology and Medical Oncology (in Medicine) at Columbia University Mailman School of Public Health in New York, investigated the prevalence of antioxidant use in women with breast cancer who participated in the population-based Long Island Breast Cancer Study Project (LIBCSP). LIBCSP, which included more than 1,500 breast cancer patients, began as a federally mandated study that investigated whether breast cancer risk was associated with environmental exposures among women in Nassau and Suffolk counties in New York State. Dr. Greenlee's study is based on the **764 patients** who completed a follow-up interview and provided information on antioxidant supplement use.

Among the 764 patients studied, 663 women (86.8 percent) reported receiving chemotherapy, radiation, or hormone therapy for breast cancer. Of these 663 women, **six in ten (60.5 percent) reported using antioxidants during breast cancer treatment,** which included chemotherapy, radiation, and tamoxifen (anti-estrogen) therapy.

About seven in ten antioxidant users (69.3 percent) used high doses, defined as higher than the dose contained in a Centrum multivitamin. Women who took high doses of antioxidants during treatment were more likely to be using tamoxifen and to have a history of eating more fruits and vegetables, using herbal products, and engaging in mind-body practices.

"Given the common use of antioxidant supplements during breast cancer treatment, often at high doses and in conjunction with other complementary therapies, future research should address the effects of antioxidant supplementation on breast cancer outcomes," including whether antioxidants affect treatment toxicities, treatment efficacy, cancer recurrence, and survival, say the authors. ("Prevalence and predictors of antioxidant supplement use during breast cancer treatment:The Long Island Breast Cancer Study Project." Heather Greenlee, Marilie D. Gammon, Page E.Abrahamson, Mia M. Gaudet, Mary Beth Terry, Dawn L. Hershman, Manisha Desai, Susan L. Teitelbaum Alfred I. Neugut, and Judith S. Jacobson. *CANCER*; Published Online: June 08, 2009 (DOI: 10.1002/cncr.24378); Print Issue Date: July 15, 2009).

1.2.2.1 Antioxidants must be good and EMODs bad

The following was excerpted from: Supplement: Free Radicals: The Pros and Cons of Antioxidants. Executive Summary Report. Harold E. Seifried, Darrell E. Anderson, Barbara C. Sorkin and Rebecca B. Costello. The American Society for Nutritional Sciences J. Nutr. 134:3143S-3163S, November 2004.

1.2.2.2 Free Radicals, Cancer Prevention, and Therapy (Ames)

Free Radicals, Cancer Prevention, and Therapy: Delaying the Oxidative Mitochondrial Decay of Aging Bruce Ames, Children's Hospital and Research Institute at Oakland

Bruce Ames, Professor and Senior Scientist, Department of Biochemistry and Molecular Biology, University of California—Berkeley, discussed the effect of oxidants on aging and metabolism, strategies for preventing oxidants from being produced during aging, and his perspective on the manner in which the scientific community views oxidants and antioxidants. (Ames, B. (2004) Supplements and tuning up metabolism. J. Nutr. 134:3164S-3168S).

Research over the past 40 y has led to a greater understanding of the aging process. Energy production occurs in the mitochondria, and these energy generators become less efficient as we age, producing greater numbers of mutagenic oxygen radicals. (**RMH Note: I believe that the increasing numbers of EMODs increase with age for the body's defense, not to injure it.**) Experimental studies indicate that there is a decrease in the level of cardiolipin, a key lipid in the mitochondrial membrane, responsible for the membrane's electrical potential, causing reduced utilization of oxygen and increased production of oxygen radicals. **Studies in rats show that young rats have ~24,000 oxidative lesions in DNA per cell, increasing to ~67,000 oxidative lesions per cell in older rats.**

Animal studies from Italy report that **old rats fed acetyl carnitine (ALC), the transporter that carries the fatty acid "fuel" into the mitochondria, have less mitochondrial damage and less DNA damage than old rats not fed ALC**. Dr. Ames's research group repeated and extended this experiment using isolated hepatocytes and confirmed the earlier findings. Cardiolipin levels and mitochondrial membrane potential in old rats fed acetyl carnitine remained as high as in young rats, although the production of oxygen radicals remained elevated. To address this conundrum, **old rats were fed the oxidized form of lipoic acid (LA), a coenzyme for mitochondrial enzymes, as a potential mitochondrial antioxidant, and the number of oxygen radicals decreased as a result**. In addition, vitamin C and glutathione levels also increased. ALC and LA may also diminish the effects of aging on the immune system and brain function. Both old and young rats fed ALC and LA showed increased T-cell stimulation, a positive sign for improved immunity. In tests of spatial memory and ambulatory activity, rats fed ALC and LA did better than rats fed a standard diet. Other research groups have conducted numerous human trials on ALC for Alzheimer's disease and cognitive impairment and on LA for diabetes. Meta-analyses of the overall study results show improvement among patients administered ALC or LA.

As life expectancy increases, there will be pressure on the scientific community to address the causes of aging with better treatments and, ideally, prevention of the aging process. Metabolic changes and the biochemistry involved in aging are emerging fields in science, but much remains to be learned. **Diet and lifestyle can be modified to decrease the effects of aging.** Diet in America has received a lot of attention in the past few decades. Much of this research shows that micronutrient deficiencies accompany caloric excess in this country. Obesity is of great concern because of the negative effects of this condition on the economy and the medical system. Obese individuals tend to be deficient in dietary micronutrients, including zinc, iron, and calcium. Vitamin and mineral deficiencies adversely affect general biochemistry. For example, 25% of menstruating women in the United States consume <50% of the recommended daily allowance (RDA) of iron. Iron deficiency destroys mitochondria, increases oxidant levels, and accelerates the aging process. Conversely, men may consume too much iron because they eat a lot of meat. Deficiencies of zinc, vitamins B-6 and B-12, and folate also are marked in the United States and can lead to chromosome breakage just as severe as that caused by radiation exposure.

Diet has been the focus of many large epidemiologic studies, and many (but not all) show that fruits and vegetables have a protective effect against cancer. In comparisons of the **quartiles of the population that consume the fewest versus the most fruits and vegetables, 24 of 25 studies show that the group that consumes the fewest servings of fruits and vegetables per day has double the risk of developing cancers of the lung, oral cavity, larynx, and esophagus. Even among cigarette smokers (smoking accounts for 90% of lung cancers), consuming fruits and vegetables cuts the risk by half.** Smoking puts a tremendous amount of oxidative stress on the body because cigarette smoke is full of nitrogen oxides, which are powerful oxidants, and evidence indicates that oxidants produced by smoking lower the body's levels of vitamin C, which leaves the cells less well defended against oxidants. *Helicobacter pylori* infection, which can cause stomach cancer, also reduces vitamin C levels. Fruits and vegetables may afford some protection by reducing the levels of oxygen radicals produced by the infection.

Mitochondrial damage is associated with an array of chronic diseases that are related to dietary deficiencies. A wealth of information shows that methyl-group deficiencies are a major contributor to DNA damage and that folate deficiency is a major cause. For example, folate and vitamin B-12 deficiency increases the level of homocysteine, which is associated with damage to endothelial cells and consequent heart disease. **Biotin deficiency is associated with an increase in oxidants, and zinc deficiency is associated with chromosome damage by oxidation. RMH Note: This may have therapeutic application for increasing oxidative capacity.**

There is a need to conduct small intervention studies on antioxidants to address many of the questions remaining about the role of diet and dietary factors on cancer and oxidative stress. The type of study envisioned would be similar to the recent study conducted in Washington State in a collaboration of the Bruce Ames group with the Terry Shultz group, which investigated whether vitamin B-6 deficiency causes chromosome breaks. This study found that there is a level of deficiency (i.e., ~50% of the RDA for vitamin B-6) that is associated with chromosome breaks. These types of studies are difficult to conduct, but they offer a level of control of the diet that cannot be satisfied in epidemiological studies.

1.2.2.3 Antioxidants Can Be Prooxidants When You Least Expect That to Be So

Frank Meyskens, University of California—Irvine

Frank L. Meyskens, M.D., Professor, Department of Medicine and Biological Chemistry, Cancer Center, University of California—Irvine, presented information on antioxidants behaving as prooxidants. **The antioxidant/prooxidant issue was highlighted recently by the results of the Alpha-Tocopherol and Beta-Carotene (ATBC) Cancer Prevention study, which reported that ß-carotene caused an increase in lung cancer among heavy smokers.** This was **contrary to predictions** from epidemiologic studies in the 1980s that reported an inverse dietary relation between many epithelial cancers and ß-carotene. There were, however, experimental studies and mechanistic data showing that **ß-carotene could be a prooxidant at high oxygen concentrations** and under special circumstances, which could have helped to predict the adverse effects noted in the more recent trials.

A further look at the **data from the ß-Carotene and Retinol Efficacy Trial (CARET) showed similar unexpected results**. Participants had a significant smoking history or were prior smokers and were randomly assigned in a 2 x 2 factorial design to treatment with ß-carotene, retinol, a combination of both, or placebo. **The cumulative incidence of lung cancer was greater among those treated with ß-carotene**, compared with placebo. In addition, the incidence of cardiovascular disease was greater for those treated with ß-carotene than for those treated with placebo. However, there was a nonsignificant decrease in lung cancer in nonsmokers, which was **teased out by later analysis**. This study supported the earlier overall results of the ATBC study, and all the ß-carotene clinical studies being conducted at that time were stopped.

The question remains as to whether ß-carotene causes or stimulates lung cancer. One possible explanation for the difference in results between epidemiological studies and the ATBC and CARET trials is that the dose of ß-carotene in the epidemiological studies ranged from 6 to 89 mg and the dose of ß-carotene in the ATBC and CARET trials was 25 to 30 mg. The high doses selected in the trials using ß-carotene supplements probably play a role in lung cancer development because they produce high serum concentrations of the vitamin that are not physiologic. These higher levels may be in the range to act oxidatively. **RMH Note: These investigators can not see or believe that antioxidants are bad in any way and any bad results or disease causation associated with an antioxidant must be due to the antioxidant acting as an oxidant.**

Another recent trial investigated the separate effects of ß-carotene, vitamins C and E, and ß-carotene plus vitamins C and E on the recurrence of colorectal adenomas. Results indicate protection among nonsmokers and nondrinkers but an increase in similar carcinogenic and cardiovascular adverse effects in smokers and drinkers as seen in the earlier lung cancer trials. This is a very important observation, supporting a marked difference in response in active smokers to ß-carotene specifically.

One potential mechanism to explain ß-carotene becoming a prooxidant is that at high doses, and in the presence of high oxygen tension, ß-carotene produces free radicals. Evidence also suggests that peroxyl radicals form after autooxidation and the consumption of ß-carotene. This produces an additional prooxidative event because another free radical is generated. **The prooxidative and antioxidative effects of many compounds, including ß-carotene, are highly dependent on the underlying redox milieu of the tissue in which they take place.** Another explanation may be the effect of ß-carotene on other carotenoids. There is some evidence that the uptake of oxycarotenoids from the gut is negatively affected by too much ß-carotene in the system. Cytokines may also interact with ß-carotene to produce oxidative stress and cause an unexpected prooxidative effect. Some people think that high levels of ß-carotene can enhance Phase I enzymes, so the compound may function as a cocarcinogen for some procarcinogens under certain conditions. More recently, there is evidence that ß-carotene can suppress RAR-ß, one of the more important retinoic acid receptors in epithelial tissue.

Melanin, contained in melanocytes in the skin, is a redox-active polymer that can serve as an antioxidant in most circumstances but as a prooxidant in others. It also can bind metals and functions as a stable semiquinone and as a free radical. Dr. Meyskens noted that most of his research on melanin has been on eumelanin, the form of melanin responsible for black and brown hair. A model of early melanoma progression has been developed that includes the production of high concentrations of reactive oxygen species (ROS) and reactive nitrogen species (RNS). **Melanin usually serves as an antioxidant, which helps to decrease the concentration of ROS.** In the intracellular milieu, there are sufficient amounts of enzymatic and nonenzymatic antioxidants to lower the overall levels of ROS. The intracellular milieu also maintains the appropriate control of transcription factors and stress responses, as well as a very strong antiapoptotic mechanism. Redox cycling of melanin may be one mechanism for reducing the potential prooxidative effects of melanin. Other antioxidants also may help to decrease ROS levels in melanocytes and slow or stop progression to melanoma, although **a study including large doses of**

vitamin C in melanoma patients showed explosive tumor growth. A downstream effect of some of the cardiovascular drugs is to lower ROS levels, which might explain some of the epidemiological findings of lovostatin, for example, which seems to protect against melanoma. It may be that the timing of antioxidant administration provides a benefit, although this needs to be investigated in much more detail.

Dr. Meyskens noted that to avoid some of the pitfalls recognized in the ß-carotene saga, there must be an assessment of all the factors that might lead to an adverse event in Phase III trials. **Mechanisms that determine when an antioxidant becomes a prooxidant are largely unknown**, and these need to be established before recommending nutritional or nutritional/pharmacologic interventions. Doses are important and the underlying oxidative properties of the tissue being looked at are extremely critical.

1.2.2.4 Signaling Pathways Activated by Oxidative Injury and Their Roles in Determining Cell Fate

Nikki Holbrook, Yale University School of Medicine

Nikki Holbrook, Ph.D., Professor, Department of Internal Medicine, Geriatrics Section, Yale University School of Medicine, Cambridge, MA, discussed signaling pathways activated by oxidative injury and their roles in determining cell fate. **Historically, ROS have been viewed in a negative light;** both **their generation and targets were presumed to be indiscriminate and random, and their consequences entirely detrimental.** We now know that **ROS serve some very important physiologic functions as second messengers in a variety of different signal transduction pathways** (most notably proliferative signaling pathways). They also provide host-defense mechanisms against microbial invaders. In these instances, **the generation of ROS is both purposeful and necessary.** However, ROS also produce a number of undesirable effects that are believed to contribute to disease and aging, including damage to DNA, proteins, and lipids and the inappropriate activation of some signaling pathways. Many of the ROS are produced as by-products of normal metabolism, but excessive ROS levels also occur as a consequence of environmental exposure. Certain toxins themselves behave as oxidants, whereas others trigger ROS production as the cell attempts to detoxify or eliminate them. Hence, for cells living in an aerobic environment, **ROS constitute a double-edged sword**. Researchers need to know how antioxidants can be used to prevent the undesirable effects of ROS without compromising normal physiologic functions.

We know that **ROS can elicit a plethora of responses ranging from proliferation, to growth arrest (transient or permanent), to senescence, to cell death (through either an apoptotic or necrotic mechanism).** Lower doses of oxidants are generally associated with mitogenesis, moderate doses with growth arrest, and higher doses with cell death. Other factors that determine oxidative effects include the nature of the ROS and the type of cell in which it is operating. On the positive side, certain ROS-activated pathways are important for normal cell growth and may be protective in cases of acute oxidative injury such as reperfusion injury. However, in the long run, they may promote tumor growth. Moreover, necrosis and apoptosis may cause the loss of physiologic function, which is considered a negative consequence, but **the removal of damaged cells is the same process the body uses for tumor suppression**. It is important to know what determines the effects that are seen, and understanding the affected signal pathways may help explain what happens in the cell. Notably, however, the same signaling pathway can be beneficial in one instance of oxidative stress and harmful in another.

The extracellular signal-regulated kinase (ERK) activation pathway serves as an example to emphasize this point and to illustrate the complexity of the response to oxidative injury. ERK is activated in response to both oxidant exposure and growth factor treatment, with similar mechanisms serving to activate the pathway in each case. In acute oxidative injury, ERK activation generally blocks apoptosis and promotes survival. The short-term beneficial effects are the prevention of tissue loss and the enhancement of host survival, but in the long term, it could lead to tumorigenesis or affect therapeutic drug sensitivity. In other situations, however, **ERK activation promotes apoptosis. For example, ERK activation increases the sensitivity of cells to cisplatin treatment and promotes apoptosis in response to the drug in many cell types. ERK activation in response to oxidative injury decreases with aging, and this contributes to the reduced tolerance of old cells to oxidative stress.** Restricting energy intake can delay the onset of many characteristics of aging. Accordingly, cells from animals fed an energy-restricted diet do not show the attenuated activation of the ERK pathway as a function of age and exhibit greater tolerance to acute oxidative injury. It remains to be determined what downstream targets of ERK might account for these effects.

1.2.2.5 Mechanisms of Pro- and Antioxidation

Homer Black, Baylor College of Medicine

Homer Black, Ph.D., Professor, Department of Dermatology, Baylor College of Medicine, Houston, TX, presented information on the mechanisms of pro- and antioxidation. Oxidation related to diet has been studied for >60 y. Dietary energy restriction reduces cancer at many sites but the mechanisms for such protection are not completely understood. Studies on (n-6) fatty acids (PUFAs) show that they increase free radical reactions, and these reactions can be exacerbated by UV light to increase the likelihood of carcinogenesis. It is assumed that a process of lipid oxidation occurs with polyunsaturated fats, in which a radical attacks a polyunsaturated fatty acid to produce free radicals. It has been assumed that supplementation with one or more free radical reaction inhibitors, such as antioxidants, would prevent lipid oxidation. (Black, H. S. (2004) Mechanisms of pro- and antioxidation. J. Nutr. 134:3169S-3170S).

Antioxidant function, however, is much more complex than just radical scavenging. To illustrate, **animal studies show that the phenolic antioxidant BHT reduces the rate of tumor growth**. It may be that the mechanism by which BHT exerts its anticarcinogenic activity involves the quenching of lipid-soluble radicals and ROS. Animals fed a high-fat diet supplemented with BHT exhibit a significant lengthening of the tumor latency period compared with animals fed a diet without BHT. As the dietary lipid level is reduced, so is the effect of BHT. At the lowest lipid level, the protective effect of BHT is almost nonexistent. This suggests that the exacerbative effect of increasing lipid levels on UV carcinogenesis, and presumably lipid peroxidation, are important parts of the carcinogenic process and that BHT is effective in blocking that process. In addition, the skin of animals fed a diet without BHT allows ~65% more UV light through the stratum corneum, which may also promote UV carcinogenesis.

ß-Carotene does not affect epidermal absorption through the stratum corneum, and although earlier studies reported that it has a photoprotective effect, this photoprotection was based on the **carotenoid-specific capacity to quench singlet oxygen** and other oxy-radicals. **Under certain dietary conditions, ß-carotene exacerbates UV carcinogenesis**. Supplementing even a semidefined diet containing ß-carotene diminishes the tumor latency period and increases tumor multiplicity. ß-Carotene can act as a prooxidant at high oxygen concentrations and under oxidative stress conditions. Many of the oxidizing species, especially peroxyl radicals, convert this carotenoid to the 1-electron oxidized form, yielding a ß-carotene radical cation.

Studies show that ß-carotene reacts not with the α-tocopherol radical but with the α-tocopherol radical cation to produce a carotenoid radical cation. This radical cation can be repaired with ascorbic acid, producing an ascorbate radical. To explore the role of ascorbate on ß-carotene radical repair, animals were fed a semidefined diet (i.e., casein, corn oil, and cornstarch or corn sugar) supplemented with ß-carotene and either no extra ascorbate or a 6-fold increase in ascorbate. The level of ascorbate did not influence the exacerbative effect of the carotenoids. These findings weaken the argument that ascorbate can repair the ß-carotene radical, which leaves it in a prooxidative state.

Before recommending that individuals take antioxidants for chemoprevention, a better understanding of free radical–mediated damage must be considered.

1.2.3.0 Iron, Free Radicals, and Oxidative Injury

Joe McCord, University of Colorado

Joe McCord, Ph.D., Professor, Department of Medicine, Webb-Waring Institute, University of Colorado—Denver, discussed the role of iron, free radicals, and oxidative injury. Iron has been studied as a human micronutrient since ancient Greece. Although iron is essential, it also may be toxic in certain forms and at high doses. The relation between iron and free radicals has been studied in many disease types because of their ability to damage cellular components and processes (i.e., DNA, proteins, aberrant signaling). **Iron can undergo single-valence changes in both directions, and, like copper and other transition metals, can interface very easily with free radical reactions because these reactions typically involve the transfer of single electrons.** If available, iron can greatly amplify the damage caused by free radical generation. There is an ongoing discussion within the scientific community concerning whether there is a healthy level of iron stores in the body. (McCord, J. M. (2004) Iron, free radicals, and oxidative injury. J. Nutr. 134:3171S-3172S).

One potential negative effect of increased iron stores is their ability to react with superoxide to form iron-loaded ferritin, which is reduced from ferric to ferrous valence and then released to participate in redox reactions. **Ferritin only binds ferric iron, but it binds it so strongly that the iron is redox inactive. When the iron is released, it becomes redox reactive and can react with hydrogen peroxide to generate another secondary radical, the hydroxyl radical**, which is the second most potent oxidizing species.

Ferritin is relatively harmless until disease strikes, when the excess iron becomes a significant liability, increasing the damage caused by heart attack or stroke and increasing the likelihood of cancer. It is estimated that most Americans are iron loaded as a result of food supplementation. In addition, ~14% of Americans carry a mutant *HFE* gene, which causes hemochromatosis. **Humans accumulate iron as they age**, which may contribute to and amplify disease processes.

An *HFE* mutation has been introduced in a mouse knockout model to produce a model of human hemochromatosis, which is extremely useful. These mice accumulate iron in their tissues just like humans with hemochromatosis. Even when fed an extremely iron-restricted diet, the *HFE* knockout mice accumulate more iron in the heart than do wild-type mice fed a normal diet. When the heart is subjected to ischemia reperfusion (triggering a heart attack in this laboratory model), it is apparent that the heart damage is in direct proportion to the amount of iron the heart has stored. Lipid peroxidation can be used as the index of damage; after a heart attack, wild-type mice increase their lipid peroxidation 4-fold, but the *HFE* knockout mice increase theirs by 10 to 15 times.

HFE is a transcriptional factor that induces the production of the hormone hepcidin, which regulates iron uptake if both of these gene products are present. The mutant *HFE* that produces hemochromatosis transcribes little or no hepcidin. In an unregulated system—one that is homozygous for hemochromatosis—iron is actively absorbed from the gut and appears in the bloodstream as iron-loaded transferrin. Iron-loaded transferrin is detected by a receptor on the surface of liver cells (the TF2 receptor), which normally binds HFE protein and ß-2 microglobulin to the cell membrane. When the liver cell detects adequate iron in the system, it releases HFE from its membrane. HFE then translocates to the cell nucleus, where it upregulates the production of hepcidin secreted by the liver cell into the bloodstream. The hepcidin goes to the intestinal cells, which have a hepcidin receptor, and shuts off the absorption of iron from the gut. This feedback system controls the absorption of iron.

A recent study in *Nature Genetics* reported that constitutive hepcidin expression in transgenic mice can prevent iron overload in *HFE* knockout mice (a better model for studying hemochromatosis). Theoretically, recombinant hepcidin may restore the normal regulation of iron in patients with hemochromatosis, although too much hepcidin may shut down iron absorption completely, which would lead to anemia.

1.2.3.1 Oxidative Stress and Human Genetic Variation

Ralf Morgenstern, Karolinska Institutet

Ralf Morgenstern, Ph.D., Professor, Institute of Environmental Medicine, Karolinska Institutet, Stockholm, Sweden, presented information on oxidative stress and human genetic variation. Single nucleotide polymorphisms (SNPs) are the most common single-base-exchange genetic variations in humans. There are 3 billion bases in the human haploid genome, and most of the variants are SNPs, but there also are insertions and deletions. **It is estimated that humans currently have 1 genetic variant per 100–300 base pairs, which means there are 10 million possible sites of such genetic variation in a typical human**. Most of the variation and allelic frequency of these variants are the result of drift; these random events may have occurred in very small tribes during human evolution. The NCI has developed a database of SNPs (see http://www.ncbi.nlm.nih.gov/SNP/), many of which are involved in oxidative stress. There also is a database of validated SNPs at the NCI Cancer Genome Anatomy Project website (see http://www.nih.gov/science/models/mouse/resources/cancer_genome.html) that includes oxidative-stress-related genes. **One example of an oxidative-stress-related gene is the catalase gene, which has been mapped**. Expression analysis of variants of the catalase promoter region (C/T) shows that the variants affect transcription factor binding sites. Carriers of the T allele have markedly more catalase than carriers of the C allele. This shows that the genetic variant affects human catalase levels. (Morgenstern, R. (2004) Oxidative stress and human genetic variation. J. Nutr. 134:3173S-3174S).

Studies of genes for glutathione peroxidase 1 show that a particular amino acid alteration is present in samples collected from participants in past studies, but there is no correlation between the SNP and glutathione peroxidase 1 levels. However, this variant correlates to lung cancer in association studies. In addition, blood glutathione peroxidase concentration is a biomarker for selenium status.

There are many variants that may have potential applications as markers of oxidative stress, including single amino acid alterations, alterations that affect the intracellular targeting of mitochondrial superoxide dismutase, and numerous variants of glutathione. There is a lack of strong evidence from association studies to show that genetic variants are directly related to disease or disease processes. In addition, there may be a lack of real benefit in studying variants that have low penetrance in the population, especially if they have no apparent negative effect on health.

There is, however, a need to find out whether genetic variants are related to cancer, and this may be one of the greatest research needs for the future. In vitro models are needed, but there also is a need for human studies. Even if the effects of a variant are small and the effect on a population is small, there may be improved statistical methods in the future that can help address the underlying questions about genetic status and oxidative stress. One example of a gene that could be studied at the present time is the 8-hydroxy deoxyguanosine (*8OHdG*) repair gene.

1.2.3.2 Session 2: Antioxidative effects—Pros and cons

Session Chair: *Richard Rivlin, Institute for Cancer Prevention*

Richard Rivlin, M.D., Senior Vice President, Medical Affairs, Naylor Dana Chair in Nutrition, Institute for Cancer Prevention, New York, NY, introduced the session on the pros and cons of antioxidative effects. **One of the most troubling aspects of antioxidant research is that clinicians do not have the information they need to make recommendations to patients regarding antioxidant supplementation.** There are very strong market forces that tell the public about supplements, but there is very little reliable advice about them. In addition, the amount of contradictory advice is confusing to consumers. Also, **physician training is inadequate on this issue; only one-quarter of the nation's medical schools have required courses in nutrition, so most physicians have no training in this area.** It is important that we understand the factors that regulate the serum levels of endogenous antioxidants and learn more about herbal products. Other areas for research include making cancer therapy more effective and safer, and understanding the dose-response relation with respect to the efficacy and toxicity of antioxidants.

1.2.3.3 Phytochemical Effects beyond Antioxidation

David Heber, University of California—Los Angeles

David Heber, M.D., Ph.D., Director and Professor, Department of Medicine, Center for Human Nutrition, David Geffen School of Medicine, University of California–Los Angeles, discussed phytochemical effects beyond antioxidation. **There may be as many as 25,000 phytochemicals in the human diet, with many having physiological antioxidative effects, but these effects are not directly related to their many other effects on cellular signaling pathways, gap junctions, and metabolic enzyme induction, which often do not follow their antioxidative potencies in rank order of comparison.** Phytochemicals occur in families; they are usually present in plants as complex mixtures and not as single purified compounds. Moreover, members of the same family of compounds may act through different mechanisms. (Heber, D. (2004) Phytochemicals beyond antioxidation. J. Nutr. 134:3175S-3176S).

Phytochemicals will interact with cells in unique ways: synergistically with related compounds as they occur in nature, with unrelated compounds, and through the activation of metabolic enzymes. What the pharmaceutical literature calls *drug-metabolizing enzymes* actually are *phytochemical-metabolizing enzymes* (i.e.,

Phase I and Phase II enzymes). Humans evolved without drugs per se, but used the environment (e.g., plant and animal products and minerals) to treat medical conditions.

Lycopene is a phytochemical antioxidant with no pro–vitamin A activity that is found in tomatoes, which have only been widespread in the human diet for ~ 500 y. **Having the highest antioxidative activity among all carotenoids, lycopene exists in tomatoes** and derived products as one of numerous phytochemicals, many with similar structures and properties. Epidemiological data suggest that lycopene may reduce the risk of prostate cancer. When consumed, phytochemicals enter the cells, where they interact with very low affinity, high-capacity receptor molecules that trigger various intracellular actions and cell signaling pathways, as well as stimulating the metabolism of these compounds. They do not act on a single pathway, but in concert with many other pathways. If supplemental lycopene is added to a cell culture of prostate or breast cancer cells and tested against tomato oil, the complex product is more effective than lycopene alone. This argues strongly for not simply studying single compounds when exploring the mechanisms behind epidemiological observations.

When phytochemicals are consumed, some of them are absorbed intact, but many are metabolized in very subtle ways. For example, **lycopene is metabolized to form the *cis*-metabolite, which is found in larger amounts in the bloodstream than in the tomato product consumed. In addition, the amount of lycopene that gets to a specific cell is often very different from what is found in the blood or the food itself. This is true for ascorbic acid as well.**

1.2.3.4 Tumor-Suppressing Effects of Antioxidants from Tea

Roderick Dashwood, Linus Pauling Institute, Oregon State University

Roderick Dashwood, Ph.D., Chief, Cancer Chemoprotection Program, and Professor, Linus Pauling Institute, Oregon State University—Corvallis, provided information on the tumor-suppressing effects of antioxidants from tea. In human colon cancer, the ß-catenin/Tcf signaling pathway is activated by mutations in *APC* or *ß-catenin*, which cause overexpression of downstream targets such as c-*myc*, c-*jun*, *cyclin D1*, PPAR-δ, and *matrix metalloproteinase*-7. Research shows that epigallocatechin-3-gallate (EGCG), an antioxidative polyphenol in tea, can inhibit the activity of the ß-catenin/Tcf signaling pathway in vitro. **More than 80% of human colon cancers have a mutation in the *APC* gene,** and those that do not have mutations in *ß-catenin*.

To investigate diet and its effect on the genetic processes that lead to colon cancer, in vitro studies were conducted in human embryonic kidney cells transfected with *ß-catenin* and *TCF-4*. A reporter (Top Flash) was introduced into this model because it binds to *TCF-4* and *ß-catenin*. Adding purified EGCG to the mix inhibited reporter activity in a concentration-dependent manner. Adding tea with EGCG more effectively inhibited reporter activity; Sulindac, a nonsteroidal anti-inflammatory drug (NSAID), had no effect at the doses tested in vitro.

In vivo studies in a mouse model using an oncogenic form of *ß-catenin* under the control of the A33 antigen promoter were conducted to determine whether EGCG or Sulindac could reduce the formation of colon polyps. Mice were pretreated with a colon carcinogen and then exposed postinitiation to white tea or Sulindac. There was no reduction in aberrant crypt foci; however, a combination of white tea and Sulindac caused a significant reduction in tumor volume, tumor number, and tumor size.

Further studies of molecular changes in the polyps showed that *ß-catenin* was more strongly expressed in the polyp than in the adjacent normal-looking tissue from the same mouse. The mice fed Sulindac expressed much lower levels of *ß-catenin*. Looking at downstream targets of ß-catenin/TCF-4 signaling, the polyps had much higher levels of the target proteins than the adjacent normal-looking tissue. Sulindac alone reduced expression of ß-catenin protein, as well as downstream targets, either in polyps and/or in the adjacent normal-looking tissue around the polyps. These results support the view that **a drug and diet combination may be more effective against colon cancer than single treatment with tea or an NSAID alone. (**Orner, G. A., Dashwood, W.-M. & Dashwood, R. H. (2004) Tumor-suppressing effects of antioxidants from tea. J. Nutr. 134:3177S-3178S**).**

1.2.3.5 Antioxidants Suppress Apoptosis: p53 increases EMOD-apoptosis

Steven Zeisel, University of North Carolina—Chapel Hill

Steven Zeisel, M.D., Ph.D., Professor and Chair, Department of Nutrition, Associate Dean, Research School of Public Health, University of North Carolina—Chapel Hill, discussed antioxidants and the mechanisms for suppressing apoptosis (cell suicide) and apoptotic signaling. There is a growing body of evidence that there are signaling systems that physiologically use ROS as intermediate signals. **ROS not only regulate the signaling for apoptosis, but are capable of activating apoptotic pathways upstream, and many of**

the drugs and treatments used to kill cancer cells (chemotherapy and radiation) work by generating ROS to activate apoptotic pathways and kill cells. These pathways involve activation of a caspase upstream, a mitochondrial depolarization that generates ROS, which can then activate the caspase, as well as activation of downstream signals that end in final common pathways for cell suicide. (Zeisel, S. H. (2004) Antioxidants suppress apoptosis. J. Nutr. 134:3179S-3180S).

Choline deficiency involves an apoptotic pathway that uses ROS as an intermediary message and a nuclear factor κ-B (NFκB) signal downstream. **If there is little antioxidant content in liver cells that are also choline deficient, apoptosis is induced. If an antioxidant is added, such as *N*-acetylcysteine, apoptosis is inhibited by blocking the ROS signal.** *N*-acetylcysteine also blocks transforming growth factor ß-1 (TGF-ß-1)–induced apoptosis, which also uses a ROS to produce an intermediary signal from the mitochondria during the signaling cascade for apoptosis.

There is a lot of research ongoing involving ROS and apoptosis, including research showing that **the activation of caspase-9, which has a cysteine-cysteine bond that is sensitive to redox state, causes apoptosis**. In addition, ***p53* activation increases ROS production and induces apoptosis. ROS production also causes induction of cytochrome-C,** which activates the caspase-3 signaling pathway. The key question is still how to make cancer cells undergo apoptosis without affecting normal cells.

RMH Note: Thus, cytochrome C, capase and p53 all increase EMODs, which induces apoptosis.

Studies using a mouse model with a mutated retinoblastoma (Rb) protein show that mice fed a diet low in vitamin E and other antioxidants have higher rates of apoptosis and decreased tumor volume. Other researchers report that **antioxidants such as vitamin E and *N*-acetylcysteine delay and inhibit apoptosis in a number of models, including pancreatic cells and PC-12 cells.** There are some data in the literature to suggest that the effective mechanism in killing cells with chemotherapy or radiation is the generation of excess levels of ROS that then induce cell death. Administration of antioxidants during these treatments would reduce the amount of cell death produced.

Studies have investigated the effects of antioxidant supplementation on cancer therapy. Studies on cisplatin indicate that it kills breast cancer cells by apoptosis and necrosis, and that the addition of vitamin E blocks much of the apoptotic process. **High-dose vitamin E reduces the efficacy of cisplatin,** although the normal cells involved would be protected by vitamin E. **Lymphoma cells treated with 5 Gy of radiation die or stop dividing, but if *N*-acetylcysteine is added to the media, the lymphoma cells keep growing. Vitamin E succinate also protects cells against the effects of radiation in vitro.**

There is no conclusive evidence to show which antioxidant doses or mixtures protect cells against DNA damage and lipid and protein oxidation but do not interfere with apoptosis signaling pathways. There may be a threshold beyond which DNA is protected against oxidants because the ROS oxidants produced are quenched and there may be a higher dose needed to suppress signaling. **Oversupplementation may actually produce an environment that is beneficial to the tumor and allow it to survive.**

1.2.3.6 Green Tea Polyphenols, EGCG: Antioxidative and Prooxidative Effects

Chung S. Yang, Rutgers, The State University of New Jersey

Chung S. Yang, Ph.D., Professor and Chair, Department of Chemical Biology, Ernest Mario School of Pharmacy, Rutgers, The State University of New Jersey—Piscataway, discussed the antioxidative and prooxidative effects of green tea polyphenols. **Green tea and green tea polyphenols inhibit tumorigenesis at different organ sites, including the skin, lung, oral cavity, esophagus, stomach, liver, pancreas, and prostate.** Studies on skin and lung demonstrate that tea is an effective inhibitor when given to animals at the initiation, promotion and progression stages of carcinogenesis. (Yang, C. S., Hong, J., Hou, J. Z. & Sang, S. (2004) Green tea polyphenols: antioxidative and prooxidative effects. J. Nutr. 134:3181S).

There is a presumption that the active ingredient in tea is EGCG, but much is unknown about the specific mechanisms involved. Other tea constituents (such as caffeine) could also be important. **EGCG is a strong antioxidant, and its antioxidative activity is stronger than that of vitamins C and E in vitro.** However, the importance of such antioxidative activity in vivo after tea consumption, has not been fully established.

Much of the published mechanistic information on the action of EGCG was obtained from studies in cell culture. When EGCG is added to different cell lines, it can inhibit growth and/or induce apoptosis, but the **results need to be interpreted with caution**, because the concentrations of EGCG used are usually much higher than those that can be reached through systemic distribution. EGCG enters the cell through passive diffusion, is methylated and glucuronidated, and is pumped out of the cell by multidrug resistance associated proteins (MRPs).

In addition, **EGCG can be oxidized to form dimers and produce H_2O_2.** EGCG can induce apoptosis at concentrations of 10 µmol/L (micromolar), and this activity becomes more prominent at 30 and 100 µmol/L. **This proapoptotic activity is at least partly mediated by H_2O_2, because catalase blocks apoptosis completely in some cells and partially in others.** The addition of EGCG to cultured cells causes the overexpression of many genes, and **some of these genes are not activated in the presence of catalase.**

It is reported that EGCG inhibits the epidermal growth factor (EGF)-induced signal transduction pathways. Many of these experiments require a preincubation period. During this period of time, a large part of the added EGCG has been oxidized (to form dimers and other derivatives). Superoxide is believed to be involved in mediating the autooxidation, because EGCG is stabilized by the addition of superoxide dismutase (SOD). SOD also prevents the inhibition of EGF-induced signaling pathways by EGCG. It is possible that the superoxide generated during autooxidation of EGCG contributes to the inactivation of EGF receptor and thus inhibits the signaling pathway. In the presence of SOD, the cell growth inhibition effects are enhanced, suggesting that the growth inhibition is caused by EGCG, not mediated by H_2O_2.

Many research groups report the inhibition of MAP kinases by EGCG (possibly through competition for the binding site with protein substrates). The inhibition of other protein kinases such as IKK and cyclin-dependent kinases as well as proteinase activities such as the chymotryptic activity of 20s proteosomes and matrix melalloproteinases (MMP2 and MMP9) could also be important mechanisms. These activities do not appear related to the antioxidative activity of EGCG.

In summary, **there is only a moderate increase in antioxidant capacity after tea consumption because the bioavailability of tea polyphenols is low.** Although antioxidative and prooxidative activities can be demonstrated in vitro, other mechanisms may be important in the anticancer activity of tea and EGCG in vivo.

1.2.3.7 Rationale for Using High-Dose Multiple Antioxidants as an Adjunct to Radiation Therapy and Chemotherapy

Kedar Prasad, University of Colorado Health Sciences Center

Kedar N. Prasad, Ph.D., Professor, Department of Radiology, University of Colorado Health Sciences Center, Denver, presented information on the use of high-dose multiple antioxidants as an adjunct to radiotherapy and chemotherapy. The use of antioxidants in cancer therapy is driven by two opposing hypotheses. One hypothesis states that the use of dietary multiple antioxidants and micronutrients improves the efficacy of treatment; the opposing hypothesis states that the use of antioxidants and micronutrients protects cancer cells against free radical damage. These opposing hypotheses have grown out of generalized experimental data. (Prasad, K. N. (2004) Rationale for using high-dose multiple dietary antioxidants as an adjunct to radiation therapy and chemotherapy. J. Nutr. 134:3182S-3183S).

No data exist to clearly show that antioxidants protect cancer cells at doses that reduce the growth of the tumor cell but not the growth of the normal cell. At these doses, there is a selective effect of antioxidants on growth inhibition, apoptosis, or cell differentiation in cancer cells but not in normal cells. Given these facts, it seems that antioxidants might enhance the effects of radiation and chemotherapy on tumor cells but not on normal cells, but **supporting data are scant**.

There is a difference between dietary antioxidants and endogenous antioxidants. Studies indicate that endogenous antioxidants, such as glutathione-elevating agents and *N*-acetylcysteine or α-lipoic acid, always protect both normal cells and cancer cells. Thus, there should not be a recommendation to supplement endogenous antioxidants or compounds that will increase the levels of endogenous antioxidants. In addition, there are data that show that **cancer cells transfected with the SOD enzyme become resistant to radiation and therefore should not be used as an adjunct in radiotherapy**.

When dietary antioxidants are used at low doses, they do not affect the growth of either cancer cells or normal cells. It is not recommended that low doses of antioxidants be given in any therapeutic situation.

Some experimental studies provide information on the use of antioxidants and cancer therapy. In a rat melanoma cell line, cells treated with vitamin E succinate converted to a normal phenotype. Studies in human melanoma cell lines indicate that vitamin E succinate just inhibits growth or induces apoptosis.

In a study of hormone-insensitive breast cancer cells pretreated with vitamin E succinate, the cells became hormone sensitive after radiation treatment. Vitamin E succinate did not affect the mitotic accumulation of human fibroblasts in vitro, but slowed down the cell cycle.

Human parotid acinar carcinoma cells exposed to vitamin C do not show growth inhibition, but conversely, human melanoma cells respond to vitamin C. Acinar carcinoma cells are extremely sensitive to ß-carotene, but the vitamin has no effect on melanoma cell proliferation. These effects can be dose dependent. Often, different cell lines require different doses to respond. Vitamin E succinate also affects one of these cell lines and not the other, as does retinoic acid. Determining the dose of a nutrient that is necessary to produce an inhibitory effect is very important before beginning a clinical trial. At certain doses, nutrients can enhance the growth of cancer cells instead of inhibiting it.

Although it is difficult to extrapolate from one experimental condition to another or from one dose to another, it is clear that dose is important. In a human neuroblastoma cell line, 2 µg of vitamin E succinate does not affect growth, but 20 µg markedly inhibits growth. The gene expression profile is also entirely different between the two doses, which should be an area of interest to clinicians and cancer researchers.

Experimental studies also show that combinations of antioxidants often are more effective than single antioxidants. A single antioxidant did not affect the growth of human melanoma cells, but when a combination of antioxidants was added to the media, it inhibited the growth of the cell line by 50%. Increasing the dose of vitamin C in this mixture from 50 to 100 µg enhanced the inhibitory effect dramatically, even though vitamin C by itself did not affect growth.

In another experiment, vitamin E succinate inhibited the growth of neuroblastoma cells more effectively than radiation, but the two together produced an even more powerful effect. In addition, a water-soluble preparation of vitamin E inhibited the growth of colon cancer cells transplanted to athymic mice better than 5-fluorouracil, but the two together produced almost no growth. Vitamin C enhances the effect of 5-fluorouracil on cancer cells but not on normal cells, and enhances the effect of adriamycin on HeLa cells but not on normal cells.

1.2.5.0 Section 3: biomarkers

Session Chair: *Steven Clinton, Ohio State University, Arthur G. James Cancer Hospital*

1.2.5.1 Biomarkers of Oxidative Stress: Fact or Artifact?

James Swenberg, University of North Carolina

James Swenberg, D.V.M., Ph.D., Professor, Department of Environmental Science and Engineering, University of North Carolina—Chapel Hill, described research on biomarkers of oxidative stress. **Oxidative damage is the most common form of DNA damage, with ~1 x 10^6 nucleotides damaged by oxidation at any one time.** Damage can arise from both endogenous and exogenous sources, which can complement each other. Most studies in the literature focus on adducts of *8OHdG*, although there are newer studies focused on oxidized bases, oxidized abasic sites, and cyclic DNA adducts. Slot blot electrophoresis is used to analyze intact DNA, and mass spectrometry is used to analyze nucleosides and bases.

One of the most complex issues regarding antioxidants is the dose response to hydrogen peroxide. At low concentrations, iron associates with DNA around the *N-7* position of guanine, which is readily available for Fenton chemistry and is responsible for a steep increase in oxidation early in the process. Iron also associates with the deoxyribose moiety of DNA, where it is tightly bound and it is not readily available for Fenton chemistry, which results in a descending slope of activity. This decrease in oxidation damage is seen **because hydrogen peroxide is not only a prooxidant; it can also be an antioxidant under certain conditions.**

The efficiency of oxidant-induced DNA damage is highest at low concentrations, such as 0.6 μmol/L. As the concentration goes up, there is a smaller effect on the DNA per unit of exposure, which is not the dose response that is normally seen in the laboratory. Using base-excision repair enzymes, it is possible to look at oxidized purines, such as 8-hydroxydeoxyguanosine (*8OHdG*), and pyrimidines as targets of oxidation. From 1983 to 2003, the same complex dose response for hydrogen peroxide was seen with 4 different endpoints being measured. This is the result of iron being present in different intracellular pools, with differential availability for Fenton chemistry, and **hydrogen peroxide acting as both an anti- and a prooxidant.**

In experiments using *8OHdG* formation as an endpoint biomarker, it is important to avoid artifacts, which can change the results of the experiment. The use of TEMPO, a free radical trapping agent, or desferal, an iron chelator, during the tissue workup helps to reduce artifacts. It is also important to understand the amount of background *8OHdG* found in the specific tissues and cells used in specific experiments. A large study conducted by the European Standards Committee on Oxidative DNA Damage (ESCODD) found that the average amount of *8OHdG* present in the lymphocytes of a normal, healthy, 25- to 30-y-old is ~0.6 to 6 per 10^6 guanines, depending on the method used for isolation and analysis. Additional assays are being developed to improve the accuracy of measurements of direct oxidative damage and lipid peroxide-induced DNA damage, and to determine whether adducts are produced from exogenous or endogenous exposure.

1.2.5.2 Plasma Antioxidant Measurements

Ronald Prior, Arkansas Children's Nutrition Research Center

Ronald L. Prior, Ph.D., Research Chemist and Nutritionist, Agricultural Research Service, USDA, Arkansas Children's Nutrition Research Center, Little Rock, discussed plasma antioxidant measurements. **There are several antioxidant defense mechanisms, such as free radical–scavenging enzyme systems and nonenzymatic systems that include antioxidant compounds, compounds that are active in the lipid domain, water-soluble compounds, flavonoid compounds, the carotenoids, uric acid, and plasma proteins.** Antioxidant capacity assays essentially are inhibition methods. A free radical species is generated, and the inhibition of the free radical action by an added antioxidant is designated as the antioxidant capacity. Antioxidants can produce either a total inhibition of free radical action that is detected as a lag phase or a partial inhibition of free radical action, in which no lag phase will be detected unless a very high concentration of free radicals is involved. Inhibition of free radical action by an antioxidant has 2 components: the inhibition time and the degree of inhibition.

Measures of in vivo antioxidant status are important in understanding the role of oxidative events in the initiation and progression of numerous diseases, including cancer, atherosclerosis, and diabetes. Measurement of individual plasma or tissue levels of antioxidants such as vitamin C, vitamin E, or the carotenoids can assess in vivo antioxidant status. However, it is a much more difficult task when one considers the numerous other compounds, including flavonoid and polyphenol-like compounds, that may influence in vivo antioxidant status. In this case, measures of antioxidant capacity are an important tool in the assessment of antioxidant status. Numerous techniques, often utilizing quite different free radical sources, have been developed and used to assess antioxidant capacity (AOC) in plasma. AOC is evaluated in terms of the levels of low-molecular-weight antioxidants in plasma or tissue. However, **AOC assays do not address the role of various antioxidant enzymes in protecting against free radical action.** Advantages of AOC measurement are that individual analysis of each antioxidant component is not necessary and an estimate of the total AOC can be obtained. However, until recently, no true measure of total AOC (hydrophilic and lipophilic AOC) was available. A useful assay should be able to use a biologically relevant radical source, such as peroxyl, hydroxyl, or singlet-oxygen- and peroxynitrate-containing compounds. **Radicals from different sources produce different estimates, so it is important which radical is utilized.** The ideal assay should measure both lipophilic and hydrophilic antioxidants and measure both inhibition time and the degree of inhibition.

The **oxygen radical absorbance capacity (ORAC) assay can determine antioxidant activity against peroxyl radicals and measures most of the well-known antioxidants, including ascorbic acid, glutathione, bilirubin, α-tocopherol, ß-carotene, uric acid, melatonin, and flavonoids.** The ORAC assay measures a total of the antioxidants that are present in a sample, which can be from biological fluids, or tissue, or food. The advantages of ORAC is that it takes into account the time and degree of inhibition. ORAC can be adapted to analyze both hydrophilic and lipophilic antioxidants and can be automated for large studies in which a large number of samples must be processed.

A limitation of ORAC is that it often is restricted to measurement of events in the blood, and these measurements may not reflect what is happening in the target tissue. Another potential question revolves around the response to oxidative stress. Immediately after exposure to an oxidative stressor, there is a decrease in antioxidant capacity using the available antioxidants, but over time there may be a response in the tissue, so that antioxidant capacity increases. This complicates interpretation of the results. The assay gives a snapshot in time of the potential antioxidant status.

The literature reports lower antioxidant capacity in preterm infants, patients with HIV (37% reduction), Alzheimer's patients (24% reduction), patients with sepsis, and patients with diabetes (50% reduction). Of course, I believe that all of these conditions are directly related to an EMOD insufficiency.

Preliminary studies indicate that the intake of total antioxidants from the diet is reflected in higher serum concentrations of antioxidants. For example, in a study of antioxidant levels after consuming a meal high in antioxidants, serum levels increased after consumption of blueberries, strawberries, spinach, red wine (phenolics), and ascorbic acid. Further analysis of the meal with blueberries showed that the hydrophilic antioxidant levels peaked at 2 h and then declined, but the lipophilic antioxidants peaked at 2 h and remained stable. Cherries produced an oxidative effect for hydrophilic antioxidants, but also produced a very strong rise in the level of lipophilic antioxidants. **It is not clear why most fruits have relatively low lipophilic components.** Prune juice contains a high level of antioxidants, but very low levels of them were found in serum. **All of these fruits have high antioxidant levels but very different phytochemical composition, absorption profiles, and metabolism, which produce highly varied in vivo responses.**

A European study used the ferric-reducing antioxidant power (FRAP) assay to investigate serum antioxidant levels after consuming cranberries, blueberries, and control foods. Results indicate that serum concentrations were highest with cranberries and lowest with the controls.

Plasma antioxidant measurements seem to be stable over a 2- to 3-mo period, and certain clinical disease states can alter plasma antioxidant capacity. Increased consumption of fruits and vegetables can increase antioxidant levels, depending on the food's metabolism and absorption profile. This elevation is transient and returns to baseline in 4 to 6 h after the meal.

Measurement of serum antioxidant capacity is a research tool that can be used to assess oxidative stress. **A battery of assays should be performed, not just one**, to fully explore antioxidant status. Relations between dietary antioxidant intake and plasma antioxidant capacity, and how they affect cancer and other health problems, remain to be determined. (Prior, R. L. (2004) Plasma antioxidant measurements. J. Nutr. 134:3184S-3185S).

1.2.5.3 DNA Oxidation Products, Antioxidant Status, and Cancer Prevention

Henry Thompson, Colorado State University

Henry Thompson, Ph.D., Professor and Director, Cancer Prevention Laboratory, Colorado State University—Fort Collins, discussed the challenges encountered when laboratory data on DNA oxidation products are used to design clinical intervention studies on antioxidant status and cancer risk. (Thompson, H. J. (2004) DNA oxidation products, antioxidant status, and cancer prevention. J. Nutr. 134:3186S-3187S) **The direct evidence of an antioxidant effect on DNA oxidation is inconsistent at best,** although most researchers think that antioxidants should affect DNA oxidation based on indirect evidence.

Several gaps in knowledge appear critical in addressing the antioxidant–cancer prevention hypothesis, which can only be resolved through well-designed studies to specifically answer this question. The study should last at least 2 to 8 wk and include specific markers of oxidative stress, such as *8OhdG*. It should also use both direct and indirect measurement approaches. The tissue of choice could be the lymphocyte, although some have considered urine and specific target organs. Measurements should be taken at weekly intervals to assess differences in treatment effects, and attention should be paid to the methods used for sample collection, storage, and the number of analytical runs necessary to produce good data. Measurements of antioxidant concentrations, scavenging activity, ROS, and oxidation products (DNA, lipids, proteins, or downstream events) would make the study valuable in addressing the many questions that still remain about oxidative stress and antioxidants.

To address the need to correlate this research with cancer risk factors, DNA oxidation could be assessed, because the oxidation of bases produces promutagenic events, promutagenic events increase the potential for mutagenic events, and more mutagenic events increase the risk of cancer. Although *8OHdG* would be the oxidative marker of choice, as it seems to be the most prevalent, other markers should be simultaneously assessed. There are many methods to measure oxidation products; LC tandem mass spectrometry is used in many studies, as is HPLC.

There must be some method to minimize ex vivo DNA oxidation, such as isolation of the nuclei, adding an iron ion chelator, or using a precipitating agent such as sodium iodide. The results from different laboratories encompass differences of several orders of magnitude if these methods are not used. Variance and random error are other methodologic barriers to consider.

In a study of an intervention on women at risk for breast cancer, 50% of the participants had *8OHdG* levels that were higher than the target value. To address this finding, participants were randomly assigned to a lower– or higher–fruit and vegetable diet group (3.5 vs. 12 servings/d, respectively, for 2 wk). Levels of *8OHdG* decreased 16% in the high–fruit and vegetable diet group.

The neutral single-cell microgel electrophoresis assay (comet assay), a simple, rapid, sensitive, indirect technique that can be performed on hundreds of cells at a time, can be applied to investigate oxidized pyrimidines using endonuclease-3 and oxidized purines using formamidopyrimidine *N*-glycosylase (Fpg). The assay uses a small sample and the cells can be frozen for months, which is an advantage when conducting large-scale experiments or complex human trials. However, intralaboratory variability is high with this qualitative assay, and intraindividual variability is equal to the variability between different individuals. Calibration of interlaboratory data is also difficult due to the semiquantitative nature of the assay.

ELISA can also be used to assess urinary *8OHdG*, although there are problems with correlation to intake of antioxidants, as there are with almost all methods described in this presentation.

There are many gaps in our knowledge on this topic. Questions about the relation between different target tissues and appropriate markers of DNA, lipid, and protein oxidation remain unanswered. Markers need to be validated to improve correlation so information gained in these studies can be used to tailor antioxidant treatment to individual genotypes. The overall question remains, however, about what role DNA oxidation plays with specific genetic mutations and how this affects carcinogenesis.

1.2.5.4 Use of Biomarkers of Oxidative Stress in Research Studies

Jeffrey Blumberg, Tufts University

Jeffrey B. Blumberg, Ph.D., Professor, Friedman School of Nutrition Science and Policy and Jean Mayer USDA Human Nutrition Research Center on Aging, Tufts University, Boston, MA, discussed the use of biomarkers of oxidative stress in research studies (Blumberg, J. (2004) Use of biomarkers of oxidative stress in research studies. J. Nutr. 134:3188S-3189S).

Biomarkers can be employed to reflect environmental prooxidant exposures and dietary antioxidant intake or serve as a surrogate measure of a disease process. **To be truly useful, the biomarker must have some degree of predictive validity, but full substantiation of this relation is still lacking. A number of challenges must be overcome to obtain not only a better understanding of the contributions of reactive species to the carcinogenesis**

process but a rational application of biomarkers of oxidative stress to observational studies and clinical trials of antioxidants and cancer. Nonetheless, without measuring parameters relevant to the status of antioxidant defenses and oxidative stress, it is not possible to determine whether the selection, dose, and duration of an antioxidant intervention achieves its intended biochemical or physiological endpoint or whether the enrolled subjects even present with oxidative stress.

Exposure to endogenous and environmental carcinogens causes DNA damage indicative of oxidative stress, with consequences for cytotoxic and mutagenic activity, as well as aberrant changes to cell cycle progression and replication. Moreover, oxidation of cellular lipids and proteins can adversely affect several steps of the carcinogenic process through changes in a variety of cell regulatory functions, including signal transduction and gene expression. Thus, **biomarkers of oxidative stress have the potential to help** establish pathogenic stages of and risk for disease and should be employed to inform the design and outcome measures of clinical trials. Identification and application of suitable biomarkers should shorten the time it takes to demonstrate that an agent has a beneficial, untoward, or null effect on health promotion and disease prevention or a therapeutic value in disease treatment. However, **some proposed biomarkers of oxidative stress might prove simply to be general markers of oxidative damage and relatively poor indicators of disease process and outcome.**

New research studies must address whether and how biomarkers adequately measure relevant physiologic functions or relate to established pathological signs, particularly with regard to their **accuracy, precision, and reliability**. Such efforts must consider the potential for artifacts produced during sample collection, processing, storage, and instrumental analyses, as well as confounding by the presence of related factors such as the status of facets of the antioxidant defense network that are not under direct study. The validation of biomarkers must include an assessment of the degree of bias in their measurement, especially the characterization of their prevalence and variability within large-scale population studies. An important issue for study will be determining whether specific biomarkers reflect short- or long-term exposure to an antioxidant status or oxidative stress.

When establishing the Dietary Reference Intakes, the Institute of Medicine (IOM) used biomarkers of oxidative stress to define dietary antioxidants. The IOM definition of dietary antioxidant includes the ability to significantly decrease the adverse effects of reactive species, such as reactive oxygen and nitrogen species, on normal physiologic function in humans. However, **it is not clear whether**

sufficient scientific agreement yet exists regarding the validity of these biomarkers as a reflection of the action and efficacy of dietary antioxidants. This issue is confused by the apparent difficulty, in many studies, of demonstrating an antioxidant effect unless oxidative stress is first markedly elevated, as found, for example, in smokers or patients with marked inflammatory conditions.

One common working definition of oxidative stress is the disturbance in the pro-oxidant–antioxidant balance, in favor of the former, leading to potential cellular damage. However, **measuring oxidative stress can be difficult due to the presence of complex endogenous systems for correction and repair**, as may occur, for example, when a brief elevation in oxidative stress rapidly induces various antioxidant defenses, particularly antioxidant enzymes such as superoxide dismutase, catalase, and glutathione peroxidase, that quickly reduce the stress and limit the researcher's ability to detect a change. Oxidative stress can result from diminished antioxidant protection as well as increased free radical production. Therefore, investigating antioxidant depletion as a biomarker of oxidative stress may involve determining decreases in concentrations of antioxidants or increases in levels of their metabolites. However, such changes may not reflect a clinically significant or pathogenic event but merely indicate that the antioxidant defense system is functioning.

DNA, lipid, and protein oxidation products provide an extensive and growing array of potential biomarkers, although our understanding of the relation between their status in cells and tissues, including plasma and urine, remains to be elucidated. Development of a broader panel of biomarkers to examine both pro- and antioxidant reactions should be pursued. This might include the capacity of a biological sample to resist oxidation in vitro or ex vivo and modulation of redox-sensitive transcription factors or related alterations in signal transduction pathways.

In practice, single elements or combined parameters from these approaches are currently employed, although, not infrequently, only **one analyte** is measured. **The conclusion may then be incorrectly drawn that the single measurement satisfactorily reflects overall oxidative stress.** Although the capability to adequately assess genomic factors relevant to antioxidant defenses and oxidative stress is limited, this facet added to new research approaches will become increasingly important in determining which individuals are most likely to respond to antioxidant interventions. Further elucidation of the relation between antioxidants and cancer risk will require validation of existing biomarkers of oxidative stress as well as the creation of new indices and their further evaluation.

There may come a time when entry into a clinical trial could be determined by biomarkers of oxidative stress, although that is not now possible. An even better approach would be to develop the ability to stratify individuals at risk in clinical trials through a panel of biomarkers.

1.2.5.5 Manganese Superoxide Dismutase: Genetic Variation and Regulation

Daret St. Clair, University of Kentucky

Daret St. Clair, Ph.D., Professor, Department of Toxicology, University of Kentucky—Lexington, discussed manganese superoxide dismutase (MnSOD) and genetic variation and regulation (St. Clair, D. (2004) Manganese superoxide dismutase: genetic variation and regulation. J. Nutr. 134:3190S-3191S).

MnSOD is the primary antioxidant essential for the survival of aerobic life. Its relation to cancer is well documented in cell cultures and animal models. MnSOD activity is altered in cancer cells compared to normal cells, which makes a difference in cell function because MnSOD reduces radiation-induced neoplastic transformation, protects against the cytotoxicity of chemotherapy, promotes cellular differentiation, suppresses cancer phenotypes and metastatic potential, and alters the expression of oncogenes. **RMH Note: SOD is the primary producer of hydrogen peroxide and is therefore a prooxidant!**

The gene that regulates MnSOD is a single-copy gene consisting of 5 exons and 4 introns. One of the unique characteristics of this gene is its intronic enhancer element, which is absolutely essential for the induction of the gene by cytokines and tumor necrosis factors. The promoter region is extremely G-C rich, and consists of a cluster of Sp1 and AP2 transcription factor binding sites, which overlap extensively.

Sp1 upregulates the transcription activity of the human MnSOD promoter, and mutations to the Sp1 binding sites decrease *MnSOD* transcription. AP2 downregulates the transcription activity of the human MnSOD promoter, and mutations of the AP2 binding sites increase such transcription and promoter activity. A set of 3 unique mutations that cause these problems occur in the promoter region of *MnSOD* in many types of cancer.

Polymorphisms in the leader sequence of *MnSOD* are associated with an increased risk of lung and breast cancer. Premenopausal women who are homozygous for the AA allele have a 4-fold greater risk of developing breast cancer than women with 1 or 2 V alleles. The risk is greatest among women who consume low levels of dietary antioxidants. Women who consume high levels of antioxidants have a minimal risk of developing the disease. Menopause does not alter these risks. Polymorphisms in exon 3 of the mature protein are associated with an increased sensitivity to, and inactivation by, thiol reagents.

1.2.6.0 Session 4: Clinical aspects of antioxidant usage

Session Chair: *Rebecca Costello, Office of Dietary Supplements, NIH*

Rebecca Costello, Ph.D., F.A.C.N., Deputy Director, Office of Dietary Supplements, NIH, Rockville, MD, presented goals for Session 4. The session served to set the stage and describe what is known about dietary supplement use among Americans as well as by individuals at risk for or diagnosed with cancer. Topics included types of supplements, frequency of consumption, how they are consumed (i.e., single or multiple supplements), and how they are purchased (i.e., over the counter or prescription). In addition, behaviors and motivations related to supplement use were discussed. The session presented information on oxidative biomarkers of disease, the utility of biomarkers in studying population groups, and the methodological approaches currently available for assessing exposure to antioxidant nutrients for epidemiologic research, with an emphasis on the use of biomarker-based approaches.

1.2.7.0 Consumer Perspectives about Antioxidants

Cheryl Toner, International Food Information Council

Cheryl Toner, M.S., R.D., Director of Health Communications, International Food Information Council (IFIC), Washington, DC, discussed consumer perspectives about antioxidants (Toner, C. (2004) Consumer perspectives about antioxidants. J. Nutr. 134:3192S-3193S).

IFIC conducted telephone surveys in 1998, 2000, and 2002, of 1004 adults in the United States. Results of the survey indicated that Americans have a positive attitude about nutrition and health and want to know more about the health benefits of food, with an increasing need for information on "functional foods." ***Functional foods* were defined as foods that may provide a health benefit beyond basic nutrition, and may include fortified foods as well as fruits and vegetables.** In general, consumers are focused on the role of foods in cardiovascular disease and cancer and are becoming more aware of the associations between specific food health claims and disease. For example, in 2002, 79%

of consumers were aware of the association between calcium and osteoporosis; **54% for antioxidants and cancer;** and 35% for soy protein and heart disease.

According to the survey, **consumers tend to increase consumption of foods that carry a health claim if they believe in the efficacy of the claim. For antioxidants, consumers understand the health claims but are not sure which foods contain the antioxidants that could be beneficial.** In addition, a significant barrier to increasing use of antioxidants for health benefits may be a lack of confidence in the claims; **many consumers do not seem convinced that antioxidants are as great a health benefit as reported in the media.**

Factors for health message effectiveness include the seriousness of the disease expressed in the claim (e.g., cancer is more serious than osteoporosis), the knowledge of the component (e.g., fruits and vegetables have many benefits), the association with supplements (e.g., consumers do not know what foods contain vitamin E), and the availability of the component (e.g., calcium is perceived to be in many foods; therefore, supplements are not as necessary).

When consumers were asked whether they had heard of an individual's genetic variability as a factor to consider when determining the right foods or supplements to use for health benefits, they expressed some awareness of the concept, but were cautious about privacy concerns surrounding information on their personal genetic makeup. The word *nutrigenomics* was not perceived to be a consumer-friendly term, and researchers should be aware of the sensitivity of such technical terms.

1.2.8.0 Antioxidant Supplement Use in Cancer Survivors and the General Population

Cheryl Rock, University of California—San Diego

Cheryl Rock, Ph.D., R.D., Professor, Department of Family and Preventive Medicine, University of California—San Diego, reported on antioxidant supplement use in cancer survivors and the general population (Rock, C. L., Newman, V. A., Neuhouser, M. L., Major, J. & Barnett, M. J. (2004) Antioxidant supplement use in cancer survivors and the general population. J. Nutr. 134:3194S-3195S).

Approximately one-half of the general population takes dietary supplements, and use is higher among individuals with health concerns, especially those diagnosed with cancer. Researchers have suggested that there may be both beneficial and adverse effects of supplement use among individuals diagnosed with cancer.

Two recent studies, the Olestra Post-Marketing Surveillance Study (OPMSS) and the Women's Healthy Eating and Living (WHEL) Study, collected data on supplement use. Results from OPMSS indicate that predictors of antioxidant use are age, education, sex, and region of the United States. OPMSS participants reported taking multivitamins (41%), vitamin E (9.5%), vitamin C (17%), and ß-carotene (2%). Among users of supplements, the median dosage of vitamin C was 500 mg and that of vitamin E was 34 mg; Dr. Rock commented that each of these represents relatively modest intake from supplements.

The WHEL study examined data on women diagnosed with stage I, II, or IIA invasive breast cancer within the past 48 mo and after treatment. Results indicated that at baseline (1995–2002), there was a wide range of antioxidant dietary supplement use. At baseline, 91% of women used dietary supplements. Specific antioxidant dietary supplements used included multivitamins (59%), **antioxidant mixtures (9.8%),** selenium (10.1%), vitamin A and carotenoids (10.6%), vitamin C (41.6%), and vitamin E (45.8%). Positive predictors of supplement use included older age (vitamins E and C), high levels of physical activity (vitamins E and C and multivitamins), and education and stage at diagnosis (multivitamins). Negative predictors of supplement use included race or ethnicity and BMI (vitamins E and C and multivitamins) and time since diagnosis (vitamins E and C). Motivations for supplement use included beliefs that vitamin C and E increase general health, that vitamin E decreases menopausal symptoms, and that vitamin C improves immune functions.

Conclusions drawn from these studies suggest that the prevalence of antioxidant dietary supplement use is higher among cancer survivors than among the general population, and that the supplements being used are increasingly complex mixtures of ingredients.

1.2.9.0 Efficacy of Dietary Antioxidants to Prevent Oxidative Damage

Balz Frei, Linus Pauling Institute, Oregon State University

Balz Frei, Ph.D., Director and Endowed Chair, Linus Pauling Institute, and Professor, Department of Biochemistry and Biophysics, Oregon State University, Corvallis, OR, presented data on antioxidant protection and oxidative damage in human plasma (Frei, B. (2004) Efficacy of dietary antioxidants to prevent oxidative damage and inhibit chronic disease. J. Nutr. 134:3196S-3198S).

He reviewed the levels of defense against oxidative damage, which can be categorized into proteinaceous and small-molecule antioxidants. There are antioxidant proteins that are nonenzymatic defense systems (e.g., iron- and copper-binding proteins such as transferrin, ferritin, and albumin), which prevent metal ions from producing free radicals in solution. **Antioxidant enzymes, including superoxide dismutase, catalase, and peroxidases, are primarily intracellular enzymes and are absent or found only in small concentrations in extracellular fluids.**

Among the small-molecule water-soluble antioxidants in plasma, urate is found in high concentrations, followed by vitamin C (ascorbate) and bilirubin, whereas glutathione is present only in low concentrations, usually <2 µmol/L. Lipid-soluble small-molecule antioxidants in plasma include α-tocopherol, which is present at a level of about 10 molecules per low-density lipoprotein particle, and ß-carotene, lycopene, and other carotenoids and oxycarotenoids, which are found in considerably lesser amounts.

To investigate the relative importance of the endogenous antioxidants in plasma, fresh human plasma was exposed at 37°C to 50 mmol/L 2,2'-azobis(2-amidinopropane) hydrochloride (AAPH), which causes oxidative stress by producing aqueous peroxyl radicals at a rate of ~3 µmol $\cdot L^{-1} \cdot min^{-1}$; the consumption of endogenous antioxidants in relation to the formation of lipid hydroperoxides was measured as a marker of oxidative damage. Vitamin C is the first line of defense and is used up in the first 60 min of the experiment; no lipid peroxidation occurs during this time. **After the vitamin C is consumed, different classes of lipid hydroperoxides are formed, and bilirubin, urate, and α-tocopherol are consumed, in that order. These data suggest a defined sequence of antioxidant defense.**

Further studies of other types of oxidative stress, (e.g., activated neutrophils, the gas phase of cigarette smoke, superoxide radicals and hydrogen peroxide generated by the xanthine-xanthine oxidase system, and excess copper or iron), show that vitamin C always forms the first line of antioxidant defense and is the only antioxidant in plasma that can completely prevent lipid peroxidation. **Interestingly, copper or iron ions and ascorbate act as prooxidants in vitro because ascorbate reduces the metal ions, leading to production of hydroxyl radicals from hydrogen peroxide. This does not, however, happen in biological systems**

such as plasma, where ascorbate appears to act only as an antioxidant, even in the presence of excess copper or iron and hydrogen peroxide.

Identified biomarkers of oxidative stress in vivo include F_2-isoprostanes, 8-oxo-2'-deoxyguanosine, and protein carbonyls. For example, F_2-isoprostanes are validated biomarkers of lipid oxidative damage. F_2-isoprostanes are oxidation products of arachidonic acid and are elevated in humans with many conditions, including Alzheimer's disease, hepatic cirrhosis, and atherosclerosis, and with coronary risk factors such as cigarette smoking, diabetes, obesity, hypercholesterolemia, and hyperhomocysteinemia. **A gap in knowledge exists because of the lack of prospective studies and clinical trials to clearly establish a link between oxidative stress (assessed by validated oxidative biomarkers) and increased disease risk.**

Studies in healthy subjects indicate that there is no relation between vitamin C dose and lower F_2-isoprostane levels in urine. In addition, vitamin E supplementation does not appear to affect urinary levels of F_2-isoprostanes in healthy subjects. In patients with elevated F_2-isoprostane levels at baseline, however (e.g., smokers), vitamin C (2.0 g for 5 d) markedly decreases F_2-isoprostane levels. Very similar results are reported in patients with liver cirrhosis administered vitamin C supplementation (2.5 g for 10 d). Furthermore, patients with type 2 diabetes have elevated levels of F_2-isoprostanes, which are markedly decreased by vitamin E supplementation (0.6 g/d for 2 wk).

The European Prospective Investigation of Cancer (EPIC) Trial, a multinational survey on diet, lifestyle, and physical activity involving >500,000 volunteers, found a strong inverse association between plasma vitamin C levels and total, cardiovascular, and cancer mortality. However, **whether this is a beneficial effect of vitamin C itself or fruit and vegetable consumption in general (for which plasma vitamin C serves as a marker) remains unclear.**

The MRC/BHF Heart Protection Study, a large secondary prevention trial in patients with cardiovascular disease or diabetes, found that a daily cocktail of 250 mg vitamin C, 600 mg vitamin E, and 20 mg ß-carotene does not reduce mortality from, or incidence of, any type of vascular disease, cancer, or other chronic disease.

In addition, pooled analyses of prevention trials of vitamin E and ß-carotene did not show significant benefits for these antioxidants with

respect to cancer, cardiovascular disease, or all-cause mortality. In fact, the results of the ATBC and CARET trials showed that ß-carotene supplements have a markedly adverse effect among active smokers.

The question regarding the role of oxidative stress in chronic disease remains unanswered. Clinical trials have not investigated oxidative stress, nor has the relation between risk factors for disease and oxidative stress been adequately addressed. It is not known whether certain risk factors increase disease through oxidative stress mechanisms or whether oxidative stress increases independently of disease risk or as a consequence of disease. Future clinical trials need to assess oxidative stress (i.e., validated oxidative biomarkers) before and after antioxidant supplementation; otherwise, it is impossible to know whether antioxidants fail to prevent or treat disease because they do not lower oxidative stress or because oxidative stress does not have a causal role in disease.

1.3.0.0 Biomarkers for Assessing Antioxidant Nutrient Intakes and Status

Susan T. Mayne, Yale University School of Medicine

Susan Mayne, Ph.D., Associate Professor, Department of Epidemiology and Public Health, Yale University School of Medicine, New Haven, CT, discussed the challenges in assessing antioxidant intake and status (Mayne, S.T., Wright, M. E. & Cartmel, B. (2004) Assessment of antioxidant nutrient intake and status for epidemiologic research. J. Nutr. 134:3199S-3200S).

She focused on exposure assessment for carotenoids, vitamin E, vitamin C, and selenium.

Although there are >600 identified carotenoids, the following carotenoids account for most intake in humans: α- and ß-carotene, lycopene, lutein and zeaxanthin, and ß-cryptoxanthin. Food-composition data for these compounds have improved in the past decade, which is a benefit to epidemiologists attempting to estimate intake of these compounds. The database developed by the USDA is available online [www.nal.usda.gov/fnic/foodcomp]. Researchers also can use HPLC technology to assess carotenoids in plasma and in other tissues. Dr. Mayne discussed issues regarding the best method to quantify nutrient status and how this can be related to health messages for the public were discussed. She also presented emerging noninvasive technologies, including skin reflection spectrophotometry and Raman resonance spectroscopy (RRS).

Carotenoids accumulate in skin, which makes these methods attractive. Validation studies of these technologies are underway.

Vitamin E includes 4 tocopherols and 4 tocotrienols, although the USDA food-composition database uses α-tocopherol equivalents as the standard metric for intake assessment. Bioequivalency in the current USDA database is based on activity in the rat fetal resorption assay. A 2000 IOM report concluded that **vitamin E forms are not interconvertible in humans and recommended the use of 2*R*-stereoisomeric forms of α-tocopherol to meet vitamin E requirements in humans.** With this change, food-composition databases and nutrient requirements are based on different systems. Biochemical assessment of the various vitamin E forms (e.g., HPLC) is another approach for exposure assessment. The α:γ tocopherol ratio can be used as a biomarker of vitamin E supplement use.

Plasma ascorbate can also be measured by HPLC as a biomarker for vitamin C status, although these values may not correlate with intake estimates at very high levels of intake. **Dietary estimates of selenium based on food-composition data are not accurate because the amount of selenium in food varies as a function of the selenium content of the soil, which differs markedly geographically**. Biomarkers of selenium intake, such as selenium content in toenail clippings and plasma selenium levels, are preferred to assessments of dietary intake, given the uncertainties in intake assessment.

Most epidemiologic studies of antioxidant nutrients focus on one or two specific compounds, with little research on synergism and interactions among antioxidants. There is a need to develop more comprehensive indices of antioxidant nutrient intake and status. Dr. Mayne discussed various approaches for creating indices, such as principal component analyses of dietary antioxidants, or using ORAC scores to weight foods based on their antioxidant score. All of the more comprehensive approaches require further development and validation prior to routine use in human studies of antioxidant nutrients.

1.3.1.0 Session 5a: Chemotherapy-antioxidant reactions

Session Chair: *David Rosenthal, Harvard University Health Sciences Center Cancer*

1.3.2.0 Chemotherapy and Antioxidants: An Overview

Kenneth Conklin, David Geffen School of Medicine, University of California—Los Angeles

Kenneth A. Conklin, M.D., Ph.D., Clinical Professor, Jonsson Comprehensive Cancer Center, David Geffen School of Medicine, University of California—Los Angeles, discussed the controversy surrounding the use of antioxidants during chemotherapy (Conklin, K.A. (2004) Cancer chemotherapy and antioxidants. J. Nutr. 134:3201S-3204S).

Approximately 300 to 400 preclinical studies have been published on this topic, and most show that antioxidants do not interfere with the mechanism of action of therapeutic agents. However, **too few clinical studies have been done to draw any definitive conclusions.**

Antioxidants (e.g., vitamins C and E) act as reducing agents to neutralize free radicals. If a therapeutic agent works by releasing free radicals, it is possible that antioxidants may interfere with its action. **Some antioxidants are also strong nucleophiles (e.g., GSH, *N*-acetyl cysteine, and α-lipoic acid), and they may interfere with the anticancer effects of platinum coordination complexes (e.g., cisplatin and carboplatin) and alkylating agents.**

Doxorubicin (Adriamycin), a very versatile antineoplastic agent, is an anthracycline that is reduced to a semiquinone that can generate superoxide radicals. Anthracyclines are important in the study of antioxidant effects because they form large amounts of free radicals and induce oxidative stress. Regarding the mechanism of action of anthracyclines, the most compelling evidence shows that at clinically relevant concentrations they intercalate with double-stranded DNA and inhibit the function of topoisomerase II. Free radicals produced by doxorubicin may play a role in cancer therapy, but preclinical studies suggest that antioxidants do not interfere with the anticancer actions of the drug.

The side effect of greatest concern when doxorubicin is administered is cardiac toxicity. **In heart cells, doxorubicin forms a deoxyaglycone that can replace coenzyme Q10 (CoQ10) in the electron transport chain and act as an electron acceptor.** This disrupts the energetics of cardiac mitochondria, leading to reduced generation of ATP, and accounts for the commonly seen side effects of acute cardiac toxicity (arrhythmias and reduced ejection fraction). The effect of doxorubicin on cardiac mitochondria is uniquely different from its effect on mitochondria of other cells. This is most likely due to the unique structure of cardiac mitochondria, which contain an NADH dehydrogenase on the outer surface of the inner membrane; this organization is not found in noncardiac mitochondria. Animal studies show that **doxorubicin generates ROS in cardiac mitochondria for at least 1 wk after the drug is administered.** This causes the formation of mitochondrial DNA-adducts that can suppress gene expression and reduce synthesis of critical components of the mitochondrial electron transport systems. This may irreversibly damage cardiac mitochondria and be responsible for the development of chronic cardiac toxicity (congestive heart failure that is not responsive to digitalis).

The platinum coordination complexes also generate free radicals that can damage the kidney. **Animal model studies with antioxidants (reducing agents) show that they do not reduce the toxicity of platinum drugs such as cisplatin.** However, several studies suggest that the nucleophilic antioxidant GSH, administered intravenously, ameliorates renal toxicity without interfering with the antineoplastic action of the drug.

Oxidative stress induced by many antineoplastic agents may interfere with cell-cycle progression and reduce the cytotoxicity of drugs that exhibit activity on specific time points in the cell-cycle phase. The aldehydes generated from PUFAs during oxidative stress may also interfere with drug-induced apoptosis, possibly by interference with death receptor pathways or by inhibition of caspase activity.

Future studies could include CoQ10 supplementation as a potential means for reducing cardiac toxicity of anthracyclines and study of certain nucleophilic antioxidants such as GSH for lowering or preventing toxicity of platinum coordination complexes. Such studies may lead to valuable information on reducing toxicity without interfering with the action of these widely used drugs.

1.3.3.0 Redox and Vitamin C in Cell Signaling and Genomic Protection

David Golde, Memorial Sloan-Kettering Cancer Center

David W. Golde, M.D., Enid A. Haupt Chair in Hematologic Oncology, Department of Medicine, Memorial Sloan-Kettering Cancer Center, New York, NY, reviewed basic laboratory data on vitamin C. **Ascorbic acid is oxidized to dehydroascorbate (DHA) outside cells and then transported intracellularly by the facilitative glucose transporters. Inside the cell, DHA is quickly reduced back to ascorbate, where it serves as an antioxidant to protect the cell from oxidation.** Another mechanism for the cell to accumulate vitamin C is through the sodium-ascorbate cotransporter system, which allows vitamin C to be directly transported into the cell. Studies in mice show that vitamin C crosses the blood-brain barrier in the form of DHA through the glucose transporters. The therapeutic importance of this finding is that DHA injections provide significant neuroprotection in a stroke model in mice.

Experimental studies with vitamin C show that it inhibits signaling pathways associated with human granulocyte macrophage colony-stimulating factor (GM-CSF). At the molecular level, loading the cells with vitamin C inhibits GM-CSF phosphorylation of mitogen-activated protein (MAP) kinase, JAK-2, and ßGMR. Likewise, vitamin C loading suppresses TNFα-induced NfκB activation. A study in human monocytes shows that DHA inhibits FAS-mediated apoptosis and the amount of ROS generated in the cell as a result of signaling. The mechanism acts largely through inhibition of caspase-8 activation. The implication is that vitamin C may enhance the immune system because it may increase the life of FAS-sensitive cells.

Cancer cells have an increased number of glucose transporters; therefore, intracellular vitamin C can protect them from hypoxia as well as increase their resistance to chemotherapy and radiation. In addition, vitamin C can reduce apoptosis, increase resistance to oxidative stress, inhibit mutation, and influence signaling involving ROS.

1.3.4.0 Drugs, Glutathione, and ROS in Regulation of Proliferation

Kenneth Tew, Fox Chase Cancer Center

Kenneth Tew, Ph.D., D.Sc., Chair, Department of Pharmacology, Fox Chase Cancer Center, Philadelphia, PA, presented data on a 10-y drug development project related to phase II detoxification enzymes (Tew, K. D., Boyd, J. T., Chen, Z. J., Davis, W., Jr, Fazilev, F., Findlay, V., Gaté, L., Ile, K., Soulika, A. & Townsend, D. M. (2004) Glutathione and ABC transporters as determinants of sensitivity to oxidative and nitrosative stress. J. Nutr. 134:3205S-3206S).

The glutathione *S*-transferase (GST) family is very commonly seen in many solid tumors and is overexpressed in drug-resistant tumors that have been exposed to toxic anticancer drugs. Dr. Tew said it would be accurate to extend the definition of GSTs as ligand-binding proteins in addition to enzymes and that human polymorphisms will undoubtedly influence the drug resistance phenotype.

A drug to inhibit GSTπ, designated TLK199, was studied in animals. Results show that TLK199 treatment increases white blood cell levels in animals. TLK199 is designated a small-molecule myeloproliferative agent. Mechanisms were investigated and there is a connection between GSTπ and c-Jun-*N*-terminal kinase (JNK), in which the GST acts as an endogenous suppressor of kinase activity. Treatment of cells with TLK199 causes a disassociation of the protein:protein interaction with subsequent activation of the kinase cascade.

Another novel drug is TLK286, which is a GSTπ-activated prodrug. Although less is known about the mechanisms of TLK286, preliminary investigations identified DNA-dependent protein kinase as a potential target for the drug. Studies in human ovarian cancer cell lines indicate that TLK286 has significant activity in cisplatin-resistant cells, which makes this a promising drug for phase II and III clinical trials in this disease.

1.3.5.0 Session 5b: Radiation-antioxidant interactions

Session Chair: *Norman Coleman, Center for Cancer Research, NCI Antioxidants and Radiation Therapy Carmia Borek, Tufts University School of Medicine*

Carmia Borek, Ph.D., Professor of Community Health, and Director, Nutrition and Infectious Diseases, Tufts University School of Medicine, Boston, MA, reviewed background material on antioxidants and radiation therapy (Borek, C. (2004) Antioxidants and radiation therapy. J. Nutr. 134:3207S-3209S).

Approximately 60% of cancer patients in the United States receive radiotherapy, mostly ionizing radiation (IR) or to a lesser extent particle beam radiation (PR). Radiotherapy is a local treatment confined to the area of affected cells and activates a variety of genes, including NfκB, thereby activating cytokines and causing inflammation. **An important goal of radiotherapy is to administer enough radiation to kill tumor cells without killing adjacent normal cells.**

DNA is the primary target of radiotherapy; damage to DNA occurs through a direct effect but mostly (two-thirds of damage) through an indirect effect, by free radicals [superoxide, hydroxyl radical (the most toxic), and nitric oxide metabolites]. Cells are most sensitive to radiation damage in the G1-mol/L phase of the cell cycle; **oxygen concentration and cyclins will modify radiation response.** Irradiation of nondividing or slow-dividing cells causes apoptotic death.

Antioxidants, including vitamins, help normal cells to withstand oxidative stress and may modify tumor-cell response to radiation. Depending on the tissue and the presence and level of free radicals, specific vitamins may be of greater benefit. To illustrate, ß-carotene is an effective antioxidant at low levels of pO_2, and vitamin E is more effective at high levels of pO_2. Radiation reduces tissue antioxidant levels; in animals, radiation exposure reduces vitamin E levels in cells. In other studies, bone marrow vitamin C and E levels are reduced, and in breast cancer studies, vitamin A, C, and E and selenium levels fall during cancer radiotherapy. **Whether supplementing antioxidants during radiotherapy is beneficial to cancer patients or has an adverse effect is not known.**

Studies of antioxidants in radiation therapy provide interesting insights into the amount of protection that is possible with supplementation. **Selenium increases the number of antioxidant enzymes in normal cells but not in cancer cells.** A study using ultraviolet light as the source of radiation on human cell lines indicates that functional *p53* increases, causing increased DNA repair in these cells.

Vitamin E protects cells from radiation-induced chromosome damage, reduces side effects of radiotherapy, reduces the expression of *ras* oncogenes, prevents apoptosis in normal cells by increasing *bcl2* and decreasing *bax*, and induces apoptosis in cancer cells. In the brain, vitamin E plays an important role in protecting neurons and acetylcholine receptors from free radical damage and prevents apoptosis in neural cells. In glioblastoma, vitamin E may help increase apoptosis and activates capsase-3 enzyme activity.

Cancer is generally an age-related disease, and **plasma antioxidant levels decrease with age;** it is important to take this into consideration during radiotherapy. Recent human experiments show that plasma proteins containing thiols are radioprotective and there is an inverse relation between plasma radioprotective ability and age.

Phytochemicals found in fruits and vegetables include many with antioxidant potential (e.g., flavonoids and carotenoids) that also have an important role in reducing oxidative stress. For example, *S*-allyl cysteine is a water-soluble compound in garlic that increases glutathione in cells and stimulates apoptosis in prostate cancer cells. A trial in England is investigating a compound in grape-seed extract that may protect against fibrosis after radiation treatment for breast cancer. Tea compounds are also a rich area of investigation in the search for agents to increase apoptosis in cancer cells.

It is important to remember that radiation does cause cancer and that vitamin E and selenium protect against radiation-induced malignancy in vitro. This may be the direction of future research because radiotherapy will remain a part of cancer therapy. The use of antioxidant combinations can help decrease damage expected from radiotherapy, especially high-dose radiotherapy.

1.3.6.0 Novel Functional Imaging for Tissue Oxygen Concentration and Redox Status

James Mitchell, Center for Cancer Research, NCI

James B. Mitchell, Ph.D., Branch Chief, Radiation Biology Branch, Center for Cancer Research, NCI, NIH, Rockville, MD, discussed noninvasive functional and molecular imaging and what they can tell us about the role of antioxidants (Mitchell, J. B., Yamada, K., Devasahayam, N., Cook, J. A., Subramanian, S. & Krishna, M. C. (2004) Novel functional imaging for tissue oxygen concentration and redox status. J. Nutr. 134:3210S).

Electron paramagnetic resonance (EPR) has been used in investigations of free radical chemistry for some time; however, new techniques are being developed with the potential for imaging electrons. Nitroxides—stable free radicals—are used as the contrast agents in EPR. **Tempol and Tempol-H are the nitroxides that act as antioxidants and protect against superoxide, pO_2, and hydroperoxide-induced cytotoxicity**. Investigations are under way to determine whether these agents can be used with EPR imaging.

One study investigating whether Tempol protects tumor cells, as it does normal cells during localized radiation, found no protective effect on tumor cells. Analysis of the results suggests that tumor cells reduce the nitroxide at a faster rate than normal tissue. A trial at the University of Pennsylvania is investigating whether timing is important in the topical application of nitroxide. Results indicate that nitroxide applied 15 min before radiotherapy decreases hair loss. If these results can be applied to humans, it may be possible to limit hair loss in patients undergoing full-brain radiotherapy.

Animal studies are testing the use of nitroxides in redox imaging. It appears that redox rates differ between normal and tumor cells, which lead to some interesting questions related to radiotherapy timing. It is possible to develop a redox image based on these relative redox rates. An experiment on redox rates in mouse tumors indicates that glutathione slows reduction rates, suggesting that glutathione has a role in the tissue's ability to reduce nitroxide. **Because tumors are hypoxic (i.e., low in oxygen), they represent a reducing environment compared with normal tissue. To test this hypothesis, mice were placed in an atmosphere of 95% oxygen; redox maps showed that this treatment impaired the ability of the tumor to reduce oxygen.**

Oxygen imaging is of interest because cancer researchers have long known that **tumors create a hypoxic environment.** Noninvasive low-intensity magnetic resonance (LIMR) with a free radical contrast agent is being used to develop oxygen maps. Assessments using microelectrodes show correlations between LIMR images and pO_2.

This imaging may be used to select patients with low pO_2 levels, evaluate the effectiveness of molecular targeted reagents, and see changes in tumor and normal tissue during cancer treatment. It may also be useful for angiogenesis inhibitor assessment, stroke assessment, and cardiac ischemia assessment.

1.3.7.0 Oxidative Genome Damage and the Pathogenesis of Prostate Cancer

William Nelson, Johns Hopkins University School of Medicine

William Nelson, M.D., Ph.D., Professor, Departments of Oncology, Urology, Pharmacology, Pathology, and Medicine, The Sidney Kimmel Comprehensive Cancer Center, Johns Hopkins University School of Medicine, Baltimore, MD, presented information on oxidative damage and prostate cancer (Nelson, W. G. (2004) Prostate cancer prevention. J. Nutr. 134:3211S-3212S).

An environment of elevated ROS characterizes early pathogenesis of prostate cancer. The target cell for ROS is the prostate epithelial cell; it becomes crippled by a lack of protection from chronic oxidative damage, but the disease takes many years to develop. This makes prostate cancer a good candidate for prevention and early intervention.

All prostate cancers have many somatic genome abnormalities, although the abnormalities are heterogeneous. A common abnormality is the presence of prostate cells that have lost the ability to use the GSTπ expression system, causing hypermethylation and leading to a loss of transcriptional ability. These cells are targeted for neoplastic transformation and may have unbridled JNK signaling that gives them a growth advantage. Studies of *RNASEL*- and *MSR1*-knockout mice suggest that infection (and the resulting inflammation) may be the initiating event for prostatic lesions, although more study of familial clusters is needed to verify this.

Studies of diet and prostate cancer are equivocal on an association with fat and meat consumption. There is evidence, however, that cooking red meat at high temperatures (blackened or well done) creates heterocyclic aromatic amine carcinogens, such as 2-amino-1-methyl-6-phenylimidazo[4,5-b] pyridine (PhIP). Male mice fed PhIP have higher rates of prostate cancer; female mice have higher rates of breast cancer. Cell studies show that PhIP exposure increases formation of DNA adducts, but the addition of GSTπ1 reduces the number of adducts, detoxifying the metabolically activated *N*-hydroxy PhIP. The pathway that operates in the intact prostate may be an ATP-dependent pathway, specifically in the absence of GSTπ1.

Dr. Nelson suggested that oxidation damage in the prostate might arise from infection. Epidemiologic studies have not been totally successful in connecting inflammation from prostatitis with prostate cancer, although there are many other infections that also exist at lower levels in the prostate. Recent studies report epithelial damage in prostate epithelium, possibly caused by inflammation. For example, almost all prostate cancer cells present GSTπ1 silencing; almost 70% of samples from prostatic intraepithelial neoplasia show silenced GST π1. Early in the neoplastic process, proliferative inflammatory atrophy (PIA), a lesion characterized by GSTπ1 silencing, exists in ~10% of cells. The appearance of PIA cells may indicate the potential for subsequent cancer or an early stage of the disease, although more research is needed to confirm this finding.

Case-control studies on the use of selenium to prevent prostate cancer show a clear association between higher levels of selenium and reduced risk of prostate cancer. Further analysis of these studies shows that **plasma levels of selenium tend to decrease with age;** this parallels the time when prostate cancer rates increase. This suggests that selenium supplementation for older persons may help prevent prostate cancer.

Anti-inflammatory agents also may help prevent prostate cancer. The therapeutic target may be a COX2 enzyme, and a clinical trial to test this hypothesis is planned. The most promising targetable stage of prostate neoplastic progression appears to be in PIA, where COX2 is expressed at high levels. Another possible target is inducible nitric oxide synthase, which also is found in PIA.

1.3.8.0 Redox-Sensitive Signaling Factors and Antioxidants: How Tumor Cells Respond to Ionizing Radiation

David Gius, Center for Cancer Research, NCI

David Gius, M.D., Ph.D., Chief, Molecular Radiation Oncology Branch, Center for Cancer Research, NCI, NIH, Rockville, MD, discussed the molecular aspects of redox signaling and the role of antioxidants in this process regarding radiation exposure (Gius, D. (2004) Redox-sensitive signaling factors and antioxidants: how tumor cells respond to ionizing radiation. J. Nutr. 134:3213S-3214S).

There is a paradigm that ionizing agents induce the expression of prosurvival genes and that activation of these genes can alter phenotypes in cells. A model utilizing AP-1 DNA-binding transcriptional complex, containing a protein from the *fos* family and a protein from the *jun* family, was used to illustrate this paradigm. Various outside factors that produce oxidative stress, such as ionizing radiation, activate this complex. **Hydroxyl radicals produced from water by ionizing radiation probably act as a signal that the cell has been initiated by oxidative stress.**

Many signaling cascades that redirect metabolism in response to stress are thought to sense changes in cellular oxidation–reduction (redox) status through redox-sensitive thiol-containing proteins [such as thioredoxin (TRX), Ref-1, and AP-1]. These redox-sensitive signaling proteins and downstream transcription factors might therefore play a central role in maintaining the steady-state intracellular balance between prooxidant production, antioxidant capacity, and the repair of oxidative damage. **Ionizing radiation (IR) causes the formation of reactive oxygen intermediates that are thought to initiate several redox-sensitive signaling cascades in response to the damaging and cytotoxic effects of IR.** Because IR appears to activate redox-sensitive signaling factors, it is logical to hypothesize that critical cysteine residues contained in thioredoxin and thioredoxin reductase (TRX/TR) might mediate these signaling pathways.

Antioxidants and oxidative stress activate proteins such as thioredoxin and thioredoxin reductase Ref-1 through modification of sulfur atoms on cysteines, primary targets for redox reactions. The critical redox-sensitive signaling proteins and their cysteines transport a signal from the cytoplasm to the nucleus to turn on the transcription factor. For example, thioredoxin interacts in the nucleus with a second signaling protein, Ref-1 (i.e., an endonuclease), a protein that has a 5'-critical cysteine that is necessary for its signaling activity. Investigations confirm this observation. There is a physical interaction between Ref-1 and the *fos* and *jun* proteins of the transcriptional complex of AP-1, and the DNA-binding activity of the complex increases, as does transcription.

Hydrogen peroxide stimulates many cytoplasmic signaling factors (e.g., *erk* families, *p38*, *ras*, and *raf*). Hence, it seems logical to determine whether activation of these factors by hydrogen peroxide and ionizing radiation is important in the response to the damaging effects of oxidative stress. To address this issue, cell lines that overexpress wild-type or cysteine mutant forms of TR were used. The mutant form of TR lacks critical *N*-terminal cysteine residues that presumably are involved with the transfer of electrons from NADPH to TRX, effectively inhibiting the ability of TR to reduce TRX. The results of the experiments with cells that over-express wild-type TR demonstrated constitutive increases in AP-1 DNA-binding activity and reporter gene expression (relative to vector controls), with little further induction after exposure to IR. In contrast, cell lines that overexpress mutant TR showed no increase in constitutive AP-1 DNA-binding activity and reporter gene expression (relative to vector controls), as well as no induction after IR. In addition, very similar results were observed with the permanently transfected cell lines expressing the wild-type and mutant TRX genes. Interestingly, this observed increase in AP-1 DNA-binding activity is independent of increased total TRX or c-Fos and c-Jun protein levels. Finally, preliminary results suggested that TR may regulate AP-1 activity by a mechanism involving the regulation of TRX subcellular localization. The results of these experiments, combined with earlier results, strongly support the hypothesis that after exposure to IR, TR mediates an alteration in the redox state of TRX that participates in the activation of AP-1 DNA binding activity and gene expression. In addition, it appears that the critical cysteines in TR and TRX are targets for this signaling process, further suggesting a mechanism involving alternations in the redox status of these proteins.

Based on these results, it is appealing to hypothesize that TR is a signaling factor in a cascade that begins with IR-induced free radicals in the cytoplasm, then activates transcription factors in the nucleus, which, in turn, regulate downstream genes that protect the cell from the oxidative stress induced by free radicals. This raises several interesting questions regarding the mechanisms involved in cytoplasmic signaling cascades activated by H_2O_2 or IR as well as the specific factors that pass the signal from the cytoplasm to the nucleus. The results of these studies identify the cysteine residues located in the *N*-terminal regions of TR and TRX as critical for IR-induced activation of AP-1 activity. Thus, it would appear that these critical cysteine residues are targets for the passage of redox-sensitive cellular signals to transcription factors in response to stress. In this model, subtle changes in cellular redox potential induced by a stressing agent could alter the flow of electrons through the cysteine residues of TR and TRX, causing profound changes in protein activity. These critical cysteines would appear to act as redox-sensitive "sulfhydryl switches" that reversibly modulate protein activity and allow signal transduction cascades to redirect metabolism in response to radiation-induced stress using redox-sensitive transcription factors.

To summarize the model, **hydrogen peroxide and ionizing radiation produce free radicals**; the NADP level is altered in cytoplasm and mitochondria (not proven); thioredoxin reductase is activated and passes the signal on to thioredoxin, which is transported into the nucleus; thioredoxin forms a physical interaction with REF1; REF1 passes the signal to the AP-1 transcriptional complex, which is composed of *fos* and *jun*, each of which have critical cysteine in the DNA-binding domain; and DNA-binding activity increases.

1.3.9.0 Session 6: Wrap-up

Session Chair: *John Milner, DCP, NCI*

Panel Members: *Steven Clinton, Steven Zeisel, Richard Rivlin, David Rosenthal, Susan Mayne, and William Nelson*

Dr. Milner began the session by restating the purpose of the meeting. The main purpose was to assist clinicians and researchers regarding recommendations on diet, including the use of dietary supplements, for minimizing the risk of cancer through prevention efforts and by working in concert with other types of therapy. It is clear that interindividual variability is a large issue, as is the definition of *antioxidant*. The NIH needs suggestions on how to move forward on these issues. He also noted that Dr. von Eschenbach, the new director of NCI, has requested research on discovery, development, and delivery in all areas of cancer research

Dr. Rosenthal said that, as a clinician, it is difficult to make any recommendation to a patient because the answers are not clearly known. There is a need to assimilate the available information before clinical trials are carried out. Standard measurements of intake must also be done first, which may involve the use of biomarkers.

Dr. Zeisel said that oxidants and antioxidants act in many ways, via a series of signaling pathways, as well as by causing a series of structural effects (e.g., damage to proteins, lipids, and DNA). He suggested that cell culture methods might be a place to gain information to use in the development of model systems before human trials are planned. The NIH should invest in a model system with outcome markers for each of the important signaling pathways and functional outcomes (e.g., apoptosis, necrosis, and structural damage) so that they can be measured accurately. Once the model system is implemented, dose and combinations of antioxidants can be investigated.

Dr. Clinton commented that there is a lot of information already known, although clinicians do not have the guidance necessary to make the decisions they must make. An investment in translational animal studies seems necessary to determine the outcome of antioxidant use.

Dr. Mayne reaffirmed the comments made by Dr. Clinton but added that there is a need to determine what antioxidants people are taking through data collection. In addition, there is a need to validate biomarkers and collect them for populations through observational studies.

Dr. Rivlin said that there are many challenges for scientists (e.g., understanding the mechanisms and basic science), clinicians (e.g., letting patients know how complex the issues are), and consumers who want good information.

Dr. Rosenthal added that looking at the past should be a lesson in how we could move forward in the future. The pharmaceutical industry, in the current environment, has no incentive to do any specific research in the antioxidant arena. Because natural products are not patentable in the usual sense, it is all the more important for the NCI to step in to fund development of infrastructure to conduct research and trials in order to answer many of these questions. This will give some direction as to what the industry is allowed to do and say regarding health claims it would like to make for dietary supplements.

Dr. Milner informed participants that a U54 mechanism initiative (collaborative research) will be issued soon that will ask for research applications from those interested in investigating the nutritional modulation of genes associated with cancer. There will be $28 million in funding for this collaborative research, which could be used to investigate free radicals. In addition, there is existing RO3 and R21 funding that can be used for this research.

Key comments made by participants during this session included the following:

It is difficult to make the leap from experimental studies to human clinical trials because studies in cell lines show very different responses to antioxidant exposure with regard to gene expression as opposed to responses in animals or in situ tumors in humans.

It may be hard to recruit eligible patients to clinical trials of antioxidant use because many people are already taking antioxidants. For example, at least one-half of the participants in the PCPT trial were already taking selenium and vitamin E, and many would not agree to stop taking them to participate in the SELECT trial.

If it is advisable to discontinue antioxidants before radiotherapy, is it not logical that we also tell patients to reduce their intake of fruits

and vegetables that contain antioxidants? It was stated that this comment was only meant to highlight the lack of information regarding antioxidants and radiotherapy or chemotherapy. In response, Dr. Mayne commented that the bioavailability of ß-carotene in supplements is 10 to 20 times that of ß-carotene normally found in food, implying that one must also consider the dose.

There are antioxidant enzymes that are highly efficient at removing ROS, such as superoxide and hydrogen peroxide. These are catalytic reactions to antioxidants. It may be important to understand the effects of chemotherapy and radiotherapy on antioxidant enzymes (as well as phase I and phase II enzymes), which may play a more important role in reducing oxidative stress than antioxidant compounds

Recommendations

Recommendations were developed from comments made by the panel members, speakers and from the audience during the comment period.

There is a critical need to use an evidence-based approach for summarizing data, drawing conclusions, and making recommendations about antioxidant usage and efficacy. An advisory panel approach may need to be developed to assist with this process while research continues.

This evidence-based approach should focus on the need to answer the myriad questions surrounding pro- and antioxidative mechanisms of action associated with antioxidant use, and what effects dose and environment have on these mechanisms before recommending nutritional or nutritional-pharmacologic interventions.

There is a need for additional short- and longer-term clinical trials (both small interventions with specific agents as well as larger placebo-controlled double-blind studies) that build on the substantial in vitro and preclinical data.

Biomarkers, including biomarkers of oxidative stress and damage as well as markers of exposure and consumption, must be identified and validated.

There is a need to study the relation of genetic variants to specific cancers and develop in vitro models systems to study them.

It is important to evaluate molecular targets and signals to explain what happens in the cell and why the same signaling pathway can be beneficial in one instance of oxidative stress and harmful in another.

A central database will allow easier comparison of research results related to antioxidants and help with data-mining activities and the design of probing studies.

Among those engaged in antioxidant research, there is a need to investigate, develop, and cultivate collaborations with existing NCI programs, such as the Early Detection Research Network and the Mouse Models for Human Cancers Consortium, as well as other institutes and industrial research organizations.

Presented as part of the conference "Free Radicals: The Pros and Cons of Antioxidants," held June 26–27 in Bethesda, MD. This conference was sponsored by the Division of Cancer Prevention (DCP) and the Division of Cancer Treatment and Diagnosis, National Cancer Institute, NIH, Department of Health and Human Services (DHHS); the National Center for Complementary and Alternative Medicine (NCCAM), NIH, DHHS; the Office of Dietary Supplements (ODS), NIH, DHHS; the American Society for Nutritional Science; and the American Institute for Cancer Research and supported by the DCP, NCCAM, and ODS. Guest editors for the supplement publication were Harold E. Seifried, National Cancer Institute, NIH; Barbara Sorkin, NCCAM, NIH; and Rebecca Costello, ODS, NIH.

1.4.0.0 Antioxidant (NAC) may stop pulling out of hair (trichotillomania)

7-17-09 Our brains can give rise to all manner of odd psychiatric problems, but one of the strangest is **trichotillomania - better known as hair-pulling**. The uncontrollable desire to yank out one's hair may seem like a freaky sideshow diagnosis, but the disorder is actually not so uncommon, **affecting perhaps 2 million American adults over 22**. Exact numbers are hard to come by since people with the condition often hide it - sometimes they don't even appear in public because of their embarrassing, mangy bald spots. There is no approved treatment.

But a paper published in the prestigious *Archives of General Psychiatry* offers a simple new hope for trichotillomania sufferers. In a small trial of 50 hair pullers, more than half of those who took an over-the-counter antioxidant called **N-acetylcysteine**, which is available in pill form at mainstream stores like GNC and Vitamin Shoppe, had improvement of symptoms after 12 weeks, compared with 16% of those taking a placebo.

If the findings bear out, they may herald a potential new treatment for an age-old condition. As psychiatric symptoms go, hair-pulling is among the earliest recorded. According to Dr. Jon Grant, a trichotillomania expert at the University of Minnesota School of Medicine and the lead author of the new paper, Hippocrates himself said that in order to test whether patients were faking their illness, doctors must ask whether they are pulling out their hair. The behavior is so commonly associated with distress that the stock phrase to describe **a stressful situation is that it causes you to tear your hair out**.

We seem wired to attack our hair under traumatic conditions, possibly because forcibly extracting hair is painful; it can divert attention from stress to the more immediate matter of how to solve a pressing problem. For chronic hair pullers, that diversion turns into addictive psychological relief. Some people with trichotillomania pull out hairs not only from their heads but also from their pubic areas and armpits; **as many as 20% eat their hair; a small minority pull other people's hairs**. "Many say it's not painful but more of a sense of just a tug, one that provides a calming feeling," says Grant. "Some of these people are not even aware they are pulling their hair. Their spouses will say, 'Stop that,' and they are not even aware they have a clump of hair on their lap."

Grant theorizes that trichotillomania may be a kind of grooming irregularity that falls into the obsessive-compulsive family of disorders. "Some parrots pull out all their feathers," he says. "Some mice pull out all their fur."

That may explain why the antioxidant N-acetylcysteine can help prevent it. The compound is thought to work by reducing the synaptic release of a neurotransmitter called glutamate. As Grant told me, **glutamate is the communication chemical that "tells the brain, 'Do it! Do it! Do it! Do it!'** And the rest of the brain can be overwhelmed by this drive state." Reduce glutamate and you may reduce the drive state. Previous studies have suggested the supplement may also reduce urges to use cocaine and to gamble.

Likewise, in Grant's 12-week study, **those compulsive hair pullers who were randomly assigned to receive 1,200 to 2,400 milligrams of N-acetylcysteine a day experienced a 40% reduction in scores on a test designed to measure trichotillomania. Unfortunately the patients did**

not report a substantial improvement in quality of life, but Grant believes that may be because three months is too soon for unsightly bald spots to have grown back.

Currently, most patients with trichotillomania are treated with psychotherapy or anti-depressants, including selective serotonin-reuptake inhibitors (SSRIs), like Prozac. But in recent years, four studies that looked at SSRIs in the treatment of trichotillomania showed they are not effective in relieving the condition. (Indeed, there is an emerging debate about the limitations of SSRIs, which received enormous media exposure in the '90s and have become the go-to drug to treat not only depression but, with varying success, anxiety, nicotine addiction, body-image problems, bipolar disorder, psychosis and a host of other mental disorders.) While there's been less research on drugs that manipulate glutamate - perhaps because it can be modulated fairly easily with nonprescription amino acids like N-acetylcysteine - the new study suggests the neurotransmitter may play a key role not only in the rare condition of hair-pulling but also in other obsessive-compulsive problems.

I believe that NAC is a dangerous drug because it successfully blocks EMOD-induced apoptosis of neoplastic cells.

1.4.1.0 Vitamins C and E and Beta Carotene Supplementation and Cancer Risk: A Randomized Controlled Trial

Observational studies suggested that a diet high in fruits and vegetables, both of which are rich with antioxidants, may prevent cancer development. However, **findings from randomized trials of the association between antioxidant use and cancer risk have been mostly negative.**

Methods: From **8171 women** who were randomly assigned in the **Women's Antioxidant Cardiovascular Study, a double-blind, placebo-controlled 2 x 2 x 2 factorial trial of vitamin C (500 mg of ascorbic acid daily), natural-source vitamin E (600 IU of α-tocopherol every other day), and beta carotene (50 mg every other day), 7627 women who were free of cancer** before random assignment were selected for this study. Diagnoses and deaths from cancer at a specific site were confirmed by use of hospital reports and the National Death Index. Cox proportional hazards regression models were used to assess hazard ratios (represented as relative risks [RRs]) of common cancers associated with use of antioxidants, either individually or in combination. Subgroup analyses were conducted to determine if duration of use modified the association of supplement use with cancer risk. All statistical tests were two-sided.

Results: During an average 9.4 years of treatment, 624 women developed incident invasive cancer and 176 women died from cancer. **There were no statistically significant effects of use of any antioxidant on total cancer incidence**. Compared with the placebo group, the RRs were 1.11 (95% confidence interval [CI] = 0.95 to 1.30) in the vitamin C group, 0.93 (95% CI = 0.79 to 1.09) in the vitamin E group, and 1.00 (95% CI = 0.85 to 1.17) in the beta carotene group. Similarly, no effects of these antioxidants were observed on cancer mortality. Compared with the placebo group, the RRs were 1.28 (95% CI = 0.95 to 1.73) in the vitamin C group, 0.87 (95% CI = 0.65 to 1.17) in the vitamin E group, and 0.84 (95% CI = 0.62 to 1.13) in the beta carotene group. Duration and combined use of the three antioxidants also had no effect on cancer incidence and cancer death.

Conclusions: **Supplementation with vitamin C, vitamin E, or beta carotene offers no overall benefits in the primary prevention of total cancer incidence or cancer mortality** (Vitamins C and E and Beta Carotene Supplementation and Cancer Risk: A Randomized Controlled Trial. Jennifer Lin, Nancy R. Cook, Christine Albert, Elaine Zaharris, J. Michael Gaziano, Martin Van Denburgh, Julie E. Buring, JoAnn E. Manson. JNCI Journal of the National Cancer Institute 2009 101(1):14-23).

1.4.2.0 Nutritional Prevention of Cancer: basically a failure

The prospects for cancer prevention through micronutrient supplementation have never looked worse.

Several large, randomized cancer prevention trials have recently reported no reduced risk from micronutrient supplementation (Zhang SM, Cook NR, Albert CM, et al. Effect of combined folic acid, vitamin B_6, and vitamin B_{12} on cancer risk in women. A randomized trial. JAMA (2008) 300(17):2012–2021) (Lin J, Cook NR, Albert CM, et al. Vitamins C and E and beta carotene supplementation and cancer risk: a randomized controlled trial. J Natl Cancer Inst (2009) 101(1):14–23) (Lippman SM, Klein EA, Goodman PJ, et al. Effect of selenium and vitamin E on risk of prostate cancer and other cancers. The Selenium and Vitamin E Cancer Prevention Trial (SELECT). JAMA (2009) 301(1):39–51) (Gaziano JM, Glynn RJ, Christen WG, et al. Vitamins E and C in the prevention of prostate and total cancer in men. The Physicians' Health Study II Randomized Controlled Trial. JAMA (2009) 301(1):52–62).

The short report by Figueiredo et al. in this issue of the Journal adds to a growing body of evidence that **micronutrient supplementation may be harmful**.

Figueiredo et al. have conducted a secondary analysis from a trial that reported previously that **folate (1 mg/d) increased the risk of recurrence of an advanced colorectal adenoma by 67%** (Cole BF, Baron JA, Sandler RS, et al. Folic acid for the prevention of colorectal adenomas: a randomized clinical trial. JAMA (2007) 297(21):2351–2359).

They have found that **folate increased the risk of prostate cancer by 163%.** Among studies addressing micronutrient supplementation for the prevention of cancer, **only a single randomized trial, testing 1200 mg of calcium for preventing the recurrence of colorectal polyps, has reported a statistically significant and positive result for its primary cancer outcome** (Baron JA, Beach M, Mandel JS, et al. Calcium supplements for the prevention of colorectal adenomas. N Engl J Med (1999) 340(2):101–107), whereas **large trials testing supplementation with multivitamins, folate, selenium, β-carotene, and vitamins E, C, D, B_6, and B_{12} have found no benefits.**

Even clinical trials designed to test agents that were found to reduce cancer risk in secondary analyses of previous trials, such as vitamin E and selenium for prevention of prostate cancer, have failed to find benefit from supplementation (Lippman SM, Klein EA, Goodman PJ, et al. Effect of selenium and vitamin E on risk of prostate cancer and other cancers. The Selenium and Vitamin E Cancer Prevention Trial (SELECT). JAMA (2009) 301(1):39–51).

The harmful effects of β-carotene supplementation in heavy smokers are well established (Omenn GS, Goodman GE, Thornquist MD, et al. The β-Carotene and Retinol Efficacy Trial (CARET) for chemoprevention of lung cancer in high risk populations: smokers and asbestos-exposed workers. Cancer Res. (1994) 54(7):2038s–2043s), and it **now appears that folate supplementation may increase cancer risk as well.**

Because **the likelihood that micronutrient supplementation will be included in any public health policy for cancer control has become vanishingly small**, it is a good time to step back and consider what we have learned and how we might better focus cancer chemoprevention research in the future.

The primary lesson from our experience in the nutritional prevention of cancer is that it is not simple. It was not unreasonable to test micronutrients for cancer prevention, given the findings in cohort studies that high concentrations of some serum micronutrients and high consumption of some micronutrient-rich foods were associated with reduced cancer risk.

We must remember that we were misled by the erroneous free radi-crap theory.

However, in hindsight, this approach appears excessively reductionist. If food patterns do indeed affect cancer risk, this benefit is more likely related to energy intakes, relative macronutrient density, and exposure to complex mixtures of bioactive compounds that may include not only micronutrients but also non-nutrients such as glucosinolates and cathechins. In the trial reported by Figueiredo et al., for example, high serum folate at baseline was associated with reduced prostate cancer risk; this association likely was with foods high in folate or with a dietary pattern containing high-folate foods and not with folate itself since **folate supplementation increased the risks of prostate cancer**.

Furthermore, the notion that some is good and therefore more is better has been proven wrong; it is more likely that for any given micronutrient, there is an optimal range of intake. We generally can define and understand the effects of micronutrient deficiency, and in deficient populations, **there is limited evidence that supplementation at levels found in foods can reduce cancer risk** (Blot WJ, Li JY, Taylor PR, et al. Nutrition intervention trials in Linxian, China: supplementation with specific vitamin/mineral combinations, cancer incidence, and disease-specific mortality in the general population. J Natl Cancer Inst (1993) 85(18):1483–1492) (Duffield-Lillico AJ, Dalkin BL, Reid ME, et al. Selenium supplementation, baseline plasma selenium status and incidence of prostate cancer: an analysis of the complete treatment period of the Nutritional Prevention of Cancer Trial. BJU Int (2003) 91(7):608–612).

However, the long-term effects of micronutrient supplementation at levels below those that induce acute toxicity are not as well understood. Again, using the folate supplementation trial as an example, it is not unreasonable to assume that optimal levels of folate are associated with more fidelity in DNA replication and thus a lower risk of spontaneous mutations, but high folate may also support more rapid cell growth and promote carcinogenesis in previously initiated cells. It is safe to conclude that cancer prevention is not going to be as simple as recommending high-dose micronutrient supplements for middle-aged and older adults.

The best directions for new research in the nutritional prevention of cancer are not simple to prescribe, but we suggest two areas for consideration. First, we should turn our attention back to cohort studies. Although clinical trials are certainly the most rigorous approach to test effects of dietary patterns on cancer risk, **our experience shows clearly that current dietary interventions do**

not achieve the sustained, substantial behavior change over the many years needed to complete a clinical trial with a cancer incidence endpoint (Kristal AR. Are clinical trials the "gold standard" for cancer prevention research? Cancer Epidemiol Biomarkers Prev (2008) 17:3289–3291).

But a new and substantial investment in cohort studies will be necessary because almost all past cohort studies have relied upon a very poor tool for measuring diet, **the food frequency questionnaire, which has proven to be so inaccurate that drawing conclusions about diet and cancer from studies using it is unwise** (Kristal AR, Peters U, Potter JD. Is it time to abandon the food frequency questionnaire? Cancer Epidemiol Biomarkers Prev (2005) 14(12):2826–2828).

New cohorts using improved dietary assessment methods, or the modification of existing cohorts to add better methods, is certainly one important direction for further research. Second, we need a concerted effort to develop human models for cancer prevention that do not require many thousands of study participants and many years of follow-up. This effort essentially entails the transition of mechanistic studies from in vitro and animal models to humans, which is difficult to organize and even more difficult to get funded because it requires cross-disciplinary and innovative collaboration between nutritional scientists, molecular biologists, oncologists, and statisticians. This model development can be illustrated by an example from our research, which addresses the association found in observational studies between broccoli consumption and reduced prostate cancer risk (Kristal AR, Stanford JL. Cruciferous vegetables and prostate cancer risk: confounding by PSA screening. Cancer Epidemiol Biomarkers Prev (2004) 13(7):1265) (Giovannucci E, Rimm E, Liu Y, Stampfer M, Willett W. A prospective study of cruciferous vegetables and prostate cancer. Cancer Epidemiol Biomarkers Prev (2003) 12(12):1403–1409) (Kirsh VA, Peters U, Mayne ST, et al. Prospective study of fruit and vegetable intake and risk of prostate cancer. J Natl Cancer Inst (2007) 99(15):1200–1209).

From in vitro, animal, and limited human studies, we know that sulforaphane, a compound derived from broccoli, upregulates expression of genes with an antioxidant response element, including *AKR1C1* and *AKR1C2*, the enzymes that catabolize dihydrotestosterone. In a trial requiring only 100 men, we will test whether *AKR1C1* and *AKR1C2* expressions are induced and intraprostatic dihydrotestosterone is reduced following sulforaphane supplementation and whether the kinetics of prostate cancer cell proliferation are altered favorably as a result. When a trial of this type is successful, it would be followed by additional small trials designed and powered to test alternative doses and formulations of dietary compounds, as well as identify any individual genetic characteristics that strongly modify treatment response. Ultimately, this body of knowledge could be used to motivate and more rationally design large-scale trials with cancer endpoints. These suggestions may seem controversial to some. Nevertheless, they can serve as a starting point for discussions among cancer prevention scientists about new directions we can pursue for research in human nutrition and cancer risk **(**Nutritional Prevention of Cancer: New Directions for an Increasingly Complex Challenge. Alan R. Kristal, Scott M. Lippman. JNCI Journal of the National Cancer Institute 2009 101(6):363-365**).**

1.4.3.0 Vitamin Supplements and Cancer Prevention: Where Do Randomized Controlled Trials Stand?

Cancer chemoprevention as a concept and research methodology that examines inhibition of human carcinogenesis by nutritional, phytochemical, and other pharmacological substances dates to at least the early 1980s (Sporn MB. Combination chemoprevention of cancer. Nature (1980) 287(5778):107–108) (Peto R, Doll R, Buckley JD, Sporn MB. Can dietary beta-carotene materially reduce human cancer rates? Nature (1981) 290(5803):201–208).

At that time, a flurry of chemoprevention trials was launched predicated on epidemiological observations regarding potential protective roles for a wide range of foods and nutrients, including retinoids, beta carotene, calcium, and lower dietary fat in several cancers, and on basic research that provided both corroboration of the hypotheses through tumor inhibition in experimental models and evidence relevant to the responsible biological mechanisms. However, **only a few of the randomized controlled studies, or RCT's, have demonstrated the hoped-for reductions—or even unanticipated benefits—in incidence or recurrence of neoplasia from nutrient supplementation or dietary modification.**

For example, **the Nutritional Prevention of Cancer Study, which aimed to prevent nonmelanoma skin cancers with selenized yeast, failed to do so**, but unexpected yet statistically significant reductions in prostate, lung, and colorectal cancers were observed (Clark LC, Combs GF Jr, Turnbull BW, et al. Effects of selenium supplementation for cancer prevention in patients with carcinoma of the skin. A randomized controlled trial. Nutritional Prevention of Cancer Study Group. JAMA (1996) 276(24):1957–1963).

Similarly, **the Nutritional Intervention Trial targeted a high esophageal cancer incidence area and found a 21% reduction in gastric (but not**

esophageal) cancer mortality in response to a selenium, beta carotene, and vitamin E combination (Blot WJ, Li JY, Taylor PR, et al. Nutrition Intervention Trials in Linxian, China: supplementation with specific vitamin/mineral combinations, cancer incidence, and disease-specific mortality in the general population. J Natl Cancer Inst (1993) 85(18):1483–1492).

In the Calcium Polyp Prevention Study, daily supplementation with calcium carbonate did lead to a 15% reduction in colorectal adenomatous polyp recurrence (Baron JA, Beach M, Mandel JS, et al. Calcium supplements for the prevention of colorectal adenomas. N Engl J Med (1999) 340(2):101–107).

1.4.4.0 Failed studies and harmful endpoints

The majority of similar cancer trials demonstrated no chemopreventive efficacy for their primary neoplastic endpoints [eg, (Wactawski-Wende J, Kotchen J, Anderson G, et al. Calcium plus vitamin D supplementation and the risk of colorectal cancer. N Engl J Med (2006) 354(7):684–696) (Lee I, Cook N, Gaziano J, et al. Vitamin E in the primary prevention of cardiovascular disease and cancer. JAMA (2005) 294(1):56–65) (Hercberg S, Galan P, Preziosi P, et al. The SU.VI.MAX Study: a randomized, placebo-controlled trial of the health effects of antioxidant vitamins and minerals. Arch Intern Med (2004) 164(22):2335–2342) (Hennekens CH, Buring JE, Manson JE, et al. Lack of effect of long-term supplementation with beta carotene on the incidence of malignant neoplasms and cardiovascular disease. N Engl J Med (1996) 334(18):1145–1149)], **and in some there was evidence of unexpected harmful effects, such as an increased number of lung cancers in those receiving beta carotene in the Alpha-Tocopherol, Beta-Carotene Cancer Prevention (ATBC) Study** (The Alpha-Tocopherol, Beta Carotene Cancer Prevention Study Group. The effect of vitamin E and beta carotene on the incidence of lung cancer and other cancers in male smokers. N Engl J Med (1994) 330(15):1029–1035) (Albanes D, Heinonen OP, Taylor PR, et al. Alpha-tocopherol and beta-carotene supplements and lung cancer incidence in the Alpha-Tocopherol, Beta-Carotene Cancer prevention study: effects of base-line characteristics and study compliance. J Natl Cancer Inst (1996) 88(21):1560–1570) **and Beta-Carotene and Retinol Efficacy Trial (CARET)** (Omenn GS, Goodman GE, Thornquist MD, et al. Effects of a combination of beta carotene and vitamin A on lung cancer and cardiovascular disease. N Engl J Med (1996) 334(18):1150–1155 Omenn GS, Goodman GE, Thornquist MD, et al. Risk factors for lung cancer and for intervention effects in CARET, the Beta-Carotene and Retinol Efficacy Trial. J Natl Cancer Inst (1996) 88(21):1550–1559), **and an increased number of colorectal neoplasias in participants receiving folic acid in the Aspirin/Folate Polyp Prevention Study** (Cole B,

Baron J, Sandler R, et al. Folic acid for the prevention of colorectal adenomas: a randomized clinical trial. JAMA (2007) 297(21):2351–2359).

1.4.5.0 Low fat diets fail to prevent adenomas

Other nonsupplementation trials of dietary modification including **two that assessed the effect of lower fat intake yielded statistically null results for their primary hypotheses** (Schatzkin A, Lanza E, Corle D, et al. Lack of effect of a low-fat, high fiber diet on the recurrence of colorectal adenomas. N Engl J Med (2000) 342(16):1149–1155) (Prentice R, Thomas C, Caan B, et al. Low-fat dietary pattern and cancer incidence in the woman's health initiative dietary modification randomized controlled trial. J Natl Cancer Inst (2007) 99(20):1534–1543), although the latter study showed a small breast cancer incidence reduction.

1.4.6.0 Vitamins C and E fail to prevent cancer or heart disease

The findings of Lin et al. (Lin J, Cook NR, Albert C, et al. Vitamin C and E and beta carotene supplementation and cancer risk: a randomized controlled trial. J Natl Cancer Inst (2008) 101(1):14–23) in this issue of the Journal fall into the well-populated category of null trials. Using a factorial design, the **Women's Antioxidant Cardiovascular Study**, or WACS, tested supplementation for 8–10 years with beta carotene (50 mg daily), vitamin C (as ascorbic acid, 500 mg daily), and vitamin E (as RRR-alpha-tocopherol, 600 IU every other day) in more than 7600 women who at study entry were at least 40 years old and at elevated risk of cardiovascular disease. Based on 624 cancer diagnoses (41% of which were breast cancers) and 176 cancer deaths, the investigators observed relative risks (RRs) for the beta carotene, vitamin C and vitamin E trial arms of 1.00, 1.11, and 0.93, respectively, for overall cancer incidence, and 0.84, 1.28, and 0.87, respectively, for relative mortality. **The investigators concluded that the vitamins had no effect, singly or in combination.** Duration of active supplementation within the range studied, compliance, and "drop-in" use of extrastudy supplements did not appear to account for the findings.

1.4.7.0 Vitamins C and E and B6 and B12 fail to prevent cardiovascular disease

By contrast, the "lack of complete follow-up" alluded to by the investigators as a methodological limitation [presumably the 93% follow-up completeness through January 31, 2005, and/or exclusion of approximately 40 unconfirmed cases] or the high cardiovascular disease (CVD) risk of the study population which might overshadow other health benefits may have contributed to the lack of efficacy for the cancer endpoints. **Neither the antioxidants nor the fourth intervention added later—a combination of folic acid and vitamins B_6 and B_{12} – had any statistically significant effects in terms of cardiovascular disease endpoints** (Cook NR, Albert CM, Gaziano JM, et al. A randomized factorial trial of vitamins C and E and beta carotene in the secondary prevention of cardiovascular events in women: results from the Women's Antioxidant Cardiovascular Study. Arch Intern Med (2007) 167(15):1610–1618) (Albert C, Cook N, Gaziano J, et al. Effect of folic acid and B vitamins on risk of cardiovascular events and total mortality among woman at high risk for cardiovascular disease. JAMA (2008) 299(17):2027–2036).

1.4.8.0 Folic acid, B6 and B12 fail to prevent breast cancer

Their just-reported findings for **folic acid–B vitamins and cancer were that overall rates and breast cancer rates were comparable in the active and placebo arms** (Zhang SM, Cook NR, Albert CM, Gaziano JM, Buring JE, Manson JE. Effect of combined folic acid, vitamin B6, and vitamin B12 on cancer risk in women: a randomized trial. JAMA (2008) 300(17):2012–2021). Thus, taken as a whole, **WACS provides little or no evidence that such vitamin supplementation as tested offers any measurable preventive impact on cancer in women.**

Despite the trial's conclusion that there were no overall benefits for primary cancer prevention, two of the specific findings reported by Lin et al. deserve additional mention because they corroborate previous trial results and demonstrate the potential for site-specific efficacy. The first is the possible effect of vitamin E supplementation in preventing colorectal cancer (RR = 0.63), similar to what was observed in the ATBC Study and in a pooled analysis of serum tocopherol levels in cohort studies. The second is the elevated lung cancer risk in the beta carotene arm, along with modest excess overall cancer risk in smokers and heavier drinkers. **The suggested harmful effects from vitamin C for lung and pancreatic cancers, with the former effect achieving statistical significance,** are also noteworthy and raise questions concerning the chemopreventive potential of ascorbic acid. All these observations, based on the randomized design, represent value-added data that will contribute to a better understanding of cancer etiology and prevention and the appropriate role of these micronutrient supplements.

Nutritional intervention trials inevitably test multiple biological effects that can and should be expected even with single-agent supplements such as those used in WACS. **Functionally diverse putative cancer preventive mechanisms**

have been demonstrated for vitamins C and E, beta carotene, and many other nutrients that have been tested in tumorigenesis and cell culture experiments. These mechanisms include inhibition of, or interference with, oxidative damage and free radical formation, cell proliferation, retinoic acid receptor signaling, angiogenesis, nitrosamine formation, and inflammation, as well as enhancement of apoptosis, cellular differentiation, and immune function (Longnecker MP, Martin-Moreno JM, Knekt P, et al. Serum alpha-tocopherol concentration in relation to subsequent colorectal cancer: pooled data from five cohorts. J Natl Cancer Inst (1992) 84(6):430–435).

Nutritional supplements also modulate integral cellular detoxification and other metabolic pathways, notably cytochrome p450 enzymes (e.g., CYP 1A1), that have extensive and diverse effects on metabolism. This could be one explanation for some of the findings of recent meta-analyses suggesting adverse effects in trials where dosages and the role of high-risk populations have been considered. Conversely, because cell culture experiments can demonstrate beneficial effects for thousands of compounds on myriad molecular targets they should be followed by careful examination of safety clinical and observational data before selection of interventional agents, dosages, and target populations for future trials.

WACS is but the most recently reported example of an informative, efficient, "multitasked" prevention study. Controlled trials allow for the simultaneous examination of primary and multiple secondary endpoints and thus help the research community, public health and medical practitioners, and the public gain a more comprehensive understanding of cancer preventative strategies that might be considered, including possible modifications of prevalent lifestyle behaviors such as vitamin supplement use in the United States (Albanes D. Antioxidant supplements and mortality. JAMA (2007) 298(4):400).

These RCTs are an integral and important component of nutritional epidemiological cancer research programs that test mature hypotheses in the appropriate populations. The conduct of these trials has depended on experimental, dietary, and serologic studies that allowed for rational selection of candidate micronutrients that could be ethically and safely tested in controlled settings. Consideration of supplementation dosages should be in line with observational data where evidence based on middle-level or higher (but physiological and not pharmacological) intakes suggests benefit. Vitamin E may be an example of this with WACS and many of the trials discussed here opting for 300–400 IU of alpha-tocopherol per day in the face of the ATBC Study's beneficial findings for prostate cancer (and possibly colorectal and lung cancers) based on a 50-IU dose. **Selection of study populations should also consider the possibility that persons of low or**

deficient nutritional status might be most susceptible to intervention efficacy [eg, (Duffield-Lillico AJ, Dalkin BL, Reid ME, et al. Selenium supplementation, baseline plasma selenium status and incidence of prostate cancer: an analysis of the complete treatment period of the Nutritional Prevention of Cancer Trial. BJU Int (2003) 91(7):608–612) (Blot WJ, Li JY, Taylor PR, et al. Nutrition Intervention Trials in Linxian, China: supplementation with specific vitamin/mineral combinations, cancer incidence, and disease-specific mortality in the general population. J Natl Cancer Inst (1993) 85(18):1483–1492).

The recent announcement of early termination of the Selenium and Vitamin E Cancer Prevention Trial's (SELECT) interventions because of lack of efficacy and observation of possible adverse events (ie, small and not statistically significant increases in type 2 diabetes in those receiving selenium alone and in prostate cancer incidence in the vitamin E (alone) group) should serve as a reminder that the unexpected can happen in these well-designed trials (Lippman SM, Klein EA, Goodman PJ, et al. Effect of selenium and vitamin E on risk of prostate cancer and other cancers: the Selenium and Vitamin E Cancer Prevention Trial (SELECT). [published online ahead of print December 9, 2008]*JAMA*. doi:10.1001/jama.2008.864).

Large controlled studies are perhaps more likely to reveal unanticipated outcomes owing to at least two factors. One is the intense balancing that randomization imposes such that "confounding" and case–control differences in highly correlated lifestyle characteristics and risk factors play no role in an intervention outcome in a large RCT (although effect modification of efficacy can and has occurred). The other is the highly specific "exposure" represented by the intervention(s)—not a questionnaire estimation of a self-reported nutrient intake or a one-time blood sampling. Careful, comprehensive surveillance for a wide range of potential clinical outcomes and unknown adverse effects required for efficacy and safety monitoring in trials also contributes to multifaceted and unanticipated outcomes.

Progress in the field of cancer prevention, as in most scientific pursuits, can vary from slow, incremental accumulation and synthesis of new findings relevant to a range of hypotheses, to quantum advances from much anticipated corroboration or refutation of hypotheses and pure surprises. It is easy to view unexpected RCT outcomes as failures or proof of an overly simplified or **overly sold concept**, and obviously, the most satisfying trials are those that deliver the goods; that is, they show their anticipated cancer prevention effects. Null trials or those with unexpected outcomes should not, however, be viewed as failures; they have and will continue to shed light on the causes of cancer and help us discover the means for its prevention (Vitamin Supplements and Cancer Prevention: Where Do Randomized Controlled Trials Stand? Demetrius Albanes. JNCI Journal of the National Cancer Institute 2009 101(1):2-4).

1.5.0.0 Selective Enhancement of Cellular Oxidative Stress by Chloroquine

The following was excerpted, modified from: Selective Enhancement of Cellular Oxidative Stress by Chloroquine: Implications for the Treatment of Glioblastoma Multiforme. Steven M. Toler, Pharm.D., Ph.D.; Dennis Noe, M.D.; Amarnath Sharma, Ph.D. Neurosurg Focus. 2006;21(6).

from Neurosurgical focus. Published 5/2/2007. http://www.medscape.com/viewarticle/554870_print

Chloroquine is used in the treatment of malaria, a disease caused by infection with the parasite *Plasmodium*. Although chloroquine appears to possess diverse pharmacological activity, **its plasmodicidal activity results from augmentation of parasite oxidative stress. Chloroquine also appears to augment oxidative stress in metabolically active mammalian cells, including human astroglial cells.** The authors propose that chloroquine may augment oxidative stress induced by radiotherapy in the treatment of glioblastoma multiforme, enhancing therapeutic efficacy. Such an effect would be consistent with the known pharmacological effects of chloroquine observed in *Plasmodium*. **Other selective redox agents, such as tempol and artemisinin, should be investigated clinically for therapeutic benefit when co-administered with combined radio- and chemotherapy for cancer**.

1.5.1.0 Summary

Glioblastoma multiforme is the most common and aggressive primary glial tumor, comprising 30% of all brain malignancies in adults. This is a rapidly infiltrating tumor that is resistant to current therapies, resulting in a median survival duration of approximately 1 year. Despite all efforts, few therapeutic advances have been achieved over the last decade that have significantly improved survival rates. Nevertheless, results from **two small studies support the suggestion that the addition of chloroquine to conventional therapy may improve the median survival duration in patients with GBM** (Briceno E, Reyes S, Sotelo J: Therapy of glioblastoma multiforme improved by the antimutagenic chloroquine. *Neurosurg Focus 14(2): E3, 2003)* (Sotelo J, Briceno E, Lopez-Gonzalez MA: Adding chloroquine to conventional treatment for glioblastoma multiforme: a randomized, double-blind, placebo-controlled trial. *Ann Intern Med 144:* 337-343, 2006*)*.

1.5.2.0 Advances in Treatment of GBM, glioblastoma multiforme

In an initial study, a statistically significant increase in survival time was found following conventional therapy plus chloroquine (33 ± 5 months) relative to conventional therapy plus placebo (11 ± 2 months, nine patients in each group). In a second follow-up study, the median survival time increased from 11 months following placebo plus standard therapy to 24 months following chloroquine plus standard therapy (15 patients in each group), and although these results failed to achieve statistical significance, there was a trend toward an increase in overall survival for the chloroquine treatment arm. At least two theories have been proposed to account for the apparent therapeutic benefit associated with chloroquine treatment: 1) chloroquine possesses antimutagenic properties that impede the development of treatment-resistant clones; and 2) the lysosomotrophic effects of chloroquine lead to cell necrosis. However, an alternative hypothesis, **enhancement of cellular oxidative stress, may better explain the apparent improvement** in median survival duration noted in patients undergoing concurrent chloroquine therapy.

1.5.3.0 Importance of Oxidative Stress ==

The treatment of patients with GBM typically includes surgical tumor ablation and radiotherapy with or without chemotherapy. Postoperative radiotherapy has been recognized as the standard of care for several decades, whereas the additional use of chemotherapy has been controversial. Recently, tumor ablation followed by radiotherapy and concurrent temozolomide administration has become the new standard of care. In the studies mentioned earlier (Briceno et al. and Sotelo et al.), chloroquine therapy was initiated 5 days postsurgery, prior to the start of radiotherapy (total dose 6000 Gy) or chemotherapy (four cycles of carmustine, 200 mg/m^2) in patients with GBM.

In tissues exposed to treatment, **radiotherapy produces cytotoxic free radicals and extensive oxidative stress**. (Cook JA, Gius D, Wink DA, Krishna MC, Russo A, Mitchell JB: Oxidative stress, redox, and the tumor microenvironment. *Semin Radiat Oncol 14:* 259-266, 2004) (Doroshenko N, Doroshenko P: The glutathione reductase inhibitor carmustine induces an influx of Ca2+ in PC12 cells. *Eur J Pharmacol 497:* 17-24, 2004).

Ionizing radiation produces a number of reactive oxygen species, including superoxide ion, hydroxyl radical, and hydrogen peroxide; it is currently postulated that the primary therapeutic effects from radiotherapy are mediated through the generation of cytotoxic reactive oxygen species. (Cook JA, Gius D, Wink DA, Krishna MC, Russo A, Mitchell JB: Oxidative stress, redox, and the tumor microenvironment. *Semin Radiat Oncol 14:* 259-266, 2004) (Lee HC, Kim DW, Jung KY, Park IC, Park MJ, Kim MS, et al: Increased expression of antioxidant enzymes in radioresistant variant from U251 human glioblastoma cell line. *Int J Mol Med 13:* 883-887, 2004).

Furthermore, **cancer cells accumulate iron, and radiotherapy elevates intracellular free iron concentrations that can lead to the production of cytotoxic hydroxyl radicals through the Fenton reaction** (Kwok JC, Richardson DR: The iron metabolism of neoplastic cells: alterations that facilitate proliferation? *Crit Rev Oncol Hematol 42:* 65-78, 2002) (Weijl NI, Elsendoorn TJ, Moison RM, Lentjes EG, Brand R, Berger R, et al: Non-protein bound iron release during chemotherapy in cancer patients. *Clin Sci (Lond) 106:* 475-484, 2004).

Therefore, **cells exposed to radiotherapy are subjected to heightened oxidative stress.** These cells must either adapt to such conditions or perish. Adaptation often includes induction of biochemical pathways that quench or mediate the destructive effects of reactive intermediates. **In U251 human glioblastoma cells, radiation has been shown to induce the expression of a number of antioxidant enzymes, including superoxide dismutase (twofold) and glutathione peroxidase** (fivefold) (Lee HC, Kim DW, Jung KY, Park IC, Park MJ, Kim MS, et al: Increased expression of antioxidant enzymes in radioresistant variant from U251 human glioblastoma cell line. *Int J Mol Med 13:* 883-887, 2004).

Antioxidant adaptations noted in U251 human glioblastoma cells are consistent with clinical observations of GBM resistance to radiotherapy (Lee HC, Kim DW, Jung KY, Park IC, Park MJ, Kim MS, et al: Increased expression of antioxidant enzymes in radioresistant variant from U251 human glioblastoma cell line. *Int J Mol Med 13:* 883-887, 2004).

1.5.4.0 Chloroquine Enhances Oxidative Stress

Chloroquine, a 9-aminoquinoline synthesized in 1934, is used in the treatment of malaria, a disease caused by infection with the

parasite *Plasmodium*. Although chloroquine appears to possess diverse pharmacological activities, **its plasmodicidal effect results from augmentation of oxidative stress in this parasite** (Farombi EO, Shyntum YY, Emerole GO: Influence of chloroquine treatment and Plasmodium falciparum malaria infection on some enzymatic and non-enzymatic antioxidant defense indices in humans. *Drug Chem Toxicol 26:* 59-71, 2003) (Ginsburg H, Golenser J: Glutathione is involved in the antimal arial action of chloroquine and its modulation affects drug sensitivity of human and murine species of Plasmodium. *Redox Rep 8:* 276-279, 2003) (Monti D, Basilico N, Parapini S, Pasini E, Olliaro P, Taramelli D: Does chloroquine really act through oxidative stress? *FEBS Lett 522:* 3-5, 2002).

During schizogony, *Plasmodium* subsists on amino acids derived from hemoglobin, resulting in production of the prooxidant hemeiron complex ferriprotoporphyrin IX. This heme iron complex is detoxified in *Plasmodium* through a number of glutathione-dependent pathways (including incorporation into hemozoin). Chloroquine appears to inhibit the detoxification of ferriprotoporphyrin IX, in part by diminishing the availability of **reduced glutathione. Excess iron and ferriprotoporphyrin IX, in the absence of sufficient glutathione, leads to autooxidation and parasite death**. Furthermore, chloroquine appears to interact directly with free ferriprotoporphyrin IX in an electron transfer reaction that produces highly reactive radicals.

Chloroquine also appears to augment oxidative stress in mammalian cells that have high metabolic activity, and it generates reactive oxygen species in human astroglial cells (Balo KP, Mensah A, Mihluedo H: [Chloroquine maculopathy and prevention of malaria.] *J Fr Ophtalmol 19:* 770-776, 1996 [Fr]) (Lai WW, Lam DS: Chloroquine-induced bull's eye maculopathy. *Hong Kong Med J 11:* 55-57, 2005) (Murugavel P, Pari L: Attenuation of chloroquine-induced renal damage by alpha-lipoic acid: possible antioxidant mechanism. *Ren Fail 26:* 517-524, 2004) (Pari L, Murugavel P: Protective effect of alpha-lipoic acid against chloroquine-induced hepatotoxicity in rats. *J Appl Toxicol 24:* 21-26, 2004) (Park J, Choi K, Jeong E, Kwon D, Benveniste EN, Choi C: Reactive oxygen species mediate chloroquine-induced expression of chemokines by human astroglial cells. *Glia 47:* 9-20, 2004) (Toler SM: Oxidative stress plays an important role in the pathogenesis of drug-induced retinopathy. *Exp Biol Med (May wood) 229:* 607-615, 2004) (Wielgo-Polanin R, Lagarce L, Gautron E, Diquet B, Laine-Cessac P: Hepatotoxicity associated with the use of a fixed combination of chloroquine and proguanil. *Int J Antimicrob Agents 26:* 176-178, 2005).

1.5.5.0 Therapeutic Benefit of Chloroquine: Potential Mechanisms

We propose that **chloroquine may augment oxidative stress induced by radiotherapy in cancer cells**. Such an effect would be consistent with the known pharmacological effects of chloroquine in *Plasmodium*. **Directed radiotherapy selectively produces oxidative stress in targeted cancer cells,** generating free radicals and elevating concentrations of free iron. Following such treatment, cancer cells often induce antioxidant defenses as an adaptive response to thwart cytotoxicity. Agents such as **chloroquine that promote oxidative stress** may hinder the effectiveness of these antioxidant adaptations, resulting in heightened tumoricidal activity. The therapeutic benefit noted with chloroquine appears to be the result of effective proliferation of reactive intermediates initiated by radiotherapy, resulting in increased tumor cytotoxicity.

At least two alternative theories have been proposed to explain the apparent benefit of adding chloroquine to traditional GBM therapy. One theory contends that chloroquine is antimutagenic and prevents the development of treatment-resistant clones.[2] However, there are at least two inconsistencies with this theory. First, there is little evidence that chloroquine is antimutagenic. Although quinacrine, a compound structurally related to chloroquine, has demonstrated antimutagenic properties in two cell lines, it appears to be mutagenic in others. Furthermore, most data on chloroquine support its mutagenic properties rather than antimutagenic effects, which is consistent with other 4-aminoquinolines.

Second, if chloroquine possessed antimutagenic properties, diminished rather than enhanced efficacy might be expected with concurrent radio- and chemotherapy, because treatment-induced mutations are what yield the desired tumor cytotoxicity.

Another theory states that the radiosensitization produced by chloroquine is due to its lysosomotrophic effects. The lysosomotrophic effects produced by chloroquine, a cationic amphipathic drug, result from protonation and subsequent molecular "trapping" within acidic lysosomes, which elevates lysosomal pH. However, there are vast numbers of cationic amphipathic drugs that have not been reported to induce radiosensitization. The radiosensitizing effects of chloroquine appear to be unique relative to other lysosomotrophic compounds like ammonium chloride, fluoxitine, and amitriptyline. Although lysosomal membrane rupture contributes to cell necrosis after radiation and chloroquine treatment, the cause of membrane rupture may be lysosomal membrane lipid peroxidation produced by the distinct prooxidant properties of chloroquine rather than lysosomotrophism.

Discussion

Cancer cells, including malignant glial cells, accumulate iron to a greater extent than do normal cells, producing a condition similar to that found in *Plasmodium*. (Kwok JC, Richardson DR: The iron metabolism of neoplastic cells: alterations that facilitate proliferation? *Crit Rev Oncol Hematol 42:* 65-78, 2002) (Mykhaylyk O, Dudchenko N, Cherchenko A, Rosumenko V, Zozulya Y: Dysregulation of non-heme iron metabolism in glial brain tumors. *Med Princ Pract 14:* 221-229, 2005).

After radiotherapy, protein-bound intracellular iron is released as free iron, and **chloroquine may promote oxidative stress through propagation of reactive oxygen species in a manner similar to the stress produced in *Plasmodium*.** Of interest, the antimalarial agent artemisinin has recently demonstrated activity against human glioma and breast cancer cell lines in vitro (Kim SJ, Kim MS, Lee JW, Lee CH, Yoo H, Shin SH: Dihydro artemisinin enhances radiosensitivity of human glioma cells in vitro. *J Cancer Res Clin Oncol 132:* 129-135, 2006).

Artemisinin, an endoperoxide, appears to be activated to release reactive oxygen species by elevated concentrations of intracellular free iron in both *Plasmodium* and cancer cell lines (Kamchonwongpaisan S, Meshnick SR: The mode of action of the antimalarial artemisinin and its derivatives. *Gen Pharmacol 27:* 587-592, 1996) (Lai H, Sasaki T, Singh NP: Targeted treatment of cancer with artemisinin and artemisinin-tagged iron-carrying compounds. *Expert Opin Ther Targets 9:* 995-1007, 2005).

Another **redox-active compound, tempol (a piperidine nitroxide)**, demonstrates antiproliferative effects in C6 glioma cells in vitro and in mouse xenografts (Gariboldi MB, Ravizza R, Petterino C, Castagnaro M, Finocchiaro G, Monti E: Study of in vitro and in vivo effects of the piperidine nitroxide Tempol-a potential new therapeutic agent for gliomas. *Eur J Cancer 39:* 829-837, 2003).

Tempol, a superoxide dismutase mimetic, converts superoxide into hydrogen peroxide, which in the presence of free iron is converted to the highly reactive hydroxide ion (Chen YF, Cowley AW Jr, Zou AP: Increased H(2)O(2) counteracts the vasodilator and natriuretic effects of superoxide dismutation by tempol in renal medulla. *Am J Physiol Regul Integr Comp Physiol 285:* 827-833, 2003).

Like chloroquine, **tempol has demonstrated plasmodicidal activity in vitro, further supporting theories about its role as a prooxidant agent in the presence of available iron** (Schwartz E, Samuni A, Friedman I, Hempelmann E, Gokenser J: The role of superoxide dismutation in malaria parasites. *Inflammation 23:* 361-370, 1999).

Tempol, artimisinin, and chloroquine appear to demonstrate little cytotoxicity in the absence of preexisting oxidative stress, thus sparing normal cells (Ravizza R, Cereda E, Monti E, Gariboldi MB: The piperidine nitroxide Tempol potentiates the cytotoxic effects of temozolomide in human glioblastoma cells. *Int J Oncol 25:* 1817-1822, 2004) (Gariboldi MB, Ravizza R, Petterino C, Castagnaro M, Finocchiaro G, Monti E: Study of in vitro and in vivo effects of the piperidine nitroxide Tempol-a potential new therapeutic agent for gliomas. *Eur J Cancer 39:* 829-837, 2003).

Because it appears that chloroquine serves as a promoter rather than an initiator of oxidative stress, it may also prove beneficial in cases in which oxidative stress is therapeutically induced by cytotoxic agents. **Tumor-selective chemotherapeutic regimens (such as emodin/arsenic trioxide) that preferentially induce heightened oxidative stress in cancer cells** might exhibit additional efficacy if coadministered with chloroquine (Yang J, Li H, Chen YY, Wang XJ, Shi GY, Hu QS: Anthra quinones sensitize tumor cells to arsenic cytotoxicity in vitro and in vivo via reactive oxygen species-mediated dual regulation of apoptosis. *Free Radic Biol Med 37:* 2027-2041, 2004).

Similarly, chloroquine may prove beneficial in the treatment of tumors characterized by phenotypic autooxidations, such as melanoma (Joshi G, Sultana R, Tangpong J, Cole MP, St Clair DK, Vore M: Free radical mediated oxidative stress and toxic side effects in brain induced by the anti cancer drug adriamycin: insight into chemobrain. *Free Radic Res 39:* 1147-1154, 2005) (Sander CS, Hamm F, Elsner P, Thiele JJ: Oxidative stress in malignant melanoma and non-melanoma skin cancer. *Br J Dermatol 148:* 913-922, 2003).

Both pre- and posttreatment, malignant melanoma cells exhibit heightened oxidative stress (Sander CS, Hamm F, Elsner P, Thiele JJ: Oxidative stress in malignant melanoma and non-melanoma skin cancer. *Br J Dermatol 148:* 913-922, 2003).

Preclinically, **chloroquine increases cytotoxicity in melanoma cell lines when administered alone or following radiation or hyperthermia** (Inoue S, Hasegawa K, Ito S, Wakamatsu K, Fujita K: Anti melanoma activity of chloroquine, an antimalarial agent with high affinity for melanin. *Pigment Cell Res 6:* 354-358, 1993). Therefore, chloroquine therapy might prove beneficial in the treatment of malignant melanoma.

Because of its ability to induce oxidative stress in *Plasmodium*, chloroquine has been used in the treatment of malaria for nearly half a century. Other chemically and pharmacologically diverse agents, such as artemisinin and tempol, demonstrate plasmodicidal and tumoricidal activities, providing evidence for a link between therapeutic effect and the creation of oxidative stress. These prooxidant activities probably explain the beneficial effects noted with chloroquine in the treatment of GBM with traditional radiotherapy. By selectively promoting tumor oxidative stress, chloroquine could prove beneficial in the treatment of other tumor types such as malignant melanoma, or following chemotherapy. Other selective redox agents, such as tempol and artemisinin, should be investigated clinically for their possible therapeutic benefit when coadministered with traditional GBM regimens

I believe that chloroquine should be added to my regimen to increase oxidative capacity for disease prevention and therapy.

The synthetic quinoline drug-**Chloroquine (CQ) is commonly used in treatment of malaria. CQ is used for the treatment of a wide range of disease such as inflammation, extra intestinal amebiasis or gout and rheumatoid arthritis** (Issacson D, Elgart M, Tunner ML: Antimalarial in dermatology. Int J Dermatol, 1982; 21: 379-395) (Augustijus P, Verbeke N: Stereoselective phoramacokinetic properties of chloroquine de-ethyl-chloroquine in humans. Clin Pharmacokinet, 1993; 24: 259-269).

The Structure of Chloroquine ($C_{18}H_{26}ClN_3$).

Clinical treatment with CQ is often accompanied by serious side effects such as gastrointestinal upset, pruritus, headache, visual disturbances and cardiotoxic action (Ekpechi OL, Okoro A: Chloroquine causes unpleasant pruritus in Nigerians. Arcb Derm, 1964; 89: 631).

CQ has been reported to cause liver damage and a severe life threatening toxic hepatitis at higher dosage (Pari L, Murugavel P: Protective effect of a - lipoic acid against CQ induced hepatotoxicity in rats. J Appl Toxicol, 2004; 24: 21-26) (Dass EE, Shah KK: Paracetamol and conventional antimalarial drugs induced hepatotoxicity and its protection by methionine in rats. Ind J Exp Biol, 2000; 38: 1138-1142) (Koranda FC: Antimalarials, J Am Acad Dermatol, 1981; 4: 650-655).

CQ acts directly or indirectly and alters antioxidant status that makes certain organs, more susceptible to oxidative stress. Several studies have shown that CQ causes increased lipid peroxidation and decreased enzymic and non-enzymic antioxidants (Magwere T, Saik YS, Hasler JA: Effect of chloroquine treatment on antimalarial enzymes in rat liver and kidney. Free Rad Biol Med, 1997; 22: 321-327 Murugavel P, Pari L: Attenuation of chloroquine-induced renal damage by a - lipoic acid: possible antioxidant mechanism. Ren Fail, 2004; 26: 515 - 522).

1.5.6.0 The lamentable free radical story

Free radicals are the highly unstable chemicals that attack, infiltrate, and injure vital cell structures. Most stable chemical compounds in the body possess a pair of electrons. Sometimes, one member of the electron pair gets stripped away. The resulting compound (that is short of one electron) is called a free radical.

In chemistry, the term free radical means that it is now free to combine with another element to form a new stable compound. One way to think of free radical is the way our social system work. In a family there is husband and wife. They are joined together. Both are "tied up" or not available for other partners. Let us assume that they get 'separated'. Now we have two "free" persons who are looking for other partners to partner with. The way free radicals work, one of these free spouse go and break up a stable marriage of another couple, by joining with one of the spouses. This results in the ouster of a person from that family creating a brand new "free radical" who goes around prowling to find another "compound" to attack. You can see that **free radicals can do lot of harm by forming a chain reaction.**

A similar thing happens with free radicals in the body. When a free radical is born, it goes around the body looking for another compound to steal an electron from. This breaks up the "contented" couple, that results in releasing another free radical, and so on. While on the prowl, these free radicals (which are really the oxidation products from the body) can do tremendous damage to the delicate machinery of your cells. The most studied free radical chain reaction in living things is lipid peroxidation. (The term lipid refers to any fat-soluble substance, animal or vegetable. Peroxidation means the formation of a peroxide molecule. These are the molecules with the greatest proportion of oxygen molecules. For example, a water molecule has two hydrogen atoms and one oxygen atom. Hydrogen peroxide has two Hydrogen atoms and two oxygen atoms. In other words, there is an excess oxygen atom in a hydrogen peroxide molecule.)

Ninety eight percent of the oxygen we breathe is used by tiny powerhouses within our cells called mitochondria, that convert sugar, fats and inorganic phosphate by combining with oxygen into adenosine triphosphate (ATP), the universal form of energy we need to live. This energy producing activity of the mitochondria involves a series of intricate, complex and vital biochemical processes that depends on vast numbers of enzymes (estimates vary from 500 to 10,000 sets of oxidative enzymes). These, in turn, depends on dozens of nutrient factors and co-factors. In this metabolism process, a very small amount of left over oxygen loses electrons, creating free radicals. These **free radicals burn holes in our cellular membranes**. Calcium penetrate our cells through these holes. This excess calcium results in cell death. This, in turn, weakens tissues and organs. As this damage continues, **our body become "rusty",** less able to fight other invaders such as cancer, hardening of the arteries, premature aging, and other bodily disorders.

Because of the amount of oxygen we breathe **every day (our bodies take 630 quadrillion damaging oxygen hits per day,** each of our cells takes about 10,000 hits per day and each DNA strand in the cell gets hit 5,000 times per day. This free radical bombardment causes a typical human cell to undergo thousands of changes or mutations daily. If a DNA strand gets hit and is not repaired before its twin gets hit, we will have the onset of a potentially lethal cancer.

In addition to the oxygen we breathe, the **free radicals can also come from such things as environmental pollution, radiation, cigarette smoke, chemicals, and herbicides.**

The key to having a healthy body is to repair the damages caused by the free radicals before it is too late, and to protect the body's tissue cells from the free radicals before they cause mutations. Antioxidants are substances that have free-radical chain-reaction-breaking properties. Like a bouncer, the **antioxidants** deactivate potentially dangerous free radicals before they can damage a cells' machinery. Most of these antioxidants come from plants and are called phytochemicals. **More than 60,000 of such plant chemicals are identified.** Among the most effective and dedicated antioxidants are Vitamin A, C, and E (known as the ACE trio.). Out of these, Vitamin C is the most powerful.

Each cell produces its own antioxidants. But the ability to produce them decreases as we age. That is why our diet should supply anti-oxidants, phytochemicals (fruits and vegetables are a good source for this.) and additional vitamins and minerals. (http://www.holisticonline.com/Chelation/chel_ben_free_rad.htm).

I believe that articles such as the above are clearly examples of nonscience/nonsense.

The FDA estimates that there are currently 29,000 supplements on the market, with 1,000 new ones introduced annually. The Nutrition business Journal estimated 2005 U. S. dietary supplement sales at $20.9 billion, an increase of 2.1 billion since 2003.

1.5.7.0 Vitamins C and E can undo health benefit of exercise

5-11-09 **Antioxidant vitamins can undo some of the most important health benefits of exercise,** research has shown. **Taking vitamins C and E after a workout appears to prevent physical exercise improving the body's energy regulation**, a study found.

Exercise is known to increase sensitivity to the hormone insulin, which governs the way cells use sugar as an energy source. Type 2 diabetes occurs when the body becomes resistant and less sensitive to insulin.

Some vitamins can block this beneficial effect of exercise, the new findings suggest. Ironically, it is the supplements' health-boosting properties that appear to be to blame. Allegedly, **Vitamins such as C and E neutralise destructive "free radical" molecules called reactive oxygen species that can damage cells and DNA, and speed up ageing.**

These molecules are a by-product of metabolism and generated in larger numbers during vigorous exercise. But the new research suggests that as well as causing damage, **oxygen free radicals also spur the body into becoming more sensitive to insulin.** By mopping up the molecules, antioxidant vitamins cancel out this beneficial effect.

In addition, scientists from the University of Jena in Germany found that **the vitamins weakened the body's own exercise-induced free radical defence system,** which relies on the production of natural antioxidants.

The findings add to the growing evidence that vitamins have complex effects on the body which can do harm as well as good.

Taking vitamins C and E after a workout appears to prevent physical exercise improving the body's energy regulation, a study found. **Exercise is known to increase the effects of the hormone insulin, which keeps blood sugar levels in balance which is vital for energy and it appears that supplements of vitamin C and E may block this beneficial effect of exercise,** the new findings suggest.

Destructive "free radical" molecules called reactive oxygen species (ROS) can damage cells and DNA, and speed up ageing and are produced in large numbers during vigorous exercise. However **these molecules are also used by the body to prevent cellular damage after exercising and vitamins such as C and E neutralise their effects**, it has been found.

Researchers compared two groups of 20 men who took 85-minute exercise sessions five days a week for a month. One group took daily vitamin C and E supplements during their training and the other did not.

The researchers report that men who consumed antioxidant supplements showed no changes in their reactive oxygen levels, whereas **those who did not take antioxidant showed an increase in the formation of the free radicals.**

After four weeks of training, the men who did not take antioxidant supplements were shown to be sensitive to the effects of insulin and the men on the supplements were not.

The authors show that **reactive oxygen likely has a positive effect on the body by increasing insulin sensitivity**, and **this effect is blocked by the consumption of antioxidant vitamins.**

Dr Michael Ristow, from the University of Jena in Germany, and colleagues wrote in the journal **Proceedings of the National Academy of Sciences: "We find that antioxidant supplements prevent the induction of molecular regulators of insulin sensitivity and endogenous antioxidant defence by physical exercise.**

"We propose that transiently increased levels of oxidative stress reflect a potentially health-promoting process, at least in regards to prevention of insulin resistance and Type 2 diabetes mellitus."

I discussed the relationship of EMODs to diabetes in my book on this subject.

1.5.8.0 Antioxidant stress (glutathione) leads to heart failure in mice

Reductants, sometimes referred to as antioxidants, are elements or compounds that easily give up an electron to become "oxidized," while oxidizing agents readily accept electrons. In the body, such oxidation-reduction (redox) reactions are integral to the release and storage of energy. Many cellular pathways are also sensitive to the prevailing redox condition.

Despite the popular notion that antioxidants, such as vitamins C and E, offer health-promoting benefits by protecting against damaging free radicals, a new study in the **August 10, 2007 issue of the journal Cell** reveals that, in fact, balance is the key. The researchers show in mice that **an overload of natural antioxidants can actually lead the heart to failure.**

There is plenty of evidence about the damaging effects of oxidative stress, but "there is another side to the coin," **said Ivor Benjamin of the University of Utah, Salt Lake City.** "There has been so much emphasis on free radicals to the exclusion of the potential consequences of reductants. Our study provides **the first bona fide example of the role that reductive stress can play in disease."**

Oxidative stress, which consumes reducing equivalents, has been often implicated in numerous cardiac and other diseases, Benjamin noted. However, the possibility remained that an inverse imbalance could provoke reductive stress, with the potential for similar deleterious effects. Indeed, **reductive stress had been demonstrated in simpler organisms but not in mammals and/or disease states**, he said.

In the current study, the researchers examined mice carrying a human mutation earlier linked to so-called protein aggregation skeletal myopathies and cardiomyopathies, in which weakening skeletal and heart muscle contain clumps of proteins. Although the genetic basis for the disease had been linked to mutations in one of two genes, the mechanism responsible remained mysterious.

The researchers now show that **mice with one of the mutant genes, áB-crystallin, specifically in the heart develop the same symptoms seen in human patients, including heart enlargement, progressive heart failure, and an early death. They further show that the animals' hearts are under reductive stress**.

The find initially took Benjamin by surprise, he said. They had conducted a test traditionally used to measure the level of oxidative stress in the animals, expecting they might see higher than normal levels. Instead, **they found the mice had "markedly reduced" oxidative stress levels due to an abundance of a natural antioxidant known as glutathione.**

The mutant mouse hearts exhibited a heightened stress response, including higher activity of heat shock proteins that have been documented in human heart failure, Benjamin explained. Such stress responses yield reactive oxygen species, triggering antioxidative pathways to kick in. In the diseased animals, however, that pathway—in which oxidized glutathione is recycled to its reduced, antioxidant form—soon got out of hand, producing **excess levels of the reduced glutathione and a condition of reductive stress.**

Moreover, they showed that the offspring of the heart-diseased animals and mice with lower levels of one of the antioxidant enzymes, glucose-6-phosphate dehydrogenase (G6PD), were relieved of their symptoms. That finding suggests that drugs or other treatments targeting the antioxidant pathway through G6PD "might modify the phenotype and the natural history of this inherited disorder in humans," according to the researchers.

The results found in the heart suggest that reductive stress might underlie other diseases, as well. "Our findings open up a whole new line of investigation in protein aggregation diseases," **including neurodegenerative diseases such as Alzheimer's and Huntington's disease,** Benjamin said.

The researchers include Namakkal S. Rajasekaran, Ryan P. Taylor, Andras Orosz, Xiu Q. Zhang, Tamara J. Stevenson, William H. Barry, and Shannon J. Odelberg of University of Utah, Salt Lake City; Patrice Connell, Liang-Jun Yan, and Ronald M. Peshock of University of Texas Southwestern Medical Center, Dallas; Elisabeth S. Christians of University of Texas Southwestern Medical Center, Dallas and Centre for Developmental Biology UMR5547, Toulouse; Jane A. Leopold and Joseph Loscalzo of Brigham and Women's Hospital, Harvard Medical School, Boston; Ivor J. Benjamin of University of Utah, Salt Lake City and University of Texas Southwestern Medical Center, Dallas.

(Rajasekaran et al.: "Human aB-Crystallin Mutation Causes Oxido-Reductive Stress and Protein Aggregation Cardiomyopathy in Mice." Publishing in Cell 130, 427–439, August 10, 2007. DOI 10.1016/j.cell.2007.06.044 http://www.cell.com). **I believe that this is just a glimpse into the "allowance" of disease because of EMOD insufficiency.**

1.5.9.0 Largest multivitamin study shows they do nothing

2-9-09 **Many postmenopausal women take multivitamins in the belief that they help prevent cardiovascular disease or cancer, but a large study has found that they do neither. Previous studies have had mixed results**, some suggesting that multivitamin supplements are associated with a reduced risk for some cancers, others finding little or no effect.

For the new findings, published in the February 9, 2009 issue of The Archives of Internal Medicine, researchers analyzed data from **68,132 women who were enrolled in a clinical trial and 93,676 in an observational study.** They followed the women for an average of about eight years to track the health effects of multivitamins. After controlling for age, physical activity, family history of cancer and many other factors, the researchers found that **the supplements had no effect on the risk for breast cancer, colorectal cancer, endometrial cancer, lung cancer, ovarian cancer, heart attack, stroke, blood clots or mortality.**

The scientists acknowledge that women who take vitamins also engage in other healthy behaviors, and that there may be unknown variables affecting their results.

"Consumers spend money on dietary supplements with the thought that they are going to improve their health, but there's no evidence for this," said Marian L. Neuhouser, the lead author and a nutritional epidemiologist with the Fred Hutchinson Cancer Research Center in Seattle. "Buying more fruits and vegetables might be a better choice,

Thus, the largest multivitamin study shows that they do nothing.

1.6.0.0 Women's Health Initiative study 2-9-09 Multivitamins fail

Millions of postmenopausal women use multivitamins, often believing that supplements prevent chronic diseases such as cancer and cardiovascular disease (CVD). Therefore, we decided to examine associations between multivitamin use and risk of cancer, CVD, and mortality in postmenopausal women.

Methods The study included **161 808 participants** from the Women's Health Initiative clinical trials (N = 68 132 in 3 overlapping trials of hormone therapy, dietary modification, and calcium and vitamin D supplements) or an observational study (N = 93 676). Detailed data were collected on multivitamin use at baseline and follow-up time points. Study enrollment occurred between 1993 and 1998; the women were followed up for a median of **8.0 years** in the clinical trials and 7.9 years in the observational study. Disease end points were collected through 2005.

We documented **cancers of the breast (invasive), colon/rectum, endometrium, kidney, bladder, stomach, ovary, and lung; CVD (myocardial infarction, stroke, and venous thromboembolism); and total mortality.**

Results A total of 41.5% of the participants used multivitamins. After a median of 8.0 years of follow-up in the clinical trial cohort and 7.9 years in the observational study cohort, 9619 cases of breast, colorectal, endometrial, renal, bladder, stomach, lung, or ovarian cancer; 8751 CVD events; and 9865 deaths were reported. Multivariate-adjusted analyses revealed no association of multivitamin use with risk of cancer (hazard ratio [HR], 0.98, and 95% confidence interval [CI], 0.91-1.05 for breast cancer; HR, 0.99, and 95% CI, 0.88-1.11 for colorectal cancer; HR, 1.05, and 95% CI, 0.90-1.21 for endometrial cancer; HR, 1.0, and 95% CI, 0.88-1.13 for lung cancer; and HR, 1.07, and 95% CI, 0.88-1.29 for ovarian cancer); CVD (HR, 0.96, and 95% CI, 0.89-1.03 for myocardial infarction; HR, 0.99, and 95% CI, 0.91-1.07 for stroke; and HR, 1.05, and 95% CI, 0.85-1.29 for venous thromboembolism); or mortality (HR, 1.02, and 95% CI, 0.97-1.07).

Conclusion After a median follow-up of 8.0 and 7.9 years in the clinical trial and observational study cohorts, respectively, the Women's Health Initiative study provided convincing evidence that **multivitamin use has little or no influence on the risk of common cancers, CVD, or total mortality in postmenopausal women (**Multivitamin Use and Risk of Cancer and Cardiovascular Disease in the Women's Health Initiative Cohorts. Marian L. Neuhouser et al. *Arch Intern Med.* 2009;169(3):294-304**).**

Neuhouser et al investigated multivitamin use and disease risk in the Women's Health Initiative (WHI), a large study of **161 808 postmenopausal women** participating in either a set of clinical trials or an observational study. Of the WHI participants, 41.5% used multivitamins, but after a median of 8.0 years of follow-up in the clinical trials and a median 7.9 years in the observational study, **there was no evidence that multivitamins confer meaningful benefit or harm in relation to cancer or cardiovascular disease. The risk for invasive cancers of the breast, colon/rectum, endometrium, lung, bladder, and ovary was no different among women who used multivitamin compared with those who did not use multivitamins. Similarly, risk of myocardial infarction, stroke, venous thrombosis, and death from**

any cause was no different for multivitamin users than for nonusers. Multivitamins do not appear to be effective for the prevention of cancer or cardiovascular disease.

1.6.1.0 Group disputes cancer claims on One A Day vitamins

6-18-09 A consumer advocacy group on Thursday threatened to sue Bayer Healthcare if it continues to claim its One-A-Day vitamins for men reduce the risk of prostate cancer.

The **Center for Science in the Public Interest** says the company's ubiquitous TV and radio ads misleadingly claim that a key ingredient of One-A-Day Men's Health Formula and 50+ Advantage helps prevent cancer.

The group says **a study backed by the National Institutes of Health found no evidence the ingredient selenium prevents prostate cancer in men.**

"The largest prostate cancer prevention trial has found that selenium is no more effective than a placebo," said David Schardt, the group's senior nutritionist. "Bayer is ripping people off when it suggests otherwise in these dishonest ads."

Researchers halted the study of 35,000 men last October after it became clear that selenium did not prevent prostate cancer, according to the group.

Bayer said Thursday the claims on its vitamins have been approved by the Food and Drug Administration.

"We stand behind all claims made in support of our products," said Bayer spokeswoman Trisch McKernan.

Bayer's One-A-Day brand of vitamins had sales of $191 million last year, according to the company's annual report.

The Center for Science in the Public Interest also sent a letter to the Federal Trade Commission on Thursday asking regulators to halt Bayer's marketing of the vitamins. The German conglomerate has run at least 11 television ads and 9 radio ads suggesting One-A-Day vitamins can help prevent prostate cancer, according to data from VMS advertising monitoring service.

The letter argues that Bayer's advertising violates a 2007 agreement with the FTC requiring the company to back up all claims on One-A-Day vitamins with scientific evidence. Bayer entered the agreement after paying a $3.2 million penalty to settle claims that its advertising misled the public about the weight loss benefits of its vitamins.

A spokeswoman for the FTC said Thursday the agency has not yet received the group's letter.

1.6.2.0 The great vitamin debate

3-27-09 Joe Schwarcz is known for his blunt, take-no-prisoners style when he gets fired up. For the past 25 minutes, the erudite director of McGill University's Office for Science and Society and outspoken star of the Dr. Joe Show on Toronto's CFRB radio has been on a roll, **taking shots at pseudo-science, the gullible public, "vitamin advertisers who shove things down our throat" and the biggest kahuna of them all, the $23.7-billion dietary supplements industry**.

So it's just a matter of time before he mentions **Nick Nolte**.

"Look at him!" Schwarcz directs, and sure enough, an image of the aging actor's ravaged face comes to mind. These days, Nolte eschews hard living for a **thousands-of-dollars-a-week vitamin habit** in an effort to turn back the clock. "See how sick he looks?" Schwarcz says, his voice rising in exasperation. **"He takes 60 supplements a day!"**

It's an extreme example - few of us live Nolte's life, much less endure his medical bills - but it does beg the question: If 60 pills a day doesn't make a visible difference to someone's visage, what chance does a single multivitamin have?

To Schwarcz, a food chemist who wrote **2007's An Apple a Day (Harper Perennial**) to scientifically counter consumers' worst flights of food fancy, it's the $23.7-billion question. (Schwarcz says supplements do make sense; he takes vitamin D and omega-3 fatty acids.)

"People take multivitamins as nutritional insurance," he says (Statistics Canada reported in 2004 half of Canadian women take vitamins). "Most people are eating crap and thinking that they'll take a vitamin to equalize things. It's pointless. The problem with our diet is not a lack of vitamins. It's the fat, salt and sugar. Those issues are not addressed by taking more vitamins."

Or are they? According to the World Health Organization, one-third of the world's population don't get enough micronutrients. And the deficiency is not just limited to developing nations. **A 2002 study found that 97% of Canadians are deficient in vitamin D through winter and spring, while University of Guelph researchers say 78% of Canadian children are low in omega-3 fatty acids**. Many of us are also short on iron, calcium and - depending on whether you smoke, drink too much or are overweight - vitamins C and B as well.

So why not take a pill?

"The trouble is that we had a range of epidemiological studies showing that whole grains, fruits and vegetables were beneficial for a range of health issues, so **it was assumed antioxidants and vitamins were the source and we isolated them in supplements. This is too simplistic,**" Schwarcz explains.

"There are studies that show you can't take one compound from a food and get the same result as eating it."

What's more, there are growing questions about whether most supplements do any good at all, says Ottawa Hospital urologist **Dr. John Mahoney**, who recently contributed to an international National Cancer Institute-funded study that attempted - **and failed - to prove a link between reduced prostate cancer and selenium/vitamin E supplements**. The results were repeated in a recent study by the Women's Health Initiative: **Researchers found the 41.5% of women who regularly took multivitamins were no more likely to avoid a range of cancers, heart disease, stroke or blood clots than those who didn't**.

"You think they're making people better, but there's no evidence that they are," says Mahoney. "What harm could they be giving? I think I'd say that the evidence is not showing they're doing good - and we haven't proven they're doing any harm, either."

For Schwarcz, the solution is fundamental and obvious - a healthy diet. "Food has hundreds of different compounds and each one is a cog. You need many cogs working together to get the machine going. The simple fact is that people should be making the effort to eat properly."

If only it were that straightforward, say critics.

Trans fats - the bane of our arteries - are being replaced as the villain by the even scarier spectre of compromised food safety, tainted meat supplies, salmonella scares and diminished nutritional quality through pesticides, farming practices and green-picking produce that ripens on its way to market.

Still, the situation is fraught enough to feed **the exponential growth of the supplements industry,** says Brett Waslefsky, president of Employee Vita, an Arizona-based company that makes supplements aimed at people in certain careers, such as nurses and teachers.

"My view is that a supplement should never be taken as a silver bullet to replace a healthy diet or lack of exercise," Waslefsky says. "If everyone ate perfectly, if they were active, didn't smoke or drink, our industry would diminish quite a bit. But we have to be realistic. We've been raised on fast food, high-fructose corn syrup and food that isn't local anymore."

Lifestyle also has much to answer for in our low nutrient levels, says Sherry Torkos, a Niagara-based pharmacist and author of The Canadian Encyclopedia of Natural Medicine (Wiley, 2008).

"Chronic stress depletes us in vitamin B and C, birth control depletes the B vitamins, statins deplete coenzyme Q10, antacids deplete calcium and vitamin D, smoking depletes vitamin C - I could go on," Torkos says.

"The truth is most people are not getting nearly enough fruits and vegetables. Supplements can be used to complement a healthy diet and lifestyle to make up for things that cause deficiencies, like smoking, eating food with a lower nutritional value and drinking too much.

"Swallowing 100 pills a day is not necessary, there's no need to go crazy over it. So take a multivitamin. It can't hurt you."

But will it help?

Schwarcz may not be convinced, but neither does he want to "paint a picture that a One-a-Day is dangerous."

"People think they're the cure-all and they're not. The question is, do we need more vitamins than what is available in food? My advice is stop wasting your money and spend it on healthier food."

Which vitamin for what?

Despite the controversy over diet supplements, Joe Schwarcz says some supplements make sense, including the following:

Calcium: In the five years after menopause, the risk of developing osteoporosis increases rapidly as women's absorption of calcium declines. While supplementation won't completely offset bone loss, it can help, particularly if taken with vitamin D and vitamin K, found in yogurt and dark green vegetables. A recent National Cancer Institute study also found that those subjects with the highest levels of calcium had the lowest levels of colorectal cancer.

Omega-3 fatty acids: Found in cold water fish such as salmon, flax, pumpkin seeds and fortified eggs, omega-3 fatty acids have been associated with reduced risk of heart disease, high blood pressure, osteoporosis, high cholesterol levels, depression and circulatory problems.

Folic acid: According to the Public Health Agency of Canada, the incidence of neural tube defects like spina bifida has been steadily decreasing in newborn babies, due to folic acid supplementation two to three months before and throughout pregnancy.

Vitamin D: Through winter and spring, the vast majority of Canadians - up to 97% - have a vitamin D deficiency, which is linked to everything from increased colds and rickets to greater risk of some cancers, osteoporosis and type 2 diabetes.

1.6.3.0 Arthritis alternative treatments ineffective (also vitamins A, C & E)

Most complementary therapies used by people with rheumatoid arthritis are not effective, a study has suggested. The **Arthritis Research Campaign** looked at the scientific evidence available for 40 treatments. **Two thirds of treatments for rheumatoid arthritis and a fifth of treatments for osteoarthritis were found to be ineffective** by the researchers.

The Arthritis Research Campaign said it wanted people who used the therapies to know what evidence was available. **The message is not 'don't take them'** Professor Alan Silman, Arthritis Research Campaign

Rheumatoid arthritis is caused by inflammation of the lining (synovium) of the joints.

Osteoarthritis is caused by the breakdown of protective tissue called cartilage in the joints. Inflammation results when the unprotected bones of the joint begin to rub together.

It most commonly affects the joints of the fingers, knees, hips, and spine. In total, **60% of people with arthritis are thought to use some form of complementary medicine.**

1.6.4.0 Antler velvet

The researchers looked at compounds taken by the mouth or applied to the skin.

Effectiveness is measured by improvements in pain, movement or general well-being.

When the researchers examined treatments for rheumatoid arthritis, they found 13 out of 21 complementary medicines were shown to have no or little effect based on the available evidence.

The 13 were: antler velvet powder, blackcurrant seed oil, collagen, eazmov (a herbal mixture), feverfew (herb), flaxseed oil, green-lipped mussels, homeopathy, reumalex herbal mixture, selenium, the Chinese herb tong luo kai bi, vitamins A, C and E, and willow bark.

However, **fish body oil was given five out of five in the report, for being effective in reducing joint pain and stiffness.**

In addition, six out of 27 treatments for osteoarthritis were shown to have little or no effect based on the available evidence

Capsaicin gel, made from chilli peppers, proved most effective in relieving pain and joint tenderness.

But the effectiveness of glucosamine, a popular supplement used by people with OA which costs around $10 a month, which researchers have previously said was ineffective, again called into question.

For fibromyalgia, which causes widespread pain in muscles and joints, only four products were assessed, none were found to be highly effective with three medicines scoring two out of five, and the fourth just one.

The researchers also examined how safe compounds were. **One - thunder god vine, a traditional Chinese medicine - was given a "red" classification, meaning there were serious safety concerns.**

A quarter of the compounds were given an "amber" safety classification, because there were some reported side-effects.

The team said they were unable to evaluate the effectiveness of 36 therapies, including basil, green tea, sarsaparilla and St John's Wort because there was insufficient data.

Professor Gary Macfarlane, from the University of Aberdeen, said while different things worked for different people, "it is useful to also have the scientific evidence available and just as important to know how safe we think they are to use." Professor Alan Silman, the Arthritis Research Campaign's medical director, added: "We didn't start this saying this was our opportunity to knock complementary medicines. **"The message is not 'don't take them'. The message is 'if you are going to take them, be aware of what the level of evidence is'."**

Dr Peter Fisher, clinical director of the Royal London Homeopathic Hospital, said the report focused on tablets and preparations applied to the skin, missing out therapies such as acupuncture and osteopathy. "I think what really comes across in this report is how sorely under-researched this area is," he said.

Jane Gray, president, of the National Institute of Medical Herbalists added: "This report is a commendable attempt to provide information on self help products for osteo and rheumatoid arthritis."

1.6.5.0 Brain generates most EMODs

According to Dr. Jimmy Gutman, "The brain is particularly susceptible to free radical attack because **it generates more oxidative by-products per gram of tissue than any other organ."**

1.6.6.0 Patients with major CNS disease showed a 50% reduction in cerebral oxygen utilization

Cerebral oxygen and glucose metabolism have been **studied in 8 patients with biochemically defined mitochondrial myopathies** and 7 normal control subjects using positron emission tomography. Four patients had myopathy alone and 4 had predominantly central nervous system (CNS) disease. Cerebral oxygen and glucose metabolism were measured concurrently in the two groups of patients with ^{15}O, ^{11}C and ^{18}F labelled tracers and positron emission tomography (PET). Patients with major CNS disease showed an uncoupling of glucose and oxygen metabolism when compared with patients without cerebral disease and normal subjects. The mean ratio between oxygen and glucose utilization was 3.8 moles of oxygen per mole of glucose in patients with CNS disease, compared with 5.6 for controls and 6.4 for patients with myopathy alone. The altered stoichiometry in CNS cases indicates aerobic glycolysis to lactate and/or other intermediate metabolites. **Patients with major CNS disease showed a 50% reduction in cerebral oxygen utilization compared with cerebrally unaffected patients and normal subjects.**

These findings indicate that in patients with a mitochondrial encephalopathy the defect identified in skeletal muscle is also expressed in the brain (THE CEREBRAL METABOLISM OF GLUCOSE AND OXYGEN MEASURED WITH POSITRON TOMOGRAPHY IN PATIENTS WITH MITOCHONDRIAL DISEASES. R. S. J. FRACKOWIA·, S. HEROLD, R. K. H. PETTY and J. A. MORGAN-HUGHES. Brain, Vol. 111, No. 5, 1009-1024, 1988). **I believe that this clearly illustrates the crucial role of EMODs in normal brain function.**

1.7.0.0 NAC

N Acetyl l cysteine (also spelled acetylcysteine, N Acetyl L Cysteine or N-acetylcyteine) is made from the amino acid cysteine joined to an acetyl group. Acetylcysteine (sometimes abbreviated as N-A-C or NAC) is a strong antioxidant. It donates the amino acid cysteine to help form the antioxidant glutathione. Glutathione is a powerful antioxidant normally found in the body. N Acetyl Cysteine is an amino acid and antioxidant. **N Acetyl l cysteine is a precursor in the body to the critical antioxidant glutathione,** which is produced within cells, particularly by the liver. Acetylcysteine is significantly more cost effective than taking glutathione.

Some have suggested that antioxidants could theoretically interfere with the effectiveness of chemotherapy. Since chemotherapy kills cancer cells, at least in part, by creating oxidative stress, taking antioxidants could weaken the cancer-fighting ability of chemotherapy drugs. **A recent analysis of past studies found that antioxidants do not diminish the effectiveness of chemotherapy. Metabolic Brain Disease, September 2008**.

NAC is a hydrophobic derivative of amino acid cysteine. It is only this hydrophobic derivative that can cross the blood brain barrier to enter into the brain. Other hydrophobic polyphenols, such as curcumin, can also do this. This is why high dietary intakes of curcumin are related to reduced incidence of Alzheimer's.

1.7.1.0 NAC toxicity

Researchers at the University of Virginia reported in 2007 study using very large doses in a mouse model that acetylcysteine, which is found in many bodybuilding supplements, **could potentially cause damage to the heart and lungs** (Palmer LA, Doctor A, Chhabra P, *et al* (September 2007). "S-nitrosothiols signal hypoxia-mimetic vascular pathology". *J. Clin. Invest.* 117 (9): 2592–601).

They found that **acetylcysteine was metabolized to *S*-nitroso-*N*-acetylcysteine (SNOAC), which increased blood pressure in the lungs and right ventricle of the heart (pulmonary artery hypertension) in mice treated with acetylcysteine.** The effect was similar to that observed following a 3-week exposure to an oxygen-deprived environment (**chronic hypoxia**). The authors also found that SNOAC induced a hypoxia-like response in the expression of several important genes both *in vitro* and *in vivo*.

The implications of these findings for long-term treatment with acetylcysteine have not yet been investigated. The dose used by Palmer and colleagues (2007) was dramatically higher than that used in humans (Palmer LA, Doctor A, Chhabra P, Sheram ML, Laubach VE, Karlinsey MZ, Forbes MS, Macdonald T, Gaston B. "S-nitrosothiols signal hypoxia-mimetic vascular pathology." *Journal of Clinical Investigation* 2007 Sep;117(9): 2592-601).

Nonetheless, the drug's effects on the hypoxic ventilatory response have been observed previously in human subjects at more moderate doses (Hildebrandt W, Alexander S, Bärtsch P, Dröge W. "Effect of N-acetyl-cysteine on the hypoxic ventilatory response and erythropoietin production: linkage between plasma thiol redox state and O(2) chemosensitivity." *Blood* 2002 Mar 1;99(5):1552-5. Accessed November 12, 2007).

1.7.2.0 Chemo-brain/mental fog blocked by NAC

A new animal study suggests that antioxidant therapy may prevent the memory and attention problems that plague many cancer patients undergoing chemotherapy.

Often called "chemo-brain," such mental side effects are seen in up to 70 percent of chemotherapy patients by some estimates.

In the new study, researchers at West Virginia University School of Medicine in Morgantown looked at whether injections of a powerful antioxidant called N-acetyl cysteine, or NAC, could prevent chemo-related memory changes in rats.

The researchers first exposed one group of rats to two drugs commonly used to treat cancer, Adriamycin and Cytoxan. They found that compared with a group of control animals, the chemo-exposed rats showed a decline in standard tests of rodent memory.

However, that mental fog was completely prevented when the researchers gave the rats NAC injections three times per week during chemotherapy administered four times per week.

The findings, published in the **September 2008 journal Metabolic Brain Disease**, are promising. But it is far too soon for chemotherapy patients to turn to antioxidants for preventing chemo-brain, according to lead researcher Dr. Gregory W. Konat.

"I wouldn't suggest that patients do anything now," he told Reuters Health. More lab research is needed before NAC can even be moved into human clinical trials, let alone be given to patients, Konat said.

Chemotherapy patients should also not take large doses of other commonly available antioxidants, like vitamin C, according to the researcher. Konat noted that a long-standing concern with antioxidants is that they could theoretically interfere with the effectiveness of chemotherapy.

Antioxidants protect cells by neutralizing cell-damaging substances called oxygen free radicals; it's thought that this damage, known as oxidative stress, may be what's responsible for the mental side effects of chemotherapy.

However, **it's also thought that chemotherapy kills cancer cells, at least in part, by creating oxidative stress**. So in theory, taking antioxidants could weaken the cancer-fighting ability of chemotherapy drugs.

A recent analysis of past studies suggests that antioxidants do not, in fact, diminish the effectiveness of chemotherapy, Konat said. Still, he added, caution is in order. "We're dealing with a very serious condition here," he pointed out. Given the unknowns, Konat advises chemotherapy patients to not self-treat with antioxidants or take any supplement without talking to their doctors first. (SOURCE: Metabolic Brain Disease, September 2008).

1.7.3.0 Are Antioxidants Safe During Chemotherapy and Radiation Treatment?

A *Healthnotes Newswire* Opinion. By Alan R. Gaby, MD

Healthnotes Newswire (September 29, 2005)—A new report concluded that cancer **patients should avoid antioxidant supplements while receiving chemotherapy or radiation treatment** (D'Andrea GM. Use of antioxidants during chemotherapy and radiotherapy should be avoided. *CA* 2005;55:319–21), prompting a feature article in the *Wall Street Journal (*Parker-Pope, Tara. Cancer and Vitamins: Patients Urged to Avoid Supplements During Treatment; *The Wall Street Journal* 2005 Sep 20 Sect. D:1*)* which argues that **antioxidants could block the beneficial effects of standard cancer therapy**; however, the available scientific evidence does not support the view that people undergoing cancer treatment should always avoid antioxidant supplements.

The authors of the new report pointed out that radiation therapy and some chemotherapy drugs act by producing free radicals—highly reactive chemicals that can damage both cancer cells and normal cells. **Antioxidants such as vitamin C, vitamin E, coenzyme Q10, glutathione, and selenium can reduce the toxicity of free radicals** (Weijl NI, Cleton FJ, Osanto S. Free radicals and antioxidants in chemotherapy-induced toxicity. *Cancer Treat Rev* 1997;23:209–40).

While supplementing with antioxidants might, therefore, protect healthy cells from the negative effects of radiation or chemotherapy, the authors expressed concern that **taking these supplements might protect cancer cells even more than normal cells**, thereby inhibiting the beneficial effect of standard treatment.

There are situations in which antioxidant supplementation would be undesirable for cancer patients, but the issue is actually a lot more complicated than the article indicated. **Although many chemotherapy drugs do induce the formation of free radicals, their anticancer effects do not, in general, seem to depend on the formation of these free radicals.** Consequently, antioxidant supplementation may in some circumstances help prevent free-radical-induced side effects without inhibiting the positive effects of the chemotherapy.

In animal studies, giving antioxidants along with certain chemotherapy drugs did not reduce the anticancer effects of the drugs and it increased survival times, compared with the survival of animals that received chemotherapy alone. In studies in humans with cancer, coenzyme Q10 prevented the heart damage that often occurs with the cancer drug adriamycin without inhibiting its anticancer effect (Cortes EP, Gupta M, Chou C, et al. Adriamycin cardiotoxicity: early detection by systolic time interval and possible prevention by coenzyme Q10. *Cancer Treat Rep* 1978;62:887–91) (Judy WV, Hall JH, Dugan W, et al. Coenzyme Q10 reduction of adriamycin cardiotoxicity. In: Folkers K, Yamamura Y, eds. *Biomedical and Clinical Aspects of Coenzyme Q*, Vol. 4, Elsevier, 1984:231–41).

In another study of women with ovarian cancer, supplementation with selenium along with chemotherapy (cisplatin plus cyclophosphamide) prevented the loss of appetite, hair loss, vomiting, and decline in white blood cell counts that occurred when the chemotherapy was given by itself (Sieja K, Talerczyk M. Selenium as an element in the treatment of ovarian cancer in women receiving chemotherapy. *Gynecol Oncol* 2004;93:320–27).

Intravenously administered glutathione prevented cisplatin-induced nerve damage in people with stomach cancer (Cascinu S, Cordella L, Del Ferro E, et al. Neuroprotective effect of reduced glutathione on cisplatin-based chemotherapy in advanced gastric cancer: a randomized double-blind placebo-controlled trial. *J Clin Oncol* 1995;13:26–32).

Furthermore, glutathione did not interfere with the anticancer effect of cisplatin; on the contrary, there was a trend toward a better treatment response and longer survival in people given glutathione group than in those receiving chemotherapy alone.

With regard to mixing antioxidants and radiation therapy, there is very little research in humans, and the recommendation made in the article was based primarily on theory and test tube studies. However, **one preliminary study in women with cancer of the cervix suggested that antioxidants (vitamin C plus bioflavonoids) might enhance the effects of radiation therapy.** Of the women who received antioxidants along with radiation therapy, 100% had a favorable response to the treatment, whereas only 59% of women receiving radiation therapy by itself had a positive response (Cheraskin E, Ringsdorf WM Jr, Hutchins K, et al. Effect of diet upon radiation response in cervical carcinoma of the uterus: a preliminary report. *Acta Cytologica* 1968;12:433–38).

We still have a great deal to learn about the interactions between cancer treatments and antioxidant supplements. Whether or not an antioxidant supplement would be helpful, harmful, or neutral presumably depends in part on the specific antioxidant (and its dose), the chemotherapy drugs being used, the type of cancer being treated, and the type of diet the patient is consuming. **We simply do not know enough at the present time to make a categorical statement that antioxidants should never be taken along with standard cancer therapy.** However, since there is at least theoretical potential for harm, people who are undergoing cancer therapy should seek the advice of a qualified professional before supplementing with antioxidants.

1.7.4.0 If you are having Chemotherapy or radiotherapy, should you take anti-oxidants like vitamin C?

Riordan's research seems to say clearly that with vitamin C you should.

In 1999 Gotlieb went further. With Kedar Prasad, Professor of Radiology at the University of Colorado, Denver, they showed that high dose vitamin C, as well as other antioxidants, can protect healthy cells which regulate their uptake levels during treatment. Whereas Prasad is quite clear, cancer cells cannot regulate uptake and this aids their death. Whilst he is actually against high doses of vitamin C because of possible toxicity in the liver, he believes C, E or beta-carotene are highly protective.

UCLA confirmed this theory in 2004, and MD Anderson have also stated that people should take their antioxidants during radiotherapy and chemotherapy. Indeed, MD Anderson have gone further and in clinical trials have shown vitamin C and vitamin K3 enhance the effects of Bladder Cancer drugs. Other US research shows that vitamin E enhances the effects of Tamoxifen. In fact women taking vitamin E need 25 per cent less Tamoxifen.

1.7.5.0 Chemotherapy and Radiation Therapy: antioxidants O.K.

4/18/07 For nearly a decade, oncologists have been telling patients undergoing chemotherapy or radiation therapy that they should not take antioxidants and other nutritional supplements because they interfere with treatment. However, a two-part article published in the most recent issues of **Alternative Therapies**, should lay this myth to rest.

Oncologist **Charles B. Simone, MD**, and colleagues searched MEDLINE (the National Library of Medicine's database of more than 16 million medical journals dating back to the 1950s), and CANCERLIT (the National Cancer Institute's database of articles related to cancer) and came up with 280 peer- reviewed studies on the concurrent use of chemo and/or radiation and dietary supplements. These included 50 human studies involving a total of **8,251 patients.**

They found that **antioxidants and other nutritional supplements did not interfere with conventional cancer treatments and actually enhanced the killing effects of chemotherapy and radiation therapy**. In 47 of the human studies, supplements were also found to protect normal tissues and reduce the often-serious side effects of chemotherapy and radiation. **And in 15 human studies, 3,738 patients actually had increased survival -- a finding that is rare for any cancer outcome**.

Dr. Simone reports that the negative slant on supplements originated from an erroneous statement made in a 1997 New York Times by a physician from Memorial Sloan Kettering Cancer Hospital, who contended that vitamin C interfered with chemotherapy and radiation in humans. This statement had absolutely no scientific backing, yet without even reviewing the evidence, the entire oncology community adopted and continues to spread this harmful, biased misconception.

There is no downside to taking supplements while undergoing chemotherapy, but there is a tremendous upside. The immune systems of cancer patients are highly compromised, and a majority of them suffer with malnutrition. Antioxidants and other vitamins and minerals restore deficiencies in essential nutrients and enhance immune function. Furthermore, antioxidants have direct anti-tumor effects, protect against the toxic effects of conventional cancer treatments, and prolong the lives of patients.

If you'd like more information on this topic, or to schedule an interview with Charles B. Simone, MD, please call (609) 896-2646 or email Dr. Simone at mail@drsimone.com

1.7.6.0 Cancer stem cell antioxidants protect cancers against oxidants and death

2-4-09 U.S. researchers think they now understand why some cancers grow back after radiation treatment. They said a specialized type of cell known as a **cancer stem cell** has a protective mechanism that keeps radiation from damaging the DNA and proteins inside the cell. And by jamming this protective mechanism, they think they may be able to make cancer treatments work better, the team reported on **2-4-09 in the journal Nature**. "Our ultimate goal is to come up with a therapy that knocks out the cancer stem cells," said Dr. Robert Cho of Stanford University School of Medicine, who worked on the study published in the journal **Nature**.

Several research teams are focusing on **cancer stem cells, a kind of master cell that appears to have the ability to replenish tumor cells**. Finding ways to destroy these cells could make cancer far easier to treat. "It's like battling weeds," Cho said of cancer stem cells' ability to regenerate. "You can go through a big field with a weed whacker, but the weeds are going to come back unless you get the roots."

Cancer stem cells appear to resist conventional cancer treatments like radiation, and Cho and colleagues wanted to know why. In a series of experiments using cells from mice and humans, the Stanford team found that **breast cancer stem cells make much higher levels of protective proteins known as antioxidants than other cancer cells.**

These antioxidants can protect the DNA and proteins from the effects of harmful substances known as reactive oxygen species, otherwise called oxidative stress.

The researchers believe this protective mechanism helped explain why breast cancer stem cells were less likely than other cancer cells to succumb to radiation. **When the team used a drug to block an antioxidant protein called glutathione, the cancer stem cells became far more vulnerable to radiation.**

"Essentially, it inactivated the cancer stem cells' protective mechanism," team-member Michael Clarke of Stanford University said in a telephone interview. The team now hopes to find drugs that can specifically disarm that protective mechanism in cancer stem cells while sparing normal cells.

This is the same old story of antioxidants protecting cancer cells from EMOD-induced apoptic cell death.

1.7.7.0 Antioxidants May Affect Chemotherapy

By June Chen M.D. J Natl Cancer Inst. 2008. The use of antioxidant supplements during chemotherapy and radiation is a controversial topic, and clinical studies have reported **conflicting evidence.** The *Journal of the National Cancer Institute* recently published a review of randomized trial data, which suggested that cancer patients should avoid the routine use of antioxidant supplements because they may potentially decrease the efficacy of cancer therapy by protecting the tumor and reducing survival.

The researchers looked at clinical trials investigating the impact of antioxidants on radiation therapy and found evidence suggesting that antioxidant supplementation reduced overall survival. However, they also found evidence that **a particular antioxidant called amifostine might protect healthy tissues from radiation damage without increasing the radiation-resistance of cancerous tissues.**

The researchers also looked at sixteen trials that focused on the effects of antioxidant supplements on the efficacy of chemotherapy. **They found no evidence that antioxidant use adversely affected response to treatment. However, they also did not find compelling evidence that antioxidant supplementation provided any additional benefit** in treatment response.

It is still not clear whether antioxidant supplements are safe or how they might affect cancer therapy, but further research on the topic is warranted, especially with the widespread availability of, and food advertising associated with, antioxidants. (J Natl Cancer Inst. 2008;100:1-11).

1.7.8.0 Vitamin C supplements reduce benefits of anticancer drugs

In pre-clinical studies, **vitamin C appears to substantially reduce the effectiveness of anticancer drugs, say researchers at Memorial Sloan-Kettering Cancer Center.** These new findings, published in the **October 1 issue of Cancer Research,** a publication of the American Association of Cancer Research (AACR), came from studying laboratory cancer cells and mice, but the study's authors say the same mechanism may affect patient outcomes, although they add this premise needs to be tested.

"**The use of vitamin C supplements could have the potential to reduce the ability of patients to respond to therapy**," said Heaney, an Associate Attending Physician at Memorial Sloan-Kettering Cancer Center.

Use of vitamin C during cancer treatment has been **controversial**. Some studies have suggested that because vitamin C is an antioxidant it might be beneficial to cancer patients. But some classes of chemotherapy drugs produce "oxygen free radicals," unpaired oxygen molecules that can fatally react with other molecules in a cell, forcing cell death. In this theory, vitamin C could sop up the radicals, keeping the cancer cell alive despite chemotherapy treatment.

Heaney and his colleagues tested a wide variety of chemotherapy drugs – those that produce reactive oxygen and those that work in other ways – on cancer cells in the laboratory, that were pretreated with **dehydroascorbic acid (DHA), the form that ascorbic acid (vitamin C) takes to enter cells.**

They found to their surprise that every chemotherapy drug they tested – which included targeted agents **like Gleevec – did not work as well if cells were pretreated with vitamin C,** as they did on untreated cancer cells. **In the cell culture experiments, 30 to 70 percent less cancer cells treated with vitamin C were killed depending on the drug tested.**

They then checked these findings by implanting the cancer cells into mice, and again found that, in an animal model system, while chemotherapy kept untreated cancer in check, **tumors grew more rapidly in mice that were given cancer pretreated with vitamin C.**

The research team, which **includes researchers from Columbia University**, then delved into the mechanism by which vitamin C may be protecting these cells, and discovered that it wasn't because the nutrient was neutralizing oxygen-free radicals.

They found instead that **DHA was restoring viability to the cancer cell's damaged mitochondria –** the cell's all-important power plant that, when injured, sends signals to force a cell to die.

"Vitamin C appears to protect the mitochondria from extensive damage, thus saving the cell," Heaney said. "And whether directly or not, all anticancer drugs work to disrupt the mitochondria to push cell death."

Heaney says that the amount of DHA used in the experiments resulted in an intracellular buildup similar to what could be seen in cancer patients using large supplemental doses of vitamin C.

Researchers at Memorial Sloan-Kettering Cancer Center have long been researching the connection between vitamin C and cancer therapy, and these new findings expand on their earlier observation that **vitamin C seems to accumulate within cancer cells more than in normal cells.**

"We recognized that DHA is the form of vitamin C that gets into cells, and that the tumor microenvironment allows cancer cells to convert more vitamin C into DHA," he said. **"Inside the cell, DHA is converted back into ascorbic acid**, and it gets trapped there and so is available to safeguard the cell."

Heaney says that he suspects that vitamin C is good for the cells of normal tissue because it provides more protection for the mitochondria, and thus probably extends cell life. "But that isn't what you want when you are trying to eliminate cancer cells," said Heaney, who notes that cancer patients should eat a healthy diet, which includes foods rich in vitamin C. It is use of large doses of over-the-counter vitamin C that is worrisome, he says.

1.8.0.0 Apoptosis controlled by p53 gene

1.8.1.0 Cancer protection secret revealed

2-1-09 Scientists say they have discovered a missing link in the way cells protect themselves against cancer. They have uncovered how cells switch a gene called **p53, which can block the development of tumours, on and off.** The researchers say the finding has important implications for cancer treatment and diagnosis.

The study, published in Genes And Development, was carried out by teams of scientists in Singapore and the University of Dundee. The p53 gene, first discovered

30 years ago, plays a vital role in keeping the body healthy by ordering damaged cells to commit suicide, or by stopping them dividing while key repair work is carried out. **In half of all cancers the gene is either damaged or inactive, giving damaged cells a free rein to keep dividing and form cancer.**

In the latest study, the scientists used a genetic trick to make zebrafish turn green when the p53 gene was switched on to explore the way it was regulated. They found that the p53 gene makes not only the well-established p53 protein, but also an alternative "control switch" variation of the p53 protein - known as an isoform.

1.8.2.0 Radiation doses

Normally zebrafish, which carry the same p53 gene as humans, can survive low doses of radiation, which causes damage to the DNA, because the gene steps in to repair that damage. But **no such repair took place in zebrafish without the isoform switch, and they died after radiation exposure.** The researchers said **this proved that the switch played a crucial role in enabling p53 to do its repair work.**

Lead researcher Professor Sir David Lane, said: "The function of p53 is critical to the way that many cancer treatments kill cells since radiotherapy and chemotherapy act in part by triggering cell suicide in response to DNA damage. "So understanding more about how this gene is controlled in cells is really important in finding ways to prevent cells from turning cancerous."

Lesley Walker, Cancer Research UK's director of cancer information, said: "This is a really exciting study which improves our understanding of how the p53 gene works. "Discovering how it is regulated will have incredibly important implications in the development of better drugs and ways to diagnose cancer." http://news.bbc.co.uk/go/pr/fr/-/2/hi/health/7861474.stm

1.8.3.0 Hepatitis C Virus: From Oxygen Free Radicals to Hepatocellular Carcinoma

Epidemiological evidence clearly identifies chronic infection with hepatitis C virus (HCV) as a major risk factor for the development of hepatocellular carcinoma (HCC). Among the mechanisms that have been implicated in the pro-carcinogenic effect of HCV infection, an increased production of reactive oxygen species in the liver seems to have a major pathogenetic role in leading from chronic inflammation to cancer. Recent data have also demonstrated that HCV is capable of inducing this active production of free radicals *per se*, not just through inflammation, a feature peculiar to this virus and the specific activity of its core protein. This paper provides an overview of the inter-relationships between HCV, liver damage, free radical production and HCC, describing at least in part the complex network involving DNA oxidative damage, cytokine synthesis, proto-oncogene activation and oestrogen receptor expression, that may all be deeply involved in liver carcinogenesis.

1.8.3.1 Hepatitis C Virus and Chronic Liver Damage

Hepatitis C virus (HCV) is currently the most important cause of chronic viral hepatitis in the Western world. At least 85% of individuals acquiring HCV infection will develop chronic hepatitis, which will evolve into cirrhosis in 20-30% of cases over a variable, usually lengthy period of time.[1,2] Chronic HCV infection is also associated with a greater risk of developing hepatocellular carcinoma (HCC), a risk recognized as being similar or even greater than is observed for chronic hepatitis B virus (HBV) infection.[3]

Apart from the well-established mechanisms of necro-inflammation and nodular proliferation specific to cirrhosis, several pathways have been thought to underlie the pro-carcinogenic effect of HCV infection, including modulation of the balance between cell proliferation and death by core or nonstructural proteins (NS3-NS5), interaction with anti-oncogenes such as p21 and/or p73,[4-6] or modulation of p53 or its co-activators by the NS5A protein.[7,8]

A number of papers have recently been published[9,10] that clearly demonstrate that the carcinogenic pathways differ between HCV and HBV, the former being characterized by Wnt activation and inactivation of E-cadherin (changes consistent with the highly invasive potential of these tumours) and different signalling pathways. In these papers, oxidative stress has been identified as a major determinant of HCC development in HCV-mediated liver damage.

This review aims to summarize what we know about the relevance of oxidative damage in carcinogenesis, the link between chronic HCV-related liver damage and reactive oxygen species (ROS) production, the role of cytokines in modulating this damage, the impact of host factors in this model, and the molecular mechanisms involved.

1.8.3.2 Reactive Oxygen Species Production, DNA Oxidative Damage and Cancer

Reactive oxygen species are known to be implicated in a number of gastrointestinal pathologies, including inflammatory diseases of the gastrointestinal tract,[11,12] alcoholic liver damage[13] and several other types of toxic liver injury,[14] as well as cancer. ROS production in the cells is controlled by numerous antioxidant extra- and intracellular defence mechanisms, which include superoxide dismutase, catalase, glutathione peroxidase and ascorbic acid. Under certain conditions, however, ROS overproduction may exceed the cellular defence needs and damage cell macromolecules,[15] including nucleic acids (DNA and RNA). When ROS attack DNA, stable covalent bonds are produced, leading to the formation of DNA adducts.[16-18]

A considerable amount of data indeed suggests that ROS may have a pathogenetic role in carcinogenesis.[19] In the initiation/promotion phase of this process, ROS may interact directly with genomic DNA,[20] damaging specific genes that control cell growth and differentiation, among others.[21] Alternatively, they may increase the activity of carcinogenic xenobiotics by facilitating their activation to reactive compounds.[22] In the subsequent progression of carcinogenesis, ROS may directly stimulate the growth of malignant cells.[23] Among the many ROS produced during the inflammatory process, the most damaging is the hydroxyl radical, which has proved responsible for a number of base modifications, including the formation of thymine and thymidine glycol,[16] 5-hydroxylmethyluracil,[17] and 8-hydroxy-deoxyguanosine (8-OHdG).[18] Eight-OHdG is a modification of guanine that induces a point mutation in the daughter DNA strands and is consequent ly used as a reliable sign of DNA damage.[24]

Like any other type of DNA damage, 8-OHdG undergoes a specific repair process. A human DNA glycosylase/AP lyase encoded by the OGG I gene removes 8-OHdG directly from DNA and suppresses its mutagenic effect. Among multiple OGG I isoforms, OGG I-type la is expressed mainly in human cells and it repairs chromosomal DNA. Inactivation of the OGG I gene in yeast and mice leads to high rates of spontaneous mutation in the cells. The human OGG I gene maps to chromosome 3p26.2 and allelic deletions of this region frequently occur in a variety of human cancers. The OGG I gene is also somatically mutated in certain cancer cells and is highly polymorphic among human populations. The repair activity levels of mutated and polymorphic OGG I proteins are lower than those of the wild-type OGG I protein and may consequently be involved in human carcinogenesis, although not everyone takes this view.[25,26] Repaired or not, the outcome of DNA oxidative damage *in vivo* remains unknown, while studies using DNA templates containing 8-OHdG indicate that this oxidatively modified residue persists, accumulating in cell DNA and causing mispairing, thus suggesting that this lesion is mutagenic and therefore potentially carcinogenic.[20]

DNA damage can be measured in urine[18,27] as the amount of adducts repaired and eliminated, but this test provides no information on the actual amount of DNA damage in the cell because urine levels depend on two factors; the quantity of adducts formed per unit of time and the enzymatic capacity of the cell to repair them during a said time. Measuring the steady-state levels of damage directly in cellular DNA definitely gives us a more specific indication of oxidative damage and the method that we and other authors use[28-30] enables even low levels of oxidatively damaged DNA to be detected with great sensitivity and specificity.

1.8.3.3 Hepatitis C Virus, Reactive Oxygen Species and DNA Oxidative Damage

Since the beginning of HCV and liver damage, it was tempting to link HCV-related infection with chronic liver damage and ROS formation. HCV-related chronic hepatitis was characterized by marked liver steatosis[31] and there were other situations in which viral infections could induce massive liver steatosis by exacerbating oxidative mechanisms, as in Reye's syndrome and other virus-related diseases.[32,33] Among the many papers published on the topic, we too suggested in our earliest reports that HCV-related liver damage was characterized by a greater free radical formation, revealed by higher liver and serum levels of products of lipid peroxidation and/or protein oxidation.[34,35] This increased ROS production was definitely related, at least to some degree, with cell death and lipid peroxidation in the liver - but was it linked in any way with liver carcinogenesis too?

In an attempt to address this topic, we had the chance, in collaboration with others, to examine a large population of anti-HCV positive subjects with varying degrees of HCV-related liver damage involved in the Dionysos Project.[36,37] Our own and other authors' findings (obtained by assessing 8-OHdG levels in DNA from circulating leucocytes) suggested a progressive build-up of genomic oxidative damage not only in patients with chronic hepatitis and cirrhosis, but also in anti-HCV positive patients with persistently normal ALT levels.[38] HCV infection was in itself associated with an almost fourfold increase in 8-OHdG levels, even in cases with 'silent' infection. This supports data showing that subjects with 'normal' transaminases may nonetheless have variable degrees of liver damage,[39,40] and confirms the presence of tissue damage linked to free radical formation. HCV-related DNA oxidative damage is, therefore, an early event in the development of liver damage, accumulating as the disease progresses, and implying that it is deficiently repaired.

Our data on 8-OHdG have been confirmed by many others, such as Shimoda *et al.*,[41] who reported increased levels of 8-OHdG in DNA extracted from liver tissues of individuals with chronic HCV-related liver disease. Indirect data on the relationship between HCV infection, free radicals and liver cancer also came from a study by Koike *et al.*[42] in a transgenic mouse model for HCV core. The expression of several cellular genes was deranged in the animal and the core protein interacted with intracellular proteins, such as tumour necrosis factor (TNF) and interleukin-1 (IL-1), leading to transcriptional activation; all said effects correlated with an overproduction of free radicals.

As mentioned earlier, various HCV structural and nonstructural proteins, such as Core and NS3, may reportedly have a role to play in cell transformation and possibly in hepatocarcinogenesis too,[43-46] but the whole picture of the scenario linking HCV and liver cancer remains to be fully elucidated. Koike and others suggest that ROS accumulation prompted by the HCV core protein may help trigger the chain of genomic events eventually leading to HCC. ROS overproduction to such an extent as to overwhelm the liver's physiological scavenging capacity may indeed be a pivotal event in HCV-related liver carcinogenesis.[47]

Oxidative genomic damage thus came to mind as a putative factor in this process of virus-induced carcinogenesis, as shown in experiments *in vitro*[48] and recognized by several authors.[49,50] But is free radical formation in the liver justified by the inflammatory reaction elicited by the presence of HCV alone, or does HCV itself have the potential to trigger ROS accumulation? This question has been addressed by Moriya *et al.*,[51] who reported oxidative stress in the absence of inflammation in a mouse model of HCV-associated hepatocarcinogenesis, showing that inflammation was not necessary for free radical production in HCV infection. A more recent study based on a similar mouse model, transgenic for HCV polyprotein,[52] showed that co-factors may affect ROS formation: iron overloading, for instance, promoted liver carcinogenesis in the presence of increased 8-OHdG formation. Iron accumulation is a frequent finding in HCV hepatitis and both we and other authors have already reported that both serum ferritin and liver tissue iron are increased in patients with chronic, HCV-mediated liver damage.[34]

Is this oxidative damage detectable in sensitive liver targets? Studying intrahepatic oxidative DNA damage by *in situ* 8-OHdG detection using immunohistochemistry in controls and patients with various stages of chronic liver disease showed that 8-OHdG expression in hepatocytes was nuclear in chronic hepatitis and particularly abundant in the periportal areas, with piecemeal necrosis and prominent cell infiltration.[50]

In the last two decades, we have learned very well that HCV is by no means a straightforward pathogenic agent. For instance, whether genotype I HCV-related infection coincides with more severe liver damage and, in the long run, a higher risk of HCC is still debated. Even recently, some authors have presented data confirming the more clear-cut pathogenicity of genotype 1b liver infection,[53] while others suggest that the presence of genotype 1b is merely the sign of a long-standing infection, which is naturally characterized by more severe liver damage and a higher risk for HCC.[54] We know that increased liver cell proliferation is a potent risk factor for cancer onset,[55] but there are no data to confirm whether or not genotype 1b infection boosts liver cell proliferation. Dutta *et al.* [56] failed to demonstrate any association between HCV genotype and Ki67-assessed liver proliferation, p53 or BCl-2 expression, or other potential markers of a higher cancer risk, and Donato *et al.*[55] obtained similar results. On the other hand, our own data support the conviction that genotype I is a risk factor for more severe liver damage, in biological terms at least, since the presence of genotype Ib HCV infection was associated in our series with significantly worse oxidative damage. These findings were documented both when we assessed the levels of oxidative DNA damage in circulating white blood cells in an open population and when we considered 8-OHdG levels in livers with different degrees of liver damage.[38] The genotype specificity of these biochemical events is also confirmed for other changes characterizing HCV infection. It has recently emerged that genotype 3 HCV has a stronger direct role in inducing liver steatosis than other genotypes,[57,58] and we confirmed this specific 'pro-steatotic' activity of genotype 3 HCV, which was also linked to specific molecular effects. For example, we observed a less pronounced upregulation of c-myc (a common phenomenon in HCC)[59] in genotype 3 than in genotype 1b HCV infection, and an upregulation of Fas/Fas-ligand, a potential mechanism underlying progression to fibrosis, was observed in association with steatosis in patients with genotype 3 HCV hepatitis.[60]

1.8.3.4 Hepatitis C Virus, DNA Damage and Host Factors

As in many other diseases,[61] it is now clear that host factors determine the extent of HCV-mediated liver damage,[62,63] e.g. by modulating inflammatory response, and it has been shown that polymorphisms in TNF or IL-10 are linked to a differing severity and outcome of the infection.

This is true also for other mechanisms. For instance, DNA oxidative damage is counteracted by several intra- and extra-cellular mechanisms and efficiently repaired, as mentioned earlier. Recent data that we obtained on OGG1 polymorphisms in HCV-related chronic liver damage seem to suggest that a somatic heterozygosity for the gene is frequent (in about 60% of patients in our experience), while homozygosity for the mutated gene is rare. The importance of OGG1 in liver damage is confirmed by a very recent paper by Russo *et al.*,[64] who demonstrated, in mice at least, that the liver is the only organ in which OGG1 inactivation suffices to alter steady-state 8OHdG levels. Whether or not the presence of mutations correlates with a higher tendency for evolution to cirrhosis or HCC in humans remains to be seen. There are several data, however, to suggest that OGG1 plays an important part in modulating the process of liver damage and carcinogenesis. Albeit in a different model, it has been reported that pre-S HBV mutant surface antigens greatly induce OGG1[49] and, even more interestingly, that a loss of heterozygosity in the gene, accompanied by genomic instability (LOH3), occurs in the early stages of liver cancer.[65]

1.8.3.5 DNA Oxidative Damage, Cytokines and Molecular Targets

Which molecular and genomic mechanisms lie behind and link an event such as DNA oxidative damage (which may well be the first hit in the general mechanism of carcinogenesis) with the onset of cancer? Although ROS induction is known to derive from a complex network of tissue and inflammatory responses involving the expression of cytokines, growth factors and oncogenes, this network has not been thoroughly investigated in HCV-related liver disease.

Liver injury is reportedly associated with a chronic inflammatory response involving, for instance, TNF-α and IL-1β. The former has a central role in liver injury, triggering the production of other cytokines that, in turn, recruit inflammatory cells, promote fibrogenesis and further activate oxidative burst.[66] Among the many effects of TNF-α,[67] however, we must also consider the initiation of a number of intracellular signalling pathways involving apoptotic and/or anti-apoptotic signals. HCV infection is associated with an increased TNF-α production and the expression of viral proteins apparently results in more severe liver injury and hepatocyte death.[68-70]

Interleukin-1β gives rise to the inflammatory response cascade. Recent reports have shown that its levels are higher in HCV-related liver disease than in other forms of liver damage,[71] and its polymorphisms have been correlated with the risk of progression to HCC.[72,73] These data point to a specific role for oxidative DNA damage, prompted by pro-inflammatory cytokines and/or a specific effect of HCV core protein,[74,75] and associated with an imbalance between apoptosis and cytoproliferation,[76] in the activation of the basic mechanisms of liver carcinogenesis.

A number of additional mediators are involved in liver carcinogenesis, including oncogenes such as c-myc, which controls hepatocyte proliferation,[77] and growth factors such as TGF-α, again involved in controlling liver regeneration and tumour progression,[78] particularly when co-expressed.[79] We recently sought correlations between oxidative DNA damage and the levels of pro-inflammatory cytokines, TGF-α and c-myc in chronic HCV-related liver damage. Our first results concern TNF-α and IL-1β.[80] As mentioned earlier, IL-1β, prompts the cascade of the inflammatory response and reportedly has a direct effect in causing growth arrest, but it also has a chronic effect in inducing TNF-α expression.[72] This last effect was not confirmed in our study, however, since no correlation emerged between IL-1β and TNF-α. On the other hand, IL-1β expression was higher in the later stages of HCV-related liver disease, as already demonstrated by Gramantieri *et al.*,[81] while the opposite was true of TNF-α, whose levels of expression were higher in chronic active hepatitis.

It is worth stressing that both TNF-α and IL-1β are involved in controlling the balance between cell proliferation and apoptosis, and consequently take part in determining the liver cells' fate and progression to liver cancer. TNF-α and IL-1β binding to their receptors leads to the activation of transcriptional factors, such as NFkB and AP-1, again involved in controlling cell proliferation.[72] But how does persistent oxidative stress fit into the picture? The overproduction of oxidative species linked to the over-expression of inflammatory cytokines may be responsible for inhibiting the apoptotic process, probably by activating the NFkB-dependent pathway.[82]

Oxidative damage may also be related to the expression of proto-oncogenes, such as c-myc,[83] that was significantly more expressed in cirrhotic than in non-cirrhotic tissues in our experience too. This means that the progression of tissue damage from hepatitis to cirrhosis, and the related cell growth changes, may be mediated to some degree by c-myc, considered one of the activators of cell proliferation.[84] For instance, recent studies have demonstrated that TGF-α/c-myc double transgenic mice exhibit enhanced cell proliferation and accumulate extensive oxidative DNA damage, a phenomenon that may account for an accelerated progression to cancer.[85]

Last, but not least, the β-catenin Wnt pathway is gaining in importance in liver carcinogenesis. Enhanced Wnt-1 expression has been demonstrated in hepatocarcinogenesis,[86] β-catenin being expressed in up to 80% of liver cancer samples,[87] with a frequency of mutation ranging from 17% to 44%.[88,89] In a transgenic mouse model characterized by the lack of the functional retinoic acid receptor, Yanagitani *et al.*[90] recently described a series of events that, among others, included a tremendous amount of **H_2O_2 formation**, associated with increased 8-OHdG liver levels and upregulation of β-catenin. These events were in turn linked to cyclin D1 over-expression, thus suggesting a potential additional role for oxidative damage in liver carcinogenesis through activation of the β-catenin pathway. This aspect obviously warrants further investigation.

Oxidative damage may also occur in other sensitive molecular targets. Cell cycle gene mutation is one of the most common genetic changes in malignant tumour cells. Recent reports, for instance, have shown a strong correlation between oxidative damage and telomerase activity,[91] an essential factor in cancer cell immortalization. Oxidative guanine damage in DNA containing telomeric and nontelomeric sequences generates 8-OHdG mainly in the telomeric segment, because GGG sequences are more reactive in duplex DNA, thus confirming a selectivity of oxidative damage for sensitive targets.

Telomerase activity regulation is complex, however, and involves control at gene transcription level, with post-translational protein-protein interactions and protein phosphorylation. Proto-oncogenes and tumour suppressor genes, including c-myc, BLI2, p21/Waf1 and p53, have been implicated in the direct and indirect regulation of telomerase activity.[92] Here again, the tumour suppressor gene p53 is likely the most important of the many genes directly activated in circumstances of stress and oxidative damage, and it has been described as a universal sensor of genotoxic stress.[93] ROS are involved at multiple levels in p53 signalling and are potent activators of the tumour suppressor gene, which in turn activates the production of more ROS and induces a number of other genes.[93] Polyak *et al.*[94] has shown that many of the genes upregulated by p53 activation were predicted to encode proteins that might generate or respond to oxidative stress, in a kind of vicious circle.

1.8.3.6 The Role of Sex Hormones

Other co-factors may well be involved in modulating the process of free radical formation and carcinogenesis. One is iron overload, as already discussed, which is relatively frequent in patients with chronic HCV-related liver damage and linked to more severe disease in man[95,96] and to accelerated carcinogenesis, in animal models.[53] The other area that has attracted much attention in recent years is the role of sex hormones. To some extent, liver cell proliferation is a process controlled by sex hormones, as confirmed by reliable data obtained both *in vitro* and *in vivo*.[97-99] Sex hormone dysregulation has also been linked to the onset of HCC[100] and anti-oestrogen treatment has been used in advanced HCC in an attempt to modify its growth, with alternate but ultimately poor results.[101-103]

Prompted by data obtained by Villa *et al.*,[104,105] we also considered the possible relationship between oestrogen receptor (OR) expression, type of receptor, oxidative DNA damage and c-myc mRNA expression in chronic liver disease, to see whether HCV infection correlated with any change in this pathway. In previous *in vivo* studies, increased 8-OHdG levels were seen in the liver and kidney of hamsters exposed to oestradiol or 4-hydroxyoestradiol[106] and it was demonstrated that ethynyloestradiol-induced liver carcinogenesis is associated with increased 8-OHdG levels.

Oestrogens affect cell division rate by binding to the receptor, by transcriptional activation of the cyclin D1 gene and by increased G1 regulatory protein myc expression.[107] Two subtypes of OR have been studied, OR-α and OR-β, and the former has been found strongly expressed in many cell types and involved in oxidative damage.

It has been demonstrated that a variant form of OR lacking exon 5 of the hormone binding domain is predominantly if not exclusively expressed in some HCCs already at an early stage of the disease, especially in HBsAg positive patients. This has given rise to the hypothesis that the expression of this variant receptor may be important in liver carcinogenesis.[105] Our data confirmed a peak in the proportion of liver tissues positive for variant ORs in patients with HCC and we found that patients with both HBV- and HCV-related chronic liver disease positive for variant liver OR have higher 8-OHdG levels and express more c-myc m-RNA than patients negative for the said variant receptor.[108] In short, our own and other reported data indicate that sex hormone balance and receptor status are involved in modulating liver carcinogenesis through an oxidative-damage mediated pathway too.

1.8.3.7 Conclusions

In summary, this review describes the role of ROS in DNA damage and cancer, the link between HCV infection and oxidative DNA damage, the impact of host factors, including sex hormones, in said genomic damage and the changes in cytokine expression and in molecular targets that depend on the effects of HCV infection. Overall, although it is limited with respect to all the possible genomic or post-genomic interactions, the network linking HCV infection, inflammation, free radical production and carcinogenesis that we and other authors have described, it applies very well to HCV-mediated chronic liver damage, just as it applies to any chronic inflammatory condition.[47] Past and present in-depth investigations into the role of HCV structural and nonstructural proteins and the changes induced in oncogenes, anti-oncogenes, cytokine expression, intracellular kinases and other factors, clearly show that HCV is capable *per se*, and not just via inflammation, of inducing an active output of free radicals, an effect that is specific to this virus. This **ROS production, with oxidative genomic damage, is in turn a *primum movens* in a cascade of genomic and post-genomic events that play a relevant part in liver damage and, specifically, in carcinogenesis** (see Fig. 1). Additional data are eagerly awaited from recently introduced techniques, including micro-arrays and mass spectrometry for proteomics, that will hopefully close the gap between hypothesis and understanding (Hepatitis C Virus: From Oxygen Free Radicals to Hepatocellular Carcinoma. F. Farinati, R. Cardin, M. Bortolami, P. Burra, F. P. Russo, M. Rugge, M. Guido, A. Sergio, R. Naccarato. J Viral Hepat. 2007;14(12):821-829).

1.8.4.0 Hyperoxia causes cellular arrest and induces p53

Hyperoxia increases free radical production, leading to DNA damage. Recent studies indicate that oxygen augments the expression of p53 and p21 WAF1/CIP1, and increases apoptotic labeling of airway epithelial cells. Similar changes in regulatory gene products have not been reported in other pulmonary cells, nor have these changes been investigated in conjunction with alterations in cell-cycle distribution. The present study was conducted to determine whether oxygen alters the expression of p53 and p21

WAF1/CIP1 in human bronchial smooth-muscle cells (BSMC). BSMC placed in room air (RA), 40% O2, or 95% O2 were examined for 3 d to determine cell number, thymidine incorporation, cell-cycle distribution, and lactate dehydrogenase release. Apoptosis was assessed through the terminal deoxynucleotidyl transferase–deoxyuridine triphosphate end-nick labeling (TUNEL) technique, and p53 and p21 WAF1/CIP1 protein levels were determined through enzyme-linked immunosorbent assay. Exposure of BSMC to 95% O2 decreased proliferation and DNA synthesis within 24 h, and was accompanied by an increase in S-phase cells (72 h; RA:12.96 4.6%, versus 95% O 2: 34.66 7.0%;*P*,0.01). By comparison, exposure to 40% O2 resulted in decreased proliferation at 48 h without significant alterations in cell-cycle distribution. Both p53 and p21 WAF1/CIP1 levels were increased by 95% O2, with maximal differences noted at 24 and 48 h, respectively.

All atmospheres showed, 8% cell death and few TUNEL-positive cells. Our results indicate that oxygen-mediated alterations in BSMC proliferation are time- and concentration-dependent. Furthermore, high oxygen levels induce S-phase arrest and increased expression of p53 and p21 WAF1/CIP1. Activation of these genes may prevent replication without inducing apoptosis to allow for the repair of oxidative damage.

(Shenberger, J. S., and P. S. Dixon. 1999. **Oxygen induces S-phase growth arrest and increases p53 and p21 WAF1/CIP1 expression in human bronchial smooth-muscle cells.** Am. J. Respir. Cell Mol. Biol. 21:395–402).

Numerous studies have demonstrated the ability of oxygen to slow the proliferation of cells grown in culture. Alveolar type II cells, fibroblasts, and tracheal smooth-muscle cells all exhibit decreased growth within 24 h of exposure to O2 fractions exceeding 50% O2 (1–3, 16). This high-oxygen environment increases the generation of reactive oxygen species (ROS) and fosters the release of H2O2 from mitochondria, either of which effect may lead to DNA strand breaks, protein oxidation, and lipid peroxidation In conclusion, we have shown that oxygen produces graded reductions in DNA synthesis and mitochondrial function in BSMC, and that extremely high concentrations of oxygen induce an accumulation of cells in the S phase of the cell cycle. These changes occur in conjunction with increased expression of p53 and p21WAF1/CIP1 proteins, but without significant cell loss, suggesting that upregulation of cell-cycle regulatory genes occurs to promote cellular repair rather than apoptosis.

1.8.5.0 Ozone/Oxygen Shot Helps Heal Herniated Disk

3-9-09 A shot of ozone and oxygen may prove to be a safe, effective and less invasive way to relieve the pain of a herniated disk, U.S. researchers say.

Small spongy discs normally act as shock absorbers between the vertebrae, but when one is damaged, it may bulge or break, putting pressure on spinal cord nerves. The standard treatments for severe pain caused by herniated disks are either open diskectomy or microdiskectomy, surgeries that require the removal of disk material through an incision.

But one study of more than **8,000 patients found that injecting a gas mixture of oxygen and ozone into a herniated disk significantly relieves the pressure put on the nerves**, easing patients' pain. A second study showed that the oxygen/ozone treatment works by reducing disc volume **through ozone oxidation**; the reduced volume eases disc pressure on the nerves.

"Oxygen/ozone treatment of herniated disks is an effective and extremely safe procedure. The estimated improvement in pain and function is impressive when we looked at patients who ranged in age from 13 to 94 years with all types of disk herniations," Dr. Kieran J. Murphy, an interventional neuroradiologist and vice chair and chief of medical imaging at the University of Toronto in Canada, said in a news release issued by the conference's sponsors.

The findings were expected to be presented in San Diego at annual meeting of the Society of Interventional Radiology.

In the study of more than 8,000 patients, those who had the oxygen/ozone treatment reported their **pain lessening by an average of nearly 4 points**, based on a 10-point scale (with 0 being no pain and 10 representing the worst pain experienced). The patients' ability to conduct everyday tasks -- such a washing and dressing themselves or even just standing up -- also **improved by more than 25 percent based** on the rating scale used.

"Equally important, pain and function outcomes are similar to the outcomes for lumbar disks treated with surgical diskectomy, but the **complication rate is much less** (less than 0.1 percent)," Murphy said. "In addition, the **recovery time is significantly shorter** for the oxygen/ozone injection than for the diskectomy."

Much of the research into oxygen/ozone therapy has been done in Italy, where it is believed as many as 14,000 individuals have been treated in the past five years.

"There are millions of people with back pain who suffer and who can't work because of their pain. Undergoing invasive surgical diskectomy puts you on a path where you may be left with too little disk. Taking out a protruding disk may lose the shock absorption that naturally resides between them in the spine," said

Murphy. **He predicts that this procedure will become standard in the United States within the next five years. I believe that this another example of the importance of oxidation and of its low toxicity.**

1.8.6.0 Mannitol is an antioxidant

Besides its physiological importance in the cultivated mushroom, mannitol also plays an important role in the pharmaceutical and food industry, where it is increasingly used as a nutritive sweetener and antioxidant. Commercial production of mannitol occurs mainly through chemical reduction of fructose, a process that yields small amounts of both mannitol and its by-product sorbitol

1.8.7.0 Antioxidants increase mortality

The vitamin industry has long touted antioxidants as a way to improve health by filling in gaps in diet, but a new review of studies **found no evidence that the nutrition supplements extend life.** Worse, the review authors said that some antioxidants could increase risk for death (Bjelakovic G, et al. Antioxidant supplements for prevention of mortality in healthy participants and patients with various diseases (Review). Cochrane Database of Systematic Reviews 2008, Issue 2).

The meta-analysis of 67 randomized studies found that supplemental antioxidants do not reduce mortality and that some -- including vitamin A, beta-carotene and vitamin E -- could increase mortality. The review combined evidence from more than 200,000 people.

1.8.8.0 Antioxidant vitamin recommendations, The Medical Letter, 2005

There is no convincing evidence that taking supplements of vitamin C prevents any disease except scurvy. Women should not take vitamin A supplements during pregnancy or after menopause. No one should take highdose beta carotene supplements. A balanced diet rich in fruits and vegetables may be safer than taking vitamin supplements. No biologically active substance taken for a long term can be assumed to be free of risk.

(The Medical Letter. Volume 47. Issue 1213. July 18, 2005).

1.8.9.0 Current Patterns and Prevalence of the Public's Use of MVM Supplements

More than half of American adults take dietary supplements in the belief that they will make them feel better, give them greater energy, improve their health, and prevent and treat disease. The use of supplements has been steadily increasing, and growth appears likely to continue. Currently, users spend more than $23 billion per year on supplements, and among this supplement-using population, MVM is the major category of supplements, used by about one third of Americans. Uncertainty remains in estimating prevalence of use because of problems defining these products; increasing complexity in the formulation of supplements, including more non-MVM components and specialized formulas; and varying frequency of use. (NIH State-of-the-Science Conference Statement. Multivitamin/Mineral Supplements and Chronic Disease Prevention. 15–17 May 2006).

Conclusion

Basic food condiments like herbs and spices are extensive sources of antioxidants. The benefits of antioxidants may depend on their variety and interaction. We know that we can optimize health by encouraging the consumption of a wide variety of nutritious foods, but **we cannot, so far, be such about the risks and benefits of taking antioxidants supplements.**

1.9.0.0 Data on Food Antioxidants Aid Research

By Rosalie Marion Bliss
November 6, 2007

Measures of the antioxidant capacities of 277 selected foods were released today by Agricultural Research Service (ARS) scientists. The new database provides easy access to antioxidant values for a wide variety of foods, many of which may be excellent sources of healthful compounds.

The database will be used by scientists to help guide ongoing research into how antioxidants may correlate to health benefits. For example, many fruits and vegetables are known to be good sources of antioxidant vitamins, such as E, C, and beta carotene, a form of vitamin A. But these natural foods also contain other compounds, collectively known as phytonutrients, that may contribute to health. The database was prepared by ARS researchers at the Nutrient Data Laboratory, part of the agency's Beltsville Human Nutrition Research Center (BHNRC) at Beltsville, Md., in collaboration with colleagues at the ARS Arkansas Children's

Nutrition Center in Little Rock. ARS is the U.S. Department of Agriculture's chief scientific research agency.

Many of the fruits, nuts, vegetables and spices listed were analyzed for their Oxygen Radical Absorbance Capacity, known as ORAC, at the Arkansas center. ORAC is one of a number of methods available to evaluate the antioxidant capacities of foods. The method was developed by ARS chemist Ronald Prior with colleagues. Prior also studies the ability of antioxidants to be absorbed and utilized within the human body.

Data on foods analyzed using the ORAC method were also gathered during an extensive search of peer-reviewed, scientific literature, and screened through a USDA-developed, data-quality-evaluation system. Both the screened data and the analyzed data are listed in the database, along with data quality indicators. Antioxidant capacity measures may vary due to factors such the type of cultivar studied and its growing and harvesting conditions, as well as the methods used for a food sample's preparation, processing, and/or analysis.

The new release expands upon the 2004 data release by ARS on estimates of the antioxidant capacity of 171 foods.

To access the new database, go to:

http://www.ars.usda.gov/nutrientdata/ORAC

Last Modified: 11/06/2007

1.9.1.0 Linnane argues against the free radical theory

The overarching role of coenzyme Q(10) in gene regulation, bioenergy formation, cellular redox poise regulation, and hydrogen peroxide formation is presented. Coenzyme Q(10) has a central role acting as a prooxidant in the generation of H(2)O(2). Contrary to the dogma that superoxide and H(2)O(2) formation are highly deleterious to cell survival this premise is rejected. **Data are discussed that continuous superoxide and hydrogen peroxide formation are essential for normal cell function and that they play a major role in subcellular redox state modulation. It is the prooxidant activity of the so-called antioxidants that may be responsible for previously claimed benefits** for high doses of oxido-reduction nutritional supplements such as alpha lipoic acid and coenzyme Q(10). Oxygen-free radical formation is essential for the biological function and is not a direct causation of the mammalian aging process; aging is a multisystem stochastic process (Cellular redox regulation and prooxidant signaling systems: a new perspective on the free radical theory of aging. Linnane AW, Eastwood H. Ann N Y Acad Sci. 2006 May;1067:47-55). **RMH Note: Tony, I agree wholeheartedly.**

1.9.2.0 Linnane argues of the essentiality of EMODs

The production of reactive oxygen species (ROS) and reactive nitrogen species (RNS) has long been proposed as leading to random deleterious modification of macromolecules with an associated progressive development of age associated systemic disease. ROS and RNS formation has been posited as a major contributor to the aging process. On the contrary, this review presents evidence that superoxide anion (and hydrogen peroxide) and nitric oxide (and peroxynitrite) constitute regulated prooxidant second messenger systems, with specific sub-cellular locales of production and are essential for normal metabolome and physiological function. The role of these second messengers in the regulation of the metabolome is discussed in terms of radical formation as an essential contributor to the physiologically normal regulation of sub-cellular bioenergy systems; proteolysis regulation; transcription activation; enzyme activation; mitochondrial DNA changes; redox regulation of metabolism and cell differentiation; the concept that orally administered small molecule antioxidant therapy is a chimera. The formation of superoxide anion/hydrogen peroxide and nitric oxide do not conditionally lead to random macromolecular damage; under normal physiological conditions their production is actually regulated consistent with their second messenger roles (Healthy aging: regulation of the metabolome by cellular redox modulation and prooxidant signaling systems: the essential roles of superoxide anion and hydrogen peroxide. Linnane AW, Kios M, Vitetta L. Biogerontology. 2007 Oct;8(5):445-67. Epub 2007 Apr 6).

1.9.3.0 CoQ is an essential prooxidant - Linnane

Coenzyme Q10 plays a central role in cellular bioenergy generation and its regulation. Closed membrane systems generate a proton motive force to create transient localized bio-capacitors; the captured energy is used for the synthesis of mitochondrial ATP but also for many other processes, such as metabolite translocations, nerve conduction and a host of other bioenergy requiring processes. Coenzyme Q10 plays a key role in many of these sub-cellular membrane energy generating systems. Integral to this phenomenon is **the prooxidant role of coenzyme Q10 in generating the major superoxide anion/hydrogen peroxide second messenger system.**

This messenger system, largely but not exclusively, arises from coenzyme Q10 semiquinone function; it contributes to the regulation of sub-cellular redox potential levels; transcription/gene expression control; is essential for modulated protein turnover and activation; mediates hormone and growth factor extracellular signaling. The regulated prooxidant formation of the superoxide anion/ H_2O_2 second messenger system is essential for the normal physiological function of the metabolome. The normally functioning metabolome is the expression of a finely tuned dynamic equilibrium comprised of thousands of anabolic and catabolic reactions and all cellular signaling systems must be finely regulated. There is still much to be learnt about the up/down regulation of the H_2O_2 messenger system. **The concept that superoxide anion/ H_2O_2 cause random macromolecular damage is rebutted.** The administration of antioxidants to quench the inferred toxicity of these compounds as a therapy for age associated diseases is unsupported by extant mammalian clinical trials and should be subject to serious re-evaluation. **The role of ascorbic acid as a beneficial hydrogen peroxide prodrug is discussed** (Coenzyme Q(10)--its role as a prooxidant in the formation of superoxide anion/hydrogen peroxide and the regulation of the metabolome. Linnane AW, Kios M, Vitetta L. Mitochondrion. 2007 Jun;7 Suppl:S51-61. Epub 2007 Mar 30)

1.9.4.0 Denham Harmans' take on antioxidants and age, as of 2000

Abstract. Ingestion of antioxidant supplements by the United States (US) population has increased steadily since the mid-1950's. This review tried to determine if the supplements have contributed significantly to beneficial changes in the US during this period. Experimental animal studies have demonstrated that anti-oxidant supplements lower the incidence of a wide variety of diseases and increase life span. Anti-oxidants are associated with similar changes in man. Changes since the mid-1950's in the US population include: 1) **ingestion of antioxidant supplements has increased from one percent, or less, to 40–50 percent today. Cost: now 4–5 billion dollars per year**, 2) disproportionate increases in the percentage of older individuals as average life expectancy at birth (ALE-B) rose, 3) declining chronic disability in the elderly since 1982, 4) declining cancer mortality since 1991, and 5) the decline in the rate of reported cardiovascular disease beginning in the 1950's which significantly increased further in 1965.

The last four changes suggest that the rate of increase in physiological age with time has been slowed. This can be attributed to decreases in the rate of accumulation of free radical-induced aging changes by the joint action of antioxidant supplements/dietary measures, and improvements in conventional measures (CM) which increase ALE-B, e.g., better medical care, nutrition, housing, accident prevention. The contribution by antioxidants to decreases in physiological age is seemingly small compared to that of CM. However, it will grow relative to CM as the amount and duration of supplement use increases and improvements in CM raise ALE-B closer to 85 years, the age associated with optimal living conditions. (Antioxidant supplements: Effects on disease and aging in the United States population. Denham Harman·AGE. J. Amer. Aging Assoc. Volume 23, Number 1 / January, 2000. pp 25-31).

1.9.4.1 Origin and evolution of the free radical theory of aging: a brief personal history of Denham Harman, 1954–2009

Aging is the progressive accumulation in an organism of diverse, deleterious changes with time that increase the chance of disease and death. The basic chemical process underlying aging was first advanced by the free radical theory of aging (FRTA) in 1954: the reaction of active free radicals, normally produced in the organisms, with cellular constituents initiates the changes associated with aging. The involvement of free radicals in aging is related to their key role in the origin and evolution of life. The initial low acceptance of the FRTA by the scientific community, its slow growth, manifested by meetings and occasional papers based on the theory, prompted this account of the intermittent growth of acceptance of the theory over the past nearly 55 years.

(Origin and evolution of the free radical theory of aging: a brief personal history, 1954–2009. Denham Harman. Biogerontology. **Received:** 7 May 2009 **Accepted:** 12 May 2009 **Published online:** 24 May 2009).

The free radical theory of aging (FRTA) was first advanced by Denham Harman more than 50 years ago. The theory proceeds logically from a small number of straightforward assumptions, based on observations from radiation biology. From the Science of Aging Timeline:

1.9.5.0 Harman's logic proceeds from three observations:

(1) irradiation causes premature aging;

(2) irradiation creates oxygen radicals, which may mediate its effects; and

(3) cells produce oxygen radicals under normal conditions.

From these premises, he theorized that aging could be caused by endogenously generated oxygen radicals.

Over a half-century, the FRTA has evolved substantially (eventually focusing on the mitochondria as a major source of the initially postulated endogenous radicals), and has lately been the subject of several reviews evaluating its explanatory power and extent of current acceptance.

It's a very personal account, starting with the educational experiences that Harman credits with putting him in the right place at the right time, continuing with a description of the origins of the theory, and paying a great deal of attention to the "fits-and-starts" advancement of the theory toward broad acceptance (though not without effort and extensive modification). Pieces like these, in which the originator of a hugely influential theory provides their individual perspective on the consequences of their work, are rare indeed — hence this is a must-read for students and practitioners of biogerontology.

1.9.6.0 Number of cancer deaths wrong

A total of 549,838 cancer deaths were recorded in 1999 in the United States, up by 8,306 deaths compared with 1998. **Adjusting for changes in rules for selecting underlying cause of death** reduced the increase in the number of cancer deaths to 4,624.

Despite the yearly fanfare regarding new cancer drugs, the percentage of Americans dying from cancer in 2003 was about the same as it was in1970. But, still conventional doctors can't prescribe alternatives cancer treatments. Six hundred lobbyists paid by pharmaceutical companies are doing their best to make sure that conventional doctors never can prescribe alternative cancer treatments.

After 2003, the number of new cancer cases became artificially reduced which allowed agencies like the American Cancer Society to claim that progress is being made. In 2004 the Centers for Disease Control (CDC) reported that VA hospitals in at least 13 states are no longer reporting cancer cases and that reporting has been inconsistent in 14 additional states. **Therefore, as many as 70,000 new cancer cases (about 5% of the national total) were not reported.** Any improvement in the number of cancer cases is therefore in doubt.

In another blow to the supposed cancer-fighting powers of antioxidants, vitamins C and E, new research suggests that supplement forms of the vitamins don't prevent the disease.

At the end of 2008,Three new RCT studies verify the failure of cancer development or progression by antioxidants and it nullifies the free radical theory.

1.9.6.1 The Cancer Business

by Patrick Rattigan ND

From Truth Campaign Magazine 14

1.9.6.2 The Dark at the End of the Tunnel

In Britain, at the present time, around one third of general hospital patients are suffering from cancer. Two out of five of the population have, or will develop, the disease. If we accept the figures, for cancer incidence, of 30 percent in 1980, 40 percent now and 50 percent in the year 2010, at the present rate of increase the figure will reach 100 percent around 2080. A multitude of factors suggest that the rise is set to accelerate.

The 5-year survival figures, not to be confused with the successful treatment of the disease, for the major cancers are:

- stomach - 5 percent
- trachea, bronchus and lung - 5 percent
- breast - 50 percent
- oesophagus - 5 percent
- large intestine - 22 percent
- pancreas - 4 percent
- liver - 2 percent [1]

There has been no significant increase in survival rates since records began.

1.9.6.3 The Solid Gold Source; cancer business is second only to petrochemicals

The cancer business is second only, in size, to its big brother, petrochemicals.

In the 20 years from 1970 to 1990, in the USA alone, the cancer business was worth an estimated 1 trillion dollars ($1,000,000,000,000).[2] If the same percentage of the overall disease bill applies in Britain as in the US, the current expenditure on cancer will be 3 to 6 billion pounds per year.

With these kind of amounts involved it is quite understandable why the drug/radiation/scalpel/vivisection cancer cartel have maintained a constant, ruthless campaign to suffocate, at birth, any and all attempts to introduce rational therapeutic regimes to deal with the **species-threatening plague**.

1.9.6.4 The Enemy Within

The cancer epidemic has many **causative components**; virtually all of them either actively promoted by or ignored by the government health departments, the medical trade etc.: the lethal 'doctor's balanced diet', vaccination, antibiotics, antipyretics, analgesics, steroids, routine X-ray screening, animal-'safety-tested' pesticides, herbicides, solvents, dyes, detergents etc., fluoride-waste dumping in public drinking water, radio/chemo 'therapy', nuclear energy, electro-pollution and so on.

Ever aware of the need to protect their brethren in the petro-pharmaceutical cancer machine, the cancer P.R. boys, aided and abetted by their on-the-payroll media pals - passing themselves off as unbiased observers - faithfully maintain the line that the whole thing is down to smoking and sun-bathing. One thing that they need to explain is the canine carnage: **in a population of 7 million domestic dogs, over a million per year are dying from cancer - or the treatment.**[3] This constitutes a dog cancer death-rate 50 times that of the human rate, due to the regime of vet-approved vaccines, antibiotics, worming drugs, flea sprays, pesticides, herbicides etc. - all 'safety tested' on animals - tinned dog-meat etc. We are all - humans, dogs, cats - dying, like flies, from the synthetic deluge. The farm animals would exhibit the same syndrome if they were not killed, prematurely, for 'food'.

Cancer is, above all else, a nutritional problem. The lethal British diet of meat, dairy produce, eggs, refined carbohydrates, common salt and synthetics, with token amounts of fruit, vegetables and wholewheat bread - all saturated with pesticides - is a recipe for a vast range of maladies, cancer included.

1999 will see 700,000,000 drug prescriptions dished out by British doctors: a deluge of vaccines, antibiotics, analgesics, steroids, antipyretics, anti-inflammatories... all add up to a huge onslaught on the body's immune defences. Acute diseases, the body's efforts to regain health, are being continually suppressed by allopathic treatment.

Vaccination has reached a 98 percent uptake in some areas. The vaccines, between them, contain a mixture of animal-derived proteins and viruses, formaldehyde, mercury, aluminium, carbolic acid and so on. This is injected directly into the blood stream and thence to the cells, major organs etc. The immune defences stand no chance.

When alien material from dogs, monkeys, calves, chickens etc. is put directly into the human blood stream, the material is likely to change the genetic structure as the foreign proteins etc. are incorporated into the invaded cells, which, in their mutated form, continue to replicate. The immune defences can then no longer differentiate between self and non-self.

The body is then liable to invade its own cells with a variety of immune and auto-immune diseases, cancer included, as an inevitable end result.

Water fluoridation was first popular with the totalitarian regimes of the Soviet Union and Nazi Germany.[4] Aside from being a narcotic, fluoride is also a highly toxic, persistent waste by-product of aluminium and fertiliser production, an enzyme-inhibitor, an immuno-suppressant and a listed carcinogen. 'Fluoridated Birmingham has now been compared with non-fluoridated Manchester over the years 1971-1977. After simultaneous standardisation of all data...it was found that over 1,000 excess deaths per year are now linked with fluoridated Birmingham.'[5]

The cavalier use of routine and diagnostic X-rays by the medical trade is a major cancer threat. Prof. John Gofman M.D. PhD., as early as 1980, put the figure for the US alone at 12,000 extra fatal cancers per year. He also stated that around three quarters of breast cancer cases are caused by medical X-rays; this is apart from the huge doses from 'radiotherapy'. The use of the new X-ray toys for mass lung-screenings, head irradiation for ring worm, shoe-fitting, sore throats etc. caused incalculable amounts of cancer deaths. 'I confess that I believed in the irradiation of tonsils, lymph nodes and the thymus gland. I believed my professors when they said the doses we were using were absolutely harmless. Years later the 'absolutely harmless' radiation... was reaping a harvest of thyroid tumours.'[6]

The huge, increasing assault on the immuno-defence systems and the ever-growing deluge of carcinogens will certainly result in a considerable acceleration of the rates of cancer incidence and death. The theoretical 100 percent cancer incidence could well be here around the mid 2,000s.

1.9.6.5 The Orthodox Cure Hoax

The definition of cure in cancer is the restoration of the cancer defence mechanisms and the elimination of cancer through these mechanisms. If this restoration is not possible, the next best is the constant support, through safe, natural means, of **the body's attempts to keep the disease at bay.**

Neither of these is supplied by orthodox cancer treatment.

The cancer research fund-raisers' definition of cancer cure is the apparent lack of symptoms for five years. If, or when, a patient dies a year or two after the five years, from the effects of the treatment, they remain in the 'cure' statistics: cured and dead at the same time.

'Patients may die from secondary growths at any time from a few months to many years after the treatment. Only after a gap of as much as twenty one years does the risk of death from some other cause exceed the risk of death from the original disease.'[7] Or from the original treatment.

On June 8 1990, at Chelmsford Crown Court, a 42-year old woman was awarded £155,000 damages. She had suffered seven years of cancer treatment. 'She spent 13 months in and out of cancer wards during which she made friends and saw them die. Her hair fell out and she suffered continual nausea during six spells of painful radiological and drug treatment...Surgeons opened her stomach and removed an ovary in an unsuccessful search for breast cancer. Only then was the shattered woman told it had been a mistake.' (Times 9.6.1990)

The woman, who lost her career and her marriage, had never believed the diagnosis but had allowed herself to be rail-roaded by the white-coated cancer gods. The precise number of people who have been mis-diagnosed and have then been killed by the onslaught or who have survived and have been put in the 'cure' statistics cannot be estimated. One anonymous cancer statistician commented: 'I wouldn't be surprised if they are curing a lot of leukaemia that never existed.'[8]

In 1940, according to Prof. Hardin B. Jones:[19]

'Through re-definition of terms, various questionable grades of malignancy were classed as 'cancer'. After that date, the proportion of cancer cures

having 'normal' life-expectancy increased rapidly, corresponding to the fraction of questionable diagnosis included.'

The oldest prong of the lethal trident, cynically known as modern cancer therapy, is surgery. **The notion being that the removal of a tumour cures the patient; ignoring the fact that cancer is a whole body, systemic, constitutional disease which eventually manifests a tumour**; the location of the growth being due to individual constitutional factors, and the nature of the carcinogen. As for surgery, George Bernard Shaw was of the opinion that, 'The more appalling the mutilation, the more the mutilator is paid.' In medispeak, the more appalling the mutilation the more 'heroic' the surgery; it not being readily apparent whether the heroism is on the part of the patient or the surgeon who must know that one day he will have to stand before the Lords of Karma and explain his actions.

The hemi-corporectomy, the amputation of everything below the pelvis,[9] was one of the bravest operations carried out by the heroic cutters but the greatest scalpel heroism was the 'total exenteration' or 'hollowing out'[10] – the removal of the stomach, internal reproductive organs, pelvic floor and wall, pancreas, spleen, colon, rectum, bladder, ureter and part of the liver: far more fun than the nutritional approach to cancer.

Surgery is a massive shock to the system, uses carcinogenic anaesthesia and increases the risk of cancer in the scar tissue. It has a place only where the threat to life processes is immediate, as in digestive obstruction etc.

The routine removal of every malignant lump which is surrounded by the body with a defensive shield, is a death sentence.

Chemotherapy involves the use of extremely toxic petrochemical drugs in the hope, never realised, of killing the disease before killing the patient. The drugs are designed to kill all fast-growing cells, cancerous or not. All cells caught in the act of division are systematically poisoned. The effects include hair loss, violent nausea, vomiting, diarrhoea, cramps, impotence, sterility, extreme pain, fatigue, immune-system destruction, cancer and death.

According to the government's own figures,[11] around 2 percent of chemotherapy recipients are still alive after 5 years: the term 'alive' is used, here, in its literal sense: i.e. not yet clinically dead.

'Recently someone very dear to me, someone who can never be replaced, died a premature and totally unnecessary death. He had cancer and he was my father. Although there are safe, effective, natural treatments for this dreaded disease...my father allowed himself to be talked into having chemotherapy.

The side-effects of the drugs were horrendous and unspeakably cruel but he persevered with the treatment because he had faith and trust in his doctors and believed every word they told him. Clearly he was dying but he continued taking the awful treatments because he was repeatedly told that he was doing 'so well'. After all, the good doctors wouldn't lie to him, would they?...the truth about his real condition was not revealed to him until my mother accompanied him to the clinic for what was to be his last treatment...the prognosis was "very grim"...my father had less than a month to live... then, and only then, did my father allow us to take him elsewhere for non-toxic treatment... My husband took him to a cancer help centre where he received metabolic therapy...he was one hundred percent more comfortable and relatively free of pain...and he died a peaceful death.

He did not die of cancer, however, but of pneumonia, one of the chemotherapy's side-effects. Chemotherapy damages if not destroys the body's immune defence system...had my father been told that chemotherapy would never cure him...he would have allowed us to take him elsewhere...much sooner...I keep thinking of the Hippocratic oath, in particular, the first line, "First do no harm", and, "I will never do harm to anyone. To please no one will I prescribe a deadly drug, nor give advice which may cause his death." I loved my dad very much and to lose him in this cruel horrible unnecessary manner is certainly the heartbreak of my life.'[12]

Whilst toxic chemotherapy has killed untold millions of patients, a systemic approach, using genuine, natural, anti-cancer agents is a valid, if not ideal, approach to cancer. 'Radiotherapy', however, is devoid of any rational basis in theory or practice.

After radium was discovered it was tried out in various situations. It was inevitable that 'some enterprising medical men started a fad in using it on cancer victims.[13] The tumours were shrinking; cancer was being cured. This led to a price rise of 1,000 percent and the birth of a multi-billion dollar industry without an atom of science as its basis.

In late 1991 someone at the North Staffordshire Hospital, in Stoke, noticed that the settings on the tumour-burning machine were set too low. Various masterminds, including the local MP, went on air with dire warnings of the consequences to the 1,000 patients who had not received enough of the healing rays. An investigation was ordered.

The team undertaking the investigation faced a considerable problem. If they accepted the view of the doctor-in-charge, that the 'under-dosed' patients fared no worse than those given prescribed doses, they might have been asked why patients were, and are, given large doses of immuno-suppressive, carcinogenic radiation, when not necessary.

If they decided to preserve the virtue of radiation as a valid therapy by declaring that the UDs died quicker, they risked litigation from the relatives. If they found, as cynics strongly suspected, that the UDs lasted longer, they risked some trouble-maker wanting a further 1,000 patients treated with the radiation machine turned off altogether.

They needed to bring in the Creative Cancer Statistics Squad: pronto.

Finally, the CCSS delivered their verdict: the doctor involved was wrong; the lack of radiation adversely affected the patients. Litigation from the relatives was to be preferred to admitting that the dosage made no difference.

In the US, an anonymous National Cancer Institute scientist[14] explained:

'Look, when you've got 10,000 radiologists and millions of dollars worth of radiation equipment, you give radiation treatments, even if study after study shows that a lot of it does more harm than good. What else are they going to do?

Like surgeons, they've been trained to cut: so they cut.'

One person who chose to have treatment with the radiation machine turned off altogether was the jockey Bob Champion. Convinced by the early detectors, in spite of feeling well, that he was, '...likely to die of cancer of the lymph gland,' he decided that he did not relish the thought of a treatment that, '...could have ruined his lungs.'[15] - let alone the rest of him - and opted for drugs.

He eventually survived the treatment and the 'lymphoma'. His doctor, 'cancer specialist' Ann Barrett, declared:

'He is the only patient in my experience who has come through this disease and achieved such a high degree of physical fitness afterwards. His recovery is even more remarkable when you consider that he refused to have the conventional treatment.' !!!

The plight of the ever-increasing number of parents of child cancer victims facing 'radiotherapy' was well illustrated in October 1993:

'...after learning of the appalling side-effects of radiotherapy...her anxious mother has opted to take her to America for private treatment... "I've been told the radiotherapy will cause brain damage knocking forty points off her I.Q....Her growth would be stunted... she would need hormones to help her growth and sexual development. It is also likely she would be sterile"'[16]

Further delights include bone and nerve damage, leading to amputation of limbs, severe burns and, of course, death, at a future time, from cancer and leukaemia due to the highly carcinogenic, immuno-suppressive effects of the huge doses of radiation.

'Chemotherapy and radiotherapy will make the ancient method of drilling holes in a patient's head, to permit the escape of demons, look relatively advanced...the use of cobalt...effectively closes the door on cure.'[17]

The five year survival rates for the different onslaughts are: [11]

- Surgery - 22 percent
- Radiotherapy -12 percent
- Surgery/radiotherapy combined - 6 percent
- Chemotherapy plus others - 2.5 percent
- Chemotherapy alone - 1.6 percent

... none of which has stopped the cancer industry from carrying out the same procedures, day in, day out, for decades: with the same deadly, inevitable results.

Temporarily suppressing, with the scalpel, drug or radiation, the symptoms of cancer does nothing for the victim's chances of survival. Adding gross insult to injury, the treatment involves massive doses of carcinogens and super-poisons.

The patient is subject to a regime diametrically opposed to that which is needed for survival.

Cancer is an acceptable form of suicide for those who have lost the desire to live: this loss being a major factor in the development of the disease in the first place. The great tragedy and scandal is where the victim has a strong determination to live and fight but is then destroyed by the assault from the lethal, useless treatment and not by the cancer.

1.9.6.6 Early Detection

A boost to the early detection and cure hoax has been the improved methods used in picking up early cancer - real or imaginary.This has led to an increase in numbers of people lasting five years and being put in the cure statistics. Early stage patients are stronger and more likely to survive the assault; whereas, before the improved techniques, patients with more advanced disease succumbed to the disease/treatment before the five years were up.

On early detection and orthodox treatment, Prof. H.B. Jones, then the leading US cancer statistician, with over 30 years experience, stated, in 1975:

'It is utter nonsense to claim that catching cancer symptoms early enough will increase the patient's chances of survival: not one scientist or study has proven that in any way. My studies have proved conclusively that untreated cancer victims live up to four times longer than treated individuals. If one has cancer and opts to do nothing at all, he will live longer and feel better than if he undergoes radiation, chemotherapy or surgery, other than used in immediate life-threatening situation.'

One person who, before the reality hit him, may well have smiled at Jones' statement was US Senator Hubert Humphrey. Former vice-president Humphrey, a true believer - until it was too late - in the cancer boys and their early detection was told that he was suffering from bladder cancer.This was duly 'cured' with radiation. Later, in May 1976, the prognosis was that there was no reason for any further treatment. Six months later Humphrey was operated on for the removal of a bladder tumour. His surgeon, Willard Whitmore, declared: 'As far as we are concerned the Senator is cured.'

Whitmore added that '...to wipe out any microscopic colonies of cancer cells that may be hidden somewhere in the body' treatment with experimental chemotherapy - 'bottled death' as Humphrey later called it - would begin. Humphrey changed from an active middle-aged man into a feeble, ageing wreck and died within one year in full view of the media who all, apparently, thought he had died of cancer.

Any doubts about the brass neck of the Syndicate, in the face of such a spectacular public defeat, were dispelled the very next year by the publication of a book which stated that Humphrey was a '...famous beneficiary of modern radiation therapy' who had '...remained well for three years until the development of a new, more advanced cancer.'[20]

The use of very expensive body scanners to detect early lumps has been a favourite source of pride with the cancer cartel and their faithful fund-raisers. A letter from an MP stated: 'I have now received the enclosed reply from the...DHSS about the value of body scanners in treating cancer. As you will read, the government does acknowledge the value of body scanners but can give no statistical evidence of this.'[21]

This is fully in keeping with the tradition of orthodox medical practices. Estimates vary from 50 percent to over 85 percent as to the degree of these practices which are, at best, unproven or, at worst, lethal.

1.9.6.7 Breast Cancer

Around 15,000 women, diagnosed with breast cancer, die each year in the UK. The medical cynics, engaged in the ongoing competition to demonstrate that it is quite impossible to insult the intelligence of the public on matters of health, have always found fertile ground in the field of breast cancer; the crowning achievement being when one of the jokers convinced healthy women to have both breasts removed to prevent breast cancer.

'The American Cancer Society and the National Cancer Institute, as a showcase project of the "war on cancer", co-sponsored a massive X-ray screening program for breast cancer - on 280,000 women - the notorious mammography follies. With kind smiles and Pollyanna counsel, women were encouraged to affirm their virtue on the altar of technology by exposing themselves to periodic radiation known to increase the risk of the disease. ...Emphasis was placed on radiating women over 50, the very age group that would be most vulnerable to induction of cancer by radiation.'

By 1989 four random-controlled mammography trials had taken place: in the USA, UK and two in Sweden. In the final, and most sophisticated, trial, in Malmo, it was found that for one woman to have a cancer avoided or delayed it would need 68,000 women to be screened. As such a figure is completely meaningless, the grave dangers of mammography are entirely without any possible counter-balancing benefits.

'Breast scanning increases cancer risks for women....middle-aged women who have regular mammograms are more likely to die from breast cancer than those who are not screened...

The largest ever trial of mass breast cancer screening was the Canadian National Breast Screening Study, involving 50,000 women and directed by Prof. Anthony Miller. Half of the women were given X-ray screening every year or 18 months and half were given just a physical examination. **Within the X-rayed group the cancer death-rate was 'significantly higher.'**

The danger, according to Miller, was from the fact that mammograms lead to surgery for tiny lumps, encouraging secondaries to grow. Also, according to Miller: '...one potential problem was that surgery, the anaesthetic and radiotherapy, involved in treating women with breast cancer, were interfering with immunity.' No kiddin'?

Dr. Irwin Bross, Director of Biostatistics, Roswell Park Memorial Institute, had his funding stopped by the National Cancer Institute when he released his figures **linking X-rays with cancer and leukaemia**. Bross said that the mammography stunt would cause four or five cancers for every one detected, leading to '..the worst epidemic of iatrogenic breast cancer in history. In my view...the NCI would be better off putting the money allocated for future screenings into a trust fund for the victims of the programme who will develop cancer in 10 to 15 years time.'

According to Prof. Jones: 'With every patient that...boosts his health to build up his natural resistance, there's a high chance that the body will find its own defence against the cancer.' Prof. Jones warned against '...being made into a hopeless invalid through radical medical intervention which has zero chance of extending his life.'

None of which has made any impression on the screeners or the knife/drug/ray tumour-zappers; or on the ever-willing multitude of females, following the camp and determined to be the next sacrifice, virgin or otherwise, at the feet of The Great God of Consensus Medicine.

1.9.6.8 Bristol

In June 1986, a study, financed by the Cancer Research Campaign and the Imperial Cancer Research Fund, began at the Bristol Cancer Help Centre. The BCHC had approached the Syndicate with a view to the evaluation of the

Centre's 'complementary' methods; methods, apparently, designed to try to stop the patients dying from **slash/burn/poison** for as long as possible.

The study involved women who had undergone or, incredibly, were still undergoing, the orthodox onslaught, and offered a golden opportunity for the cartel to deliver a decisive blow to rational cancer treatment: a blow from which the Centre and holistic medicine has yet to fully recover. The report of the study was written by C.E.D. Chilvers, T.J. McElwain, F.S. Bagenal, D.F. Easton, and E. Harris.

The opening lines of the report set the tone for the rest of the document: 'Interest in and use of alternative medicines and practices for the treatment of cancer has been growing for several years despite lack of any scientific evidence for anti-tumour effects.'[18]

Of the findings, the report stated: 'These results suggest that women with breast cancer attending the BCHC fare worse than those receiving conventional treatment only... the possibility that some aspects of the BCHC regime is responsible for their decreased survival must be faced.' The report implied that women without metastasis - cancer cells spreading - were around 3 times more likely to relapse in the BCHC group.

Without subjecting the report to the usual peer or statistical review, the triumphant cancer orthodoxy, at a press conference organised by the ICRF, could hardly conceal their glee at such an easy victory. Whilst the BCHC staff, now showing belated signs that they realised what the trial was all about, looked for holes in which to be swallowed.

Karol Sikora, of the cancer unit at the Hammersmith Hospital, had expressed doubts about the report's authenticity and had provisionally agreed to attend the press event to offer the BCHC support. He was later to contact the Centre saying that he would not attend. Walter Bodmer, one of the cancer barons behind the report and director-general of the ICRF, who were funding some of Sikora's work, repeatedly refused on camera to comment on whether he knew anything of a telephone call causing Sikora's about face.[24]

Sikora later became deputy director of clinical research at the ICRF.

After the media blitz had done the required damage, the facts about the report began to emerge: the BCHC women were much more ill than the control group. No constant check was made to see if the Bristol women kept to the regime. No-one ensured that the controls were avoiding the 'complementary' therapies available at the Royal Marsden Hospital, where half the controls were based. Lifestyle, relationships, environmental factors etc. were not taken into account. All BCHC women were classed as 'cancer-free' at the start when nearly half had active cancer, with 19% 'incurable'. 43% of BCHC cases had undergone a mastectomy compared with 36% of controls. 85% of Bristol women were under 55, a group with a worse prognosis. The controls had 73% under 55...etc.

The report found itself under a deluge of criticism, mainly in the pages of the Lancet; and a couple of months after the report publication one of the reporters, T.J. McElwain, committed suicide. None of which caused the others involved - Chilvers, Bagenal etc. - to call for official withdrawal of the report; a report which had concluded: 'Other alternative practitioners should have the courage to submit their work to this type of stringent assessment.'

1.9.6.9 Tamoxifen

Tamoxifen is a drug which is related, structurally, to the infamous DES and is used in the treatment of breast cancer. It is now being promoted as a breast cancer preventative in the UK, despite serious reservations on both sides of the Atlantic. Women are being asked to take a tablet of the drug every day for five years with regular X-rays throughout the period. According to Professor Samuel S. Epstein of the School of Public Health, University of Illinois: 'As relatively few breast cancer patients have taken the drug for more than five years tamoxifen may be a much more potent human carcinogen than is currently recognised.'

Studies have suggested an increased risk of uterine cancer, 6.4 times higher for those women taking tamoxifen.[27] The literature, sent out by the promoters states: 'Liver tumours develop in rats given large doses of tamoxifen, but not in mice so it is difficult to be sure about the effects in humans.'

This has not deterred some ladies from signing up; presumably, having reasoned that they are more like mice than rats.

'Drug maker may quit cancer trial - Healthy women taking part in a clinical trial to prevent breast cancer might have been put at a risk of developing other tumours...the drug may increase the risk of tumours in the womb, liver and bowel. The disclosure, on the eve of the launch...has led to the manufacturer threatening to pull out.'[28]

Hamish Cameron, head of medical affairs at Zeneca, the drug's makers, stated: 'Should the benefit/risk balance shift adversely, we reserve the right to withdraw that drug supply. If the evidence is quite clear I would hope the trialists themselves would realise that the game is up.'

Dr.Richard Bulbrook, one of the original proposers of the tamoxifen enterprise, voiced his concerns: 'Things have changed. There are now so many side-effects reported - there were 41 at the last count - and some of these are fatal.'

The USA abandoned the tamoxifen prevention scam on safety grounds: all in sharp contrast to Gordon McVie 'scientific director' of the 'Cancer Research Campaign': 'What we want to know is can we get more mileage out of tamoxifen, possibly by giving it for life.'

On the question of how orthodox cancer treatment 'saves' half the women with breast cancer, Dr Irwin Bross is quite unequivocal - half the women don't have breast cancer in the first place:

'If you are a woman who has been diagnosed as "early breast cancer"... there is one simple scientific fact that you need to know...more than half the time the pathologist is wrong - it is not actually breast cancer*...What most women have is a tumour which, under a light microscope, looks like a cancer to a pathologist. Chances are this tumour lacks the ability to metastasize...the hallmark of a genuine cancer...*

The world's first controlled trial of adjuvant therapies for breast cancer was centralised in my department...Dr Leslie Blumenson and I...made a surprising discovery. ***More than half of the patients...had tumours...that were more like benign lesions.***

*Our discovery was highly unpopular with the medical profession. Doctors could never afford to admit the scientific truth because the standard treatment in those days was radical mastectomy. Admitting the truth could lead to malpractice suits by women who had lost a breast because of an incorrect medical diagnosis. The furious doctors at the National Cancer Institute...took our highly successful breast cancer research program away from us...****they eventually succeeded in suppressing our findings and blocking new publications...***

Breast cancer and prostate cancer are statistical twins. When the functions of these two sexual organs diminish, the cells often become abnormal and

look like cancer cells...The Journal of the American Medical Association reported amazingly high survival rates...of untreated early prostate cancer which showed 7 out of 8 tumours were not cancers.

There is no reason for women to panic when they hear "cancer"; panic makes them easy victims.'

The patient who is wrongly diagnosed and has no cancer, and is therefore more likely to survive the 'therapy', is recorded as a 'cancer cure'.

The patient who has cancer and is in a weak state is usually killed by the treatment and recorded as having 'died of cancer'.

Those who never had cancer in the first place are made far more likely to develop the disease, in the future, from the lethal carcinogenic, immuno-suppressive effects of the surgery, drugs and radiation.

1.9.6.10 Save the Children

According to the latest Morbidity Statistics from General Practice, UK childhood cancer incidence almost tripled in ten years. In the USA, '...of the 23 children admitted to the largest paediatric ward of the University of Minnesota hospitals in a single day, 18 had cancer.'[25]

A mother, writing in a women's magazine, said:

'By the time you read this my son Michael, who is just five, will be almost at the end of a year's course of treatment for cancer... To show for it Michael has a scar from one side of his body to the other, where doctors removed a huge malignant tumour and one of his kidneys. Radiotherapy at Bart's hospital left him limp like a rag doll with all the stuffing knocked out of him. Chemotherapy has made all of his hair fall out. The drugs... make him vomit for hours on end... his face is small and mostly pale: his eyes are dark and sullen and shadowed, the way a child's eyes should never be.'

Whilst it is unknown how long this child stood up to his tormentors, **before being killed**, it is certain that none of the medical inquisitors were hung, jailed for life, thrown into a padded cell or struck off any medical register.

It is also certain that anyone approaching the torturers with a suggestion that a regime of metabolic, herbal, nutritional... etc. treatment might effect a safe, effective approach to the illness would have been ignored or ridiculed. In the USA, Food and Drug administrator Robert Young admitted:

'In Boston a hospital tested a new NCI drug...on children. Their kidneys were lost within days...this was no big deal because new... NCI drugs are given out with literally no safeguards for people who will receive them.'

Having killed one child too many for litigatory safety, the cancer boys finally decided to tone down the assault. This led, inevitably, to longer survival times, which became 'great progress in childhood cancer treatment.' Whilst any reduction at all in the level of the drug/radiation lunacy is to be greatly welcomed, the idea that these longer survival times were due to anything other than less lethal treatments is merely wishful thinking.

The Autumn 1997 edition of the Leukaemia Research News reported the views of some LRF scientists:

'The intensive therapy given to children to ensure their survival (!)...can result in longer term side effects such as intellectual impairment, heart damage, growth disorders and even second cancers.'

When the second cancers - first cancers if the original leukaemia diagnosis was wrong - and the treatment, kill the patient, the original 'leukaemia cure' still stands in the statistics - cured and dead.

1.9.7.0 The FRT and aging

There are more than 300 theories to explain the aging phenomenon. Many of them originate from the study of changes that accumulate with time. Among all the theories, **the free radical theory of aging, postulated first by Harman, is the most popular and widely tested**, and is based on the chemical nature and ubiquitous presence of free radicals (The aging paradox: free radical theory of aging. Badithe T. Ashok and Rashid Ali. Experimental Gerontology. Volume 34, Issue 3, June 1999, Pages 293-303).

Despite the fact that the free radical theory of aging is generally accepted by most biological gerontologists as the most likely mechanistic cause of aging, it is based on very little direct experimental evidence (Beckman, K.B. and Ames, B.N. (1998) Physiol. Rev. **78**, 547–581.)

After assessing the 14 years of evidence concerning the FRTA, Beckman and Ames conclude that; "...the momentum gathering behind the free radical theory is not due to any single experiment or approach, but rather derives from the extraordinary multidisciplinary nature of current research. Although no single line of reasoning alone permits definitive conclusions, together they present a compelling case.... In its broader sense ('oxidants contribute significantly to the process of degenerative senescence [aging]'), the theory has clearly been validated. In the more strict sense of the theory, ('oxidants determine maximum life span potential'), **whilst the data are not yet conclusive**, a large body of consistent data, [that tends to support the theory] has been generated." (Beckman, K. & Ames, B. (1998) "The free radical theory of aging matures" Physiol Rev 78: 548-81).

The free radical theory of aging is not just one of the oldest and still current theories of aging - it is one of the best proven. Any serious long-term anti-aging program must be based upon practical knowledge of, and disciplined use of various techniques and supplements to cope with, the reality of free radicals. And even if an antioxidant/ anti-free radical program doesn't ultimately lengthen one's life, it should still seriously reduce the risk of heart attacks, strokes, cancer, Alzheimer's disease, and many other of the "plagues" of the modern world. **WRONG!**

There are four primary sources of oxidants formed within living organisms. The major source of free radicals and oxidants is the mitochondrial generation of ATP energy using oxygen. A small percentage (2-3% or less) of oxygen in mitochondria is inadvertently converted to superoxide radical, which can in turn generate hydrogen peroxide, hydroxyl radical, and all other free radicals. A second source of oxidants, especially hydrogen peroxide, is the peroxisomes, organelles that degrade fatty acids. A third source of oxidants is cytochrome P450 enzymes. These enzymes help cells, especially in the lungs and liver, detoxify a broad range of potentially toxic food, drug and environmental pollutant molecules. Superoxide radical is a by-product of many of these detoxification reactions.

http://www.bccancer.bc.ca/PPI/UnconventionalTherapies/Vitamins.htm

1.9.7.1 Proponent/ Advocate Claims – Antioxidant Use in Treating Cancer

"Multiple antioxidant vitamin supplements together with diet and lifestyle modifications may improve the efficacy of standard and experimental cancer therapies." (Prasad KN, *et al.* High doses of multiple antioxidant vitamins: essential ingredients in improving the efficacy of standard cancer therapy. J Am Coll Nutr 1999;18:13-25)

"In our study, (Ingram et al 1992) we demonstrated strong association for beta-carotene and vitamin C consumption with a degree of improvement in differentiation [degree of improvement in grade or speed of growth] with increasing consumption of these nutrients" (Ingram D et al. Diet and subsequent survival in women with breast cancer. British Journal of Cancer 1994;69:592-595)

1.9.7.2 Professional Evaluation/ Critique - Antioxidant Use in Treating Cancer

"Neither vitamins nor other dietary supplements cure cancer." (Cassileth BR. Alternative medicine handbook: the complete reference guide to alternative and complementary therapies. New York: W.W. Norton & Co., 1998:65-71)

"There are important distinctions between dietary supplements in the form of the vitamin pill that many take each morning and products aimed at treating illness." (Cassileth BR. Alternative medicine handbook: the complete reference guide to alternative and complementary therapies. New York: W.W. Norton & Co., 1998:65-71)

There is at least a theoretical disadvantage in the use of anti-oxidants during radiation therapy (which works via oxidation processes). (Rheaume D. BC Cancer Agency verbal communication 1996)

"Oxidation reactions, which are frequently destructive to biologic molecules and involve combining a substance with oxygen, appear to initiate apoptosis and move it along. ["Apoptosis, or programmed cell death, is an intricately choreographed form of suicide by irretrievably damaged cells, including those already on their way to becoming cancerous."] **Too much antioxidant, researchers theorize, might interfere with these oxidation reactions, derailing apoptosis and leaving the precursors of cancer alive.** The implications may be particularly serious for cancer patients. Chemotherapies often act by inducing apoptosis, so antioxidant vitamins, in theory, could interfere with chemotherapy." (Holzman D. Do antioxidants promote cancer? Alternative and Complementary Therapies 1997 June:167-9).

"High doses of antioxidants that may help prevent cancer could make things worse once the disease has struck, a study by Dutch researchers hints.

Antioxidants such as vitamin C seem to prevent cancer by mopping up free radicals that can damage DNA. [However], Jurgen Karczewski and colleagues at

Nijmegen University in the Netherlands say that **free radicals can also kill cancer cells. If so, antioxidants should be bad for cancer patients because they remove radicals**." (Day M. Cancer Catch. New Scientist 1997 Sept 13;16)

1.9.8 0 Transmissible cancers (Tasmanian devils and Canine transmissible venereal tumor)

(The New York Times. Olivia Judson. "Cancer of the Devil"). October 14, 2008. Some human cancers are infectious in the sense that they are caused by infectious viruses. **Cervical cancer, for instance, is caused by human papilloma virus, which spreads from one person to another during sex.**

But **the cancer that's killing the Tasmanian devils is different. The cancer cells themselves are infectious.**

Here's what happens. The cancer causes a tumor on the animal's face. If an infected animal bites another — which happens often, as devils are aggressive creatures, especially during the mating season — some of the tumor cells get transferred. These then start growing on the other animal. It's as though you kissed someone with throat cancer, and got their cancer yourself.

Which is pretty weird. Cancers are usually part of you, a group of your own cells that begin to grow out of control. Foreign cells — such as the ones that cause the devils' cancer — are normally rejected by the immune system. That's why organ transplants are difficult: the immune system immediately recognizes that the transplanted organ is not part of you, and begins attacking it. This happens unless there's a close match between the donor and the recipient at a set of genes known as the major histocompatibility locus, or MHC. If there is a match, you may be similar enough, genetically speaking, that the immune system doesn't notice the difference between the foreign organ and you. But unless you're having a transplant from a close relation, the odds of this are low. Human MHC genes are extremely variable. Most people who get organ transplants thus have to take drugs that suppress their immune system. Otherwise, the foreign organ gets attacked and destroyed.

So it's not surprising that most of the devil-style infectious cancers known in humans have happened when someone's immune system hasn't been working. Recipients of transplanted organs occasionally receive cancer cells as well; the drugs that prevent the immune system from destroying the organ also prevent it from destroying the foreign tumor. **Because a baby's immune system**

doesn't get going until after it's born, a pregnant woman with cancer can infect her fetus. Likewise, if a mother is carrying several fetuses and one of them has a cancer, it can infect the others. But all these events are rare.

Even rarer are cases of direct transmission to someone whose immune system is robust. One example: a healthy surgeon injured his hand while operating on a cancer patient and contracted the patient's cancer. For reasons unknown, his immune system failed to respond. The resulting tumor was cut out, and the surgeon survived.

Why don't the devils reject the alien cells? There are two possibilities. The first is that the tumor somehow interferes with the immune response. (Many traditional tumors can do this.) The second is that the immune system fails to recognize the tumor as alien.

Tasmanian devils aren't the only animals to have a transmissible cancer. Dogs have one too. Theirs is transmitted during sex. **Canine transmissible venereal tumor** has been around for at least 200 years, and probably much longer. (The devils' disease, in contrast, was first spotted in 1996.) For dogs, the disease is rarely fatal. Instead, the tumor goes through an initial period of rapid growth, during which it manages to stop the dog's immune system from attacking it. But then, the immune system gets going, and kills the tumor. Having once been infected, a dog is resistant to the disease.

These cancers raise a number of questions. In particular: why aren't more cancers transmissible? After all, **there are many, many types of cancer in many different species, but only two are known to spread from one animal to another**. This suggests it isn't simply a matter of MHC diversity. After all, **animals such as beavers and cheetahs have low diversity but no cancer**; and the MHC situation of Tasmanian devils didn't suddenly change in the 1990s. Instead, it suggests that the cancer cells have to evolve in ways that makes them more likely to be transmissible. What those ways are, however, is a total mystery.

But if transmissible cancers have evolved twice, the odds are they can evolve again. The prospect is unnerving. (Even more unnerving is the idea that such cancers could be transmitted by mosquitoes, as was mooted for an infectious cancer said to be circulating among a species of hamster in the 1960s. Reports of this cancer are, however, absent from the recent scientific literature, and their significance is unclear.) Beavers and cheetahs, and other animals with low diversity at the MHC, could obviously be at risk of going the way of the devil, should a transmissible cancer evolve in these species.

What about us? Humans have lots of MHC diversity. But we have another risk factor. Owing to the failure to treat H.I.V., the virus that causes AIDS, in many parts of the world, large numbers of people have compromised immune systems. This is the sort of environment that could, perhaps, allow a transmissible cancer to evolve. Initially, it would circulate only among those who are immunocompromised. But, over time, it might evolve to infect healthy people too. It's an alarming thought — though happily, a thought is all it is. For now.

1.9.8.1 Evolution of a transmissible cancer

The transmissible agent causing canine transmissible venereal tumor (CTVT) is thought to be the tumor cell itself. To test this hypothesis, we analyzed genetic markers including major histocompatibility (MHC) genes, microsatellites, and mitochondrial DNA (mtDNA) in naturally occurring tumors and matched blood samples. In each case, the tumor is genetically distinct from its host. Moreover, tumors collected from 40 dogs in 5 continents are derived from a single neoplastic clone that has diverged into two subclades. Phylogenetic analyses indicate that CTVT most likely originated from a wolf or an East Asian breed of dog between 200 and 2500 years ago. Although CTVT is highly aneuploid, it has a remarkably stable genotype. During progressive growth, CTVT downmodulates MHC antigen expression. Our findings have implications for understanding genome instability in cancer, natural transplantation of allografts, and the capacity of a somatic cell to evolve into a transmissible parasite (Clonal origin and evolution of a transmissible cancer. Murgia C, Pritchard JK, Kim SY, Fassati A, Weiss RA. Cell. 2006 Aug 11;126(3):477-87).

1.9.8.2 Is cancer a transmittable disease?

A direct, horizontal and natural transmission of neoplasic cells has only recently been accepted by the biomedical community. **There are three known examples in mammals: the Tasmanian Devil Tumor Disease, the Canine Transmissible Venereal Tumor and a similar disease in Sirian Hamsters.** These diseases are not anecdotic cases only, but provide support for the cancer clonal evolution hypothesis (Is cancer a transmittable disease? Meléndez-Zajgla J, Maldonado V. Gac Med Mex. 2007 Jul-Aug;143(4):353-4).

1.9.9.0 Prostate cancer not warded off by supplements, selenium and E 10/27/08. The SELECT study

Selenium and vitamin E supplements do not prevent prostate cancer and may in fact be a little bit dangerous, U.S. researchers reported on 10/27/08.

The study of **35,000 men** showed the **supplements did not work together or alone to prevent prostate cancer,** the most common type of cancer in men in the United States.

"As we continue to monitor the health of these 35,000 men, this information may help us understand why two nutrients that showed strong initial evidence to be able to prevent prostate cancer did not do so," **Dr. Eric Klein of the Cleveland Clinic** in Ohio, who worked on the study, said in a statement. Other, earlier studies had suggested that the two supplements might prevent prostate cancer. **Both are antioxidants** -- compounds that interfere with chemical reactions that can damage cells and DNA.

The National Cancer Institute, which helped organize the study, said **men taking part are being told to stop taking the supplements they had been given** but will continue to have their health monitored for about three more years.

"The data also showed two concerning, but not statistically significant, trends: **there were slightly more cases of prostate cancer in men taking only vitamin E and slightly more cases of diabetes in men taking only selenium,"** the NCI, one of he National Institutes of Health, said in a statement. Neither of these findings proves an increased risk from the supplements and may be due to chance."

The men in the study were randomly assigned to take one of four sets of supplements or placebos, with one group taking both selenium and vitamin E; one taking selenium and a placebo; one taking vitamin E and a placebo; and the final group getting two dummy pills.

The American Cancer Society predicts that **in 2008, an estimated 186,320 men will be diagnosed with prostate cancer and 28,660 will die from it in the United States alone**.

Selenium: more than 750Âµg per day are associated with immune suppression.

10/27/08 National Cancer Institute release:

1.9.9.1 The SELECT study (overall description)

Key Points:

- SELECT stands for the Selenium and Vitamin E Cancer Prevention Trial, a prevention clinical trial to see if one or both of these dietary supplements prevent prostate cancer.
- SELECT is continuing to evaluate the effects of the supplements but **participants are no longer taking study supplements. The independent Data and Safety Monitoring Committee for the trial found that selenium and vitamin E, taken alone or together for an average of five years, did not prevent prostate cancer**.
- The SELECT data showed two concerning, but not statistically significant, trends: **there were slightly more cases of prostate cancer in men taking only vitamin E and slightly more cases of diabetes in men taking only selenium**. Neither of these findings proves an increased risk from the supplements and may be due to chance.

1. What is SELECT?

SELECT stands for the Selenium and Vitamin E Cancer Prevention Trial, a clinical trial to see if one or both of these substances can help prevent prostate cancer when taken as dietary supplements. The trial is funded primarily by the National Cancer Institute (NCI) and is being coordinated by the Southwest Oncology Group (SWOG), an international network of research institutions that receives NCI funding. Enrollment for the trial began in 2001 and ended in 2004. More than 400 sites in the United States, Puerto Rico, and Canada are taking part in the study. **Over 35,000 men are participating in SELECT**.

2. What is the status of SELECT?

SELECT participants are being told to stop taking their study supplements but will continue to have their health monitored by study staff for about three more years. **The independent Data and Safety Monitoring Committee (DSMC) for the trial met on September 15, 2008 to review SELECT study data and found that selenium and vitamin E, taken alone or together for an average of five years, did not prevent prostate**

cancer. They also calculated that **it was unlikely selenium and vitamin E supplementation would ever produce a 25 percent reduction in prostate cancer, as the study was designed to show.**

The data also showed two concerning, but not statistically significant, trends: there were slightly more cases of prostate cancer in men taking only vitamin E and slightly more cases of diabetes in men taking only selenium. Neither of these findings proves an increased risk from the supplements and may be due to chance. But combined with the lack of benefit of selenium and vitamin E, the DSMC recommended that the men in SELECT stop taking study supplements but continue to be monitored. **The DSMC also said that the data could not exclude a small chance that the study supplements might have effects later in the men's lives.** SELECT investigators are preparing a report of these findings for a peer-reviewed scientific journal.

3. What is happening to the men on SELECT?

Men on the study are being informed about the initial findings and told to stop taking their study supplements. Participants will continue to have their health monitored by study staff, continue to respond to the study questionnaires, and will provide a blood sample at their five-year anniversary of joining the trial (if they have not already done so). The information from the questionnaires and the blood samples will allow a complete analysis of the study, including important molecular-level research on the role of antioxidants in cancer prevention and the natural history of prostate cancer, other cancers, and diseases of male aging.

4. What if a participant has moved or otherwise lost contact with their SELECT study team?

Any participant in SELECT who has lost contact with their study team can contact the NCI's Cancer Information Service for more information and to be referred to SELECT study staff. Participants in the United States and Puerto Rico can call the CIS toll-free at 1-800-4-CANCER (1-800-422-6237), Monday-Friday, 9 a.m. - 4:30 p.m. local time or use our LiveHelp® online chat service at http://www.cancer.gov/livehelp, Monday-Friday, 9 a.m. - 11 p.m. Eastern time. E-mails can also be sent to cancer.govstaff@mail.nih.gov.

5. Who got which supplement?

Men who participated in this study took two capsules a day. Participants were randomly assigned (that is, assigned by chance) to receive:

- selenium and vitamin E
- selenium and a placebo
- vitamin E and a placebo
- two placebos

Two placebos were used in the trial: one looked like a selenium capsule; the other looked like a vitamin E capsule. Each placebo contained only inactive ingredients. Neither the participants nor the researchers know who received the selenium and vitamin E, or the placebos, a process known as 'blinding.'

6. Have the men been 'unblinded'?

Study investigators have carefully considered how to follow (monitor) participants and feel it would be most proper and useful to continue to follow SELECT participants in a blinded fashion. Men in SELECT are followed with state-of-the art care including regular prostate cancer screening tests and questions about diabetes and other health issues. Data from men who remain blinded will provide the most reliable information on which to assess prostate cancer, adult onset diabetes, or other diseases of male aging.

If a participant asks to know which supplements they were receiving, he will be told. Men who request to be unblinded will continue to be followed by study staff in the manner originally outlined in the study.

7. What are a man's chances of developing prostate cancer?

Except for skin cancer, prostate cancer is the most common type of cancer in men in the United States. In the U.S. in 2008, there will be an estimated 186,320 new cases of prostate cancer and 28,660 deaths from this disease (1). All men are at risk for prostate cancer, but those at highest risk fall into one or more of the following categories: **age 55 years or older; African-American; have a father or brother with prostate cancer.**

8. What is selenium? Why study it for prostate cancer prevention?

Our bodies need selenium, a nonmetallic trace element that we get from food-especially plant foods such as rice and wheat, seafood, meat, and Brazil nuts. **Selenium is an antioxidant** that may help control cell damage that can lead to cancer.

The Nutritional Prevention of Cancer Trial, first reported in 1996, included 1,312 men and women who had skin cancer. Results of the trial showed that men who took selenium to prevent nonmelanoma skin cancer received no benefit from selenium in preventing skin cancer.

However, **approximately 60 percent fewer new cases of prostate cancer were observed among men who had taken selenium for 6½ years than among men who took the placebo (2). In a 2002 follow-up report, the data showed that men who took selenium for more than 7½ years had about 52 percent fewer new cases of prostate cancer than men who took the placebo** (3). This trial is one of the reasons for studying selenium in SELECT.

9. What is vitamin E? Why study it for prostate cancer prevention?

We get vitamin E in a wide range of foods, especially vegetables, vegetable oils, nuts, and egg yolks. **Vitamin E, like selenium, is an antioxidant**, which may help control cell damage that can lead to cancer.

In a 1998 study of 29,133 male smokers in Finland, 32 percent fewer new cases of prostate cancer and 40 percent fewer deaths from prostate cancer were observed among men who took vitamin E to prevent lung cancer than among men who took a placebo. Some men also took beta carotene, but **neither substance helped prevent lung cancer and beta carotene did not affect prostate cancer** (4).

10. What do researchers hope to learn from SELECT?

A large trial of selenium and vitamin E was needed to substantiate earlier, separate findings from studies in which prostate cancer was not the primary outcome investigated. The primary goal of SELECT was to assess the effect of these substances on the number of new cases of prostate cancer diagnosed during routine clinical practice. **Initial analyses of SELECT data showed that selenium and vitamin E supplements do not help prevent prostate cancer.**

Other objectives of SELECT include assessments of the impact of selenium and vitamin E on the incidence of lung cancer and colon cancer, as well as on total cancer incidence and survival. SELECT will provide the basis for studying the molecular genetics of cancer risk and associations between diet and cancer. A biorepository of blood samples obtained from SELECT participants at their entry into the trial and again after five years was created for use in molecular and mechanistic studies of prostate and other cancers, and other diseases of male aging. Additionally, SELECT has been examining the impact of selenium and vitamin E supplementation on participant quality of life.

11. Who was eligible to participate in SELECT? Were there restrictions on eligibility?

Many diseases, including prostate cancer, occur more frequently in older persons. The risk of developing prostate cancer increases with age. More than 90 percent of prostate cancer cases occur in men age 55 or older (5).

African American men had to be age 50 or older to participate, and men of other races and ethnicities had to be 55 or older. The age for eligibility was lower for African American men because, on average, they get the disease at an earlier age.

12. Could men with benign prostatic hyperplasia (BPH) join SELECT?

Men with BPH, a benign enlargement of the prostate gland, could join SELECT because BPH is not a cancerous or a precancerous condition. In BPH, the prostate grows larger and presses against the urethra and bladder, interfering with the normal flow of urine. **More than half of the men in the United States between the ages of 60 and 70, and as many as 90 percent of men between the ages of 70 and 90, have symptoms of BPH.**

BPH can be treated with four different U.S. Food and Drug Administration (FDA)-approved drugs: finasteride (Proscar®), terazosin (Hytrin®), doxazosin (Cardura®), and tamsulosin (Flomax®). Men were not excluded from SELECT on the basis of taking these drugs. Instead, use of these medications was recorded by SELECT investigators.

In 2003, the SWOG-coordinated Prostate Cancer Prevention Trial, in which more than 18,000 men took either finasteride or a placebo to see if the drug reduced the risk of developing prostate cancer, showed a 25 percent reduction in prostate cancer in men taking finasteride (6). Finasteride is not currently approved by the U.S. FDA for reducing the risk of developing prostate cancer. Men in SELECT were made aware of these findings and were allowed to take the drug.

13. What tests were used to determine eligibility for SELECT? What tests are being done during the study?

The tests included a digital rectal examination (DRE) and a prostate-specific antigen (PSA) test. During a DRE, a doctor inserts a gloved finger into the rectum and feels the prostate gland through the rectal wall to check for bumps or abnormal areas. The PSA test measures the level of PSA, a protein produced by cells of the prostate gland, in the blood. A person's PSA level can rise due to cancer or benign (not cancerous) conditions. Doctors often use the PSA test and DRE as prostate cancer screening tests in men who have no symptoms of the disease.

To be eligible for the SELECT trial, participants had to have a DRE that found no signs of prostate cancer and a total PSA level less than or equal to 4.0 nanograms per milliliter (ng/ml). During the trial, DREs and PSA tests are suggested, but not required, on an annual basis throughout the course of the study. Even though supplement use is being stopped in SELECT, the participants will continue to have their health monitored by study staff, including PSA testing and DREs.

14. Who pays for these tests?

Physician, medical examination, and general clinic costs, including DREs, are charged to the participant in the same way as if he were not part of the trial. These costs may be covered by a participant's health insurance. Financial assistance may be available for some men. SELECT, however, pays for follow-up PSA tests. Men with questions about insurance coverage or reimbursement should check with their local SELECT site.

15. How much selenium was being used in SELECT? What risks were involved with taking selenium?

The amount of selenium (provided as l-selenomethionine) was 200 micrograms (μg) daily. **Although the initial results of the Nutritional Prevention of Cancer Trial showed an overall decrease in cancer incidence from selenium, a 2003 update reported 17 percent more new nonmelanoma skin cancers in the selenium group compared with the placebo group** (7). It is not clear how these results would apply to men who did not already have skin cancer when they enrolled in SELECT, or to men who are not at increased risk for skin cancer.

Since the start of SELECT, four studies have been published looking at the effect of selenium on blood glucose and risk of diabetes: two studies suggested that higher levels of selenium taken from supplements or received naturally were associated with an increased risk of diabetes. One study showed no association between the two, and one showed that people with higher levels of selenium in their blood had a reduced risk of diabetes (8-11). Starting in early 2007, the SELECT DSMC was specifically asked to review the study data for cases of diabetes because of these findings.

16. How much vitamin E was being used in SELECT? What risks were involved?

The amount of vitamin E (provided as dl-alpha-tocopherol acetate) was 400 milligrams (mg), which is equivalent to 400 International Units (IU) per day. This dose of vitamin E can thin the blood somewhat. **Men with uncontrolled high blood pressure were not eligible to take part in SELECT because taking this much vitamin E might have increased their risk of stroke.**

Vitamin E has been shown to increase the risk of some cardiovascular conditions. In a 2005 study, men and women with vascular disease or diabetes who took 400 IU of vitamin E daily for 7 years had a 13 percent increased risk of heart failure compared with participants taking a placebo (12). Heart failure is a condition in which the heart's ability to pump blood is weakened. **A 2005 analysis of several studies in which people with various medical problems took vitamin E suggested a link between high doses of vitamin E (400 IU or more) and increased mortality** (13). The continued follow up of SELECT participants will provide more information about this possible risk.

17. What other requirements were there for SELECT participants?

Upon enrollment, men were asked to have toenail clippings collected to assess selenium levels in the body because selenium concentrates in fingernails and toenails. Toenails were chosen over fingernails because they take longer to grow and thus contain more history of someone's selenium intake. Blood samples were collected upon enrollment to assess levels of vitamin E, and again at five years after a man joined the study. These blood samples are placed in the SELECT biorepository for future studies.

Also upon enrolling, men filled out a questionnaire about their diet and past supplement use. There is also an annual questionnaire that asks for updates of some of this information. Men did not have to change their diets during this study. Each man is offered a supply of a special daily multivitamin, manufactured by The Perrigo Company, Allegan, Michigan, that contains no selenium or vitamin E. Vitamin E, selenium, placebo capsules, and multivitamins were provided free of charge to enrollees. SELECT men will still be able to receive and take the multivitamin now that supplement use has been stopped.

18. What happens if a participant develops prostate cancer while involved in SELECT?

Participants diagnosed with prostate cancer during the study will be referred for treatment and will continue to be followed by the SELECT study staff, although less frequently.

Costs for diagnosis and treatment of prostate problems, prostate cancer, or other medical conditions during the study are charged to the participant in the same way as if he were not part of the trial. A participant's insurance will pay for diagnosis and treatment according to the plan's policies. If the participant has no insurance, social services may be available at the local level to cover costs for diagnosis and treatment.

19. How much did SELECT cost? Who else funded the study, and why?

NCI is the primary funding agency for SELECT, awarding about **$114 million to SWOG from 1999 through 2008, with an additional $4.5 million** contributed by the National Center for Complementary and Alternative Medicine (NCCAM), also an agency of the National Institutes of Health (NIH). NCI has been funding a substudy to see if the supplements affect colon polyp growth. In addition, ancillary studies are funded by three other NIH institutes:

- The National Institute on Aging (NIA) has provided almost $7 million for the Prevention of Alzheimer's Disease with Vitamin E and Selenium (PREADVISE) trial. This trial is NIA's add-on to SELECT. It is evaluating whether these supplements can help prevent memory loss and dementia, such as that found in Alzheimer's disease. Studies show that increased oxidative stress may damage brain cells and is linked with Alzheimer's disease. Animal and tissue culture studies of vitamin E and selenium suggest that they can protect brain cells from oxidative damage.
- The National Eye Institute (NEI) has provided almost $2 million for the SELECT Eye Endpoints Study (SEE). Age-related macular degeneration (AMD) and cataract are two leading causes of visual impairment in older Americans. AMD is a disease that affects the central vision, and is the leading cause of visual problems and blindness, with about 25 percent of

people over 65 showing some AMD. Cataract is a clouding of the eye's lens that causes loss of vision. More than 50 percent of adults in the U.S. age 75 and older suffer from visually significant cataracts. Some evidence suggests that the dietary supplements (selenium and vitamin E) being studied in SELECT might prevent these eye problems. The SELECT Eye Endpoints (SEE) study is looking at this question in a large group of SELECT participants.

- National Heart, Lung and Blood Institute (NHLBI) has given more than $3 million for the Respiratory Ancillary Study (RAS). The overall objective of RAS is to understand whether supplements being studied in SELECT impact the loss of lung function experienced with aging, which is higher in persons smoking cigarettes. This study closed to accrual in 2007. Specific SELECT Study Sites were invited to participate in RAS. All smokers at these study sites were invited to participate, as well as a random selection of former smokers.

20. What other research is being done for prostate cancer prevention?

In 2003, the Prostate Cancer Prevention Trial, in which more than 18,000 men took either finasteride or a placebo to see if the drug reduced the risk of developing prostate cancer, showed a 25 percent reduction in prostate cancer in men taking finasteride. Finasteride is not currently approved by the FDA for reducing the risk of developing prostate cancer. (See http://www.cancer.gov/pcpt for more information).

Currently, NCI has several different agents in early prevention clinical trials of men at risk for prostate cancer or who have been diagnosed with prostate cancer and have not yet received treatments. These agents include Polyphenon E, a green tea extract; di-indolylmethane (DIM), a compound found in brassica vegetables such as broccoli, kale and cauliflower; lycopene, a carotenoid found in tomatoes and other red plants; and soy.

21. Where is more information about SELECT available?

In the United States and Puerto Rico, call the NCI's Cancer Information Service at 1-800-4-CANCER (1-800-422-6237) for information in English or Spanish. People with TTY equipment can call 1-800-332-8615 for information in English.

The following Web sites provide additional information:

- http://www.swog.org - choose the SELECT option
- http://www.cancer.gov/clinicaltrials/digestpage/SELECT - from the NCI
- http://www.cancer.gov/newscenter/SELECT - provides images of the prostate, the crystalline and chemical structures of vitamin E, and selenium and vitamin E capsules

####

Selected References

1. National Cancer Institute (2008). *SEER Cancer Statistics Review 1975-2005.* Bethesda, MD: Retrieved October 24, 2008, from http://seer.cancer.gov/csr/1975_2005/results_single/sect_01_table.01.pdf
2. Clark LC, Combs GF Jr., Turnbull BW, et al. Effects of selenium supplementation for cancer prevention in patients with carcinoma of the skin. A randomized controlled trial. Nutritional Prevention of Cancer Study Group. *Journal of the American Medical Association* 1996; 276(24):1957-1963.
3. Duffield-Lillico AJ, Reid ME, Turnbull BW, et al. Baseline characteristics and the effect of selenium supplementation on cancer incidence in a randomized clinical trial: A summary report of the Nutritional Prevention of Cancer Trial. *Cancer Epidemiology, Biomarkers & Prevention* 2002; 11(7):630-639.
4. Heinonen OP, Albanes D, Virtamo J, et al. Prostate cancer and supplementation with alpha-tocopherol and beta-carotene: Incidence and mortality in a controlled trial. *Journal of the National Cancer Institute* 1998; 90(6):440-446.
5. National Cancer Institute (2008). *SEER Cancer Statistics Review 1975-2005.* Bethesda, MD: Retrieved October 24, 2008 from http://seer.cancer.gov/csr/1975_2005/results_merged/topic_age_dist.pdf
6. Thompson IM, Goodman PJ, Tangen CM, et al. The influence of finasteride on the development of prostate cancer. *New England Journal of Medicine* 2003; 349:215-224.
7. Duffield-Lillico AJ, Slate EH, Reid ME, et al. Selenium supplementation and secondary prevention of nonmelanoma skin cancer in a randomized trial. *Journal of the National Cancer Institute* 2003; 95(19):1477-1481.
8. Stranges et al. Effects of Long-Term Use of Selenium Supplements on the Incidence of Type 2 Diabetes. *Annals of Internal Medicine*; 147:217-233, 2007.

9. Bleys J et al. Serum Selenium and Diabetes in U.S. Adults. *Diabetes Care*; 30:829-834, 2007.
10. Rajpathak et al. Toenail Selenium and Cardiovascular Disease in Men with Diabetes. *Journal of the American College of Nutrition*; 24: 250-256, 2005.
11. Czernichowet et al. Antioxidant supplementation does not affect fasting plasma glucose in the Supplementation with Antioxidant Vitamins and Minerals (SU.VI.MAX) study in France: association with dietary intake and plasma concentrations. *American Journal of Clinical Nutrition*; 84:395-9, 2006.
12. Lonn E, Bosch J, Yusuf S, et al. Effects of long-term vitamin E supplementation on cardiovascular events and cancer: A randomized controlled trial. *Journal of the American Medical Association* 2005; 293(11):1338-1347.
13. Miller ER III, Pastor-Barriuso R, Dalal D, et al. Meta-analysis: High-dosage vitamin E supplementation may increase all-cause mortality. *Annals of Internal Medicine* 2005; 142(1):37-46.

1.9.9.2 Prostate Cancer Prevention: The Scoop on Supplements 1-30-09

You may have heard that taking certain vitamin or mineral supplements can lower prostate cancer risk. While some studies have found that there might be a protective benefit from some supplements, recent **results from 2 large studies didn't find any**. ("Effect of Selenium and Vitamin E on Risk of Prostate Cancer and Other Cancers." Published in the January 7, 2009 issue of the *Journal of the American Medical Association*. Corresponding Author: Scott M. Lippman, MD, Department of Thoracic and Head and Neck Medical Oncology, University of Texas M. D. Anderson Cancer Center, Houston, Texas). ("Vitamins E and C in the Prevention of Prostate and Total Cancer in Men: The Physicians' Health Study II Randomized Controlled Trial." Published in the January 7, 2009 issue of the *Journal of the American Medical Association*. Corresponding author: J. Michael Gaziano, MD, MPH, Brigham and Women's Hospital, Boston, Massachusetts).

In 2001, researchers from the National Cancer Institute (NCI) and the Southwest Oncology Group (SWOG) launched the massive **SELECT study (short for Selenium and Vitamin E Cancer Prevention Trial)** to find out whether taking selenium and vitamin E supplements could protect men from prostate cancer. **In October 2008, researchers halted the trial after early analysis showed the supplements weren't working, and in fact, in some cases, may have been doing more harm than good.**

1.9.9.3 What SELECT Revealed

More than **35,000 men** over age 50 in the US, Puerto Rico, and Canada were enrolled in the trial. Each participant was randomly assigned to take either selenium, vitamin E, a combination of the two, or a placebo for the course of the study. **After an average of 5 years, the analysis found no lower risk of prostate cancer in men taking the supplements, either alone or together.**

Men who were taking only vitamin E actually had a slightly higher risk of developing prostate cancer. And **men taking only selenium seemed to have a slightly higher risk of developing diabetes. This increased risk was not statistically significant in either case.** That means the findings could be due to chance; they don't prove the supplements raise prostate cancer and diabetes risk. Still, researchers called the findings "concerning."

The men in the study were told to stop taking their study pills. The researchers plan to continue monitoring the participants for about 3 more years to see if there are long-term effects (good or bad) from taking the supplements.

1.9.9.4 What About Vitamin C?

In another large, long-term trial, called **the Physicians' Health Study II**, researchers from Brigham and Women's Hospital and Harvard Medical School studied whether taking vitamin E or vitamin C could reduce the risk of prostate cancer. Nearly **15,000 male doctors** participated in the trial. **After an average of 8 years, neither vitamin E nor vitamin C seemed to lower the risk of prostate cancer. However, taking the supplements also did not appear to cause any harm.**

The results of **both studies were published in the January 7, 2009 issue of the *Journal of the American Medical Association***.

1.9.9.5 Controlling Your Risk

So, what can you do to reduce your risk of prostate cancer? While it now seems unlikely that specific supplements will have a major effect on risk, other factors, such as maintaining a healthy weight and eating a healthy diet, may still play a role. Following the American Cancer Society's guidelines for nutrition and physical activity may lower prostate cancer risk, and can clearly have other health benefits, including reducing the risk of some other cancers.

- Maintain a healthy weight. **While being overweight or obese has not been strongly linked to prostate cancer risk, it does seem to raise the risk of getting more aggressive forms of prostate cancer**, which could be harder to treat.
- Get at least 30 minutes of moderate to vigorous physical activity, above usual activities, on 5 or more days of the week. The effect of exercise on overall prostate cancer risk is not clear, but **some studies have suggested that getting more physical activity may reduce a man's risk of advanced prostate cancer**.
- Try to eat *at least* 5 servings of vegetables (including legumes) and fruits each day. The more brightly colored the produce, the better – it's more likely to be packed with cancer-fighting, heart-healthy nutrients.
- Aim for at least 3 servings of whole grains each day. **Eat oatmeal at breakfast, choose whole-wheat bread at lunch, or use brown rice at dinner instead of white**.
- **Cut back on red meats**, especially high-fat or processed meats – they have been linked to an increased risk.

Tomatoes (raw, cooked, or in tomato products such as sauces or ketchup), pink grapefruit, and watermelon are rich in *lycopenes*, antioxidants that help prevent damage to DNA. Some studies have suggested lycopenes may help lower prostate cancer risk, although **a more recent study found no link between blood levels of lycopene and risk of prostate cancer**. Research in this area continues.

"Effect of Selenium and Vitamin E on Risk of Prostate Cancer and Other Cancers." Published in the January 7, 2009 issue of the *Journal of the American Medical Association*. Corresponding Author: Scott M. Lippman, MD, Department of Thoracic and Head and Neck Medical Oncology, University of Texas M. D. Anderson Cancer Center, Houston, Texas.

"Vitamins E and C in the Prevention of Prostate and Total Cancer in Men: The Physicians' Health Study II Randomized Controlled Trial." Published in the January 7, 2009 issue of the *Journal of the American Medical Association*. Corresponding author: J. Michael Gaziano, MD, MPH, Brigham and Women's Hospital, Boston, Massachusetts

1.9.9.6 Antioxidants fail again in cancer prevention study

12-30-08 **Beta carotene, vitamin C and vitamin E supplements taken for years failed to lower overall cancer risk in the latest study to cast doubt on the possibility that such dietary supplements can prevent cancer**.

The findings, published on 12-30-08 in the **Journal of the National Cancer Institute**, followed **two other important studies that also did not show that various antioxidant supplements could prevent cancer**.

"Although a healthful dietary pattern rich in fruits and vegetables may lower cancer risk, such benefits cannot be mimicked by simply popping a few vitamin supplements," Dr. JoAnn Manson of Brigham and Women's Hospital and Harvard Medical School in Boston said in a statement.

Manson, Jennifer Lin and colleagues **tracked 7,627 women** who were an average 60 years old at the start of the study, who took supplements for **about 9-1/2 years.**

Some **took 500 milligrams of vitamin C daily, 600 IU (international units) of vitamin E every other day or 50 milligrams of beta carotene every other day** -- or various combinations of the three supplements. Others were given placebos.

Women who took the supplements had similar rates of cancer and cancer death compared to those who took a placebo, the researchers said. The study suggested that vitamin E supplements might reduce colon cancer risk and that beta carotene supplements might modestly raise lung cancer risk.

The researchers, however, acknowledged that while the women took the supplements for almost a decade, the study "may still be of insufficient duration to assess effects on cancer incidence, given the long latency for cancer."

"**Simply taking antioxidant supplements is insufficient to prevent cancer**. People should take more natural plant foods which are rich with many nutrients including but not limited to antioxidants," Lin said by e-mail.

Beta carotene, vitamin E and vitamin C are antioxidants thought to protect against damage caused by free radicals, substances that can harm cells, tissues and organs.

Fruits and vegetables are rich in these vitamins, and it has been shown that people who eat plenty of these foods have a lower risk of heart disease, cancer and other conditions.

The **Council for Responsible Nutrition, a dietary supplement industry group, found fault with the study.**

Andrew Shao, the group's vice president for scientific and regulatory affairs, noted in a telephone interview that the women in the study all were at high risk for heart disease, and the study's original design was to assess whether the supplements protected against cardiovascular illness.

"Supplements are just one tool that people need to incorporate into their lifestyle to stay healthy. **We can't expect just to take supplements and that's going to prevent cancer. That simply isn't the way it works," Shao added.**

In a study released in November 2008 involving about **15,000 male doctors, vitamin E and C supplements did not lower cancer risk. Another study released in October 2008 found no cancer reduction in 35,000 men taking vitamin E and selenium supplements. I believe that the thrust of these studies is the invalidation of the free radical theory, as I have been saying for years.**

2.0.0.0 Do those antioxidants in food really prevent cancer?

Not only does your body already make all the antioxidants it needs, but also none of the studies that investigated the effects of dietary antioxidants have shown any significant benefit. The reasoning went, if our natural antioxidants could be bolstered by antioxidants from food, even more oxygen could be captured and our risk for cancer should be reduced even further. In the late 1970s, researchers began to look for ways to supplement the antioxidants naturally produced by the body through a diet heavy in plant antioxidants. Immediately, newspapers began to report that these foods could prevent cancer. Newspaper headlines at the New York Times, in 1979 read as follows: "Cancer-Blocking Agents Found in Foods; Origin of New Techniques." Antioxidants were touted as newly discovered cancer cures.

Since then, research into antioxidants has followed two tracks. One examined the effects of antioxidants in a test tube, while the other looked at the effects of dietary antioxidants in live human subjects. The results of the test tube experiments led to claims that diet-supplemented antioxidants can prevent cancer or treat pulmonary fibrosis, while **the live studies reported that antioxidants have no health value or may even be dangerous**.

The discrepancy results from the differing methodology of the tests. The test tube studies just involve submitting a chemical or food product to the "oxygen radical absorbance capacity," the Food and Drug Administration standard for testing the antioxidant property of a chemical. The test involves measuring fluorescent dye decay after the target food or chemical has been exposed to oxygen.

By contrast, the live experiments have been case studies. These tests involve feeding subjects the antioxidants, monitoring them over a long period of time and comparing the results to a group that had been given a placebo.

The optimism over the potential for dietary antioxidants to prevent cancer or aging results from the test tube studies failing to consider how antioxidants are metabolized or how they act within a cell. Conversely, the live studies test all of the variables.

The test tube studies are overrepresented in antioxidant news coverage. That is because they make up the bulk of antioxidant research (as it is far cheaper and easier to conduct an experiment on a chemical than on a human) and are often well suited to mass media coverage. By presenting claims that desirable but formerly maligned foods like chocolate, wine, coffee and even martinis might be healthy, these studies tend to garner a lot of attention.

As a result of the failure of any live study to show any health benefits from antioxidant supplements, **neither the National Cancer Institute nor the American Heart Association endorse antioxidant dietary supplements as an inhibitor of heart disease or cancer.**

So, despite what the label might tell you, there's still no evidence that fancy juices, fattening sweets or any kind of booze will prevent prevent cancer. However, eating chocolate and drinking bourbon will, in my experience, cure sadness. (Scienceline. By Stuart Fox, posted March 3rd, 2008.)

2.0.0.1 Harmful effects of vitamins (references)

- Here are a number of Medline references to support the potential problems associated with overconsumption of vitamins (there are many, many more where these came from):

  Castaño G ; Etchart C ; Sookoian S

  Affiliation: Department of Internal Medicine, Hospital J.M. Penna, Buenos Aires, Argentina. castano@intramed.net

  Title: **Vitamin A toxicity in a physical culturist patient: a case report and review of the literature**.

  Source: Annals of hepatology : official journal of the Mexican Association of Hepatology (Ann Hepatol) 2006 Oct-Dec; 5(4): 293-395

  Cheruvattath R ; Orrego M ; Gautam M ; Byrne T ; Alam S ; Voltchenok M ; Edwin M ; Wilkens J ; Williams JW ; Vargas HE

  Affiliation: Division of Transplantation Medicine, Mayo Clinic Arizona, Phoenix, AZ 85054, USA. Title: **Vitamin A toxicity: when one a day doesn't keep the doctor away.** Source: Liver transplantation : official publication of the American Association for the Study of Liver Diseases and the International Liver Transplantation Society (Liver Transpl) 2006 Dec; 12(12): 1888-91

Additional Info: United States Standard No: ISSN: 1527-6465 (Print); 1527-6473 (Electronic); NLM Unique Journal Identifier: 100909185

Prakash R Title: **The acute and chronic toxic effects of vitamin A**. Source: The American journal of clinical nutrition (Am J Clin Nutr) 2006 Aug; 84(2): 462; author reply 462-3

Additional Info: United States Standard No: ISSN: 0002-9165 (Print); NLM Unique Journal Identifier: 0376027

O'Brien B ; Quigg C ; Leong T

Affiliation: Department of Anaesthesia, Our Lady's Hospital for Sick Children, Dublin, Ireland. drbobrien@hotmail.com Title: **Severe cyanide toxicity from 'vitamin supplements'.** Source: European journal of emergency medicine : official journal of the European Society for Emergency Medicine (Eur J Emerg Med) 2005 Oct; 12(5): 257-8

Additional Info: England Standard No: ISSN: 0969-9546 (Print); NLM Unique Journal Identifier: 9442482 Language: English Abstract: The use of alternative medicines is increasing and poorly regulated. We describe a case of severe cyanide poisoning arising from amygdalin, a putative vitamin supplement. A 32-year-old woman arrived in the emergency department by ambulance unresponsive, shocked and with fixed dilated pupils. She was hypothermic and tachycardic but was breathing spontaneously. Despite her age, she had documented breast cancer with hepatic metastases. Conventional treatment having failed, she only took 'vitamin supplements' bought on the Internet, her father said. Over the next 6 h she required mechanical ventilation and increasing doses of inotropes. Diabetes insipidus developed. As the appropriateness of further treatment was considered, a relative arrived with her medications including 'vitamin B 17' or amygdalin. An Internet search identified this as a debunked cancer remedy and cyanogen. Serum thiocyanate level was markedly elevated. She recovered fully over 8 h. While various antidotes to cyanide exist, in this case supportive therapy alone proved effective.

Bromley J ; Hughes BG ; Leong DC ; Buckley NA

Affiliation: Department of Clinical Pharmacology and Toxicology, The Canberra Hospital, Garran, Australia. jonathan.bromley@act.gov.au Title: **Life-threatening interaction between complementary medicines: cyanide toxicity following ingestion of amygdalin and vitamin C.** Source: The Annals of pharmacotherapy (Ann Pharmacother) 2005 Sep; 39(9): 1566-9

Additional Info: United States

Wooltorton E Title: **Too much of a good thing? Toxic effects of vitamin and mineral supplements.** Source: CMAJ : Canadian Medical Association journal = journal de l'Association medicale canadienne (CMAJ) 2003 Jul 8; 169(1): 47-8 Additional Info: Canada Standard No: ISSN: 0820-3946 (Print); 1488-2329 (Electronic); NLM Unique Journal Identifier: 9711805

2.0.0.2 Antioxidants and Cancer: Researcher admits she got it wrong

24 April 2008 It was news when it was first revealed three years ago – and it was news again last week: **antioxidant vitamins can speed up the development of cancer. But the researcher who first published the study has now admitted that she got it wrong.**

The original study – which made headlines around the world – found that cancer patients who took either vitamin A (beta-carotene) or E (alpha tocopherol) supplements were 40 per cent more likely to suffer a recurrence of their cancer than those who didn't take any supplements.

Ever since, nutritionists and alternative therapists have been on the back foot, and have tried to defend the antioxidants. But their task was made even tougher last week when **the prestigious Cochrane Collaborative released a meta-analysis that suggested that antioxidants may even shorten our life**.

But the researchers, led by Isabelle Bairati from the Quebec Research Centre, who published the 2005 study, have re-analysed their original data, and have discovered they **got it wrong. The only people in the study who were seeing their cancer return were smokers who refused to kick the habit while they were receiving radiation therapy or chemotherapy**.

Strangely, not a single newspaper has run with the story.

(Source: International Journal of Cancer, 2008; 122: 1679-83).

2.0.0.3 Time for antioxidants v2.0

The term antioxidant is a catch-all, encompassing a mind-boggling number of phytochemicals, as well as the more well-known vitamins. The message is clear: It is time for a spring-clean of the antioxidant house.

http://www.nutraingredients.com/Research/Time-for-antioxidants-V20

2.0.1.0 Antioxidants - Health Miracle or Profitable Hype?

By Stephen and Gina Antczak, authors of Cosmetics Unmasked

Without a doubt, antioxidants are the miracle discovery of the twentieth century - or ***that's what the makers of dietary supplements and cosmetics would like us to believe.*** *They seduce us with scientific words that we don't understand like 'plant polyphenols' and 'free-radical scavengers' and they promise us these 'natural herbal extracts' will keep our skin young-looking and wrinkle-free; they will keep us fit and healthy; they will protect us from heart disease and cancer; and they can even make us live up to 60% longer. It all sounds wonderful and we are told that these facts are backed up by ground-breaking scientific research. Even well known doctors writing in their Sunday newspaper columns expound on the benefits of antioxidants. But how much of it is true?*

Oxidation, we are told, is **a destructive process** that generates free radicals which play havoc with almost everything they touch. They cause the garden hose to crack in the sunshine, they dull paint and cause it to crumble and flake away, they fade the color of our wallpaper and fabrics, and they degrade the collagen in our skin, accelerating the onset of wrinkles and old age.

The free radicals have been likened to fires burning within our cells, causing damage that could eventually lead to heart disease and cancer. We are told that natural plant polyphenols are free radical scavengers that prevent the build up of free radicals and protect us from the aging process. The French, it seems, have been reaping the benefits of polyphenol antioxidants for countless years. Red wine is rich in polyphenols and there are significantly lower rates of certain cancers and cardiovascular disease in France than in Britain or the USA, where the lifestyles and diets are generally similar. Other populations such as in China and Japan, also have reduced incidences of these diseases. Here it is attributed to green tea which is also a rich source of natural antioxidants.

Public enthusiasm for these ideas has caused a boom in the sales of dietary supplements and cosmetics manufacturers have eagerly jumped on the bandwagon, filling their potions with plant polyphenols and the antioxidant vitamins, E and C. But is there any real science behind the hype or is it all just a profitable fad that is preying on our fears and scientific ignorance?

We have simplified some of the scientific ideas and words, and we have put hyphens into long words to make them easier to read. We don't have a problem with this because the article is about antioxidants and polyphenols, and neither of these words are correct scientific terms. But before we blind you with science, let's find out how much you already know about antioxidants with a quick True/False quiz.

2.0.1.1 Antioxidants quick True/False quiz

1 Vitamin C is the strongest antioxidant normally in our diet; True or False?

2 According to chemistry textbooks, there are no such things as bioflavonoids; True or False?

3 Collagen is the flexible protein found in our skin. As we age the quality and the quantity of collagen in our skin diminishes; True or False?

4 Scurvy is a disease where inferior collagen is produced by the body. This is caused by lack of vitamin C which is essential for the production of healthy collagen; True or False?

5 Pure vitamin C cannot cure scurvy; True or False?

6 The daily requirement for vitamin C is 30 milligrams. Megadoses of vitamin C (doses of 1000 milligrams or more) are probably harmful and have been shown to cause genetic damage; True or False?

7 During the production of healthy collagen, proteins must be oxidized. This involves free radicals, without which the proteins cannot be oxidized correctly; True or False?

8 The bioavailability of polyphenols in our diet is probably zero, in other words, virtually none of the polyphenols in our diet will ever get to the cells that produce collagen in our skin; True or False?

9 Polyphenols in cosmetics are unlikely to penetrate the skin and will have little effect on the skin. Those polyphenols that are readily available to cosmetics manufacturers and are known to have an effect on the skin, such as catechol and pyrogallol, have been banned from cosmetics sold within the European Union (EU); True or False?

10 Co-enzyme Q10 (ubiquinone) is said to be an important antioxidant and it has become a popular cosmetic ingredient and health supplement but in fact, its main function in the body is the exact opposite of an antioxidant; True or False?

Of course, the answer to all of these questions is True! If you answered them all correctly without guessing, you probably don't need to read the rest of this article - but you'll be missing an eye-opener.

In a nutshell, contrary to what you hear on TV or read on product labels, **oxidation is not always bad and is, in fact, vital for the formation of healthy collagen.** And **even if polyphenols could get to the right place in the body, which is doubtful, there is no good scientific evidence to show that they can prevent free radicals from doing any damage** within a living organism.

2.0.1.2 A little bit of history on vitamin C

Scurvy is a dietary-deficiency disease caused by a lack of fresh fruit and vegetables in the diet. These provide a host of nutrients, including vitamin C. **Without vitamin C and a combination of other nutrients, collagen, the most common protein in our body, is not formed correctly.** Small blood vessels become weak and bleed into all parts of the body. This is most noticeable in the skin where widespread bruising appears and trivial wounds are slow to heal. Blood can also leak into the joints, causing severe pain, and the gums bleed, resulting in loosened teeth. In other parts of the body hemorrhages can occur leading to anemia or more serious, and possibly fatal conditions, depending on where the bleeding takes place.

Today, scurvy is a relatively rare disease but it was common in sailors before the eighteenth century. During their months at sea they had little access to fresh fruit and vegetables but **in about 1750, James Lind, a British naval surgeon,**

discovered that a daily ration of lime juice would both prevent and cure this disease. Limes were chosen because they could easily stored without too much deterioration. (Thus the British became known as Limeys.)

Nearly two centuries **later in 1933, Albert von Szent-Györgi**, a Hungarian scientist, isolated vitamin C (ascorbic acid) and demonstrated its role in the prevention of scurvy. In some of his experiments he fed guinea pigs a poor diet until they developed scurvy-like symptoms. He then showed that **a combination of vitamin C and extracts from the peel of citrus fruits and peppers could quickly restore the guinea pigs to full health, but pure vitamin C administered on its own, could not.**

There was an immediate surge in scientific interest to find the mystery factors in citrus peel and peppers that worked with vitamin C to cure scurvy, and today, this research is still in full swing. Many thousands of scientific papers have been written on this subject but despite all this effort, **we are still not sure what these mystery factors are**. Polyphenols are the front-runners for this but there is still no clear scientific proof that they are. In fact, there is fair amount of evidence that says they are unlikely candidates for the mystery factor prize, but much more on this later.

2.0.1.3 What are polyphenols?

Polyphenols (pronounced polly-fee-nolls) should more correctly be called polyhydric phenols. They occur naturally in all plants and come in a huge variety of shapes and sizes. They all have two things in common; firstly, they are usually brightly colored and are used by plants to color their leaves, flowers, berries and bark, and secondly, **they all contain at least one chemical structure called a polyhydric phenol** which is very easily oxidized. It is this ease of oxidation that gives polyphenols their antioxidant properties, but more about this later.

Plant polyphenols include the tannins which are found in many leaves and especially the bark of oak trees and in gallnuts; the anthocyanins, anthocyanidins and oligomeric pro-cyanidins which are the brightly colored pigments in petals, fruits and berries; the flavonoids which include the flavones and the flavan-3-ols, again found in leaves, fruits and berries; and the theaflavins found in green and black tea leaves.

All these words seem almost unpronounceable but a good marketing team can have a field day with them using expressions like, "New antioxidant formula with natural pro-cyanidins to rejuvenate your skin and visibly reduce fine lines and wrinkles." No one understands a word of it but it sounds good and very scientific. The bottom line is, if it sells cosmetics, then use it. And if the words sound too much like vestigial organs that are removed along with your tonsils during childhood, they simply make up a new one that sounds better, hence **flavonoids become bioflavonoids** and polyphenols are mispronounced pol-if-an-ols. Presumably, if they wanted to market chocolate they would make up the word biochocolate if they thought this would boost sales (especially since it has a more healthy ring to it).

2.0.1.4 So what does all this have to do with collagen?

The collagens are a family of fibrous proteins that make up a quarter of all the proteins in your body. They are found in skin, muscle, tendons, ligaments, bone, cornea, eye-fluids, internal organs, blood vessels - just about everywhere, in fact.

All of the different types of collagen have a similar chemical structure and are formed in a similar way. They start their lives as single strands of proteins called **alpha-chains.** Three of these chains line up and spiral around each other in the same way that three cords can be wound together to make a rope. The collagen-rope (which is called **a triple helix**) forms the tough fibres which are responsible for the strength of muscles and the elasticity of skin.

These alpha-chains want to spiral together in such a symmetrical way because they have a remarkably regular structure. The alpha-chains, like all human proteins, are made from about twenty different smaller molecules called amino acids. Many hundreds of these amino acids thread together like beads on a necklace. The amino acid-beads can be threaded together in any order allowing billions of different combinations of amino acids so a countless range of different proteins can be made.

Collagen is rich in three particular amino acids called glycine, proline and hydroxy-proline. Every third amino acid in the alpha-chains is glycine. Any two of the twenty possible amino acids can go in between the glycine units but they are quite often proline and hydroxy-proline. The **hydroxy-proline is essential**. It acts like protein-Velcro which holds the three alpha-chains in their regular spiral structure.

This is where the antioxidants come in. While the alpha-chains are being formed, some of the proline units must be oxidized to hydroxy-proline. **This oxidation is vital for the formation of healthy collagen.** The oxidation process takes place in several steps. Early in the process **oxygen, in the form of a free**

radical, joins onto the proline unit. (Surely not! We've always been told that oxidation and free radicals destroy proteins, not that they build healthy ones, we hear you say.) The formation of this free radical and its subsequent conversion to hydroxy-proline involves an enzyme called a **dioxygenase,** which has an iron atom at its heart. Just like in all iron compounds, the iron in this enzyme can be in one of two forms called iron(II) (pronounced *iron two* from the Roman numerals) and iron(III) (*iron three*). (The old names for these forms of iron are ferrous iron and ferric iron. These went out of use nearly forty years ago so you should be a little suspicious of people who still use them. Their chemistry is a little out of date.)

The dioxygenase enzyme is only useful if it contains iron(II). The iron(II) helps the proline-oxygen free radical change and eventually form hydroxy-proline. During this change, the iron(II) in the enzyme is changed to iron(III) and the enzyme is now completely useless. **It cannot be used again until the iron(III) is changed back to iron(II). An antioxidant is needed for this and vitamin C is ideal** for the job but it is possible that other antioxidants could also be used.

Vitamin C converts the useless iron(III) in the enzyme back to the iron(II) state and the enzyme can now make some more hydroxy-proline. Unfortunately the vitamin C becomes oxidized and useless, so the body needs a regular supply of fresh vitamin C in the diet. **A lack of vitamin C means the enzymes cannot be 'recharged' and inferior collagen is formed with too little hydroxy-proline to 'Velcro' the alpha-chains together firmly. The collagen rope becomes loose and frayed forming weak collagen which is the primary cause of the symptoms of scurvy.**

2.0.1.5 Can polyphenols recharge the iron-enzyme?

In theory, yes they can but they are all inferior to vitamin C. **The correct name for an antioxidant is a reducing agent.** To a chemist, reduction is the opposite of oxidation. The word, antioxidant, is seldom, if ever, seen in a chemistry textbook. Vitamin C and all polyphenols are reducing agents and their reducing power can be measured. These measurements show that **all plant polyphenols are much weaker reducing agents than vitamin C.** This means that vitamin C will be much more effective at recharging the iron-enzyme than any polyphenol. It also means that the polyphenols will not be able to 'repair' the vitamin C once it has done its job. Does this mean that polyphenols are not the mystery factors that work with vitamin C? We still don't know.

2.0.1.6 What do we know about polyphenols in the body?

A glass of full bodied, young, red wine contains about 500 milligrams of polyphenols. As the wine matures, it often throws down a sediment which is rich in tannins and the amount of polyphenols left in the wine is much reduced. When you drink red wine, your mouth feels dry. This is because the polyphenols in the wine cling tightly to **proline-rich proteins (PRPs)** in your saliva. These PRPs normally act as a lubricant to keep your mouth moist and to help you to swallow. The polyphenols effectively deactivate the lubricating properties of the PRPs and your mouth puckers and feels dry.

The polyphenols in black or green tea, taken without milk, have the same drying effect. When milk is added to tea, the polyphenols cling to the milk proteins so **when you drink it, the polyphenols are not available to deactivate your saliva PRPs,** and your mouth stays moist. It is reasonable to assume that any polyphenols that get past your mouth will cling to proteins in your digestive system and any that are absorbed into the bloodstream will cling to blood proteins. **Between 6 to 8 percent of you blood consists of protein, mainly globulins, albumins and fibrinogen.** Any polyphenols that find their way into the bloodstream are likely to cling tightly to these.

Can the polyphenols separate themselves from proteins and get to the right parts of the body to do some good? The answer is no and yes. We know that polyphenols remain tightly attached to PRPs and other proteins within the digestive system. These are not available to the body so we say their **bioavailability is zero**. Recent experiments on polyphenols attached to blood proteins showed that a powerful solvent called dimethyl sulphoxide (DMSO) which is known to be able to separate polyphenols from other substances, was only able to separate a tiny fraction of polyphenols attached to blood proteins. This evidence suggests that **polyphenols in our diet stand very little chance of getting to the places where collagen is made.**

But they may do some good. Some fatty-proteins called lipoproteins are particularly prone to free radical oxidation. If a polyphenol attaches itself to a lipoprotein it will be in exactly the right place to scavenge the free radicals and protect the protein. Vitamin E working with vitamin C can also protect these lipoproteins.

The next obvious question must be, **if polyphenols cannot get to the skin-collagen factories via the bloodstream, can they get there via cosmetics that we rub into our skin? Probably not.** Skin is rich in PRPs and the polyphenols will cling to them like superglue and not get through. In fact, **tannins are plant polyphenols that are used to tan leather. That is where their name comes from.** During the tanning process the tannin-polyphenols cling to the PRPs in the animal hides and there they remain forever. Of course there is no evidence that **using polyphenols on your skin will turn it to leather**, but there again, these things have only recently been added to our cosmetics and no one knows what the long term effects of using them regularly, will be.

A good scientist should question everything and one question we have not yet asked is, **can polyphenols scavenge free radicals inside living cells? The answer is that real scientific evidence for this is sparse.** We can do test-tube experiments in the laboratory and apply chemical theories, and come up with schemes that prove polyphenols can scavenge artificially produced free radicals in test-tubes but we are not sure about what they do inside the plant cells where they are made.

Now it is time for some lateral thinking. Why do leaves change color in the autumn? Leaves contain large amounts of a green pigment called chlorophyll and they also contain colorful polyphenols and other pigments. The high levels of the green pigment usually mask the other colors. **Chlorophyll is rich in nitrogen and magnesium.** In the autumn the tree breaks down its chlorophyll and absorbs the nitrogen and magnesium, which is then stored in its trunk over winter, ready to be used next year. As the levels of green pigment falls, the other colors show through in a blaze of autumn color.

The sun's energy is normally absorbed by the chlorophyll and used to produce food for the plant. **When the levels of chlorophyll fall, the sunlight can potentially produce free radicals in the leaves that would damage them and cause them to drop before the tree has a chance to reabsorb the essential nutrients.** Recent research at the University of Aukland suggests that the colorful polyphenols and other pigments protect the leaves by absorbing the ultraviolet rays before they can produce free radicals. This suggests that the main role of plant polyphenols is not to scavenge free radicals but to prevent them from forming in the first place. Does this mean that polyphenols cannot scavenge free radicals inside the human body? No, it simply means we have no evidence that they can.

So what is the mystery factor that works with vitamin C?

We don't really know but the next section examines the history of the so called, **vitamin P,** which we now know does not exist. It is possible, although unlikely, that polyphenols are involved with vitamin C in collagen formation and there is some evidence to suggest that vitamin E, another antioxidant vitamin, could be involved. Minerals like selenium have also been suggested but the long and the short of it is, we simply don't know.

And if we don't know, why do the supplement sellers sound so sure of themselves? They seem to be able to quote scientific paper after scientific paper to prove their claims. But is it good science? In August 2001 the UK Advertising Standards Authority (ASA) told a manufacturer of a health supplement to withdraw their advertisement. The advert claimed that their product **contained a combination of eighteen antioxidants, vitamins and minerals that would combat the aging process.** They submitted 171 scientific papers and documents to the ASA in support of their claims but the ASA rejected all of them. It seems that much of the science is not good science or it is insufficiently conclusive for anyone to say positively that plant polyphenols actually do any good.

So why does all that red wine make the French healthier? **The French themselves laugh at the antioxidant theory.** They put it down to good food and good sex in combination with good wine, all contributing to a national sense of wellbeing. The moral being, stop worrying about your health and have some fun. Forget the bioflavonoid pills and pro-retinol face creams, and spend your money on a bottle of red wine instead.

So if this is all rubbish, where do these ideas about bioflavonoids and antioxidants come from?

To answer this question we have to go back to the discovery of vitamin C and the hunt for the elusive vitamin P, also known as bioflavonoid. In fact, **the word, bioflavonoid, has no well defined meaning and no agreed common usage amongst scientists** or health supplement manufacturers. It is often used interchangeably with the words flavonoid, citrin and a host of other chemical curiosities that occur in plants, and it has even been used as the chemical name of vitamin P. If scientists were to interpret chemical names in different ways we would have a sure recipe for disaster. Imagine what could happen if a prescription for "Co-proxamol" meant different things to different pharmacists.

It is for precisely this reason that the International Union of Pure and Applied Chemistry (IUPAC) set up a system for naming chemicals to ensure that there would be no ambiguous chemical names and no confusion over their meaning. As far as we are aware, **bioflavonoid is not part of the IUPAC naming system**

and we have never seen this word in any text book on advanced organic chemistry. In fact the word "flavonoid" is quite rare in these books, the favored system being to name each compound individually using the IUPAC system or by using well established, unambiguous trivial names such as "eugenol". We can conclude from this that these fancy sounding words are only favored by people who want to sell something.

As far as we can tell, "bioflavonoid" first appeared at the height of the race to patent the elusive vitamin P. You will recall that **Albert Szent-Györgi isolated vitamin C in 1933 and by 1936 he had demonstrated that it could not treat the symptoms of scurvy in its pure form.** When mixed with an extract of lemon peel, which was a mixture of natural chemicals he called citrin, vitamin C's therapeutic activity sometimes returned, but not always. He assumed that citrin contained another vitamin which he called vitamin P, and he assumed that this new vitamin was essential for the correct absorption of vitamin C. But vitamin P never achieved true vitamin status because no one was able to demonstrate that a lack of this substance caused a deficiency disease. The word 'vitaminoid' was coined to describe its vitamin-like action but this word seemed to disappear by the late sixties.

Another problem with Szent-Györgi's work on citrin was that his experiments were not **reliably repeatable**. Some samples of citrin worked and some didn't. This meant that some samples of citrin contained vitamin P and some didn't, presumably because the fruits from which citrin was extracted were in a different state of ripeness with a different chemical make up. The race was now on to separate citrin into its component parts in order to isolate and patent vitamin P.

The first attempts to separate and classify these chemicals were based on color. A separation process called paper chromatography showed that two families of chemicals were present, yellow compounds which were named flavonoids from the Latin word **"flavus" which means yellow**, and red compounds which were called anthocyanidins. These compounds were found in all citrus fruits and in many other plants as well. New words, such as citroflavonoids, were quickly coined to increase the number of patents and to maximize profits. But it was soon demonstrated that the flavonoids and anthocyanidins were not bioavailable and could not have any therapeutic effect. (Remember, **bioavailable means you can absorb it into your bloodstream by eating it.**) But since some citrin extracts worked it was assumed that there must be a bioavailable flavonoid in those extracts. The word bioflavonoid was probably coined to describe the bioavailable flavonoids.

Much poor science was done to prove the existence of bioavailable flavonoids and in 1944, Lavollay published results that proved red wine had a vitamin P effect. He claimed that 2 to 3 millilitres of red wine would double the resistance of guinea pigs' blood vessels in just 1 to 2 hours. So far, four biologists have not been able to explain to us exactly what "resistance" means in terms of blood vessels but if the experiment was scaled up to an adult's weight, it would be the equivalent of drinking between half and three quarters of a bottle of wine. That might have a measurable effect on your blood vessels as well and after drinking it you probably wouldn't care what word was used to describe it.

The red wine was fed to the guinea pigs rather than injected so Lavollay concluded that it contained a bioavailable compound, probably vitamin P, which had a major effect on vascular protection. This opened the floodgates for patent applications for plant extract-based cardiovascular drugs. Incidentally, most of this work was done in the USA because it was the only country that would allow patents on everything from plants and spring water to human genes and breeds of cats. It is also worth commenting here that many of the patented extracts were obtained from the waste generated by other industries such as the peel left over from the orange juice industry, the seeds and skins from grapes from the wine industry, peanut skins and the bark of trees from the timber industry to name but four.

Lavollay decided that the active ingredient in his wine experiments was a colorless compound called catechin. This had been overlooked in the original classification because it was invisible on the paper chromatography experiments. Catechin was chemically similar to flavonoids and is now known as a flavan-3-ol, despite it being colorless. A new word was coined for the flavanols - you guessed it - bioflavanols (which is sometimes spelt, bioflavonols).

2.0.1.7 The demise of vitamin P

In 1947 Jack Masquelier, a colleague of Lavollay, told Szent-Györgi that there was no such thing as vitamin P in citrin and that "no one in the US believed in bioflavonoids any more." In 1950 he announced that catechin was not the active compound but only a component of the elusive vitamin C co-factor. He decided that the active compounds were formed when two or three catechin molecules joined together. He called these compounds **oligomeric pro-anthocyanidins (OPCs)** and declared them to be fully bioavailable and the true co-factor that worked with vitamin C to treat scurvy. Between 1948 and 1951 he had registered several patents in the USA for various plant extracts that contained his OPCs and he made many claims about their beneficial effects on the cardiovascular system.

Between the late thirties and the late sixties there were many patented health supplements and prescribed licensed drugs based on flavonoids and anthocyanidins which were widely used to treat a host of cardiovascular diseases. **In 1968 the FDA declared that these substances, including citrin, citrus flavonoids, citroflavonoids and bioflavonoids were barely active, if not completely inactive in humans and did not warrant the description of vitamin or health supplement and they also proposed to revoke the licenses for their use as drugs.**

A new angle was needed if these extracts were to remain profitable and Masquelier was up to the challenge. He carried out numerous in-vitro experiments that showed OPCs were antioxidants and free radical scavengers and quickly assumed that they would have the same action when taken orally, although we have seen no experimental data that would make this a valid assumption. Now that he was no longer claiming to have found the vitamin C co-factor, **in 1987 he was granted US patent number 4698360, the first patented free radical scavenging antioxidant plant extract.**

2.0.1.8 A miracle drug is discovered - the anti-aging vitamin.

Masquelier claimed that his new discovery could treat cerebral involution, hypoxia following atherosclerosis, cardiac and cerebral infarction, tumour promotion, inflammation, ischemia, alteration of the synovial fluids, collagen degradation, sun-damaged skin, cataracts, etc., etc., etc. He should have stopped here but he later went on to claim that his OPCs would prevent aging, hence **it would cure "an almost full spectrum of diseases". In fact he called his discovery the anti-aging vitamin**.

From our point of view it seems quite remarkable that before the free radical scavenging antioxidant behavior was observed **OPCs were merely able to increase cardiovascular health, a claim disputed by the FDA**, but after this observation exactly the same extracts can now cure everything. Others have latched onto this bandwagon and all of the flavonoids, bioflavonoids, citroflavonoids, bioflavanols, and so on, have rocketed back into fashion. Not only can they do all of the above but they are claimed to have antibacterial effects and can also prevent bruising, increase athletic power, prevent fluid accumulation (swollen legs), prevent night cramps, relieve pain, treat oral herpes, promote circulation, stimulate bile production,... and the list goes on **ad nauseam**. The labels and advertising materials for some of these health supplements still tell us that they contain "bioflavonoid", which is "another name for vitamin P".

Our personal conclusion from this brief history of plant extract health supplements is that **this entire sector of the health industry is driven by market forces and not by medical science.** Simply because they sound scientific and roll off the tongue easily, words and ideas that were abandoned decades ago have been dug up, dusted off and put through the marketing department for a final polish-up before being used to **con an unsuspecting public.** We don't expect everybody to be completely literate in IUPAC chemical nomenclature but we do expect regulating authorities to step forward and tell the public exactly what these substances can and cannot do. On that point there is a new website at http://www.nelh.nhs.uk/hth/archive.asp It looks at newspaper and magazine articles about medical breakthroughs and health scares, and spells out the exact science behind the articles, and experts state in simple terms whether the conclusions are valid or not. Excellent! We need many more sites like this.

'*Cosmetics Unmasked*' by Dr Stephen and Gina Antczak, published by Thorsons (HarperCollins) price £9.99.

ISBN 0007105681

2.0.2.0 Free radicals: general info

Free radicals are chemicals with an unpaired electron in the outer shell of the molecule. Free radicals are allegedly highly reactive due to the presence of this unpaired electron but this is not always the case. Free radicals are capable of independent existence. That they can be highly reactive led to the erroneous belief that they have low chemical specificity, capable of reacting with most molecules near them including proteins, lipids, carbohydrates, and DNA.

They can be short-lived and turn the attacked antioxidant molecule into a free radical in the process. It was erroneously thought that once this process begins, it becomes a dangerous chain reaction disrupting the functioning of our cells and our entire body. In reality, this does not occur. Free radicals were believed to play a key role causing human disease, such as cancer, and in making some drugs toxic to our body, and they have been implicated in the aging process. They were accused of causing certain eye, brain, and mental disorders.

The radical derivatives of oxygen are the most essential free radicals in the body. They are also known as reactive oxygen species and include oxygen in its triplet state (3O2) or singlet state (1O2), superoxide anion (O2•-), hydroxyl radical (•OH), nitric oxide (NO•), peroxynitrite (ONOO-), hypochlorous acid (HOCl), hydrogen peroxide (H2O2) alkoxyl radical (LO•), and the peroxyl radical (L-•2).

There are also carbon-centered, hydrogen-centered, and sulphur-centered free radicals.

Free radicals are produced in our bodies by a process referred to as auto-oxidation, which is part of our normal breathing that results in the reduction of the oxygen diradical and the formation of reactive oxygen species, primarily superoxide, in route to the formation of water and ATP.

Free radicals are also formed in our body in others ways including by a variety of enzyme systems capable of generating large amounts of free radicals, including NADPH oxidase, xanthine oxidase, and via other metabolic activities in our body. We also get free radicals from a number of sources outside our body including via drugs, such as antibiotics that depend on quinoid groups or bound metals for their action such as nitrofurantoin, and anti-cancer drugs such as bleomycin and methotrexate.

Radiation treatment, smoking tobacco, inhalation of inorganic particles such as asbestos and silica, and ozone inhalation, even fever, are sources of free radicals. So-called oxidative stress is defined as the state in which the level of toxic reactive oxygen intermediates (ROI) overcomes our internal antioxidant defenses. This is a flawed concept. **Exercise is a great way to prevent or delay age-related diseases such as heart disease, cancer, and Alzheimer's and I believe that it is due to its increase in our overall oxidative capacity**.

2.0.2.1 Elderly who exercise 1X/wk 30% more likely to maintain cognitive function

A study published in June 2009 in the journal *Neurology* found that older people who exercise at least once a week are 30% more likely to maintain cognitive function than those who exercise less.

2.0.2.2 Oxidative stress and cancer: have we moved forward?

'Reactive species' (RS) of various types are formed in vivo and many are powerful oxidizing agents, capable of damaging DNA and other biomolecules.

Increased formation of RS can promote the development of malignancy, and the 'normal' rates of RS generation may account for the increased risk of cancer development in the aged. Indeed, **knockout of various antioxidant defense enzymes raises oxidative damage levels and promotes age-related cancer development in animals.** In explaining this, most attention has been paid to direct oxidative damage to DNA by certain RS, such as hydroxyl radical (OH*).

However, **increased levels of DNA base oxidation products such as 8OHdg (8-hydroxy-2'-deoxyguanosine) do not always lead to malignancy**, although malignant tumors often show increased levels of DNA base oxidation.

Hence additional actions of RS must be important, possibly their effects on p53, cell proliferation, invasiveness and metastasis. Chronic inflammation predisposes to malignancy, but the role of RS in this is likely to be complex because **RS can sometimes act as anti-inflammatory agents** (Oxidative stress and cancer: have we moved forward? B. Halliwell. Biochem J (2007) 401: 1-11).

2.0.2.3 Soy sauce antioxidant gives unpredicted reaction in vivo

Dark soy sauce (DSS) is a powerful antioxidant in vitro. We investigated whether this effect could occur in vivo and improve vascular function. Healthy human subjects were given DSS or placebo meals in a randomized, crossover study. Blood and urine were sampled before and 1, 2, 3, and 4h after the meal for F(2)-isoprostanes (total, free, and esterified) and 8OHdG measurements. Blood pressure, vascular augmentation index (AIx), and heart rate (HR) were also measured. **Plasma total F(2)-isoprostanes significantly decreased 3h after placebo and the decrease was greater for DSS.** Plasma free and esterified F(2)-isoprostanes were also significantly decreased after DSS. **Both placebo and DSS meals increased urinary F(2)-isoprostanes at 1h** but not thereafter, and lowered urinary 8OHdG levels, DBP and AIx, and increased HR. We conclude that DSS decreases lipid peroxidation in vivo. However, **oxidative damage biomarkers changed after the placebo meal, a phenomenon to consider when designing interventional studies** (Cautions in the use of biomarkers of oxidative damage; the vascular and antioxidant effect. CY Lee, HB Isaac, H Wang, SH Huang, LH Long, AM Jenner, RP Kelly, B Halliwell. Biochem Biophys Res Commun (2006) 344: 906-11). **This shows the unpredictability of oxidative marker studies.**

2.0.2.4 Ischemia decreases SOD

Oxidative stress is a condition in which oxidant metabolites exert their toxic effect because of an increased production or an altered cellular mechanism of protection. **The heart needs oxygen avidly** and, although it has powerful defense mechanisms, it is susceptible to oxidative stress, which occurs, for instance, during post-ischemic reperfusion. **Ischemia causes alterations in the defense mechanisms against oxygen free radicals, mainly a reduction in the activity of mitochondrial superoxide dismutase and a depauperation of tissue content of reduced glutathione.** At the same time, production of oxygen free radicals increases in the mitochondria and leukocytes and toxic oxygen metabolite production is exacerbated by re-admission of oxygen during reperfusion. Oxidative stress, in turn, causes oxidation of thiol groups and lipid peroxidation leading first to reversible damage, and eventually to necrosis. In man, there is evidence of oxidative stress (determined by release of oxidized glutathione in the coronary sinus) during surgical reperfusion of the whole heart, or after thrombolysis, and it is related to transient left ventricular dysfunction or stunning. Data on oxidative stress in the failing heart are scant. **It is not clear whether the defense mechanisms of the myocyte are altered or whether the production of oxygen free radicals is increased, or both. Recent data have shown a close link between oxidative stress and apoptosis.** Relevant to heart failure is the finding that **tumor necrosis factor, which is found increased in failing patients, induces a rapid rise in intracellular reactive oxygen intermediates and apoptosis.** This series of events is not confined to the myocytes, but occurs also at the level of endothelium, where tumor necrosis factor causes expression of inducible nitric oxide synthase, production of the reactive radical nitric oxide, oxidative stress and apoptosis. It is therefore, possible that the immunological response to heart failure results in endothelial and myocyte dysfunction through oxidative stress mediated apoptosis. Clarification of these mechanisms may lead to novel therapeutic strategies (Oxidative stress during myocardial ischaemia and heart failure. R Ferrari, G Guardigli, D Mele, GF Percoco, C Ceconi, S Curello. Curr Pharm Des (2004) 10: 1699-711). **The decreased SOD would result in decreased peroxide formation or an EMOD insufficiency.**

The proapoptotic transcription factor and gene, JNK-1 and c-Jun are involved in oxidative apoptosis. Bcl 2 is also a proapoptotic gene.

2.0.3.0 Vitamin C wards off gout in men

3-9-09 **Men with a higher intake of vitamin C from food or supplements have a lower risk of developing gout**, a form of arthritis from uric acid build-up that causes inflamed joints, researchers said on Monday.

"Vitamin C intake may provide a useful option in the prevention of gout," Dr. Hyon Choi and colleagues at the University of British Columbia in Vancouver said in a paper published in the Archives of Internal Medicine.

Gout victims are typically men age 40 and older, although the malady can also strike women. Vitamin C appears to lower the levels of uric acid in the blood, the research team said.

Gout can lead to permanent joint damage and is linked to alcohol abuse, obesity, high blood pressure and a diet heavy in meat and cheese. It is increasingly common and **afflicts 3 million people in the United States**.

A look at nearly 47,000 U.S. men studied from 1986 to 2006 for a variety of health issues found that every 500 milligram increase of daily vitamin C intake produced a 17 percent decrease in the risk for gout.

An orange has about 70 mg of the vitamin. Higher concentrations come in pill form.

Among the men studied those with daily intake of 1,500 supplemental mg a day had a 45 percent lower risk of gout than those who took in less than 250 mg a day, said the team headed by Choi, who is now at Boston University. **I believe that this effect is due to the prooxidant properties of vitamin C in high doses.**

2.0.3.1 Vitamin E does not reduce AOM-induced cancer in mice

Vitamin E, part of the body's primary lipid-soluble defense against free radicals and reactive oxygen molecules, has been suggested to reduce the risk for some cancers. However, the role of vitamin E in the etiology and prevention of colon cancer, especially in the highest risk group, the aged, is not clear. Thus, this study was conducted to elucidate the effect of vitamin E supplementation on susceptibility to colon cancer by examining **azoxymethane**

(AOM)-induced aberrant crypt foci (ACF) formation, a surrogate biomarker of colon cancer. Young (3–4 mo) and old (19–20 mo) C57BL/6JNIA mice were fed either a control diet (30 mg *dl*-α-tocopheryl acetate/kg diet) or a vitamin E-supplemented diet (500 mg *dl*-α-tocopheryl acetate/kg diet) for 16 wk. After 6 wk of dietary supplementation, young and old mice were injected with saline or AOM weekly for 5 wk to receive the same total dose of AOM (2.2 mg) and killed 10 wk after the first AOM injection. **Vitamin E supplementation had no effect on the number of AOM-induced ACF in young or old mice.** In addition, vitamin E supplementation did not have an effect on splenocyte interferon-γ, interluekin-6 and tumor necrosis factor-α levels, natural killer cell killing activity or colonic cell proliferation in young or old mice. **Thus, α-tocopherol does not seem to affect the initiation and early promotion stages of AOM-induced colon carcinogenesis in young or old mice.** Whether vitamin E supplementation might be effective in reducing AOM-induced colon tumors is unclear (Vitamin E Supplementation Does Not Alter Azoxymethane-Induced Colonic Aberrant Crypt Foci Formation in Young or Old Mice. H. Chung, D. Wu, S. N. Han, R. Gay, B. Goldin, R. E. Bronson, J. B. Mason, D. E. Smith, and S. N. Meydani. J. Nutr., February 1, 2003; 133(2): 528 - 532).

2.0.3.2 Vitamins E and C do not Prevent Cancer in Men

Discouraging results: Big study finds vitamin C or E pills do not help prevent cancer in men.

By MARILYNN MARCHIONE, Associated Press. Last update: November 16, 2008.

Vitamin C or E pills do not help prevent cancer in men, concludes the same big study that last week found these supplements ineffective for warding off heart disease.

The public has been whipsawed by good and bad news about vitamins, much of it from test-tube or animal studies and hyped manufacturer claims. Even when researchers compare people's diets and find that a vitamin seems to help, the benefit may not translate when that nutrient is obtained a different way, such as a pill.

"Antioxidants, which include vitamin C and vitamin E, have been shown as a group to have potential benefit," but **have not been tested individually for a long enough time to know, said Howard Sesso of Harvard-affiliated Brigham and Women's Hospital** in Boston.

The Physicians Health Study, which he helped lead, was designed to do that. It involved **14,641 male** doctors, 50 or older, including 1,274 who had cancer when or before the study started in 1997. They were included so scientists could see whether the vitamins could prevent a second cancer.

Participants were put into four groups and given vitamin E, vitamin C, both, or dummy pills. The dose of E was 400 international units every other day; C was 500 milligrams daily.

After an average of eight years, there were 1,929 cases of cancer, including 1,013 cases of prostate cancer, which many had hoped vitamin E would prevent.

However, rates of prostate cancer and of total cancer were similar among all four groups.

The study was funded by the National Institutes of Health **and several vitamin makers**. Results were being reported Sunday at an American Association for Cancer Research conference in Washington

"**Well-conducted clinical trials such as this are rapidly closing the door on the hope that common vitamin supplements may protect against cancer**," said Marji McCullough, nutrition chief at the American Cancer Society. "It's still possible that some benefit exists for subgroups that couldn't be measured, but the overall results are certainly discouraging.

"The American Cancer Society recommends getting these and other nutrients by eating a mostly plant-based diet with a variety of vegetables, fruits and whole grains. A bonus is that this type of diet helps to prevent **obesity, which increases the risk of several cancers."**

About 12 percent of Americans take supplements of C and E. The new study does not mean these vitamins have no value, just that they didn't prevent cancer in this group of doctors, who may be healthier than the general population, said Dr. Peter Shields, deputy director of Georgetown University's Lombardi Comprehensive Cancer Center.

The best bet, he said, is to do **things that are known to prevent the disease — eat right, maintain a healthy weight, and exercise.**

Webmd.com Nov. 17, 2008 -- Taking vitamin E and vitamin C supplements may not make cancer less likely, a new study shows.

That finding comes from the Physicians' Health Study II, which recently showed that taking vitamin C and vitamin E supplements may not lower the risk of heart attack or stroke.

Researchers have now analyzed study data on cancer risk and found no sign of lower cancer risk in people taking vitamin E and vitamin C supplements daily during the study.

"After nearly 10 years of supplementation with either vitamin E or vitamin C, we found no evidence supporting the use of either supplement in the prevention of cancer," Howard Sesso, ScD, MPH, says in an AACR news release. Sesso, who is an assistant professor of medicine at Brigham and Women's Hospital in Boston, **adds that there was also no sign that either supplement was harmful.**

The findings are only about vitamin E and vitamin C from supplements, not foods.

"Individual vitamin supplements such as vitamin E and C do not appear to provide the same potential advantages as vitamins included as part of a healthy, balanced diet," J. Michael Gaziano, MD, MPH, says in the AACR news release. Gaziano, an associate professor of medicine at Brigham and Women's Hospital, worked with Sesso on the study

Supplements Industry Responds

The study was "well done" but has some limits, notes **Andrew Shao, PhD, vice president for scientific and regulatory affairs at the Council for Responsible Nutrition, a trade group for the supplements industry.**

Shao points out that the doctors were "probably very healthy" to begin with, and that the study started when they were already "well along, in terms of age."

The study doesn't settle questions about whether different doses might be more effective, or if starting supplementation earlier in life might make a difference, Shao says.

Beyond that, Shao says **lifestyle -- including diet, exercise, and other habits -- seems to matter more than one or two nutrients.**

"It really comes down to what is the total package," **Shao says. "We can't necessarily expect a couple of nutrients to have a magic bullet effect," especially in a healthy group of people."**

Taking vitamin A and E supplements does not lower your risk of cancer, according to the results of a large clinical trial involving nearly 15,000 men in the US.

Both vitamins are powerful antioxidants - substances that can tackle harmful byproducts of the body's metabolism which can cause DNA damage and hence trigger cancer. However, the study shows that taking the vitamins in supplement form has no effect at all on cancer.

"There have been a number of previous studies that have suggested that vitamin E and vitamin C might be important in the prevention of cancer," said Dr Howard Sesso, an epidemiologist at Brigham and Women's hospital in Boston, Massachusetts. These were mostly small lab studies or research on animals. But a 1998 study of men in Finland suggested that vitamin E supplements reduced prostate cancer cases by 32% and deaths by 41%.

"The lack of an effect that we observe for vitamin E or C on cancer does convince us that these particular doses that we tested really have no role for recommendation for cancer prevention," said Sesso

2.0.3.3 Vitamin E Supplements May Raise Lung Cancer Risk

Study found a slight but significant association

Feb. 28, 2008 (HealthDay News) -- **Vitamin supplements won't protect people against lung cancer and taking vitamin E may even heighten the risk**, a new study finds. The survey covered the supplement-taking habits and lung cancer incidence of almost **78,000** adults in the state of Washington over a four-year period.

"Our study of **supplemental multivitamins, vitamin C, vitamin E and folate did not show any evidence for a decreased risk of lung cancer,"** study author Dr. Christopher G. Slatore, a fellow in the division of pulmonary and critical care medicine at the University of Washington, said in a statement. "Indeed, **increasing intake of supplemental vitamin E was associated with a slightly increased risk of lung cancer**."

As reported in the March 2008 issue of the *American Journal of Respiratory and Critical Care Medicine*, the research focused on men and women aged 50 to 76 taking part in the four-year **VITAmins and Lifestyle (VITAL) study**. Lung cancer was diagnosed in 521 participants surveyed.

In addition to the expected association with smoking, family history and other lung cancer risk factors, there was a slight but statistically significant association with vitamin E supplementation and incidence of the disease, the researchers found.

Every increase in vitamin E of 100 milligrams per day was associated with a 7 percent rise in lung cancer risk -- translating into a 28 percent increase in risk over 10 years for someone taking 400 milligrams of vitamin E daily.

"This provides additional evidence that taking vitamin supplements does not help prevent lung cancer," said Eric Jacobs, strategic director of pharmacoepidemiology at the American Cancer Society.

The society does not currently recommend use of any vitamin supplement to prevent malignancy, Jacobs said. However, "our dietary guidelines do recommend eating five or more servings of a variety of vegetables each day," he noted.

A representative of the supplements industry called the study results "not all that surprising."

"Vitamins are essential nutrients that act to maintain health and prevent vitamin deficiency," Pamela Mason, spokeswoman for the London-based Health Supplements Information Service, said in a statement. "They were never intended to be used to prevent chronic disease such as cancer. Indeed, it would be asking a lot of a vitamin pill to expect it to prevent cancer."

Since the primary cause of lung cancer is smoking, the best preventive measure is simply not to smoke, Jacobs said. Nutrients can play an auxiliary role, he noted. Anyone who cannot quit should avoid taking beta-carotene supplements, because studies have linked them to an increased risk of lung cancer, Jacobs said.

On the other hand, "for former smokers, there is some evidence that vegetables high in carotinoids, such as carrots and sweet peas, decrease the risk," he said.

Some vitamins have been linked to a reduced risk of other cancers, added Edward Gorham, an associate professor of family and preventive medicine at the University of California at San Diego.

"We have worked with vitamin D, and we found a protective effect of vitamin D on colon cancer, breast cancer and ovarian cancer, and recently a modest effect on lung cancer," Gorham said.

But **that effect came not from supplements but from sunlight**, which causes vitamin D to be formed in the human body, he said.

"These results with multivitamins do not surprise me because there is so little vitamin D in multi-supplements, 100 or 200 International Units," Gorham said. "To achieve the effect, it takes 2,000 IU. If youre in the tropics, that amounts to 10 or 15 minutes in the sun. In southern California, it takes 10 or 15 minutes in the summer and longer in the winter because the sun angle is so low."

One study has also **associated vitamin D supplements with a decreased risk of colon and breast cancer in women**, Gorham said.

2.0.3.4 Vitamin C May Interfere With Cancer Treatment

October 1, 2008 Tara Parker-Pope on Health the New York Times

Many people gobble big doses of vitamin C in hopes of boosting their immune system and warding off illness. But new research shows that **in people with cancer, the vitamin may do more harm than good.**

Researchers at Memorial Sloan-Kettering Cancer Center in New York studied the effects of vitamin C on cancer cells. As it turns out, **the vitamin seems to protect not just healthy cells, but cancer cells, too.** The findings were published today in the journal Cancer Research.

"The use of vitamin C supplements could have the potential to reduce the ability of patients to respond to therapy," said Dr. Mark Heaney, an associate attending physician at the cancer center.

Dr. Heaney and his colleagues tested five different chemotherapy drugs on cancer cells in the laboratory. Some of the cells were first treated with vitamin C. In every case, including a test of the powerful

new cancer drug Gleevec, chemotherapy did not work as well if cells had been exposed to vitamin C. The chemotherapy agents killed 30 to 70 percent fewer cancer cells when the cells were treated with the vitamin.

A second set of experiments implanted cancer cells in mice. They found that the tumors grew more rapidly in mice that were given cancer cells pretreated with vitamin C.

The researchers found that just like healthy cells, **cancer cells also benefit from vitamin C.** The vitamin appeared to repair a cancer cell's damaged mitochondria, the energy center of cells. When the mitochondria is injured, it sends signals that force the cell to die, but vitamin C interrupts that process.

"Vitamin C appears to protect the mitochondria from extensive damage, thus saving the cell," Dr. Heaney said. "And whether directly or not, all anticancer drugs work to disrupt the mitochondria to push cell death."

Dr. Heaney measured the buildup of vitamin C levels in cells and said that the levels of vitamin C used in the experiments were similar to those that would result if a patient took large doses of the vitamin in supplement form. Earlier research at the cancer center showed that **vitamin C seems to accumulate within cancer cells more than in normal cells.**

Patients should eat a healthy diet that includes foods rich in vitamin C, Dr. Heaney said, but **it's the large doses of vitamin C in tablet form that are worrisome**.

2.0.3.5 Antioxidants Vitamin C and Vitamin E for the Prevention and Treatment of Cancer

Thirty-eight studies showed scant evidence that vitamin C or vitamin E beneficially affects survival. In the ATBC Cancer Prevention Study Group, no statistically significant effect of treatment was seen for any cancer individually, and our pooled relative risk (regardless of tumor type) for α-tocopherol alone was 0.91 (95% confidence interval [CI]: 0.74, 1.12). All cause mortality was not significant. In the Linxian General Population Trial, the relative risks for cancer death for vitamin C (combined with molybdenum) was 1.06 (95% CI: 0.92, 1.21) and for vitamin E (combined with β-carotene and selenium) was 0.87 (95% CI: 0.76, 1.00).

We identified only 3 studies that reported statistically significant beneficial results: vitamin C (in combination with BCG) was found to be beneficial in a single trial of bladder cancer and vitamin E (in combination with ω-3 fatty acid) increased survival in patients with advanced cancer. In the ATBC trial, in analyses of 6 individual cancers, the prevention of prostate cancer in subjects treated with α-tocopherol was statistically significant (RR = 0.64, 95% CI: 0.44, 0.94).

CONCLUSIONS

The systematic review of the literature does not support the hypothesis that the use of supplements of vitamin C or vitamin E in the doses tested helps prevent and/or treat cancer in the populations tested. There were isolated findings of benefit, which require confirmation (Antioxidants Vitamin C and Vitamin E for the Prevention and Treatment of Cancer. Ian D Coulter et al. J Gen Intern Med. 2006 July; 21(7): 735–744).

The results of our literature synthesis show generally disappointing results for the efficacy of these antioxidant supplements in these doses to prevent, modify risks or treat cancer in these populations. The exceptions to this conclusion are a study in which vitamin C (along with other vitamins) was found to be beneficial in preventing new tumors in a single trial of bladder cancer when used in conjunction with BCG. (Lamm, D; Riggs, DR; Shriver, JS; vanGilder, PF; Rach, JF; DeHaven, JI. Megadose vitamins in bladder cancer: a double-blind clinical trial. *J Urol.* 1994;151:21–6); a study in which vitamin E when used in conmbination with omega-3-fatty acide increased survival in patients with advanced cancer (Gogos, CA; Ginopoulos, P; Salsa, B; Apostolidou, E; Zoumbos, NC; Kalfarentzos, F. Dietary omega-3 polyunsaturated fatty acids plus vitamin E restore immunodeficiency and prolong survival for severely ill patients with generalized malignancy: a randomized control trial. *Cancer.* 1998;82:395–402); and a study in which vitamin e for prevention of new tumors in subjects with prostate cancer. (Heinonen, OP; Albanes, D; Virtamo, J, et al. Prostate cancer and supplementation with alpha-tocopherol and beta-carotene: incidence and mortality **in a** controlled trial. *J Natl Cancer Inst.* 1998;90:414–5)

But, in the same study on reduction in new prostate cancer, **no effect** was seen when vitamin E and β-carotene were given together, and there was no effect on death from prostate cancer.

A number of issues potentially limit the effectiveness of this review. Methodologically, there was marked heterogeneity in the size of the population, the intent of the trial, the types of outcomes, and follow-up times. We identified a number of large primary prevention trials (α-Tocopherol, β-Carotene Group, Linxian General Population and Linxian Dysplasia Trials and the Heart Protection Study Collaborative Group) that each reported on a number of separate outcomes. The majority of remaining trials were studies of much smaller numbers of people. They included not only secondary prevention trials but also treatment trials. In addition, the populations varied greatly. The observed heterogeneity in study populations and designs deterred us from conducting a meta-analysis in 2 of our outcome domains—death and new tumors—and also excluded some studies from our colonic polyps analysis. In the face of this heterogeneity, we provide individual study risk ratios and discuss the studies descriptively. With only 2 studies in our primary analysis reporting statistically significant beneficial results, we could not perform any meaningful sensitivity analysis using study quality. Similarly, we cannot assess the relationship between the possible heterogeneity in treatment effects and study or population characteristics with such small numbers of studies available.

Clinically, a number of potential limitations could be identified as well. Few studies evaluated single agents for efficacy. There was no standard amount of vitamin C or E given, nor were the multivitamin formulas consistent from study to study. Some of this variation may be because of differences in the populations assessed; however, it also reflects lack of consensus on recommended doses of these vitamins to be used therapeutically. Given the small number of studies and the differences in doses and formulas, no assessment could be made regarding effectiveness of varying dosage levels or combinations of individual supplements.

During the submission and review of this paper, 2 new major randomized-controlled trials (RCTs) have been published. The first was a study by Lonn et al. of more than 4,000 patients randomized to receive a daily dose of 400 IU of vitamin E or placebo and followed for a median of 7 years. **No evidence of beneficial effect was observed** (incidence RR = 0.94, 95% CI: 0.84–1.06; death RR = 0.88, 95% CI: 0.71–1.09). (Lonn, E; Bosch, J; Yusuf, S, et al. HOPE and HOPE-TOO Trial Investigators. Effects of long-term vitamin E supplementation on cardiovascular events and cancer: a randomized controlled trial. *JAMA*. 2005;293:1338–47)

The second paper was part of the Women's Health Study by Lee et al. in which 40,000 women were randomized to receive vitamin E (600 IU on alternative days), aspirin or placebo in a factorial design trial. (Lee, IM; Cook, NR; Gaziano, JM, et al. Vitamin E in the primary prevention of cardiovascular disease and cancer: the women's health study: a randomized controlled trial. *JAMA*. 2005;294:56–65) **There was**

no significant effect on the incidence of total cancer (RR = 1.01), or for breast cancer (RR = 1.00), lung cancer (RR = 1.09), or colon cancers (RR = 1.00). These findings support the results of our review and metaanalysis.

In trying to resolve the randomized trial results with the cellular/molecular and the epidemiologic data there are several possible explanations: the type of antioxidants used in the trials was different (synthetic vs natural); the dose used was wrong; the results were because of something other than the single antioxidants or combinations that were tested in the trials; the duration of treatment was too short; and unaccounted for confounding means the observed epidemiologic association is not causal.

We conclude that **there is no evidence that the antioxidants tested, in the doses tested, and for the populations tested, help prevent cancer**. This does not constitute "proof" that antioxidants do not influence cancer, especially in light of the fact that some of the risk ratios were clinically significant but lacked power. This suggests, for these outcomes at least, further studies are needed. However, **the generally negative results from the randomized trials do place the burden of proof on the proponents of antioxidant supplements to identify the specific supplement, the dosage, and the population combination that is efficacious** (Antioxidants Vitamin C and Vitamin E for the Prevention and Treatment of Cancer. Ian D Coulter et al. J Gen Intern Med. 2006 July; 21(7): 735–744).

2.0.3.6 Vitamins E and C do not Prevent Cardiovascular Disease in Men

2.0.3.7 The Physicians' Health Study II Randomized Controlled Trial 11/09/08

Howard D. Sesso, ScD, MPH; Julie E. Buring, ScD; William G. Christen, ScD; Tobias Kurth, MD, ScD; Charlene Belanger, MA; Jean MacFadyen, BA; Vadim Bubes, PhD; JoAnn E. Manson, MD, DrPH; Robert J. Glynn, ScD; J. Michael Gaziano, MD, MPH.

JAMA. 2008;300(18):(doi:10.1001/jama.2008.600).

Basic research and observational studies suggest vitamin E or vitamin C may reduce the risk of cardiovascular disease. However, few long-term trials have evaluated men at initially low risk of cardiovascular disease, and no previous trial in men has examined vitamin C alone in the prevention of cardiovascular disease.

Objective. To evaluate whether long-term vitamin E or vitamin C supplementation decreases the risk of major cardiovascular events among men.

Design, Setting, and Participants. The Physicians' Health Study II was a randomized, double-blind, placebo-controlled factorial trial of vitamin E and vitamin C that began in 1997 and continued until its scheduled completion on August 31, 2007. There were **14 641 US male physicians** enrolled, who were initially aged 50 years or older, including 754 men (5.1%) with prevalent cardiovascular disease at randomization.

Intervention. Individual supplements of 400 IU of vitamin E every other day and 500 mg of vitamin C daily.

Main Outcome Measures. A composite end point of major cardiovascular events (nonfatal myocardial infarction, nonfatal stroke, and cardiovascular disease death).

Results. During a mean **follow-up of 8 years**, there were 1245 confirmed major cardiovascular events. Compared with placebo, vitamin E had no effect on the incidence of major cardiovascular events (both active and placebo vitamin E groups, 10.9 events per 1000 person-years; hazard ratio [HR], 1.01 [95% confidence interval {CI}, 0.90-1.13]; *P* = .86), as well as total myocardial infarction (HR, 0.90 [95% CI, 0.75-1.07]; *P* = .22), total stroke (HR, 1.07 [95% CI, 0.89-1.29]; *P* = .45), and cardiovascular mortality (HR, 1.07 [95% CI, 0.90-1.28]; *P* = .43). There also was no significant effect of vitamin C on major cardiovascular events (active and placebo vitamin E groups, 10.8 and 10.9 events per 1000 person-years, respectively; HR, 0.99 [95% CI, 0.89-1.11]; *P* = .91), as well as total myocardial infarction (HR, 1.04 [95% CI, 0.87-1.24]; *P* = .65), total stroke (HR, 0.89 [95% CI, 0.74-1.07]; *P* = .21), and cardiovascular mortality (HR, 1.02 [95% CI, 0.85-1.21]; *P* = .86). Neither vitamin E (HR, 1.07 [95% CI, 0.97-1.18]; *P* = .15) nor vitamin C (HR, 1.07 [95% CI, 0.97-1.18]; *P* = .16) had a significant effect on total mortality but vitamin E was associated with an increased risk of hemorrhagic stroke (HR, 1.74 [95% CI, 1.04-2.91]; *P* = .04).

Conclusions. In this large, long-term trial of male physicians, neither vitamin E nor vitamin C supplementation reduced the risk of major cardiovascular events. These data provide no support for the use of these supplements for the prevention of cardiovascular disease in middle-aged and older men.

12 percent of Americans take supplements of C and E despite growing evidence that these antioxidants do not prevent heart disease and may

even be harmful. As for vitamin C, some research suggests it may aid cancer, not fight it. A previous study in women at high risk of heart problems found it did not prevent heart attacks. The Physicians Health Study, is led by Drs. Howard Sesso and J. Michael Gaziano of Harvard-affiliated Brigham and Women's Hospital in Boston.

It involved 14,641 male doctors, 50 or older, including 5 percent who had heart disease at the time the study started in 1997. They were put into four groups and given either vitamin E, vitamin C, both, or dummy pills. The dose of E was 400 international units every other day; C was 500 milligrams daily. After an average of eight years, no difference was seen in the rates of heart attack, stroke or heart-related deaths among the groups. 39 men taking E suffered bleeding strokes versus only 23 of the others, which works out to a 74 percent greater risk for vitamin-takers. Results were so clear that they would be unlikely to change if the study were done in women, minorities, or with different formulations of the vitamins, Howard said. "In these hard economic times, maybe we can save some money by not buying these supplements," she said.

A second study found **that vitamins B-12 and B-9 (folic acid) did not prevent heart disease either, supporting the results of previous trials.** That study involved more than 12,000 heart attack survivors and was led by Dr. Jane Armitage of the University of Oxford in England.

2.0.3.8 US Vitamin supplement sales

Despite uncertainty regarding long-term health benefits, **most US adults have taken a vitamin supplement in the past year** (Timbo BB, Ross MP, McCarthy PV, Lin CT. Dietary supplements in a national survey: prevalence of use and reports of adverse events. *J Am Diet Assoc.* 2006;106(12):1966-1974).

In the 1999-2000 National Health and Nutrition Examination Survey, 12.7% and 12.4% of US adults took vitamin E and C supplements, respectively (Radimer K, Bindewald B, Hughes J, Ervin B, Swanson C, Picciano MF. Dietary supplement use by US adults: data from the National Health and Nutrition Examination Survey, 1999-2000. *Am J Epidemiol.* 2004;160(4):339-349).

With **annual vitamin supplement sales in the billons of US dollars**, vitamin supplementation has broad public health implications (Muth MK, Anderson DW, Domanico JL, Smith JB, Wendling B. *Economic Characterization of the Dietary Supplement Industry.* Washington, DC: Center for Food Safety and Administration, Food and Drug Administration; 1999).

2.0.4.0 One-third of US kids take vitamins

2-3-09 About a third of U.S. children and teens take vitamins, even though most of those taking the pills are healthy, active kids who probably don't need them, a new study suggests. Youngsters who could benefit the most from vitamins — kids in fair or poor health with the worst eating habits — were the least likely to take them, researchers reported.

The survey of parents of children aged 2 to 17 was done from 1999-2004. The results show **a decline in vitamin use from the 1970s when roughly half of all American children took vitamins**, the study's lead author said.

The study highlights a question doctors often get from parents: Should I give my kids vitamins? Stacy Fournier, of Gainesville, Fla., says it's often on her mind even though her daughter is a great eater. I probably bring it up every other time we visit the pediatrician because it is looming on my mind and I want to make sure that she's healthy," said Fournier, whose daughter is almost 3. For now, Fournier has heeded her doctor's advice against it, but she still wonders, "Why not? **It can't hurt."**

The study's lead author, Dr. Ulfat Shaikh, a pediatrician at the University of California-Davis Children's Hospital in Sacramento, says taking daily multivitamins in the dose recommended on the label **probably is harmless**. However, they often aren't needed for healthy children with a varied diet, she said.

Shaikh said kids in the study "who had the ideal profile — higher dietary fiber intake, higher milk intake, lower total fat and cholesterol intake, lower computer use, greater physical activity, lower obesity, kids that had insurance coverage, had good health care access, whose parents said that they were in good health — these kinds of kids were the highest users."

She noted that **vitamin and mineral supplements aren't cheap.** A bottle of 100 multivitamin-mineral tablets for kids can cost around $10, depending on the brand. **Almost $2 billion is spent on them annually.**

Also, some parents and teens may mistakenly think taking a daily pill will make up for a lousy diet, Shaikh said. **Pediatricians generally agree that the best source for vitamins and minerals is a varied diet that includes fresh fruit, vegetables and fiber — not pills.**

Still, there's mounting evidence about important potential benefits from a vitamin that can be hard to get enough of from food, particularly for kids who don't drink much milk. That's vitamin D.

The American Academy of Pediatrics last year doubled the amount of vitamin D it recommends for all children, from newborns to teens. It now advises 400 international units daily of vitamin D, which kids can get by drinking four cups a day of fortified milk. But many don't drink that much, and eat little of the few foods containing the vitamin, including tuna and other oily fish. So the academy recommends 400 IU supplements for kids lacking adequate vitamin D in their diets.

The vitamin can keep bones strong, but also has been linked to other possible health benefits, including preventing some cancers and heart disease.

Some physicians think kids and adults should be getting even more vitamin D, and an Institute of Medicine panel begins a series of meetings in March to discuss whether to revise recommendations for both vitamin D and calcium, which work together to keep bones healthy.

The new study, released Monday in the February issue of Archives of Pediatrics & Adolescent Medicine, asked about use of vitamin and mineral supplements in general, not about specific ones including vitamin D. It found supplement use was most common among frequent milk drinkers and those with varied diets — children who likely are meeting the academy's latest recommendations.

The study is based on data from 10,828 kids whose parents took part in a national health survey that included interviews about diet and supplement use. **Overall, 34 percent of the children had recently taken vitamin/mineral supplements and almost half of users took them daily.**

Vitamin/mineral use was highest among 2- to 4-year-olds — 43 percent, and lowest in 12- to 17-year-olds — 27 percent.

Among children in excellent health, 37 percent used the supplements, versus 28 percent of those in fair or poor health. The breakdown was similar when comparing frequent milk drinkers to those who generally avoided dairy products. Lower-income children were less likely to take vitamins and minerals than those from wealthier families. Shaikh said it's possible the healthy kids were healthy at least partly because of vitamin/mineral use. But she said it's also possible vitamin-using kids simply have more health-conscious parents.

Dr. Ronald Kleinman, editor of the pediatrics academy's nutrition handbook, said the study bolsters previous evidence that children who may need vitamins the most don't take them. "Most of us would do that by recommending a better meal plan" rather than vitamin supplements, he said.

I believe that this high vitamin use in children may be related to the increased incidence of ear infections and RSV in kids. It may also be partially to blame for the increase in type 1 diabetes and obesity.

2.0.4.1 Vitamin and Mineral Supplement Use Among US Adults After Cancer Diagnosis

Vitamin and mineral supplement use is thought to be common among the 10 million adults in the United States who have been diagnosed with cancer; however, well-conducted studies of this topic are sparse. Moreover, the biologic effects of supplement use among cancer survivors are not well established and not necessarily beneficial. We present a systematic summary of studies published between 1999 and 2006, 32 in total, addressing vitamin and mineral supplement use among US adult cancer patients and survivors. **Supplement use is widespread among cancer patients and longer-term survivors. In studies combining different cancer sites, 64% to 81% of survivors reported using any vitamin or mineral supplements and 26% to 77% reported using any multivitamins. In contrast, approximately 50% of US adults use dietary supplements and 33% use multivitamin/multimineral supplements. Between 14% and 32% of survivors initiate supplement use after diagnosis, and use differs by cancer site.** Breast cancer survivors reported the highest use, whereas prostate cancer survivors reported the least. Higher level of education and female sex emerged as factors most consistently associated with supplement use. **Up to 68% of physicians are unaware of supplement use among their cancer patients.** These results highlight the need for further studies of the association between dietary supplement use and cancer treatment toxicity, recurrence, survival, and quality of life to support evidence-based clinical guidelines for dietary supplement use among cancer patients and longer-term survivors (Vitamin and Mineral Supplement Use Among US Adults After Cancer Diagnosis: A Systematic Review. Christine M. Velicer, Cornelia M. Ulrich. *Journal of Clinical Oncology*, Vol 26, No 4 (February 1), 2008: pp. 665-673).

2.0.5.0 Avoid antioxidants in cancer patients

Many patients being treated for cancer use dietary supplements, particularly antioxidants, in the hope of reducing the toxicity of chemotherapy and radiotherapy.

Some researchers have claimed, furthermore, that antioxidants also increase the effectiveness of cytotoxic therapy and have explicitly recommended their use. However, mechanistic considerations suggest that antioxidants might reduce the effects of conventional cytotoxic therapies. Preclinical data are currently inconclusive and a limited number of clinical studies have not found any benefit. Clinicians should advise their patients against the use of antioxidant dietary supplements during chemotherapy or radiotherapy. Such caution should be seen as the standard approach for any unproven agent that may be harmful.

It is estimated from survey data that 50% of cancer patients use some kind of dietary supplementation. Patients often understand in a general sense that supplements "help protect the body," and the mechanism for protection against chemotherapy and radiotherapy toxicity is well understood. **Radiotherapy and many chemotherapy agents act by producing free radicals; some vitamins and supplements, including vitamins C and E, are antioxidants and bind to free radicals, preventing oxidative damage**. (Use of Antioxidants During Chemotherapy and Radiotherapy Should Be Avoided. Gabriella M. D'Andrea. CA Cancer J Clin 2005; 55:319-321)

2.0.5.1 Can antioxidants block chemo or radiation therapy?

In September 2005, CA: A Cancer Journal for Clinicians published a warning by Gabriella D'Andrea, MD, against the concurrent use of antioxidants with radiotherapy and chemotherapy. However, several deficiencies of the CA article soon became apparent, not least the selective omission of prominent studies that contradicted the author's conclusions. While acknowledging that only large-scale, randomized trials could provide a valid basis for therapeutic recommendations, the author sometimes relied on laboratory rather than clinical data to support her claim that harm resulted from the concurrent use of antioxidants and chemotherapy. She also sometimes extrapolated from chemoprevention studies rather than those on the concurrent use of antioxidants per se. The article overstated the degree to which the laboratory data diverged in regard to the safety and efficacy of antioxidant therapy: **in fact, the preponderance of data suggests a synergistic or at least harmless effect with most high-dose dietary antioxidants and chemotherapy.** The practical recommendations made in the article to avoid the general class of antioxidants during chemotherapy are inconsistent, in that **if antioxidants were truly a threat to the efficacy of standard therapy, antioxidant-rich foods, especially fruits and vegetables, ought also be proscribed during treatment. Yet no such recommendation is made.** Furthermore, the wide-scale use by both medical and radiation oncologists of **synthetic antioxidants (eg, amifostine)** to control the adverse effects of cytotoxic treatments is similarly overlooked. In sum, this CA article is incomplete: there is far more information available regarding antioxidant supplements as an appropriate adjunctive cancer therapy than is acknowledged. Patients would be well advised to seek the opinion of physicians who are adequately trained and experienced in the intersection of 2 complex fields, that is, chemotherapeutics and nutritional oncology. Physicians whose goal is comprehensive cancer therapy should refer their patients to qualified integrative practitioners who have such training and expertise to guide patients. **A blanket rejection of the concurrent use of antioxidants with chemotherapy is not justified by the preponderance of evidence at this time and serves neither the scientific community nor cancer patients** (Should Patients Undergoing Chemotherapy and Radiotherapy Be Prescribed Antioxidants? Ralph W. Moss. Integrative Cancer Therapies, Vol. 5, No. 1, 63-82 (2006).

2.0.5.2 Do Antioxidants Interfere With Radiation Therapy for Cancer?

Despite recent comprehensive review articles concluding that supplemental antioxidants do not undermine the effectiveness of cytotoxic therapies, **the use of antioxidants during cancer treatment remains controversial.** Many oncologists take the position that antioxidants by their nature undermine the free radical mechanism of chemotherapy and radiotherapy and should therefore generally be avoided during treatment. For their part, many integrative practitioners believe that antioxidants taken during cancer treatment not only alleviate some of the adverse effects of that treatment but also enhance the efficacy of cancer therapy. Until recently, research attention has focused primarily on the interaction of antioxidants with chemotherapy; relatively little attention has been paid to the interaction of antioxidants with radiotherapy. This article reviews the clinical literature that has addressed whether antioxidants do in fact interfere with radiation therapy. Studies have variously investigated the use of α-tocopherol for the amelioration of radiation-induced mucositis; pentoxifylline and vitamin E to correct the adverse effects of radiotherapy; melatonin alongside radiotherapy in the treatment of brain cancer; retinol palmitate as a treatment for radiation-induced proctopathy; a combination of antioxidants (and other naturopathic treatments) and external beam radiation therapy as definitive treatment for prostate cancer; and the use of synthetic antioxidants, amifostine, dexrazoxane, and mesna as radioprotectants. **With few exceptions, most of the studies draw positive conclusions about the interaction of antioxidants and radiotherapy**. Although further studies are needed, the preponderance of evidence supports a provisional conclusion that **dietary antioxidants do not conflict with the use of radiotherapy in the treatment of a wide variety of cancers**

and may significantly mitigate the adverse effects of that treatment (Do Antioxidants Interfere With Radiation Therapy for Cancer? Ralph W. Moss. Integrative Cancer Therapies, Vol. 6, No. 3, 281-292 (2007).

2.0.5.3 Should Supplemental Antioxidant Administration Be Avoided During Chemotherapy and Radiation Therapy?

(Brian D. Lawenda, Kara M. Kelly, Elena J. Ladas, Stephen M. Sagar, Andrew Vickers, Jeffrey B. Blumberg. Should Supplemental Antioxidant Administration Be Avoided During Chemotherapy and Radiation Therapy? JNCI Journal of the National Cancer Institute 2008 100(11):773-783)

Despite nearly two decades of research investigating the use of dietary antioxidant supplementation during conventional chemotherapy and radiation therapy, controversy remains about the efficacy and safety of this complementary treatment. Several randomized clinical trials have demonstrated that the concurrent administration of antioxidants with chemotherapy or radiation therapy reduces treatment-related side effects. Some data indicate that antioxidants may protect tumor cells as well as healthy cells from oxidative damage generated by radiation therapy and some chemotherapeutic agents. However, other data suggest that antioxidants can protect normal tissues from chemotherapy- or radiation-induced damage without decreasing tumor control. We review some of the data regarding the putative benefits and potential risks of antioxidant supplementation concurrent with cytotoxic therapy. **On the basis of our review of the published randomized clinical trials, we conclude that the use of supplemental antioxidants during chemotherapy and radiation therapy should be discouraged because of the possibility of tumor protection and reduced survival.**

In the absence of good evidence of benefit, it is contrary to the principle of primum non nocere to advise patients to continue a potentially harmful intervention.

Several clinical studies (Sieja K. Protective role of selenium against the toxicity of multi-drug chemotherapy in patients with ovarian cancer. Pharmazie (2000) 55(12):958–959) (Pace A, Savarese A, Picardo M, et al. Neuroprotective effect of vitamin E supplementation in patients treated with cisplatin chemotherapy. J Clin Oncol (2003) 21(5):927–931) (Conklin KA. Coenzyme q10 for prevention of anthracycline-induced cardiotoxicity. Integr Cancer Ther (2005) 4(2):110–130) (Branda RF, Naud SJ, Brooks EM, Chen Z, Muss H. Effect of vitamin B12, folate, and dietary supplements on breast carcinoma chemotherapy—induced mucositis and neutropenia. Cancer (2004) 101(5):1058–1064) (Bairati I, Meyer F, Gelinas

M, et al. Randomized trial of antioxidant vitamins to prevent acute adverse effects of radiation therapy in head and neck cancer patients. J Clin Oncol (2005) 23(24):5805–5813) (Ferreira PR, Fleck JF, Diehl A, et al. Protective effect of alpha-tocopherol in head and neck cancer radiation-induced mucositis: a double-blind randomized trial. Head Neck (2004) 26(4):313–321) **have reported modest decreases in treatment-related side effects when supplemental antioxidants—either dietary or pharmaceutical—are administered concurrently with cytotoxic regimens.**

However, **concern has been expressed** (D'Andrea GM. Use of antioxidants during chemotherapy and radiotherapy should be avoided. CA Cancer J Clin (2005) 55(5):319–321) (Seifried HE, McDonald SS, Anderson DE, Greenwald P, Milner JA. The antioxidant conundrum in cancer. Cancer Res (2003) 63(15):4295–4298 **that the action of supplemental antioxidants might not be restricted to reducing the oxidative damage to normal tissues generated by radiation therapy and certain chemotherapeutic agents.**

Theoretically, **antioxidants can exert their effects on all tissues to some degree, thereby protecting tumor cells as well as healthy ones. Experimental and clinical studies** (Bairati I, Meyer F, Gelinas M, et al. Randomized trial of antioxidant vitamins to prevent acute adverse effects of radiation therapy in head and neck cancer patients. J Clin Oncol (2005) 23(24):5805–5813) (Ferreira PR, Fleck JF, Diehl A, et al. Protective effect of alpha-tocopherol in head and neck cancer radiation-induced mucositis: a double-blind randomized trial. Head Neck (2004) 26(4):313–321) (Fantappie O, Lodovici M, Fabrizio P, et al. Vitamin E protects DNA from oxidative damage in human hepatocellular carcinoma cell lines. Free Radic Res (2004) 38(7):751–759) (Sakamoto K, Sakka M. Reduced effect of irradiation on normal and malignant cells irradiated in vivo in mice pretreated with vitamin E. Br J Radiol (1973) 46(547):538–540) (Mothersill C, Moriarty MJ, Seymour CB. Radiobiologic response of CHO-KI cells treated with vitamin A. Acta Radiol Oncol (1986) 25(4–6):275–280) (Wiernik PH, Yeap B, Vogl SE, et al. Hexamethylmelamine and low or moderate dose cisplatin with or without pyridoxine for treatment of advanced ovarian carcinoma: a study of the Eastern Cooperative Oncology Group. Cancer Invest (1992) 10(1):1–9) (Lesperance ML, Olivotto IA, Forde N, et al. Mega-dose vitamins and minerals in the treatment of non-metastatic breast cancer: an historical cohort study. Breast Cancer Res Treat (2002) 76(2):137–143) (Lawenda BD, Smith DE, Xu L, et al. Do the dietary supplements epigallocatechin gallate or vitamin e cause a radiomodifying response on tumors in vivo? A pilot study with murine breast carcinoma. J Soc Integr Oncol (2007) 5(1):11–17) (Salganik RI. The benefits and hazards of antioxidants: controlling apoptosis and other protective mechanisms in cancer patients and the human population. J Am Coll Nutr (2001) 20(5 suppl):464S–472S. discussion 473S–475S) **lend support to this hypothesis, with some clinical data also suggesting that cancer patients who use antioxidant supplements during radiation or chemotherapy have worse survival than those who do not** (Bairati I, Meyer F, Gelinas M, et al. Randomized trial of antioxidant vitamins to prevent acute adverse effects of radiation therapy in head and neck cancer patients. J Clin Oncol (2005) 23(24):5805–5813) (Ferreira PR, Fleck JF, Diehl A, et al. Protective effect of alpha-tocopherol in head and neck cancer radiation-induced mucositis: a double-blind randomized trial. Head Neck (2004) 26(4):313–321) (Lesperance ML, Olivotto IA, Forde N, et al. Mega-dose vitamins and minerals in the treatment of non-metastatic breast cancer: an historical cohort study. Breast Cancer Res Treat (2002) 76(2):137–143) (Bairati I, Meyer F, Jobin E, et al. Antioxidant vitamins supplementation and mortality: a randomized trial in head and neck cancer patients. Int J Cancer (2006) 119(9):2221–2224).

Here, we present the available data on the use of supplemental antioxidants during chemotherapy or radiation therapy and highlight the reasons why this combined treatment approach should be avoided until it is shown to be safe.

2.0.5.4 Effects of Oncological Treatment and Mechanisms of Action of Antioxidants

The principal therapeutic effect of radiation occurs indirectly via the ionization of water molecules in the cytoplasm to reactive oxygen species, for example, superoxide and hydroxyl radicals. These free radicals react with nuclear DNA, thereby creating structural bonds that are potentially fatal to cells. Some of this radiation damage can be repaired, leaving a cell that remains viable and that can proliferate. **It takes only a millisecond for the free radical–DNA reaction to occur, and a normal cell that is not killed outright can repair the damage in as few as 6 hours** (Hall E. Repair of radiation damage and the dose-rate effect. In: In: John J-R, sutton P, Marino D, eds. Radiobiology for the Radiologist (2000) 5th ed. Philadelphia, PA: Lippincott Williams and Wilkins. 67–90).

Antioxidants are compounds that can counteract free radicals and prevent them from causing tissue and organ damage (Ratnam DV, Ankola DD, Bhardwaj V, Sahana DK, Kumar MN. Role of antioxidants in prophylaxis and therapy: a pharmaceutical perspective. J Control Release (2006) 20(113):189–207).

They function through a variety of mechanisms: as preventative agents that suppress the formation of free radicals, as radical scavenging agents that inhibit chain initiation and/or propagation, as repair and de novo enzymes that repair and reconstitute cell membranes, and as adaptation agents that generate appropriate antioxidant enzymes and transfer them to the necessary site of action (Papas AM. Antioxidant Status, Diet, Nutrition, and Health (1999) Boca Raton, FL: CRC Press).

Antioxidants—whether produced endogenously (eg, α-lipoic acid, ubiquinone) or consumed in the diet (eg, α-tocopherol, ascorbic acid)—must be present in the cell during the free radical–DNA reaction, and at a sufficient concentration, to be effective in blocking free radical–mediated DNA damage. **Although antioxidants, by definition, scavenge free radicals, it is important to recognize that most also act via other mechanisms to affect cell proliferation, apoptosis, angiogenesis, and other processes relevant to tumor growth and metastasis.**

Although antioxidants may play a role in the primary prevention of cancer in part by reducing the oxidative modification of DNA, the same action might be expected to be counterproductive against radiation therapy and chemotherapeutic agents that **act solely via the production of reactive oxygen species and induction of apoptosis** (Ratnam DV, Ankola DD, Bhardwaj V, Sahana DK, Kumar MN. Role of antioxidants in prophylaxis and therapy: a pharmaceutical perspective. J Control Release (2006) 20(113):189–207).

These agents include the **anthracyclines (eg, doxorubicin), platinum-containing complexes (eg, cisplatin, carboplatin), alkylating agents (eg, cyclophosphamide, ifosfamide), and cytotoxic antibiotics (eg, bleomycin, mitomycin-C).**

Dietary antioxidants comprise a variety of chemical classes, **including carotenoids, polyphenols, tocols, and triterpenes**, and they display an array of biologic activities. Thus, it is not possible to make broad generalizations about whether or how they might interact with oncological treatments. Nonetheless, **these nutrients are defined by their shared capacity for quenching reactive oxygen and nitrogen species** even though their in vivo potency and selectivity can vary substantially by class, bioavailability, dose, and duration, as well as by route of administration (Ratnam DV, Ankola DD, Bhardwaj V, Sahana DK, Kumar MN. Role of antioxidants in prophylaxis and therapy: a pharmaceutical perspective. J Control Release (2006) 20(113):189–207).

For example, the most readily bioavailable form of **the antioxidant lycopene is in cooked rather than raw foods, and ascorbic acid acts as an antioxidant when taken orally but as a prooxidant when administered**

intravenously at high doses (Ratnam DV, Ankola DD, Bhardwaj V, Sahana DK, Kumar MN. Role of antioxidants in prophylaxis and therapy: a pharmaceutical perspective. J Control Release (2006) 20(113):189–207) (Padayatty SJ, Sun H, Wang Y, et al. Vitamin C pharmacokinetics: implications for oral and intravenous use. Ann Intern Med (2004) 140(7):533–537).

Individual variations (eg, polymorphisms) in the expression of antioxidant enzymes such as superoxide dismutase and catalase further complicate potential interactions between oncological treatments and the antioxidant defense network. For example, some polymorphisms in the gene encoding glutathione-S-transferase, an antioxidant enzyme, can decrease the antioxidant activity of the enzyme.

Laboratory evidence indicates that the effect of dietary antioxidants on tumors is dose dependent. **In the absence of radiotherapy or chemotherapy, high doses of dietary antioxidants often inhibit the growth of cancer cells without affecting the growth of normal cells** (Salganik R. The benefits and hazards of antioxidants: controlling apoptosis and other protective mechanisms in cancer patients and the human population. J Am Coll Nutr (2001) 20(5 Suppl):4645–4725) (Prasad KN, Kumar A, Kochupillai V, Cole WC. High doses of multiple antioxidant vitamins: essential ingredients in improving the efficacy of standard cancer therapy. J Am Coll Nutr (1999) 18(1):13–25) (Prasad KN, Cole WC, Kumar B, Prasad KC. Scientific rationale for using high-dose multiple micronutrients as an adjunct to standard and experimental cancer therapies. J Am Coll Nutr (2001) 20(5 suppl):450S–463S. discussion 473S–475S).

However, data from some studies indicate that **antioxidant supplementation at doses that are intermediate to dietary intakes (relatively low doses) and high supplemental doses may reduce the efficacy of x-irradiation against cancer cells** (Sakamoto K, Sakka M. Reduced effect of irradiation on normal and malignant cells irradiated in vivo in mice pretreated with vitamin E. Br J Radiol (1973) 46(547):538–540) (Witenberg B, Kletter Y, Kalir HH, et al. Ascorbic acid inhibits apoptosis induced by X irradiation in HL60 myeloid leukemia cells. Radiat Res (1999) 152(5):468–478) or stimulate tumor cell growth (Prasad KN, Kumar R. Effect of individual and multiple antioxidant vitamins on growth and morphology of human nontumorigenic and tumorigenic parotid acinar cells in culture. Nutr Cancer (1996) 26(1):11–19).

Interpretation of these experimental data is difficult because the doses that inhibit tumor cell growth vary between species and tumor types and the distribution of antioxidants varies between tumor cells and normal cells (Prasad KN, Kumar R. Effect of individual and multiple antioxidant vitamins on growth and morphology of human nontumorigenic and tumorigenic parotid acinar cells in culture. Nutr Cancer (1996) 26(1):11–19) (Hanck AB. Vitamin C and cancer. Prog Clin Biol Res (1988) 259:307–320) (Liede KE, Alfthan G, Hietanen JH, Haukka JK, Saxen LM, Heinonen OP. Beta-carotene concentration in buccal mucosal cells with and without dysplastic oral leukoplakia after long-term beta-carotene supplementation in male smokers. Eur J Clin Nutr (1998) 52(12):872–876) (Agus DB, Vera JC, Golde DW. Stromal cell oxidation: a mechanism by which tumors obtain vitamin C. Cancer Res (1999) 59(18):4555–4558) (Piyathilake CJ, Bell WC, Johanning GL, Cornwell PE, Heimburger DC, Grizzle WE. The accumulation of ascorbic acid by squamous cell carcinomas of the lung and larynx is associated with global methylation of DNA. Cancer (2000) 89(1):171–176) (Picardo M, Grammatico P, Roccella F, et al. Imbalance in the antioxidant pool in melanoma cells and normal melanocytes from patients with melanoma. J Invest Dermatol (1996) 107(3):322–326) (Langemann H, Torhorst J, Kabiersch A, Krenger W, Honegger CG. Quantitative determination of water- and lipid-soluble antioxidants in neoplastic and non-neoplastic human breast tissue. Int J Cancer (1989) 43(6):1169–1173).

We attempted to identify all published randomized clinical trials that have investigated the possible radiomodifying effects (ie, increasing or decreasing radiosensitivity) of concurrent administration of supplemental antioxidants on normal tissues and tumors.

Bairati et al. (Bairati I, Meyer F, Gelinas M, et al. A randomized trial of antioxidant vitamins to prevent second primary cancers in head and neck cancer patients. J Natl Cancer Inst (2005) 97(7):481–488) reported that among 540 head and neck cancer patients who were randomly assigned to receive either α-tocopherol with or without β-carotene vs placebo concurrent with their radiation therapy, **those who received both antioxidants had a statistically significant 38% reduction in severe, acute side effects**. However, this benefit appeared to be offset by reductions of 29% and 56% in the local tumor control rates for α-tocopherol and α-tocopherol plus β-carotene, respectively. It is interesting to note **that in a recently reported subgroup analysis of these patients** (Meyer F, Bairati I, Fortin A, et al. Interaction between antioxidant vitamin supplementation and cigarette smoking during radiation therapy in relation to long-term effects on recurrence and mortality: a randomized trial among head and neck cancer patients. Int J Cancer (2008) 122(7):1679–1683), **the interactions between antioxidant supplementation and cigarette smoking during radiation therapy were associated with an increase in both disease and cancer-specific mortality.** There was no increase in either of these outcome measures for the nonsmokers.

The most concerning data are presented in a subsequent publication by Bairati et al. (Bairati I, Meyer F, Jobin E, et al. Antioxidant vitamins supplementation and mortality: a randomized trial in head and neck cancer patients. Int J Cancer (2006) 119(9):2221–2224) on the same cohort of patients. In this article, **they demonstrate that the patients who received antioxidants had statistically significant poorer overall survival.** This study is the most important randomized clinical trial, to date, on the use of a supplemental antioxidant and radiation therapy.

Several other studies have provided evidence that antioxidants can decrease the effectiveness of radiation therapy. For example, Ferreira et al. randomly assigned 54 head and neck cancer patients who were undergoing radiation therapy to receive an oil-based oral rinse that contained either vitamin E or placebo before and after each daily dose of radiation. **Although the vitamin E supplementation was associated with a 36% reduction in symptomatic mucositis, the authors also reported a decrease in 2-year overall survival** (32% with supplemental vitamin E vs 63% with placebo; $P = .13$). This concerning decrease in overall survival, albeit **not statistically significant**, may have been confounded by the greater percentage of patients with stage 3 and 4 tumors found in the vitamin E group. (Ferreira PR, Fleck JF, Diehl A, et al. Protective effect of alpha-tocopherol in head and neck cancer radiation-induced mucositis: a double-blind randomized trial. Head Neck (2004) 26(4):313–321)

In another study, **Lesperance et al.** investigated a historical cohort of 90 patients with nonmetastatic breast cancer who received conventional treatment (eg, surgery, chemotherapy, radiation therapy, and hormonal therapy) either alone or in combination with high doses of β-carotene, vitamin C, niacin, selenium, coenzyme Q10, and/or zinc. (Lesperance ML, Olivotto IA, Forde N, et al. Mega-dose vitamins and minerals in the treatment of non-metastatic breast cancer: an historical cohort study. Breast Cancer Res Treat (2002) 76(2):137–143). **Breast cancer–specific survival (ie, patients censored only at death from breast cancer) and disease-free survival were shorter in the nutrient-supplemented group than in the nonsupplemented group, but the differences were not statistically significant** (hazard ratio of breast cancer death = 1.75, 95% CI = 0.83 to 2.69, and hazard ratio of relapse = 1.55, 95% CI = 0.94 to 2.54, respectively). Despite the substantial limitations of these studies, **it is troubling that both reported results suggesting poorer survival with concurrent administration of antioxidants and cytotoxic therapy**, even though these results are at odds with other studies.

For example, **two randomized trials—Misirlioglu et al**. (Misirlioglu CH, Erkal H, Elgin Y, Ugur I, Altundag K. Effect of concomitant use of pentoxifylline and alpha-tocopherol with radiotherapy on the clinical outcome of patients with stage IIIB non-small cell lung cancer: a randomized prospective clinical trial. Med Oncol (2006) 23(2):185–189), **testing pentoxifylline and α-tocopherol in patients with non–small cell lung cancer, and Lissoni et al**. (Lissoni P, Meregalli S, Nosetto L, et al. Increased survival time in brain glioblastomas by a radioneuroendocrine strategy with radiotherapy plus melatonin compared to radiotherapy alone. Oncology (1996) 53(1):43–46), **testing melatonin in patients with brain glioblastomas—found that radiotherapy combined with α-tocopherol or melatonin supplementation increased survival.**

However, **this suggestion of radiosensitization of tumors was not confirmed by Berk et al.** (Berk L, Berkey B, Rich T, et al. Randomized phase II trial of high-dose melatonin and radiation therapy for RPA class 2 patients with brain metastases (RTOG 0119). Int J Radiat Oncol Biol Phys (2007) 68(3):852–857) **in a randomized trial of radiation therapy and high-dose melatonin in brain metastases.**

Despite concerns about current recommendations supporting the use of antioxidant supplementation during oncological treatments, some antioxidants, such as amifostine (WR-2721), a thiol-containing antioxidant that has been approved by the Food and Drug Administration to increase the radioresistance of salivary gland tissues, show promise as cotherapies. Although some preclinical studies have shown that amifostine increases the radioresistance of tumors, neither the randomized clinical trials nor the meta-analyses of this agent have provided conclusive evidence of increased radioresistance of tumors.

Mell et al. (Mell LK, Malik R, Komaki R, et al. Effect of amifostine on response rates in locally advanced non-small cell lung cancer patients treated on randomized controlled trials: a meta-analysis. Int J Radiat Oncol Biol Phys (2007) 68(1):111–118) **stated that their "...results suggest that any effect of amifostine on reducing overall response [to radiation therapy], if it exists, is no larger than a 3% relative risk reduction.**

We identified **16 randomized clinical trials that studied the concurrent use of antioxidant supplements and chemotherapy**; 6 of those trials included a placebo control. Although no decrements in tumor response rates or survival rates were observed in the studies that reported response data, none of those studies were powered to evaluate these endpoints. For example, Pathak et al. (Pathak AK, Bhutani M, Guleria R, et al. Chemotherapy alone vs. chemotherapy plus high dose multiple antioxidants in patients with advanced non small cell lung cancer. J Am Coll Nutr (2005) 24(1):16–21) examined whether the concurrent administration of a high-dose antioxidant mixture containing vitamins C and E and β-carotene with paclitaxel and cisplatin improved tumor response and survival in 136 patients with advanced non–small cell lung cancer and observed no survival or tumor response benefits with the antioxidants. However, **the authors' conclusion that the antioxidant supplementation was safe is not warranted because the study was not sufficiently powered to evaluate a reduction in survival or tumor response.**

In a systematic review of the randomized trials of antioxidants and chemotherapy, Ladas et al. (Ladas EJ, Jacobson JS, Kennedy DD, Teel K, Fleischauer A, Kelly KM. Antioxidants and cancer therapy: a systematic review. J Clin Oncol (2004) 22(3):517–528) found such a wide range of cancer diagnoses, chemotherapy regimens, and antioxidant supplementation that they could not draw definitive conclusions about the safety and efficacy of the antioxidant interventions.

2.0.5.5 Simone concludes that antioxidants increase cancer patient survival

We find it surprising that a recent review (Simone CB 2nd, Simone NL, Simone V, Simone CB. Antioxidants and other nutrients do not interfere with chemotherapy or radiation therapy and can increase kill and increase survival, part 1. Altern Ther Health Med (2007) 13(1):22–28) (Simone CB 2nd, Simone NL, Simone V, Simone CB. Antioxidants and other nutrients do not interfere with chemotherapy or radiation therapy and can increase kill and increase survival, part 2. Altern Ther Health Med (2007) 13(2):40–46) **definitively concludes that antioxidants (and other supplemental nutrients), when given concurrently with chemotherapy and/or radiation therapy, 1) do not interfere with chemotherapy and/or radiation therapy, 2) enhance the cytotoxic effects of chemotherapy and radiation therapy, 3) protect normal tissues, and 4) increase patient survival.**

In the concluding sentence of this review, the authors recommend that "Antioxidant and other nutrient food supplements are safe and can help to enhance cancer patient care" (Simone CB 2nd, Simone NL, Simone V, Simone CB. Antioxidants and other nutrients do not interfere with chemotherapy or radiation therapy and can increase kill and increase survival, part 2. Altern Ther Health Med (2007) 13(2):40–46).

2.0.5.6 Others caution antioxidant use in cancer patients

Such a recommendation merits close examination of the evidence because it is at odds with other authoritative reviews on this topic (D'Andrea GM. Use of antioxidants during chemotherapy and radiotherapy should be avoided. CA Cancer J Clin (2005) 55(5):319–321) (Ladas EJ, Jacobson JS, Kennedy DD, Teel K, Fleischauer A, Kelly KM. Antioxidants and cancer therapy: a systematic review. J Clin Oncol (2004) 22(3):517–528) (Block KI, Koch AC, Mead MN, Tothy PK, Newman RA, Gyllenhaal C. Impact of antioxidant supplementation on chemotherapeutic efficacy: a systematic review of the evidence from randomized controlled trials. Cancer Treat Rev. (2007) 33(5):407–418) (Dennert G, Horneber M. Selenium for alleviating the side effects of chemotherapy, radiotherapy and surgery in cancer patients. Cochrane Database Syst Rev (2006) 3. CD005037) (Sagar S. Should patients take or avoid antioxidant supplements during anticancer therapy? An evidence-based review. Curr Oncol (2005) 12:44–54).

Of the 52 clinical studies Simone et al. reviewed, 36 were observational, a study design that is limited by selection bias and unknown confounders. Of the 16 randomized controlled trials they reviewed, 10 included fewer than 50 patients, a sample size too small to inspire confidence in findings of equivalent survival. Indeed, if antioxidant supplements interfered completely with an agent associated with an absolute increase in survival of 5%, a suitably powered trial would require approximately 2000 patients. The six remaining reports reviewed by Simone et al were randomized trials with at least 50 patients, and, of these, **only one** (Cascinu S, Cordella L, Del Ferro E, Fronzoni M, Catalano G. Neuroprotective effect of reduced glutathione on cisplatin-based chemotherapy in advanced gastric cancer: a randomized double-blind placebo-controlled trial. J Clin Oncol (1995) 13(1):26–32) **tested an antioxidant**. In this trial (n = 50), **glutathione improved response rates and decreased neurotoxicity in advanced gastric cancer patients who received cisplatin.** This is an interesting result, but it must be confirmed in a larger study.

A challenge to these considerations is the absence of any consistent pattern of serum status of vitamins C and E, β-carotene, or selenium in patients with cancer receiving chemotherapy (Ladas EJ, Jacobson JS, Kennedy DD, Teel K, Fleischauer A, Kelly KM. Antioxidants and cancer therapy: a systematic review. J Clin Oncol (2004) 22(3):517–528).

It is noteworthy that although the initiation of anticancer therapies may lower plasma antioxidant concentrations by altering dietary intakes**, an increase in**

plasma antioxidant levels has been associated with a reduction in the cancer burden (Jonas CR, Puckett AB, Jones DP, et al. Plasma antioxidant status after high-dose chemotherapy: a randomized trial of parenteral nutrition in bone marrow transplantation patients. Am J Clin Nutr (2000) 72(1):181–189).

2.0.5.7 When a Potential for Harm Exists, Primum non nocere

Our view on the use of complementary antioxidant therapy with chemotherapy or radiation therapy can be summarized in the following two points. First, **data from a limited number of randomized controlled trials have shown that high-dose antioxidant supplementation during radiotherapy decreases local tumor control and shortens the survival of cancer patients.** Although the potential for harm from this adjunctive therapy may be limited to a few antioxidants, the uncertainty about what doses and which compounds are clearly safe demands that **high doses of any antioxidant should be avoided during radiation therapy unless clear evidence is available that the benefits outweigh the potential risk**.

Second, limited data and theoretical understanding regarding the mechanisms of action of dietary antioxidants suggest that at high doses, some of these compounds, alone or in combination, may enhance the effects of some cytotoxic regimens and/or decrease their toxicity without reducing oncological efficacy. As such, continuing research on the use of concurrent supplemental antioxidants with chemotherapy and/or radiation therapy is warranted.

2.0.5.8 Antioxidants Including Vitamin C Do Not Decrease the Efficacy of Chemotherapy

Editor:

The idea that the use of antioxidants decreases the efficacy of chemotherapy is being used more and more by orthodox oncologists. It is based upon their hypothesis that anything which decreases the oxidant effect of drugs will decrease the efficacy of chemotherapy. More and more I hear this from my patients after they are diagnosed and chemotherapy is discussed with them by their oncologists. This opinion is not universal, but my guess is that about 75% of oncologists hold this view.

Their view is that chemotherapy destroys tumor tissue because it introduces powerful oxidation products, free radicals, and that anything which

decreases that must interfere with treatment. They know they are using sub-lethal amounts of toxic compounds which would never pass FDA standards in any different context. The aim is to kill all the tumor tissue without killing all the other tissues in the body. This is always a close call. Therefore, since vitamin C is a good antioxidant it must not be given with chemotherapy. One of my patients was told by his oncologist that if he took vitamin C he would not be given any chemotherapy.

Well, what are the facts? The first fact is that **there are no clinical series which show that patients given vitamin C and chemotherapy fare worse than those not given this vitamin.** On the contrary, all the published series show just the opposite. I have treated over 1,100 cases with large doses of vitamin C and most of them had chemotherapy.[1-4] I have examined the follow up data and find that **the mean difference on prolongation of life was heavily *in favor* of the use of the vitamins.** In the first series I published with Linus Pauling those patients on my program lived 10 to 20 times as long as the patients not receiving the vitamin.

Recently Kedar N. Prasad et al.[5] after reviewing 71 scientific papers, found no evidence that antioxidants did interfere with the therapeutic effect of chemotherapy and, on the contrary, suggest the hypothesis that it would increase the efficacy. He is properly cautious, but anyone reading his paper knows that it is clear the probability that these antioxidants prevent the therapeutic activity of chemotherapy is very low, and the probability that they do the opposite, i.e enhance the action of these toxic drugs, is relatively high. **Prasad et al.[6]** concluded, "**Antioxidants such as retinoids, vitamin E, vitamin C and carotenoids inhibit the growth of cancer cells.** These antioxidants individually, and in combination, enhance the effects of x-irradiation, chemotherapeutic agents, and certain biological response modifiers such as hyperthermia, sodium butyrate and interferon, on cancer cells. Antioxidants individually protect normal cells against some of the toxicities produced by these therapeutic agents. Therefore, the fear of oncologists and radiation therapists that these antioxidants may protect cancer cells against free radicals that are generated by these agents is unfounded. It should be pointed out that **other antioxidants such as sulfhydryl compounds will protect cancer cells at least against radiation damage.** This is not true for any of the proposed antioxidant vitamins and carotenoids."

Even earlier **Charles B. Simone et al.**[7] on the basis of a large number of clinical studies (he also examined 71 scientific papers) came to the same conclusion. He reported, "In a recent study of 50 patients with early-stage breast cancer I evaluated the treatment side effects of radiation alone, or radiation combined with chemotherapy, while the patients took therapeutic doses of nutrients. Patients also followed the **Simone Ten Point Plan**. Patients were asked to evaluate their own response to the treatment in terms of its impact on their quality of life. The results of the study were impressive: "More than 90% of both groups noted improvement in their physical symptoms, cognitive ability, performance, sexual function, general well-being and life satisfaction. Not one subject in either group reported a worsening of symptoms." He concluded, "...cancer patients should modify their lifestyles using the Ten Point Plan, which included modifying nutritional factors and taking certain vitamins and minerals **especially if they are receiving chemotherapy, and/or radiation**." (my emphasis)

Labriola et al.[8] concluded that vitamin C may prevent the therapeutic effect of chemotherapy if given concurrently and recommended that antioxidants be withheld until after the chemotherapy is completed. It is not clear whether they meant that the antioxidants should be withheld throughout the entire series of chemotherapy sessions or that it should be withheld only for the day that chemotherapy is being given. If the latter is his suggestion, there is no harm done to the patients. Most of them cannot take anything, including vitamins, during these sessions. He based his conclusion on one case which suggested this had happened and upon a hypothetical examination of the role of free radicals and antioxidants on the action of chemotherapy on cancer cells.

His report elicited two rebuttals, Reilly[9] and Gignac.[10] I will not repeat the arguments, but it was evident that Dr. Labriola was not convinced by the points put forward by Reilly and Gignac. I think the factoid repeated by Dr. Labriola would have a much better chance of becoming a fact if he had **considered the following points:**

(1) What is the therapeutic value of chemotherapy without any antioxidants? Even within the field of standard oncology **there is a debate whether chemotherapy has any merit except for a small number of cancers (Moss).**[11] Before one can claim that a treatment has been inhibited, surely there must be pretty good evidence that the treatment has any merit to begin with. It is possible (we do not know the probability for this) that chemotherapy interferes with the therapeutic value of the antioxidants. Almost all the studies testing large doses of vitamin C yielded positive results while there is no such unanimity with respect to chemotherapy.

(2) The difference between possibility and probability. Most people do not distinguish between these two. Theoretically anything is possible, and it is certainly

possible that taking vitamin C might prevent the toxic "beneficial" effect of chemotherapy. In the same way when one buys a lottery ticket, it is possible they may win. People confuse these two terms, which is why lotteries are so popular. The real statistic is the probability. What is the probability that patients receiving vitamin C during their chemotherapy will not fare as well? The lottery ticket may give one a probability of winning of one in a million, and the possibility that vitamin C may prevent the therapeutic effect of chemotherapy may be equally low. We can only assume from **the literature reviewed by Simone, by Prasad, by Lamson and Brignall, and more recently by Moss**[12] that the real probability must be extremely low. As I have pointed out earlier, I have seen no evidence that adding vitamin C inhibited the therapeutic effect of chemotherapy. Just the opposite. Patients on my orthomolecular program live substantially longer and about 40% achieved over four year cure rates.[13]

(3) If he had not tried to bolster his argument by referring so frequently to the peer-reviewed journal in which his paper appeared. This is certainly no guarantee of fact. The first factoid that vitamin C caused kidney stones appeared in eminently peer-reviewed journals. All the factoids regarding vitamins appeared first in peer-reviewed journals. **You may recall Linus Pauling's joke that peers are people who pee together**. I can assure you that articles attacking the use of vitamins have very ready access to peer-reviewed journals, but they would not have accepted their report had they tried to conclude from one patient that vitamin C taken during chemotherapy was therapeutic. This would not even be sent to the peer review committee because they do not accept anecdotes - unless of course they become scientific when they contain something adverse against vitamins.

(4) Moss points out that oncologists have no objection to using **xenobiotic antioxidants** during chemotherapy. This includes **Amifostine** which decreases the toxicity of radiation but is too toxic on its own and is not used; **Mesna,** a drug used around the world to protect against the toxic side effects of ifosfamide which damages the urinary system; and **Cardiozane**, which counters Adriamycin's toxicity. There are over 500 papers showing the safety of the latter drug. In one clinical trial using a drug similar to Adriamycin, one-quarter of the patients suffered damage to their hearts. When given Cardiozane concurrently only 7% did. Thus it appears that only orthomolecular or natural antioxidants are potentially dangerous. **Synthetic antioxidants protect against the toxic effect of drugs but do not increase their therapeutic value**. In sharp contrast, natural antioxidants not only protect against the toxic effect of drugs but *also* increase their efficacy in destroying cancer cells.

(5) Dr. Labriola emphasizes that long term studies must be used. I agree, and for this reason I followed up my patients since 1977. In my series, hardly any patients receiving chemotherapy but not antioxidants survived very long. But chemotherapy is used by many oncologists who know it will not extend life, because there is nothing else that they can do and they feel they have to do something.

A. Hoffer MD PhD FRCP(C)

Suite 3 - 2727 Quadra Street

Victoria, British Columbia V8T 4E5 Canada

250-386-8756

Fax 250-386-5828

References

1. Hoffer A & Pauling L: Hardin Jones biostatistical analysis of mortality data for cohorts of cancer patients with a large fraction surviving at the termination of the study and a comparison of survival times of cancer patients receiving large regular oral doses of vitamin C and other nutrients with similar patients not receiving those doses. *J Orthomolecular Medicine* 5:143-154, 1990. Reprinted in, *Cancer and Vitamin C*, E Cameron and L Pauling, Camino Books, Inc. P.O. Box 59026, Phil. PA, 19102, 1993.

2. Hoffer A & Pauling L: Hardin Jones biostatistical analysis of mortality data for a second set of cohorts of cancer patients with a large fraction surviving at the termination of the study and a comparison of survival times of cancer patients receiving large regular oral doses of vitamin C and other nutrients with similar patients not receiving these doses. *J of Orthomolecular Medicine*, 8:1547-167, 1993.

3. Hoffer A: Orthomolecular Oncology. In, *Adjuvant Nutrition in Cancer Treatment*, Eds. P Quillin & RM Williams. 1992 Symposium Proceedings, Sponsored by Cancer Treatment Research Foundation and American College of Nutrition. Cancer Treatment Research Foundation, 3455 Salt Creek Lane, Suite 200, Arlington Heights, IL 60005-1090, 331-362, 1994.

4. Hoffer A. One Patient's Recovery From Lymphoma. *Townsend Letter for Doctors and Patients* #160:50-51, 1996.

5. Prasad KN, Kumar A, Kochupillai V & Cole WC. High Doses of Multiple Antioxidant Vitamins: Essential Ingredients in Improving the Efficacy of Standard Cancer Therapy. *Journal American College of Nutrition* 18:13-25, 1999.

6. Prasad KN, Cole WC & Prasad JE. Multiple Antioxidant Vitamins as an Adjunct to Standard and Experimental Cancer Therapies. *Z.Onkol/J. of Oncol* 31:1201-1078, 1999.

7. Simone CB, Simone NL & Simone CB. Nutrients and Cancer Treatment. *International Journal of Integrative Medicine* 1:20-24, 1999.

8. Labriola D & Livingston R. Possible Interactions Between Dietary Antioxidants and Chemotherapy. *Oncology* 13:1003-1008, 1999, and Editorial to *Townsend Letter for Doctors and Patients*, November 1999.

9. Reilly P. Dr. Labriola's Editorial on Antioxidants and Chemotherapy, *Townsend Letter for Doctors and Patients* Feb/Mar 2000, 90-91.

10. Gignac MA. Antioxidants and Chemotherapy. What You Need to Know Before Following Dr. Labriola's Advice. *Townsend Letter for Doctors and Patients* Feb/March 2000, 88-89.

11. Moss RW. *Questioning Chemotherapy*. Equinox Press, Brooklyn, New York.

12. Moss RW. *Antioxidants Against Cancer*. Equinox Presss Inc. Brooklyn, New York, 1999.

13. Hoffer A. *Vitamin C and Cancer*. Quarry Press, Kingston, ON 2000.

The following was taken from the website of Dr. Michael Murray: the naturally living newsletter

2.0.5.9 Should antioxidants be avoided during chemotherapy treatments?

One of the most controversial recommendations to support chemotherapy (as well as radiation therapy) is the recommendation to use antioxidant nutrients during the active phase of the treatment. While there is little concern with using antioxidant nutrients after the completion of a course of chemotherapy or radiation treatment the concern that many oncologists have is that antioxidant nutrients will interfere with the effectiveness of conventional therapies. Is this fear valid? According to many experts, the answer is no. (Prasad KN, Kumar A, Kochupillai V, Cole WC. High doses of multiple antioxidant vitamins: essential ingredients in improving the efficacy of standard cancer therapy. J Am Coll Nutr 1999;18(1):13-25) (Lamson DW, Brignall MS. Antioxidants in cancer therapy; their actions and interactions with oncologic therapies. Altern Med Rev 1999;4(5):304-29).

Dr. Kedar Prasad and his colleagues at the Center for Vitamins and Cancer Research at the University of Colorado Health Science Center's Department of Radiology in Denver are among the most knowledgeable experts in this field. Dr. Prasad has stated that the concerns over the use of high dosage antioxidants during chemotherapy and radiation "are not valid." **Dr. Prasad** feels that "based on results of our studies and others, we have proposed a hypothesis that **supplementation with high doses of multiple antioxidant vitamins, together with diet modification and lifestyle changes may improve the efficacy of standard and experimental cancer therapies by reducing their toxicity on normal cells and by enhancing their growth-inhibitory effects on cancer cells.**"

The bottom line is that in addition to countless animal studies, the majority of human studies have shown patients treated with antioxidants during chemotherapy and/or radiation tolerate standard treatment better, have a better quality of life, and most importantly, live longer than patients receiving no supplements. For example, **the conclusion in a study in patients with small-cell lung cancer using combination chemotherapy of cyclophosphamide, Adriamycin (doxorubicin), and vincristine with radiation and a combination of antioxidants, vitamins, trace elements, and fatty acids was that the nutritional support significantly prolonged the survival time of patients.** (Jaakkola K, Lahteenmaki P, Laakso J, et al. Treatment with antioxidant and other nutrients in combination with chemotherapy and irradiation in patients with small-cell lung cancer. Anticancer Res 1992;12:599-606).

But, my oncologist told me scientific evidence shows that antioxidants interfere with chemotherapy, what should I do?

When oncologists cite "scientific evidence" that antioxidants interfere with chemotherapy and radiation, they tend to ignore the fact that the majority of these sorts of studies show predominantly beneficial effects. The scientific evidence that oncologists often refer to consist primarily of animal studies where they fed animals (usually via an injection into the intestines) dosages of an antioxidant that far exceed the amount normally recommended or in vitro (test tube) studies that used concentrations of antioxidants not achievable in living systems. For example, when vitamin E is given to mice at dosages not likely to be achieved with normal supplementation in humans (e.g., dosage greater than 35,000 IU) it can reduce the effectiveness of radiation therapy. (Sakamoto K, Sakka M. Reduced effect of irradiation on normal and malignant cells irradiated in vivo in mice pretreated with vitamin E. Br J Radiology 1973;46:538-540)

However, based upon human and animal studies, vitamin E at commonly used dosages does not interfere with radiation therapy or chemotherapy and actually appears to enhance the success of these treatment. (Kagreud A, Peterson HI. Tocopherol in irradiation of experimental neoplasms. Acta Radiol Oncol 1981;20:97-100) (Perez Ripoll EA, Rama BN, Webber MM. Vitamin E enhances the chemotherapeutic effects of adriamycin on human prostatic carcinoma cells in vitro. J Urol 1986;136:529-531)

The same can be said with CoQ10 and many other antioxidants. **The only real exception is N-acetylcysteine - a derivative of the naturally occurring amino acid cysteine. NAC has not been shown to significantly effect treatment outcome and carries with it some risk of inhibiting chemotherapy agents** (e.g., cisplatin). (Olson RD, Stroo WE, Boerth RC. Influence of N-acetylcysteine on the antitumor activity of doxorubicin. Semin Oncol 1983;10:S29-S34) (Roller A, Weller M. Antioxidants specifically inhibit cisplatin cytotoxicity of human malignant glioma cells. Anticancer Res 1998;18:4493-4497)

So, I do not recommend it being used during active treatment with any chemotherapy agent. After chemotherapy is over, then NAC may be of benefit in reversing any kidney or nerve damage.

2.0.6.0 Should patients undergoing chemotherapy and radiotherapy be prescribed antioxidants?

In September 2005, CA: A Cancer Journal for Clinicians published a warning by Gabriella D'Andrea, MD, against the concurrent use of antioxidants with radiotherapy and chemotherapy. However, several deficiencies of the CA article soon became apparent, not least the selective omission of prominent studies that contradicted the author's conclusions. While acknowledging that only large-scale, randomized trials could provide a valid basis for therapeutic recommendations, the author sometimes relied on laboratory rather than clinical data to support her claim that harm resulted from the concurrent use of antioxidants and chemotherapy. She also sometimes extrapolated from chemoprevention studies rather than those on the concurrent use of antioxidants per se. The article overstated the degree to which the laboratory data diverged in regard to the safety and efficacy of antioxidant therapy: in fact, the preponderance of data suggests a synergistic or at least harmless effect with most high-dose dietary antioxidants and chemotherapy. The practical recommendations made in the article to avoid the general class of antioxidants during chemotherapy are inconsistent, in that if antioxidants were truly a threat to the efficacy of standard therapy, antioxidant-rich foods, especially fruits and vegetables, ought also be proscribed during treatment. Yet no such recommendation is made. Furthermore, the wide-scale use by both medical and radiation oncologists of synthetic antioxidants (eg, amifostine) to control the adverse effects of cytotoxic treatments is similarly overlooked. In sum, this CA article is incomplete: there is far more information available regarding antioxidant supplements as an appropriate adjunctive cancer therapy than is acknowledged. Patients would be well advised to seek the opinion of physicians who are adequately trained and experienced in the intersection of 2 complex fields, that is, chemotherapeutics and nutritional oncology. Physicians whose goal is comprehensive cancer therapy should refer their patients to qualified integrative practitioners who have such training and expertise to guide patients. A blanket rejection of the concurrent use of antioxidants with chemotherapy is not justified by the preponderance of evidence at this time and serves neither the scientific community nor cancer patients (Should patients undergoing chemotherapy and radiotherapy be prescribed antioxidants? Moss RW. Integr Cancer Ther. 2006 Mar;5(1):63-82).

2.0.6.1 Selenium for alleviating the side effects of chemotherapy

Selenium supplements are frequently used by cancer patients. **Selenium is an essential trace element and is involved in antioxidant protection and redox-regulation in humans**. Several adverse effects of radiotherapy and chemotherapy in cancer patients as well as cellular processes that maintain chronic lymphoedema have been linked to oxidative cell damage in the human body. Selenium has recently been investigated as a remedy against chemotherapy and radiotherapy-associated side effects as well as its effects on lymphedema. OBJECTIVES: This review assessed the effects of supplementary selenium on adverse effects of conventional radiotherapy, chemotherapy, or surgery, in oncologic patients and on quality of life or performance status during and after oncologic treatment. SEARCH STRATEGY: We searched the Cochrane Pain, Palliative & Supportive Care Trials Register, the Cochrane Database of Systematic Reviews (The Cochrane Library, Issue 2, 2004), Medline (1966

- Sep 2004), Embase (1980 - 2004 week 12), SIGLE (October 2004), Cancerlit (October 2004), Clinical Contents in Medicine CCMed (October 2004), the German Register of Cancer Studies (October 2004), the NCI Clinical Trials Register (October 2004), the International Standard Randomized Controlled Trial Number Register ISRCTN (October 2004) and the Meta-Register of Controlled Trials mRCT (October 2004), reference lists and the archive of our working group. We contacted manufacturers of selenium supplements and investigators. SELECTION CRITERIA: Randomized-controlled trials of selenium mono-supplements in cancer patients undergoing tumor specific therapy such as chemotherapy, radiotherapy or surgery. DATA COLLECTION AND ANALYSIS: Two review authors independently checked trials for eligibility, extracted data and assessed trial quality. We sought additional information from investigators when required. MAIN RESULTS: Two trials have been included, a randomized controlled trial with **60 participants** at the beginning of the study investigating secondary lymphedema and an ongoing trial with preliminary results of **63 participants** investigating radiotherapy induced diarrhea as a secondary outcome. Both trials had drawbacks with regard to study quality and reporting. The trial on secondary lymphedema reported a decreased number of recurrent erysipela infections in the selenium supplementation group compared to placebo. However, results must be interpreted with caution and cannot be generalized to other populations. The ongoing trial on radiotherapy associated diarrhea preliminarily reported a lower incidence of diarrhea in patients receiving selenium supplementation concomitant to pelvic radiation, however, no data were presented. Publication of final results must be awaited to discuss these findings in detail. **No randomized controlled trials were found studying the effect of selenium supplementation on other therapy-associated toxicities or quality of life or performance status in cancer patients.** AUTHORS' CONCLUSIONS: **There is insufficient evidence at present that selenium supplementation alleviates the side effects of tumor specific chemotherapy or radiotherapy treatments. Or, that it improves the after effects of surgery, or improves quality of life in cancer patients or reduces secondary lymphedema.** To date research findings do not provide a basis for any recommendation in favor or against selenium supplementation in cancer patients. Potential hazards of supplementing a trace mineral should be kept in mind (Selenium for alleviating the side effects of chemotherapy, radiotherapy and surgery in cancer patients. (Selenium for alleviating the side effects of chemotherapy, radiotherapy and surgery in cancer patients. Dennert G, Horneber M. Cochrane Database Syst Rev. 2006 Jul 19;3:CD005037)

2.0.7.0 LINUS PAULING INSTITUTE SPRING/SUMMER 2005 RESEARCH REPORT

A number of controversial studies on vitamin C or E have been published recently, and some of these that attracted media attention are discussed in the following sections. Several are meta-analyses, which are statistical studies that pool the results of selected previous studies that share similar research objectives. **Meta-analyses are generally highly regarded and can provide an excellent overview of complicated subjects.** The relationship between micronutrients and health and disease is so complex and difficult to study in humans that few definitive studies have been published, and none of the following studies should be considered definitive. I thank Drs. Balz Frei, Jane Higdon, and Maret Traber for their helpful comments.

2.0.7.1 Diabetes and supplemental vitamin C

A study published in the *American Journal of Clinical Nutrition* in 2004 on supplemental vitamin C and the risk of cardiovascular disease reported that the use of vitamin C supplements was associated with an increased risk of mortality from cardiovascular disease in postmenopausal diabetic women. The study was part of the **Iowa Women's Health Study and enrolled 1,923 women** who, at baseline, reported diabetes but were free from cardiovascular disease. Their intake of dietary and supplemental vitamin C was assessed by food-frequency questionnaires at the beginning of the study, and the group was followed for 15 years. Deaths from cardiovascular disease, coronary artery disease, and stroke were analyzed at the end of the study, revealing that **the risk of mortality from these causes was not significantly affected by the intake of vitamin C from food, but significantly increased in the group that consumed at least 300 mg/day of supplemental vitamin C.** As the authors noted, the study has several serious limitations. Diabetes was self-reported at baseline and no attempt was made to verify the diagnosis. Blood levels of lipids or vitamins were never measured, nor was blood pressure. Information on supplemental vitamin use was obtained only at the beginning of the study, and participants' behavior may have changed appreciably over 15 years. **The authors speculated that the increased risk for mortality may be due to a pro-oxidant activity of vitamin C, but most studies have found that vitamin C acts as a powerful antioxidant in the body.** Moreover, **a larger study of 85,000 women followed for 16 years found that the risk of fatal and non-fatal coronary heart disease was reduced**

in women—including 2% who were diabetic—who consumed at least 400 mg/day of vitamin C from supplements. This study was published in the *Journal of the American College of Cardiology* in 2003. It has been proposed that genes may affect the influence of antioxidants on the risk of cardiovascular disease in diabetic women. **In one study published in *Diabetes Care* in 2004, diabetic women with two copies of the haptoglobin 1 gene benefited from supplementation with 1,000 mg/day of vitamin C plus 800 IU/day of vitamin E, whereas the supplements were detrimental in those with two copies of the haptoglobin 2 gene.**

• ***The verdict:*** These studies are inconclusive and surprising, but present a possible cause for concern in some diabetic women, possibly depending on genotype. LPI generally recommends consuming at least 400 mg/day of vitamin C, but diabetic individuals may want to refrain from taking more than 300 mg/day of supplemental vitamin C until more is known about its health effects in diabetes.

2.0.7.2 Gastrointestinal cancers and antioxidants

Headlines like "Vitamins can't fight cancer" on CBS, "Vitamin pills do not stop cancer" on the BBC, and "Vitamins 'may raise death risk from cancer'" in Britain's *The Guardian* emerged after publication in 2004 of a study in the British medical journal *The Lancet* claiming that **antioxidant vitamin supplements not only didn't prevent gastrointestinal cancers, their use actually increased mortality.** As usual, the headlines over-simplified a complicated story and unfairly indicted all vitamins. *The Lancet* study was a meta-analysis of 14 placebo-controlled, randomized trials involving over **170,000 subjects** who were supplemented with vitamin A (1.5-15 mg), vitamin C (120-2,000 mg), vitamin E (30-600 mg), beta-carotene (15-50 mg), and selenium (0.05-0.23 mg) alone or in various combinations. Subjects were supplemented either daily or on alternate days for 1 to 12 years, depending on the study. Four trials used selenium alone, while only two trials used vitamin C or vitamin E alone. **Only selenium reduced the risk of gastrointestinal cancers, while the use of beta-carotene in combination with either vitamin A or vitamin E resulted in an increased risk of mortality**.

Only 9 of the 14 trials reported mortality data. Most of the trials reported a slightly increased or slightly decreased risk of death associated with antioxidant supplement use. **According to *The Lancet* meta-analysis, the trial reporting the highest increased risk of mortality involved supplementation with beta-carotene and vitamin C.** This small, placebo-controlled, randomized trial, published in the *Journal of the National Cancer Institute* in 2000, evaluated the effect of an anti-*Helicobacter pylori* drug, vitamin C, and beta-carotene, alone and in combinations, on the precancerous process in the gastric system. It enrolled **976 subjects,** 631 of whom completed the 6-year trial. Infection with **the bacterium *Helicobacter pylori* is associated with gastric lesions that can lead to cancer. In this study, 18 subjects in the various groups receiving beta-carotene, vitamin C, and/or the drug died, while no one died in the placebo group. However, the authors noted that *none of the deaths in the treatment groups were related to gastric cancer*, although no specific causes were reported. Subjects who took 30 mg of beta-carotene or 2,000 mg of vitamin C daily had significant regression of premalignant lesions.**

• ***The verdict:*** **The use of beta-carotene supplements has not generally been demonstrated to provide substantial protection against gastrointestinal or other cancers, and may actually increase the risk of lung cancer in smokers or those exposed to asbestos. This meta-analysis indicates that supplemental beta-carotene in combination with vitamins A or E also does not protect against gastrointestinal cancers and may increase mortality risk.** However, the evidence mainly suggests that supplemental beta-carotene, and not antioxidant vitamins, may be the culprit. Additionally, gender may influence the effect of antioxidants on cancer risk. For example, many studies have reported that a low intake of vitamin C is associated with increased cancer risk, particularly lung cancer, in men. **LPI does not make a recommendation for supplemental beta-carotene because of the generally weak evidence of benefit and possible detrimental effects.**

2.0.7.3 Antioxidant vitamins and cancer chemotherapy

The concomitant use of high-dose antioxidants, especially vitamin C, and chemotherapy has been debated for decades. **In their 1979 book *Cancer and Vitamin C*, Linus Pauling and Ewan Cameron speculated that high-dose vitamin C might interfere with chemotherapy by drug detoxification and that patients undergoing aggressive chemotherapy expected to cure cancer might refrain from taking high-dose vitamin C at the same time.** However, they noted that many patients taking chemotherapeutic drugs and vitamin C experienced decreased side effects. Only a few small studies have investigated the effects of chemotherapy combined with antioxidants in humans. **A Finnish study published in *Anticancer Research* in 1992 reported that the use of high-dose antioxidants in conjunction with chemotherapy and radiation significantly prolonged survival in patients with small-cell lung cancer.** A randomized, double-blind, placebo-controlled Dutch study, published in 2004 in the *European Journal of Cancer*, investigated the effect of antioxidant supplementation in 50 cancer patients undergoing cisplatin chemotherapy. Half received placebo, and half were supplemented twice a day with 1,000 mg of vitamin C, 400 mg of synthetic vitamin E, and 0.1 mg of selenium. Although the antioxidant supplements did not significantly prevent kidney or inner ear toxicity, supplemented **patients had less loss of high-tone hearing**.

The latest study, published in **February 2005 in the *Journal of the American College of Nutrition*, was conducted in 136 patients with stage III or IV non-small-cell lung cancer**. About half the patients received chemotherapy (paclitaxel/carboplatinum) alone; the other half received chemotherapy and daily high-dose antioxidants, including about 6 grams of vitamin C, 1 gram of synthetic vitamin E, and 60 mg of beta-carotene. Although **not statistically significant**, there was a trend toward improved response in those who received both chemotherapy and antioxidants. A recent paper in the *Journal of Nutrition* suggested that oxidative stress, while generated by many chemotherapeutic drugs, may not play a crucial role in killing cancer cells and, therefore, antioxidant vitamins may help ameliorate this unwanted side effect. Of the wide array of chemotherapeutic drugs, only a few, such as bleomycin and mitomycin-C, have been definitively shown to depend on free radicals to kill cells.

• ***The verdict:*** While **too few clinical studies have been published to conclude that high-dose antioxidants, such as vitamins C and E, would never interfere with any specific chemotherapeutic drug**, the available evidence suggests that, for at least a few commonly prescribed drugs, especially those that do not depend on free radicals for their effectiveness, concern may be unwarranted. Cancer patients should be careful to discuss the use of antioxidants with their physician.

2.0.8.0 Vitamin C May Reduce Response to Chemotherapy

October 2, 2008 — **Large supplemental doses of vitamin C could interfere with the therapeutic cytotoxic effects of a wide range of chemotherapy agents**, suggests a new preclinical study. Although the finding comes from **research conducted in cancer cell lines and mice**, the authors say the conditions they created are similar to those found in the body, and speculate that the same mechanism might affect patient outcomes.

"It is possible that vitamin C supplementation may alter the effectiveness of commonly used chemotherapeutic agents and adversely

influence treatment outcome," the researchers write in the October 1, 2008 issue of *Cancer Research*.

Lead author Mark Heaney, MD, PhD, from Memorial Sloan-Kettering Cancer Center, in New York, New York, told *Medscape Oncology* **that he advises his cancer patients to avoid supplemental vitamin C during chemotherapy.** "I recommend that my patients continue to eat a well-balanced diet that includes fruits and vegetables that contain vitamin C."

"Such a diet could be expected to have moderate amounts of vitamin C as well as other important nutrients. There are no data to suggest that vitamin C obtained from fruits and vegetables is intrinsically different from vitamin C supplements. Given that our research was done in experimental model systems and was not a clinical trial, I am reluctant to predict a dose of supplemental vitamin C that could be extrapolated to our work. That said, oral vitamin C supplementation with doses as low as 250 mg over a 1-month period resulted in intracellular vitamin C concentrations in normal white blood cells that were close to those that we studied in white blood cell cancers," Dr. Heaney said.

2.0.8.1 Reduction in Cytotoxic Effect ==

Dr. Heaney and colleagues found that **pretreatment with dehydroascorbic acid, which is the form that vitamin C takes within the body, produced a dose-dependent attenuation of cytotoxicity for 5 unrelated chemotherapy agents: doxorubicin, cisplatin, vincristine, methotrexate, and imatinib.**

The cell culture studies showed that the cytotoxicity was reduced by 30% to 70%, depending on the drug. A similar effect was seen in the animal studies; cancer cells transplanted into mice were held in check by doxorubicin, but **grew more rapidly when they had been pretreated with vitamin C.**

"It was notable that the concentration of vitamin C measured in the tumors of the mice in this study was similar to what can be achieved in human leucocytes with oral vitamin C supplementation, suggesting that our study conditions were relevant to clinical conditions," the researchers write.

2.0.8.2 Wide Variety of Chemotherapeutics Affected

"The finding that vitamin C antagonized the cytotoxic effects of such a wide range of antineoplastic agents was unexpected," the researchers comment.

Dr. Heaney and colleagues explain that they had originally hypothesized that vitamin C, being a potent antioxidant, would antagonize the cytotoxic effects of antineoplastic agents that use reactive oxygen species, such as cisplatin and doxorubicin.

However, the finding that the cytotoxicity of other chemotherapeutic agents was also affected suggests that other mechanisms are involved. The researchers speculate that the effects might be mediated by mitochondrial membrane depolarization. All of the chemotherapeutic agents, even the highly targeted product imatinib, appear to act through this pathway. Previous studies, and some of the current results, show that **vitamin C stabilizes the mitochondria. In this way, vitamin C antagonizes 1 of the cytotoxic actions of the chemotherapeutic drugs.**

2.0.8.3 Many Cancer Patients Take Vitamin C ==

"Our study is a preclinical model that addresses only the situation when vitamin C is given in the setting of chemotherapy treatment," Dr. Heaney emphasized. There have been no clinical studies of this topic so far, he said.

However, **the finding could be of potential concern because "many people, cancer patients included, take supplemental vitamin C,"** Dr. Heaney pointed out. Clinical studies of vitamin C supplementation in patients with advanced cancers have had mixed results. There are conflicting hypotheses, he explained. One theory is that vitamin C supplementation protects the cancer and is therefore detrimental to the patient. But there is also the opposite view, that vitamin C supplementation enhances the immune system or prevents indolent cancers from mutating more and becoming aggressive, which would be beneficial for the patient.

Asked to comment on this study, Len Lichtenfeld, MACP, deputy chief medical officer at the American Cancer Society said: "Vitamin C has a long history in cancer prevention and treatment. Although there is no evidence to demonstrate that vitamin C improves the outlook for patients with cancer, there are still reported observations that cancer patients continue to believe in the potential benefits of vitamin C. Although oncologists do not routinely recommend that patients with cancer take excessive doses of vitamin C, there are reports that cancer patients are being treated with vitamin C by alternative practitioners."

"Recently, there have been research papers [indicating] that intravenous vitamin C may be beneficial in reducing the growth rates of cancers in laboratory animals. There are human clinical trials underway to determine whether or not this approach will be helpful in patients being treated for cancer," Dr. Lichtenfeld added.

However, he points out that **the current report suggests that in laboratory experiments, adding vitamin C to cancer cells may reduce the effectiveness of cancer chemotherapy drugs.**

"Clearly, there remains an open question as to whether or not vitamin C supplementation is helpful or harmful in the treatment of patients with cancer. Until those questions are resolved with further clinical studies, **it would be inappropriate to recommend that patients take large quantities of vitamin C if they have cancer**," Dr. Lichtenfeld told *Medscape Oncology*.

The researchers have disclosed no relevant financial relationships.

Cancer Res. 2008;68:8031-8038

2.0.9.0 EMOD selective kill of cancer cells with beta-phenylethyl isothiocyanate (PEITC) ==

Oncogenic transformation usually leads to increase of cellular reactive oxygen species (ROS) level that renders the cells vulnerable to additional ROS production. By targeting ROS, a naturally occurring ROS-inducing compound, beta-phenylethyl isothiocyanate (PEITC), selectively kills the transformed cells but not normal cells (Targeting ROS: Selective Killing of Cancer Cells by a Cruciferous Vegetable Derived Pro-Ox. XJ Wu, X Hua. Cancer Biol Ther (2007) 6(1):5).

2.0.9.1 Ascorbate generated H_2O_2 kills cancer cells (Human lymphoma cells) ==

Human pharmacokinetics data indicate that i.v. ascorbic acid (ascorbate) in pharmacologic concentrations could have an unanticipated role in cancer treatment. Our goals here were to test whether ascorbate killed cancer cells selectively, and if so, to determine mechanisms, using clinically relevant conditions. Cell death in 10 cancer and 4 normal cell types was measured by using 1-h exposures. Normal cells were unaffected by 20 mM ascorbate, whereas 5 cancer lines had EC(50) values of <4 mM, a concentration easily achievable i.v. **Human lymphoma cells** were studied in detail because of their sensitivity to ascorbate (EC(50) of 0.5 mM) and suitability for addressing mechanisms. Extracellular but not intracellular ascorbate mediated cell death, which occurred by apoptosis and pyknosis/necrosis. Cell death was independent of metal chelators and absolutely dependent on **H_2O_2** formation. **Cell death from H_2O_2 added to cells was identical to that found when H_2O_2 was generated by ascorbate treatment.** H_2O_2 generation was dependent on ascorbate concentration, incubation time, and the presence of 0.5-10% serum, and displayed a linear relationship with ascorbate radical formation. Although ascorbate addition to medium generated H_2O_2, ascorbate addition to blood generated no detectable H_2O_2 and only trace detectable ascorbate radical. Taken together, these data indicate that **ascorbate at concentrations achieved only by i.v. administration may be a pro-drug for formation of H_2O_2,** and that blood can be a delivery system of the pro-drug to tissues. These findings give plausibility to i.v. ascorbic acid in cancer treatment, and have unexpected implications for treatment of infections where H_2O_2 may be beneficial (Pharmacologic ascorbic acid concentrations selectively kill cancer cells: action as a pro- drug. Q Chen, MG Espey, MC Krishna, JB Mitchell, CP Corpe, GR Buettner, E Shacter, M Levine. Proc Natl Acad Sci U S A (2005) 102: 13604-9). **I believe that this shows that peroxide, either directly or by ascorbate generation, selectively kills human cancer cells. This is the basis of my singlet oxygen tumoricidal system.**

In normal state of a cell, endogenous antioxidant enzyme system maintains the level of reactive oxygen species generated by mitochondrial respiratory chain. Mitochondrial superoxide dismutase [SOD; manganese SOD (MnSOD) or SOD2] neutralizes highly reactive superoxide radical (O(*-)(2)), the first member in the plethora of mitochondrial reactive oxygen species. A polymorphism in the target sequence of MnSOD enzyme, Val(16)Ala, is known to disrupt proper targeting of the enzyme from cytosol to mitochondrial matrix where it acts on O(*-)(2) to dismutate it to hydrogen peroxide (H(2)O(2)). **A change in the level of O(*-)(2) and of H(2)O(2) in mitochondria modulates the molecular mechanisms of apoptosis, cellular adhesion, and cell proliferation and thus play key role in cancer development.** Previous studies investigating the association between MnSOD Val(16)Ala polymorphism and cancer risk have revealed **inconsistent results.** We conducted a meta-analysis on these studies. Our meta-analysis on total of **7,366 cancer cases and 9,102 controls from 13 published case-control studies showed no overall association of this polymorphism either with breast cancer risk or for cancer risk as such** (for Ala homozygous odds ratio, 0.98; 95% confidence interval, 0.90-1.07 and odds ratio, 1.02; 95%

confidence interval, 0.91-1.14, respectively). **Also, there was no major effect in either recessive or dominant model for the MnSOD Val(16)Ala**. However, a proper evaluation of this polymorphism with cancer link demands experiments involving large sample size, cross-tabulation of gene-gene, gene-environment interactions, and linkage studies, as cell biological experiments clearly correlate critical levels of mitochondrial O(*-)(2) and H(2)O(2) to carcinogenesis. (Target Sequence Polymorphism of Human Manganese Superoxide Dismutase Gene and Its Association with Cancer Risk: A Review. A Bag, N Bag. Cancer Epidemiol Biomarkers Prev 2008;17(12):3298-305).

2.1.0.0 Failed antioxidant studies

Basic research studies suggest that vitamin E, vitamin C, and other antioxidants reduce cardiovascular disease by **trapping organic free radicals**, **by deactivating excited oxygen molecules, or both**, to prevent tissue damage (Packer L. Protective role of vitamin E in biological systems. *Am J Clin Nutr.* 1991;53(4)(suppl):1050S-1055S).

Antioxidants may slow or prevent atherosclerotic plaque formation by inhibiting low-density lipoprotein cholesterol oxidation (Steinberg D, Lewis A. Conner memorial lecture: oxidative modification of LDL and atherogenesis. *Circulation.* 1997;95(4):1062-1071), **modifying platelet activity** (Steiner M. Vitamin E, a modifier of platelet function: rationale and use in cardiovascular and cerebrovascular disease. *Nutr Rev.* 1999;57(10):306-309) (Mabile L, Bruckdorfer KR, Rice-Evans C. Moderate supplementation with natural alpha-tocopherol decreases platelet aggregation and low-density lipoprotein oxidation. *Atherosclerosis.* 1999;147(1):177-185), **reducing thrombotic potential** (Mehta J, Li D, Mehta JL. Vitamins C and E prolong time to arterial thrombosis in rats. *J Nutr.* 1999;129(1):109-112), **and modifying vascular reactivity** (Andrews TJ, Laight DW, Anggard EE, Carrier MJ. Investigation of endothelial hyperreactivity in the obese Zucker rat in situ: reversal by vitamin E. *J Pharm Pharmacol.* 2000;52(1):83-86) (Koh KK, Blum A, Hathaway L; et al. Vascular effects of estrogen and vitamin E therapies in postmenopausal women. *Circulation.* 1999;100(18):1851-1857).

Some (Rimm EB, Stampfer MJ, Ascherio A, Giovannucci E, Colditz GA, Willett WC. Vitamin E consumption and the risk of coronary heart disease in men. *N Engl J Med.* 1993;328(20):1450-1456) (Stampfer MJ, Hennekens CH, Manson JE, Colditz GA, Rosner B, Willett WC. Vitamin E consumption and the risk of coronary disease in women. *N Engl J Med.* 1993;328(20):1444-1449) (Kushi LH, Folsom AR, Prineas RJ, Mink PJ, Wu Y, Bostick RM. Dietary antioxidant vitamins and death from coronary heart disease in postmenopausal women. *N Engl J Med.*

1996;334(18):1156-1162), **but not all** (Klipstein-Grobusch K, Geleijnse JM, den Breeijen JH; et al. Dietary antioxidants and risk of myocardial infarction in the elderly: the Rotterdam Study. *Am J Clin Nutr.* 1999;69(2):261-266), **prospective cohort studies support a role for vitamin E in cardiovascular disease prevention.**

Dietary and supplemental vitamin C has been inconsistently associated with cardiovascular disease, including significant (Enstrom JE, Kanim LE, Klein MA. Vitamin C intake and mortality among a sample of the United States population. *Epidemiology.* 1992;3(3):194-202) **and nonsignificant** (Ascherio A, Rimm EB, Hernan MA; et al. Relation of consumption of vitamin E, vitamin C, and carotenoids to risk for stroke among men in the United States. *Ann Intern Med.* 1999;130(12):963-970) **inverse associations as well no association** (Messerer M, Hakansson N, Wolk A, Akesson A. Dietary supplement use and mortality in a cohort of Swedish men. *Br J Nutr.* 2008;99(3):626-631) (Buijsse B, Feskens EJ, Kwape L, Kok FJ, Kromhout D. Both alpha- and beta-carotene, but not tocopherols and vitamin C, are inversely related to 15-year cardiovascular mortality in Dutch elderly men. *J Nutr.* 2008;138(2):344-350).

In a pooled analysis of 9 cohorts, **vitamin C supplement use exceeding 700 mg/d was significantly associated with a 25% reduction in coronary heart disease risk** (Knekt P, Ritz J, Pereira MA; et al. Antioxidant vitamins and coronary heart disease risk: a pooled analysis of 9 cohorts. *Am J Clin Nutr.* 2004;80(6):1508-1520).

Initial clinical trials of vitamin E alone among male smokers in the Alpha-Tocopherol Beta-Carotene Cancer Prevention (ATBC) trial **showed both possible benefits on prostate cancer** (Alpha-Tocopherol, Beta Carotene Cancer Prevention Study Group. The effect of vitamin E and beta carotene on the incidence of lung cancer and other cancers in male smokers. *N Engl J Med.* 1994;330(15):1029-1035) **and risks on hemorrhagic stroke** (Leppälä JM, Virtamo J, Fogelholm R; et al. Controlled trial of alpha-tocopherol and beta-carotene supplements on stroke incidence and mortality in male smokers. *Arterioscler Thromb Vasc Biol.* 2000;20(1):230-235), **in addition to secondary prevention trials such as the Cambridge Heart Antioxidant Study (CHAOS)** (Stephens NG, Parsons A, Schofield PM, Kelly F, Cheeseman K, Mitchinson MJ. Randomised controlled trial of vitamin E in patients with coronary disease: Cambridge

Heart Antioxidant Study (CHAOS). *Lancet.* 1996;347(9004):781-786), **which indicated possible cardiovascular disease reductions.**

Yet even as largely negative trials of vitamin E later emerged among patients with multiple coronary risk factors or preexisting cardiovascular disease (Virtamo J, Rapola JM, Ripatti S; et al. Effect of vitamin E and beta carotene on the incidence of primary nonfatal myocardial infarction and fatal coronary heart disease. *Arch Intern Med.* 1998;158(6):668-675) (Gruppo Italiano per lo Studio della Sopravvivenza nell'Infarto miocardico. Dietary supplementation with n-3 polyunsaturated fatty acids and vitamin E after myocardial infarction: results of the GISSI-Prevenzione trial. *Lancet.* 1999;354(9177):447-455) (Boaz M, Smetana S, Weinstein T; et al. Secondary Prevention with Antioxidants of Cardiovascular Disease in Endstage Renal Disease (SPACE): randomised placebo-controlled trial. *Lancet.* 2000;356(9237):1213-1218) (Yusuf S, Dagenais G, Pogue J, Bosch J, Sleight P, Heart Outcomes Prevention Evaluation Study Investigators. Vitamin E supplementation and cardiovascular events in high-risk patients. *N Engl J Med.* 2000;342(3):154-160) (Lonn E, Bosch J, Yusuf S; et al. Effects of long-term vitamin E supplementation on cardiovascular events and cancer: a randomized controlled trial. *JAMA.* 2005;293(11):1338-1347) (Cook NR, Albert CM, Gaziano JM; et al. A randomized factorial trial of vitamins C and E and beta carotene in the secondary prevention of cardiovascular events in women: results from the Women's Antioxidant Cardiovascular Study. *Arch Intern Med.* 2007;167(15):1610-1618), **vitamin E and other supplement use has remained surprisingly prevalent among healthy individuals who report its regular use as part of their routine health regimen** (Blendon RJ, DesRoches CM, Benson JM, Brodie M, Altman DE. Americans' views on the use and regulation of dietary supplements. *Arch Intern Med.* 2001;161(6):805-810).

There have been fewer long-term primary prevention trials of vitamin E alone among participants at initially low risk of cardiovascular disease, for which there has been **no effect on cardiovascular disease** (de Gaetano G. Low-dose aspirin and vitamin E in people at cardiovascular risk: a randomised trial in general practice: Collaborative Group of the Primary Prevention Project. *Lancet.* 2001;357(9250):89-95) (Lee IM, Cook NR, Gaziano JM; et al. Vitamin E in the primary prevention of cardiovascular disease and cancer: the Women's Health Study: a randomized controlled trial. *JAMA.* 2005;294(1):56-65), **with comparatively less data in men** (de Gaetano G. Low-dose aspirin and vitamin E in people at cardiovascular risk: a randomised trial in general practice: Collaborative Group of the Primary Prevention Project. *Lancet.* 2001;357(9250):89-95).

Vitamin C has typically been incorporated into antioxidant combinations with vitamin E, beta carotene, and other vitamins and minerals in large-scale clinical trials that reported no significant cardiovascular effects (Blot WJ, Li JY, Taylor PR; et al. Nutrition intervention trials in Linxian,

China: supplementation with specific vitamin/mineral combinations, cancer incidence, and disease- specific mortality in the general population. *J Natl Cancer Inst.* 1993;85(18):1483-1492) (Brown BG, Zhao XQ, Chait A; et al. Simvastatin and niacin, antioxidant vitamins, or the combination for the prevention of coronary disease. *N Engl J Med.* 2001;345(22):1583-1592) (MRC/BHF Heart Protection Study of antioxidant vitamin supplementation in 20,536 high-risk individuals: a randomised placebo-controlled trial. *Lancet.* 2002;360(9326):23-33) (Hercberg S, Galan P, Preziosi P; et al. The SU.VI.MAX Study: a randomized, placebo-controlled trial of the health effects of antioxidant vitamins and minerals. *Arch Intern Med.* 2004;164(21):2335-2342).

Vitamin C alone has only been evaluated among 8,171 women at high risk for cardiovascular disease, and no effect on cardiovascular disease was found with use of 500 mg/d of vitamin C (Cook NR, Albert CM, Gaziano JM; et al. A randomized factorial trial of vitamins C and E and beta carotene in the secondary prevention of cardiovascular events in women: results from the Women's Antioxidant Cardiovascular Study. *Arch Intern Med.* 2007;167(15):1610-1618).

Therefore, the clinical utility of vitamin C alone in preventing cardiovascular disease among those at low initial risk of cardiovascular disease remains uncertain. Further, because vitamin C may potentially interact with vitamin E, it is important to evaluate the effect of their interaction on cardiovascular disease (Niki E. Interaction of ascorbate and alpha-tocopherol. *Ann N Y Acad Sci.* 1987;498:186-199).

Given these persistent gaps in knowledge and the ongoing debate regarding the roles of vitamin E and vitamin C for cardiovascular disease prevention, we designed the **Physicians' Health Study II (PHS II)** to provide novel and clinically relevant information on the individual effects of vitamin E and vitamin C supplementation on the risk of major cardiovascular events over a median **follow-up of 8 years among 14,641 male physicians** at lower initial risk of cardiovascular disease compared with participants in most previous trials.

Expanding the definition of baseline cardiovascular disease to add angina pectoris or revascularization among 1419 men taking vitamin E still had no effect on major cardiovascular events (HR, 0.88 [95% CI, 0.70-1.10]; *P* = .26).

We also evaluated whether coronary risk factors and each of the other randomized interventions from PHS II modified the effect of vitamin E on major cardiovascular events (Table 3). Parental history of MI before age 60 years significantly modified (*P* for interaction = .04) the effect of vitamin E on major cardiovascular events, with nonsignificant reductions among men who took vitamin E and had a parental history of MI before age 60 years. Otherwise, no other significant effect modification by coronary risk factors was found on major cardiovascular events. In addition, **there was no effect modification by randomized beta carotene or the ongoing multivitamin treatment assignment.**

2.1.0.1 Vitamin C and Major Cardiovascular Events

The overall rates of major cardiovascular events for the active and placebo vitamin C groups were 10.8 and 10.9 per 1000 person-years, respectively. There was no effect of vitamin C on the primary end point of major cardiovascular events (HR, 0.99 [95% CI, 0.89-1.11]; *P* = .91; Table 2). The cumulative incidence curves showed no difference between groups in the HRs over time (log-rank *P* = .86; Figure 2). Vitamin C also had no effect on individual cardiovascular end points, including total MI (HR, 1.04 [95% CI, 0.87-1.24]; *P* = .65), total stroke (HR, 0.89 [95% CI, 0.74-1.07]; *P* = .21), and cardiovascular mortality (HR, 1.02 [95% CI, 0.85-1.21]; *P* = .86), as well as total mortality (HR, 1.07 [95% CI, 0.97-1.18]; *P* = .16). There also was no effect of vitamin C on hemorrhagic stroke. Censoring for nonadherence with vitamin C did not appreciably affect our findings for major cardiovascular events (HR, 0.98 [95% CI, 0.86-1.13]; *P* = .81).

When vitamin C use was examined among 13 887 men without and 754 men with a baseline history of cardiovascular disease, **the lack of effect of vitamin C on major cardiovascular events remained.** Vitamin C had no effect on the primary prevention of major cardiovascular events (525 events in those receiving active vitamin C and 527 events in those receiving placebo vitamin C) (HR, 1.00 [95% CI, 0.88-1.13]; *P* = .98), total MI (HR, 1.47 [95% CI, 0.82-2.63]; *P* = .19), total stroke (HR, 0.86 [95% CI, 0.69-1.07]; *P* = .18), cardiovascular mortality (HR, 0.99 [95% CI, 0.81-1.20]; *P* = .88), and total mortality (HR, 1.08 [95% CI, 0.97-1.20]; *P* = .15). In the 754 men with a history of cardiovascular disease at baseline, vitamin C did not affect incident major cardiovascular events (HR, 0.96 [95% CI, 0.72-1.27]; *P* = .77). For total MI, there were 18 and 31 cases in the active and placebo vitamin C groups, respectively (HR, 0.57 [95% CI, 0.32-1.02]; *P* = .06). Adding angina and revascularization to our definition of baseline cardiovascular disease did not change the lack of effect on major cardiovascular events (HR, 1.03 [95% CI, 0.82-1.29]; *P* = .81), and the effect on total MI weakened somewhat (HR, 0.71 [95% CI, 0.47-1.07]; *P* = .10).

We then considered whether the effect of vitamin C on major cardiovascular events was modified by baseline coronary risk factors or other PHS II randomized interventions (Table 3). No significant effect modification was found between vitamin C and various baseline factors, randomized beta carotene, or the ongoing multivitamin treatment assignment on major cardiovascular events. When we examined the 2-way interaction between randomized vitamin E and vitamin C assignments, no significant interactions were found for major cardiovascular events (*P* for interaction = .99), total MI (*P* for interaction = .12), total stroke (*P* for interaction = .26), or cardiovascular disease mortality (*P* for interaction = .80) (Figure 3). Men assigned to active vitamin E only had a lower risk of total MI than those assigned to placebo vitamins E and C (HR, 0.74; 95% CI, 0.58-0.96), but no reduction was seen in those receiving both active vitamins E and C (HR, 0.94; 95% CI, 0.74-1.19).

In this large-scale, randomized controlled trial among middle-aged and older men, long-term vitamin E and vitamin C supplement use did not reduce the primary end point of incident major cardiovascular events. We also found that neither vitamin E nor vitamin C reduced total MI, total stroke, cardiovascular death, congestive heart failure, total mortality, angina, or coronary revascularization. We did find an increase in hemorrhagic stroke with vitamin E use.

2.1.0.2 Randomized Trials of Vitamin E

Our finding that vitamin E has no effect on major cardiovascular events, including among a small subgroup of 754 men with a baseline history of cardiovascular disease, is **consistent with the majority of previous clinical trials conducted among higher risk individuals with** (Stephens NG, Parsons A, Schofield PM, Kelly F, Cheeseman K, Mitchinson MJ. Randomised controlled trial of vitamin E in patients with coronary disease: Cambridge Heart Antioxidant Study (CHAOS). *Lancet.* 1996;347(9004):781-786) (Gruppo Italiano per lo Studio della Sopravvivenza nell'Infarto miocardico. Dietary supplementation with n-3 polyunsaturated fatty acids and vitamin E after myocardial infarction: results of the GISSI-Prevenzione trial. *Lancet.* 1999;354(9177):447-455) (Yusuf S, Dagenais G, Pogue J, Bosch J, Sleight P, Heart Outcomes Prevention Evaluation Study Investigators. Vitamin E supplementation and cardiovascular events in high-risk patients. *N Engl J Med.* 2000;342(3):154-160) (Cook NR, Albert CM, Gaziano JM; et al. A randomized factorial trial of vitamins C and E and beta carotene in the secondary prevention of cardiovascular events in women: results from the Women's Antioxidant Cardiovascular Study. *Arch Intern Med.* 2007;167(15):1610-1618) **or without** (Yusuf S, Dagenais G, Pogue J, Bosch J, Sleight P, Heart Outcomes Prevention Evaluation Study Investigators. Vitamin E supplementation and cardiovascular events in high-risk patients. *N Engl J Med.* 2000;342(3):154-160) (Cook NR, Albert CM, Gaziano JM; et al. A randomized factorial trial of vitamins C and E and beta carotene in the secondary prevention of cardiovascular events in women: results from the Women's Antioxidant Cardiovascular Study. *Arch Intern Med.* 2007;167(15):1610-1618) (Alpha-Tocopherol, Beta Carotene Cancer Prevention Study Group. The effect of vitamin E and beta carotene on the incidence of lung cancer and other cancers in male smokers. *N Engl J Med.* 1994;330(15):1029-1035) (Boaz M, Smetana S, Weinstein T; et al. Secondary Prevention with Antioxidants of Cardiovascular Disease in Endstage Renal Disease (SPACE): randomised placebo-controlled trial. *Lancet.* 2000;356(9237):1213-1218)' **preexisting cardiovascular disease**.

Although some of these trials report possible reductions in composite cardiovascular end points, **meta-analyses indicate no overall benefit for vitamin E in the secondary prevention of cardiovascular disease** (Bjelakovic G, Nikolova D, Gluud LL, Simonetti RG, Gluud C. Mortality in randomized trials of antioxidant supplements for primary and secondary prevention: systematic review and meta-analysis. *JAMA.* 2007;297(8):842-857) (Bjelakovic G, Nikolova D, Gluud LL, Simonetti RG, Gluud C. Antioxidant supplements for prevention of mortality in healthy participants and patients with various diseases. *Cochrane Database Syst Rev.* 2008;(2):CD007176) (Miller ER III, Pastor-Barriuso R, Dalal D, Riemersma RA, Appel LJ, Guallar E. Meta-analysis: high-dosage vitamin E supplementation may increase all-cause mortality. *Ann Intern Med.* 2005;142(1):37-46).

The strength of PHS II is that the majority of participants (94.9%) were of low initial risk of cardiovascular disease, a previously understudied population. **Primary prevention trials such as the Chinese Cancer Prevention Study** (Blot WJ, Li JY, Taylor PR; et al. Nutrition intervention trials in Linxian, China: supplementation with specific vitamin/mineral combinations, cancer incidence, and disease-specific mortality in the general population. *J Natl Cancer Inst.* 1993;85(18):1483-1492) **and the Supplementation en Vitamines et Minéraux Antioxydants (SU.VI.MAX)** study included 30 mg/d of vitamin E as part of a combination of vitamins and minerals, with no effect found on cardiovascular disease. The Primary Prevention Project examined the individual effect of 300 mg/d of vitamin E among 1912 men and 2583 women (mean age, 64.4 years) with at least 1 cardiovascular risk factor for 3.6 years, and **found no effect on prespecified cardiovascular end points** (de Gaetano G, Collaborative Group of the Primary Prevention Project. Low-dose aspirin and vitamin E in people at cardiovascular risk: a randomised trial in general practice. *Lancet.* 2001;357(9250):89-95).

The Women's Health Study tested 600 IU of vitamin E every other day among 39 876 women at low or usual risk of cardiovascular disease for 10 years and also reported **no overall effect on major cardiovascular events** (Lee IM, Cook

NR, Gaziano JM; et al. Vitamin E in the primary prevention of cardiovascular disease and cancer: the Women's Health Study: a randomized controlled trial. *JAMA.* 2005;294(1):56-65).

Moreover, **results in PHS II did not corroborate the significant 24% reduction in cardiovascular death or the significant 26% reduction in major cardiovascular events among women aged 65 years or older in the Women's Health Study.** At present, the Selenium and Vitamin E Cancer Prevention Trial (SELECT) is the only ongoing, large-scale clinical trial testing 400 IU/d of vitamin E, with cardiovascular disease as a secondary end point (Lippman SM, Goodman PJ, Klein EA; et al. Designing the Selenium and Vitamin E Cancer Prevention Trial (SELECT). *J Natl Cancer Inst.* 2005;97(2):94-102).

Although vitamin E has appeared relatively safe with few documented adverse effects (Gilman AS, Goodman LS, Rall TW, Murad F. *The Pharmacological Basis of Therapeutics.* 7th ed. London, England: MacMillan; 1985:1586-1589), **we observed a 74% increase in the risk of hemorrhagic stroke in the vitamin E treatment group consistent with results among the male smokers in the ATBC trial,** but not observed in other primary and secondary prevention trials testing individual vitamin E supplement use. Vitamin E did not increase the incidence of reported congestive heart failure in PHS II, in contrast to increased risk reported by HOPE-TOO (Lonn E, Bosch J, Yusuf S; et al. Effects of long-term vitamin E supplementation on cardiovascular events and cancer: a randomized controlled trial. *JAMA.* 2005;293(11):1338-1347).

While meta-analyses of clinical trials have reinforced the lack of effect between vitamin E and cardiovascular disease (Bjelakovic G, Nikolova D, Gluud LL, Simonetti RG, Gluud C. Mortality in randomized trials of antioxidant supplements for primary and secondary prevention: systematic review and meta-analysis. *JAMA.* 2007;297(8):842-857)**, possible slight but significant increases in total mortality have been reported** (Bjelakovic G, Nikolova D, Gluud LL, Simonetti RG, Gluud C. Mortality in randomized trials of antioxidant supplements for primary and secondary prevention: systematic review and meta-analysis. *JAMA.* 2007;297(8):842-857). (Bjelakovic G, Nikolova D, Gluud LL, Simonetti RG, Gluud C. Antioxidant supplements for prevention of mortality in healthy participants and patients with various diseases. *Cochrane Database Syst Rev.* 2008;(2):CD007176) (Miller ER III, Pastor-Barriuso R, Dalal D, Riemersma RA, Appel LJ, Guallar E. Meta-analysis: high-dosage vitamin E supplementation may increase all-cause mortality. *Ann Intern Med.* 2005;142(1):37-46)

However, **in PHS II we found no significant effect between vitamin E and total mortality after up to 10 years of treatment and follow-up**.

The source, type, and dose of vitamin E used in PHS II warrant discussion. We used synthetic vitamin E (all-rac-alpha-tocopheryl acetate) in PHS II, similar to earlier trials, whereas more recent trials have used natural source vitamin E (*d*-alpha-tocopheryl acetate). However, **neither form of vitamin E appears more or less associated with cardiovascular disease, consistent with the observation that both vitamin E sources have similar antioxidant properties** (Traber MG, Atkinson J. Vitamin E, antioxidant and nothing more. *Free Radic Biol Med.* 2007;43(1):4-15).

Moreover, PHS II and other prevention trials have used α-tocopherol, whereas the γ-tocopherol isomer also may have a role in cardiovascular disease prevention because it has greater efficacy than α-tocopherol to inhibit lipid peroxidation[51] and it may be suppressed in the presence of α-tocopherol. In addition, our dose of 400 IU/d of vitamin E is lower than that used in some other trials of vitamin E alone, but remains far greater than usual dietary levels and can only be achieved through supplementation.

2.1.0.3 Randomized Trials of Vitamin C

The PHS II represents the first large-scale, long-term trial of individual vitamin C supplementation in the prevention of cardiovascular disease in men. The Women's Antioxidant Cardiovascular Study (WACS) also tested 500 mg/d of vitamin C in 8171 women at higher risk of cardiovascular disease, and **there was no effect on major cardiovascular end points** (Cook NR, Albert CM, Gaziano JM; et al. A randomized factorial trial of vitamins C and E and beta carotene in the secondary prevention of cardiovascular events in women: results from the Women's Antioxidant Cardiovascular Study. *Arch Intern Med.* 2007;167(15):1610-1618).

Other primary and secondary prevention trials have considered vitamin C as part of a vitamin combination, in which no cardiovascular benefits were observed (Blot WJ, Li JY, Taylor PR; et al. Nutrition intervention trials in Linxian, China: supplementation with specific vitamin/mineral combinations, cancer incidence, and disease- specific mortality in the general population. *J Natl Cancer Inst.* 1993;85(18):1483-1492) (Brown BG, Zhao XQ, Chait A; et al. Simvastatin and niacin, antioxidant vitamins, or the combination for the prevention of coronary disease. *N Engl J Med.* 2001;345(22):1583-1592) (MRC/BHF Heart Protection Study of antioxidant vitamin supplementation in 20,536 high-risk individuals: a randomised placebo-controlled trial. *Lancet.* 2002;360(9326):23-33) (Hercberg S, Galan P, Preziosi P; et al. The SU.VI.MAX Study: a randomized, placebo-controlled trial of the health effects of antioxidant vitamins and minerals. *Arch Intern Med.* 2004;164(21):2335-2342).

Trials of intermediate cardiovascular end points have yielded inconsistent results. **A combination of vitamins that included vitamin C had no effect on the rate and severity of restenosis in one trial** (Tardif JC, Cote G, Lesperance J; et al, Multivitamins and Probucol Study Group. Probucol and multivitamins in the prevention of restenosis after coronary angioplasty. *N Engl J Med.* 1997;337(6):365-372).

In contrast, **500 mg/d of vitamin C given to patients with percutaneous transluminal coronary angioplasty reduced restenosis rates** (Tomoda H, Yoshitake M, Morimoto K, Aoki N. Possible prevention of postangioplasty restenosis by ascorbic acid. *Am J Cardiol.* 1996;78(11):1284-1286).

In 520 patients with hypercholesterolemia, 6 years of a combination of vitamin C and E reduced the progression of atherosclerosis (Salonen RM, Nyyssonen K, Kaikkonen J; et al. Six-year effect of combined vitamin C and E supplementation on atherosclerotic progression: the Antioxidant Supplementation in Atherosclerosis Prevention (ASAP) Study. *Circulation.* 2003;107(7):947-953).

Yet among postmenopausal women, a combination of vitamin E and vitamin C provided no cardiovascular benefits (Waters DD, Alderman EL, Hsia J; et al. Effects of hormone replacement therapy and antioxidant vitamin supplements on coronary atherosclerosis in postmenopausal women: a randomized controlled trial. *JAMA.* 2002;288(19):2432-2440).

Our observation that vitamin C use among 754 men with preexisting cardiovascular disease nonsignificantly reduced total MI by 46% was interesting, but confined to a small subgroup. **Among 5238 women with prior cardiovascular disease in WACS, there was no effect of vitamin C on major cardiovascular disease** (HR, 1.05 [95% CI, 0.93-1.18]; $P = .43$) (Cook NR, Albert CM, Gaziano JM; et al. A randomized factorial trial of vitamins C and E and beta carotene in the secondary prevention of cardiovascular events in women: results from the Women's Antioxidant Cardiovascular Study. *Arch Intern Med.* 2007;167(15):1610-1618).

Moreover, **in PHS II long-term vitamin C supplementation had no significant effect on total and cardiovascular mortality.**

The dose of vitamin C used in PHS II, 500 mg/d, greatly exceeds usual dietary vitamin C levels and can only be achieved through supplementation. While even higher doses of vitamin C, generally tolerated up to a level of 2000 mg/d, may be considered for cardiovascular disease prevention, limits in gastrointestinal tract absorption and other physiological restrictions may hinder vitamin C bioavailability attainable by dietary and supplemental vitamin C intake (Li Y, Schellhorn HE. New developments and novel therapeutic perspectives for vitamin C. *J Nutr.* 2007;137(10):2171-2184).

Despite **the lack of effect for vitamin C on cardiovascular disease in PHS II**, more comprehensive clinical trial data on vitamin C alone at different doses and in other populations remain lacking.

2.1.0.4 Potential Limitations

Adherence is of potential concern in any clinical trial. However, adherence remained high in PHS II during up to 10 years of follow-up, with low drop-in use in all of the study groups. Sensitivity analyses that censored follow-up time based on non-adherence did not alter our findings. Although PHS II represents one of the longest trials to date of individual vitamin E and vitamin C use on cardiovascular disease, an even longer period of vitamin supplementation may be necessary to cover the critical etiologic window or provide a sufficient cumulative dose capable of preventing cardiovascular disease. Vitamins E and C represent 2 parts of a broader spectrum of essential vitamins and minerals with possible roles in cardiovascular disease prevention. The randomized multivitamin component of PHS II still continues, with total treatment and follow-up planned to last more than a decade.

2.1.0.5 CONCLUSION

In this large-scale trial, after a mean of 8 years of treatment and follow-up in 14 641 men, neither vitamin E nor vitamin C supplementation reduced the risk of major cardiovascular events. These data provide no support for the use of these supplements in the prevention of cardiovascular disease in middle-aged and older men.

This is another quality RCT supporting my theories on the flawed free radical theory, with the subsequent failed antioxidant trials for CVD.

2.1.1.0 Effect of Combined Folic Acid, Vitamin B_6, and Vitamin B_{12} on Cancer Risk in Women. A Randomized Trial. Shumin M. Zhang, MD, ScD; Nancy R. Cook, ScD; Christine M. Albert, MD, MPH; J. Michael Gaziano, MD, MPH; Julie E. Buring, ScD; JoAnn E. Manson, MD, DrPH. JAMA. 2008;300(17):2012-2021.

Folate, vitamin B_6, and vitamin B_{12} are thought to play an important role in cancer.

Objective To evaluate the effect of combined folic acid, vitamin B_6, and vitamin B_{12} treatment on cancer risk in women at high risk for cardiovascular disease.

Design, Setting, and Participants In the Women's Antioxidant and Folic Acid Cardiovascular Study, 5442 US female health professionals aged 42 years or older, with preexisting cardiovascular disease or 3 or more coronary risk factors, were randomly assigned to receive either a daily combination of folic acid, vitamin B_6, and vitamin B_{12} or a matching placebo. They were treated for 7.3 years from April 1998 through July 31, 2005.

Intervention Daily supplementation of a combination of 2.5 mg of folic acid, 50 mg of vitamin B_6, and 1 mg of vitamin B_{12} (n = 2721) or placebo (n = 2721).

Main Outcome Measures Confirmed newly diagnosed total invasive cancer or breast cancer.

Results A total of **379 women** developed invasive cancer (187 in the active treatment group and 192 in the placebo group). Compared with placebo, **women receiving the active treatment had similar risk of developing total invasive cancer** (101.1/10 000 person-years for the active treatment group vs 104.3/10 000 person-years for placebo group; hazard ratio [HR], 0.97; 95% confidence interval [CI], 0.79-1.18; *P* = .75), breast cancer (37.8/10 000 person-years vs 45.6/10 000 person-years, respectively; HR, 0.83; 95% CI, 0.60-1.14; *P* = .24), or any cancer death (24.6/10 000 person-years vs 30.1/10 000 person-years, respectively; HR, 0.82; 95% CI, 0.56-1.21; *P* = .32).

Conclusion Combined folic acid, vitamin B_6, and vitamin B_{12} treatment had no significant effect on overall risk of total invasive cancer or breast cancer among women during the folic acid fortification era. **(Effect of Combined Folic Acid, Vitamin B_6, and Vitamin B_{12} on Cancer Risk in Women. A Randomized Trial.** Shumin M. Zhang, MD, ScD; Nancy R. Cook, ScD; Christine M. Albert, MD, MPH; J. Michael Gaziano, MD, MPH; Julie E. Buring, ScD; JoAnn E. Manson, MD, DrPH. *JAMA*. 2008;300(17):2012-2021).

2.1.1.1 Singlet oxygen

2.1.1.2 Singlet oxygen background

US Patent 4986921 - Cellulose acetate bound photosensitizer for producing singlet oxygen

Diatomic oxygen in its ground state is a paramagnetic molecule because it has a triplet ground state. Electronic excitation can produce either of two excited states, both of which are diamagnetic singlet states. The lower excited state, $^1\Delta_g$, has an energy of 22.5 kcal/mol above the ground state while the higher excited state, $^1\Sigma_g$, has an energy of 37.5 kcal/mol. Only the lower excited state has a long enough lifetime to be chemically active in solution and is normally referred to as "singlet oxygen", $^1O_2$.

Singlet oxygen has been found to be a much stronger oxidizing agent than ground state molecular oxygen. **Singlet oxygen has a calculated reduction potential of 1.7 V which makes it a better oxidizing agent (in non-acidic conditions) than ozone, hydrogen peroxide, sodium hypochlorite and chlorine dioxide.** Thus, **singlet oxygen can be used in a number of oxidation reactions such as synthesis of organic compounds, removal of humic acid from water, removal of phenols from waste streams, removal of cyanide from electroplating waste, oxidation of mercaptans in hydrocarbon streams and destruction of bacteria in various streams**.

The usual method of generating singlet oxygen is by energy transfer from light and a photosensitizer. The role of the photosensitizer is to absorb the light and transfer its energy to the oxygen thereby forming singlet oxygen. The mechanism for producing singlet oxygen is well known in the art and the photosensitizers which can be used to produce singlet oxygen are also well known. Illustrative of these **photosensitizers are rose bengal, methylene blue, eosin, chlorophyll, fluorescein, pyrene, acridine orange, porphyrins, phthalocyanines, etc.**

The prior art teaches that these photosensitizers are usually used in a homogeneous phase; that is, the photosensitizer is dissolved in the reaction medium. This has the disadvantage that the photosensitizer must be separated from the reaction product. Even if separation is possible, complete separation is usually not achieved which means that fresh photosensitizer must be added to the fresh reaction medium. Since photosensitizers are expensive, the loss of photosensitizer may make the overall process uneconomical. Moreover, the effective concentration of photosensitizer which can be employed is limited not only owing to the increased difficulty of separating the photosensitizer from the products, but also owing to the fact that at higher concentrations the photosensitizers tend to form dimers and higher aggregates which reduce their effectiveness as photosensitizers.

2.1.1.3 Viruses susceptible to EMODs (H_2O_2, singlet oxygen)

Recent studies have shown that the virus suspected of causing Acquired Immune Deficiency Syndrome (AIDS), as well as herpes, hepatitis, Epstein Barr, and cytomegalovirus, join the group of viruses that are lipid coated. It has also been shown that many lipid-enveloped viruses are destroyed in the presence of concentrated oxygen, including singlet oxygen.

To enhance its applicability, chemical methods for the generation of singlet oxygen have been developed. The most well-known source is based on **the oxidation of hydrogen peroxide by sodium hypochlorite.** A more recent method involves **the disproportionation of hydrogen peroxide catalyzed by molybdate ions to yield quantitatively singlet oxygen and water.**

In contrast to oxygen, both ozone and singlet oxygen are molecules in the singlet state. Accordingly, singlet oxygen should be available from ozone by formal transfer of one oxygen to a suitable substrate. Consequently various reactions of this type have been found: Murray *et al.* have described phosphite ozonides, which form by low-temperature reaction of phosphites with ozone and are cleaved to form phosphate and singlet oxygen.

Water that has been exposed to the air is "oxygenated" to a small extent— about 8 milligrams of O_2 per liter of water at room temperature— and this can be increased by pressurizing the water with oxygen gas; each additional atmosphere of oxygen pressure pumps an additional 40 mg into each liter.

2.1.1.4 Ascorbate reacts with singlet oxygen to produce hydrogen peroxide

Singlet oxygen is a highly reactive electrophilic species that reacts rapidly with electron-rich moieties, such as the double bonds of lipids, thiols, and ascorbate

(AscH-). The reaction of ascorbate with singlet oxygen is rapid (k = 3 x 10(8) M(-1) s(-1)). Here we have investigated the stoichiometry of this reaction. Using electrodes to make simultaneous, real-time measurements of oxygen and hydrogen peroxide concentrations, we have investigated the products of this reaction. We have demonstrated that hydrogen peroxide is a product of this reaction. The stoichiometry for the reactants of the reaction (1 1O2 + 1AscH--->1H2O2 + 1dehydroascorbic) is 1:1. The formation of H2O2 results in a very different oxidant that has a longer lifetime and much greater diffusion distance. Thus, locally produced singlet oxygen with a half-life of 1 ns to 1 micros in a biological setting is changed to an oxidant that has a much longer lifetime and thus can diffuse to distant targets to initiate biological oxidations (Kramarenko Galina G; Hummel Stephen G; Martin Sean M; Buettner Garry R. **Ascorbate reacts with singlet oxygen to produce hydrogen peroxide.** Photochemistry and photobiology 2006;82(6):1634-7).

2.1.1.5 Singlet oxygen therapy

Singlet Oxygen Therapy was developed by Tony Van der Valk (see his website http://www.polyvalk.com). Air passes first through water, so as to be saturated with water vapour, and then passes a red (634nm) LED that shines on a phthalocyanine compound. This catalyses the conversion of atmospheric oxygen to the extremely reactive singlet oxygen. The singlet oxygen immediately donates its energy to the water vapour, which can then be breathed through a loose nasal cannula. **The energy is of a grade high enough (about 1 eV) to generate light in the body.** None of the usual biochemical reactions can reach such an energy. It thus performs the same function as the other Oxygen Radicals, which are obtained normally with negative ions, UV light, etc., and can be therapeutically supplied by ozone, hydrogen peroxide, etc. Tony Van der Valk's method is, however, more effective, more convenient and safer than these last. **The question of the essential function of Oxygen Radicals has been thoroughly researched by Prof. Vladimir Voekov (V.L. Voekov and V.L. Naletov: "Weak Photon Emission of Non-Linear Chemical Reactions of Amino Acids and Sugars in Aqueous Solutions". 1998. In Biophotons: J.-J. Chang, J. Fisch and F.-A. Popp Eds. Kluwer Academic Publishers. Dordrecht pp. 93-108)** and the fundamental role of light energy in the maintenance of quantum wholeness in the living organism has been researched by Dr Fritz Popp, and many other authors over the last thirty years (see Dr Mae-Wan Ho's excellent book "The Rainbow and the Worm", World Scientific, 2nd Ed. 1998). http://www.subtleenergies.com/ormus/tw/singlet.htm accessed 2-2-09.

2.1.1.6 Singlet oxygen toxicity is cell line-dependent

Singlet oxygen (1O2) can be quenched by water, lipids, proteins, nucleic acids and other small molecules. **Polyunsaturated fatty acids (PUFA) of cells principally quench 1O2 by chemical mechanisms, producing lipid hydroperoxides, while proteins physically and chemically quench 1O2.** Because cell lines can have different PUFA and protein levels, we hypothesized that 1O2 toxicity will vary between cell lines. We used Photofrin as a source of 1O2. Exposure of nine different leukemia cell lines (CEM, HEL, HL-60, K-562, KG-1, L1210, Molt-4, THP-1 and U-937) to Photofrin and light results in changes in membrane permeability (trypan blue) that vary with cell line. **The greater the lipid content of the cell line, the less susceptible they are to membrane damage.** When the cell media was supplemented with docosahexaenoic acid (DHA, 22:6), the overall unsaturation of cellular lipids increased. Photofrin and light resulted in increased radical formation in these supplemented cells compared to controls; however, there was no difference in membrane permeability between DHA-supplemented and control cells. Lipid-derived radical formation (electron paramagnetic resonance spin trapping) was cell line dependent; but no correlation between lipid content of cells and radical formation was found. However, we found that the greater the protein content of cells the more they were protected against membrane damage induced by Photofrin photosensitization. This suggests that cellular proteins are a key target for 1O2-mediated toxicity. **A remarkable observation is that cell size correlates inversely with ability of cells to cope with a given flux of 1O2.** (Schafer F Q; Buettner G R. **Singlet oxygen toxicity is cell line-dependent: a study of lipid peroxidation in nine leukemia cell lines.** Photochemistry and photobiology 1999;70(6):858-67). **The fact that lipids quench singlet oxygen is consistent with my arguments for the increase of cancer and atherosclerosis seen in obese patients. The lipids serve as sinks for EMODs, including single oxygen, which would eventually produce an EMOD insufficiency and allow for disease manifestation.**

2.1.2.0 Methylene blue to treat Alzheimer's and Parkinson's diseases

Aug. 18, 2008 — A new study conducted by researchers at Children's Hospital & Research Center Oakland shows that a century-old drug, **methylene blue, may be able to slow or even cure Alzheimer's and Parkinson's disease**. Used at a very low concentration – about the equivalent of a few raindrops in four Olympic-sized swimming pools of water – the drug slows cellular aging and enhances mitochondrial function, potentially allowing those with the diseases to live longer, healthier lives. **I know that methylene blue is capable of producing singlet oxygen, when exposed to light (634 nm) and I believe that this is its mechanism of action or that it is combined with ascorbate and produces peroxide.**

A paper on the methylene blue study, conducted by Hani Atamna, PhD, and a his team at Children's, was published in the **March 2008 issue of the Federation of American Societies for Experimental Biology (FASEB)** Journal. Dr. Atamna's research found that **methylene blue can prevent or slow the decline of mitochondrial function, specifically an important enzyme called complex IV**. Because mitochondria are the principal suppliers of energy to all animal and human cells, their healthy function is critical.

One of the key aspects of Alzheimer's disease is mitochondrial dysfunction, specifically complex IV dysfunction, which methylene blue improves. Our findings indicate that methylene blue, by enhancing mitochondrial function, expands the mitochondrial reserve of the brain. Adequate mitochondrial reserve is essential for preventing age-related disorders such as Alzheimer's disease."

Also impressed is one of Dr. Atamna's co-authors, **Bruce Ames, PhD, a senior scientist at Children's and world-renowned expert in nutrition and aging. (Really?) "What we potentially have is a wonder drug." said Dr. Ames.** "To find that such a common and inexpensive drug can be used to increase and prolong the quality of life by treating such serious diseases is truly exciting."

Methylene blue, first discovered in 1891, is now used to treat methemoglobinemia, a blood disorder. But because **high concentrations of methylene blue were known to damage the brain,** no one thought to experiment with low concentrations. Also, drugs such as methylene blue do not easily reach the brain.

Dr. Atamna's research is the first to show that **low concentrations of the drug have the ability to slow cellular aging in cultured cells in the laboratory and in live mice**. He believes methylene blue has the potential to become another commonplace low-cost treatment like aspirin, prescribed as a blood thinner for people with heart disorders.

Dr. Atamna's research, funded by the Bruce and Giovanna Ames Foundation, was conducted at Children's research institute and will continue when Dr. Atamna assumes a position as a professor of Neuroscience at The Commonwealth Medical College in Pennsylvania. (Atamna et al. **Methylene blue delays cellular senescence and enhances key mitochondrial biochemical pathways.** *The FASEB Journal*, 2007; 22 (3): 703 DOI: 10.1096/fj.07-9610com).

Methylene blue (MB) has been used clinically for about a century to treat numerous ailments. We show that **MB and other diaminophenothiazines** extend the life span of human IMR90 fibroblasts in tissue culture by >20 population doubling (PDLs). MB delays senescence at nM levels in IMR90 by enhancing mitochondrial function. **MB increases mitochondrial complex IV by 30%, enhances cellular oxygen consumption by 37–70%,** increases heme synthesis, and **reverses premature senescence caused by H_2O_2 or cadmium.**

I believe that this must be confusing to followers of the FRT, such as Ames, because it is well known that methylene blue is a superb photosensitizer for the formation of singlet oxygen. That being the case, with the FRT, the singlet should be destructive to the mitochondrion but it is not.

MB also induces phase-2 antioxidant enzymes in hepG2 cells. Flavin-dependent enzymes are known to use NAD(P)H to reduce MB to leucomethylene blue (MBH_2), whereas cytochrome *c* reoxidizes MBH_2 to MB. Experiments on lysates from rat liver mitochondria suggest the ratio MB/cytochrome *c* is important for the protective actions of MB. **We propose that the cellular senescence delay caused by MB is due to cycling between MB and MBH_2 in mitochondria**, which may partly explain the increase in specific mitochondrial activities.

Cycling of MB between oxidized and reduced forms may block oxidant production by mitochondria (RMH Note: Actually, it likely increases the prooxidant environment.). Mitochondrial dysfunction and oxidative stress are thought to be key aberrations that lead to cellular senescence and aging. MB may be useful to delay mitochondrial dysfunction with aging and the decrease in complex IV in Alzheimer disease.—(Atamna, H., Nguyen, A., Schultz, C., Boyle, K., Newberry, J., Kato, H., Ames, B. N. Methylene blue delays cellular senescence and enhances key mitochondrial biochemical pathways. *The FASEB Journal*, 2007; 22 (3): 703 DOI: 10.1096/fj.07-9610com).

2.1.2.1 Methylene blue produces hydrogen peroxide as a redox cycler (malaria)

Methylene blue (MB) has experienced a renaissance mainly as a component of drug combinations against Plasmodium falciparum malaria.

Investigators reported biochemically relevant pharmacological data on MB such as rate constants for the uncatalyzed reaction of MB at pH 7.4 with cellular reductants like NAD(P)H (k = 4 M(-1) s(-1)), thioredoxins (k = 8.5 to 26 M(-1) s(-1)), dihydrolipoamide (k = 53 M(-1) s(-1)), and slowly reacting glutathione. As the disulfide reductases are prominent targets of MB, optical tests for enzymes reducing MB at the expense of NAD(P)H under aerobic conditions were developed. The product leucomethylene blue (leucoMB) is auto-oxidized back to MB at pH 7 but can be stabilized by enzymes at pH 5.0, which makes this colorless compound an interesting drug candidate. **MB was found to be an inhibitor and/or a redox-cycling substrate of mammalian and P. falciparum disulfide reductases**, with the kcat values ranging from 0.03 s(-1) to 10 s(-1) at 25 degrees C. Kinetic spectroscopy of mutagenized glutathione reductase indicates that MB reduction is conducted by enzyme-bound reduced flavin rather than by the active-site dithiol Cys58/Cys63. The enzyme-catalyzed reduction of MB and subsequent auto-oxidation of the product leucoMB mean that **MB is a redox-cycling agent which produces H_2O_2 at the expense of O_2 and of NAD(P)H in each cycle, turning the antioxidant disulfide reductases into pro-oxidant enzymes.** This explains the terms subversive substrate or turncoat inhibitor for MB. The results are discussed in cell-pathological and clinical contexts (Interactions of methylene blue with human disulfide reductases and their orthologues from Plasmodium falciparum. Buchholz K, et al. Antimicrob Agents Chemother. 2008 Jan;52(1):183-91). **I believe that this ties into other prooxidant methods of treating malaria, in that all effective methods utilize prooxidant systems.**

2.1.2.2 Malaria parasite has strong antioxidative defenses

The malaria parasite Plasmodium falciparum is highly adapted to cope with the oxidative stress to which it is exposed during the erythrocytic stages of its life cycle. This includes the defence against oxidative insults arising from the parasite's metabolism of haemoglobin which results in the formation of reactive oxygen species and the release of toxic ferriprotoporphyrin IX.

Central to the parasite's defences are superoxide dismutases and thioredoxin-dependent peroxidases; however, **they lack catalase and glutathione peroxidases.** The vital importance of the thioredoxin redox cycle (comprising NADPH, thioredoxin reductase and thioredoxin) is emphasized by the confirmation that **thioredoxin reductase is essential for the survival of intraerythrocytic P. falciparum. (RMH Note: this means that antioxidants are required for the survival of the malarial parasite! Obviously,**

oxidants are toxic to them.). The parasites also contain a fully functional glutathione redox system and the low-molecular-weight thiol glutathione is not only an important intracellular thiol redox buffer but also a cofactor for several redox active enzymes such as glutathione S-transferase and glutaredoxin. Recent findings have shown that in addition to these cytosolic redox systems the parasite also has an important mitochondrial antioxidant defence system and it is suggested that **lipoic acid plays a pivotal part in defending the organelle from oxidative damage** (Redox and antioxidant systems of the malaria parasite Plasmodium falciparum. Müller S. Mol Microbiol. 2004 Sep;53(5):1291-305). **I believe that this confirms the need for defensive antioxidant systems for the viability of the malaria parasite. It is killed by increasing the oxidative capacity. Also, the agent which protects the parasite, lipoic acid, is one ingredient of Ames' magic drugs, Rejuvenon, which supposedly increases longevity.**

2.1.2.3 Methylene blue has syphilitic trypanocidal prooxidant activity

Methylene blue (MB) is known to have trypanocidal activity. They tested the interactions of MB with a number of trypanosomatid-specific molecules of the antioxidant metabolism. At pH 7, trypanothione and other (di)thiols were oxidized to disulfides by the phenothiazine drug. MB inhibited Trypanosoma cruzi trypanothione reductase (TR) (K(i)=1.9 microM), and served as a significant subversive substrate of this enzyme (K(M)=30 microM, k(cat)=4.9s(-1)). With lipoamide dehydrogenase, the second thiol-generating flavoenzyme of T. cruzi, the catalytic efficiency for MB reduction was found to be almost 10(6)M(-1)s(-1). **When the system MB-enzyme-molecular oxygen acts as a NAD(P)H-driven redox cycler, a reactive oxygen species, H(2)O(2) or superoxide, is produced in each cycle.** Since MB is an affordable, available, and accessible drug it might be tested--alone or in drug combinations--against trypanosomatid-caused diseases of animal and man (Cytotoxic interactions of methylene blue with trypanosomatid-specific disulfide reductases and their dithiol products. Buchholz K, et al. Mol Biochem Parasitol. 2008 Jul;160(1):65-9). **This shows that prooxidants are also capable of killing syphilitic trypanosomes. This is also why I recommend prooxidant methods to treat the scourges of mankind, such as malaria, HIV/AIDS, cancer, atherosclerosis, infections, etc.**

2.1.2.4 Tropical diseases killed oxidatively

Trypanosomes and leishmania, the causative agents of several tropical diseases, possess a unique redox metabolism which is based on **trypanothione**. The bis(glutathionyl)spermidine is the central thiol that delivers electrons for the synthesis of DNA precursors, **the detoxification of hydroperoxides** and other trypanothione-dependent pathways. Many of the reactions are mediated by tryparedoxin, a distant member of the thioredoxin protein family. Trypanothione is kept reduced by the parasite-specific flavoenzyme trypanothione reductase. Since glutathione reductases and thioredoxin reductases are missing, the reaction catalyzed by trypanothione reductase represents the only connection between the NADPH- and the thiol-based redox metabolisms. Thus, cellular thiol redox homeostasis is maintained by the biosynthesis and reduction of trypanothione. Nearly all proteins of the parasite-specific trypanothione metabolism have proved to be essential (Redox control in trypanosomatids, parasitic protozoa with trypanothione-based thiol metabolism. Krauth-Siegel RL, Comini MA. Biochim Biophys Acta. 2008 Nov;1780(11):1236-48). **This indicates that antioxidants, like trypanothione, protect some disease causing organisms from oxidative death.**

2.1.3.0 SOD

Some of the following was taken from: http://www.lef.org/magazine/mag2005/aug2005_report_sod_01.htm

2.1.3.1 Faulty reasoning concerning oxygen and accelerated aging

Oxygen toxicity was first described in 1878, when laboratory animals were exposed to pure oxygen, and these deleterious effects were further established in 1899. (Knight JA. Free radicals: their history and current status in aging and disease. Ann Clin Lab Sci. 1998 Nov-Dec; 28(6):331-46).

During the Battle of Britain in World War II, **pilots breathing pure oxygen for several hours daily developed emphysema, scarred lungs, and the effects of greatly accelerated aging.** In some cases, the pilots looked and acted like men who were more than three times their age. One of the most tragic episodes of oxygen toxicity occurred later in the 1940s, when newborn infants were placed in oxygen-rich incubators. Some of the **newborns went blind because their eye tissue had not yet accumulated dietary antioxidant carotenoids to protect against the toxic effects of higher-than-normal oxygen concentrations.** (Reedy EA. The discovery of retrolental fibroplasia and the role of oxygen: a historical review, 1942-1956. Neonatal Netw. 2004 Mar;23(2):31-8).

When placed in hyperbaric chambers of pure oxygen with several atmospheres of pressure, laboratory animals die within a matter of

minutes. By contrast, **when the atmospheric pressure is slowly increased over a period of days, the animals manage to survive**, because their bodies have time to produce higher-than-normal levels of the antioxidant enzymes that protect against oxygen toxicity. The lungs of animals exposed to higher-than-normal oxygen concentrations reveal massive tissue damage caused by too much oxygen, a condition known as **hyperoxia. Thus, at higher-than-normal concentrations, oxygen is a toxic element. (RMH Note: this is not true as evidenced by the fact that animals grew to their largest sizes during times of increased atmospheric oxygen levels, the paleozoic era, with up to 35% oxygen.)** Oxygen utilization by aerobic (that is, oxygen-requiring) organisms such as humans is associated with the generation of potent free radicals. (Knight JA. Free radicals: their history and current status in aging and disease. Ann Clin Lab Sci. 1998 Nov-Dec; 28(6):331-46) (Huang H, Manton KG. The role of oxidative damage in mitochondria during aging: a review. Front Biosci. 2004 May 1;91100-17).

2.1.3.2 Oxygen and Accelerated Aging

Numerous studies conducted over the last 60 years demonstrate that the by-products of normal oxygen utilization, including **superoxide radicals and reactive oxygen species, may contribute to aging and degenerative diseases**. (Inoue M, Sato EF, Nishikawa M, et al. Mitochondrial generation of reactive oxygen species and its role in aerobic life. Curr Med Chem. 2003 Dec;10(23):2495-505) (Ahsan H, Ali A, Ali R. Oxygen free radicals and systemic autoimmunity. Clin Exp Immunol. 2003 Mar;131(3):398-404) (Allen RG, Tresini M. Oxidative stress and gene regulation. Free Radic Biol Med. 2000 Feb 1;28(3):463-99).

Antioxidant enzymes that naturally occur in the body—including SOD, catalase, and glutathione peroxidase—act to minimize this oxidative stress, thus protecting cell membranes, essential proteins, and DNA from damage. These endogenous (internally generated) antioxidants produced within our cells are more potent in preventing free radical damage than are dietary antioxidants. **SOD, for example, may be up to 3,500 times more potent than vitamin C in quenching the dangerous superoxide radical**.

As noted earlier, however, levels of these antioxidant enzymes decline with advancing age in humans and animals alike, leading to an accumulation of free radicals and oxidative damage. (Kashiwagi K, Shinkai T, Kajii E, Kashiwagi A. The effects of reactive oxygen species on amphibian aging. Comp Biochem Physiol C Toxicol Pharmacol. 2005 Feb;140(2):197-205) (Lishnevskaia VL. The role of free radicals oxidation in the deterioration of haemovascular homeostasis in aging. Adv Gerontol. 2004;13:52-7).

In particular, **SOD levels decline, correlating with an increased incidence of degenerative and inflammatory diseases. I believe that this is due to decreased peroxide output from decreasing SOD levels.**

Rheumatoid arthritis sufferers demonstrate lower SOD levels in their cartilage cells than do arthritis-free individuals. These lower levels of SOD may contribute to the destruction of cartilage in this inflammatory disease state. (Karatas F, Ozates I, Canatan H, et al. Antioxidant status & lipid peroxidation in patients with rheumatoid arthritis. Indian J Med Res. 2003 Oct;118:178-81) (Mazzetti I, Grigolo B, Pulsatelli L, et al. Differential roles of nitric oxide and oxygen radicals in chondrocytes affected by osteoarthritis and rheumatoid arthritis. Clin Sci (Lond). 2001 Dec;101(6):593-9). **Again, I believe that the low SOD levels produces insufficient peroxide levels and the arthritis is manifested.**

2.1.3.3 Low SOD associated with diseases

Low SOD levels in humans have also been associated with a host of degenerative diseases, including **fibromyalgia** (Bagis S, Tamer L, Sahin G, et al. Free radicals and antioxidants in primary fibromyalgia: an oxidative stress disorder? Rheumatol Int. 2005 Apr;25(3):188-90), **diabetes** (Abou-Seif MA, Youssef AA. Evaluation of some biochemical changes in diabetic patients. Clin Chim Acta. 2004 Aug 16;346(2):161-70), **cancer** (Cai Q, Shu XO, Wen W, et al. Genetic polymorphism in the manganese superoxide dismutase gene, antioxidant intake, and breast cancer risk: results from the Shanghai Breast Cancer Study. Breast Cancer Res. 2004;6(6):R647-R55) (Ough M, Lewis A, Zhang Y, et al. Inhibition of cell growth by overexpression of manganese superoxide dismutase (MnSOD) in human pancreatic carcinoma. Free Radic Res. 2004 Nov;38(11):1223-33) (Manju V, Balasubramanian V, Nalini N. Oxidative stress and tumor markers in cervical cancer patients. J Biochem Mol Biol Biophys. 2002 Dec;6(6):387-90), **multiple sclerosis** (Lund-Olesen K. Etiology of multiple sclerosis: role of superoxide dismutase. Med Hypotheses. 2000 Feb;54(2):321-2), **Alzheimer's** (Choi J, Rees HD, Weintraub ST, et al. Oxidative modifications and aggregation of Cu, Zn-superoxide dismutase associated with Alzheimer and Parkinson diseases. J Biol Chem. 2005 Mar 25;280(12):11648-55), and **Parkinson's disease** (Choi J, Rees HD, Weintraub ST, et al. Oxidative modifications and aggregation of Cu, Zn-superoxide dismutase associated with Alzheimer and Parkinson diseases. J Biol Chem. 2005 Mar 25;280(12):11648-55) (Hattori N.

Etiology and pathogenesis of Parkinson's disease: from mitochondrial dysfunctions to familial Parkinson's disease. Rinsho Shinkeigaku. 2004 Apr;44(4-5):241-62). **I believe that the low SOD levels result in low peroxide levels, which allows for the manifestation of the above diseases. After all, the purpose of SOD is to generate hydrogen peroxide!**

SOD levels in humans vary by as much as 50% owing to genetic differences, which may help to explain why some people are more prone to degenerative diseases while others lead long, disease-free lives (Ueda K, Ogata M. Levels of erythrocyte superoxide dismutase activity in Japanese people. Acta Med Okayama. 1978 Dec;32(6):393-7).

2.1.3.4 SOD produces hydrogen peroxide

The principal source of hydrogen peroxide in mitochondria is thought to be from the dismutation of superoxide via the enzyme manganese superoxide dismutase (MnSOD). However, the nature of the effect of SOD on the cellular production of H_2O_2 is not widely appreciated. **The current paradigm is that the presence of SOD results in a lower level of H_2O_2 because it would prevent the non-enzymatic reactions of superoxide that form H_2O_2** The goal of this work was to: a) demonstrate that SOD can increase the flux of H_2O_2, and b) use kinetic modelling to determine what kinetic and thermodynamic conditions result in SOD increasing the flux of H_2O_2. We examined two biological sources of superoxide production (xanthine oxidase and coenzyme Q semiquinone, CoQ(*-) that have different thermodynamic and kinetic properties. We found that **SOD could change the rate of formation of H_2O_2 in cases where equilibrium-specific reactions form superoxide with an equilibrium constant (K) less than 1.** An example is the formation of superoxide in the electron transport chain (ETC) of the mitochondria by the reaction of ubisemiquinone radical with dioxygen. We measured the rate of release of H_2O_2 into culture medium from cells with differing levels of MnSOD. We found that **the higher the level of SOD, the greater the rate of accumulation of H_2O_2.** Results with kinetic modelling were consistent with this observation; the steady-state level of H_2O_2 increases if K<1, for example CoQ(*-)+ O(2)-->CoQ+O(2)(*-). However, when K>1, e.g. xanthine oxidase forming O(2)(*-), SOD does not affect the steady state-level of H_2O_2. Thus, **the current paradigm that SOD will lower the flux of H_2O_2 does not hold for the ETC.** These observations indicate that MnSOD contributes to the flux of H_2O_2 in cells and thereby is involved in establishing the cellular redox environment and thus the biological state of the cell (Buettner Garry R; Ng Chin F; Wang Min; Rodgers V G J; Schafer Freya Q. **A new paradigm: manganese superoxide**

dismutase influences the production of H_2O_2 in cells and thereby their biological state. Free radical biology & medicine 2006;41(8):1338-50). **This confirms my belief that SOD is a prooxidant and not an antioxidant.**

CoQ is the only lipophilic antioxidant to be biosynthesized.

2.1.3.5 SOD over expression increases peroxide levels and suppresses prostate cancer cells

This study investigated the role of the antioxidant enzyme manganese superoxide dismutase (MnSOD) in **androgen-independent human prostate cancer (PC-3) cells'** growth rate in vitro and in vivo. **MnSOD levels were found to be lower in parental PC-3** cells compared to nonmalignant, immortalized human prostate epithelial cells (P69SV40T). To unravel the role of MnSOD in the prostate cancer phenotype, PC-3 cells were stably transfected with MnSOD cDNA plasmid. The MnSOD protein and activity levels in clones overexpressing MnSOD were increased seven- to eightfold. These cell lines showed elongated cell doubling time, reduced anchorage-independent growth in soft agar compared to parental PC-3 (Wt) cells, and reduced growth rate of PC-3 tumor xenografts in athymic nude mice. Flow cytometric studies showed an increase in membrane potential in the MnSOD-overexpressing clone (Mn32) compared to Wt and Neo cells. Also, **production of extracellular H(2)O(2) was increased in the MnSOD-overexpressing clones.** As determined by DNA cell cycle analysis, the proportion of cells in G(1) phase was enhanced by MnSOD overexpression. Therefore, MnSOD not only regulates cell survival but also affects PC-3 cell proliferation by retarding G(1) to S transition. Our results are consistent with MnSOD being a tumor suppressor gene in human prostate cancer (Venkataraman Sujatha; Jiang Xiaohong; Weydert Christine; Zhang Yuping; Zhang Hannah J; Goswami Prabhat C; Ritchie Justine M; Oberley Larry W; Buettner Garry R. **Manganese superoxide dismutase overexpression inhibits the growth of androgen-independent prostate cancer cells.**

Oncogene 2005;24(1):77-89). **I believe that this again confirms my theory that EMODs control and curtail cancer growth. The increased SOD resulted in increased peroxide levels, which in turn suppressed tumor growth, via EMOD-induced apoptosis.**

2.1.3.6 SOD is a virulence factor in bacteria

A *Francisella tularensis* live vaccine strain mutant (*$sodB_{Ft}$*) with reduced Fe-superoxide dismutase gene expression was generated and found to exhibit decreased *sodB* activity and increased sensitivity to redox cycling compounds compared to wild-type bacteria. The $sodB_{Ft}$ mutant also was significantly attenuated for virulence in mice. Thus, this study has identified *sodB* as an important *F. tularensis* virulence factor.

Reactive oxygen intermediates (ROI) are generated as a result of the reduction of oxygen during respiration and exposure to radiation or redox cycling compounds and phagocytosis (Halliwell, B., and J. M. C. Gutteridge. 1990. Role of free radicals and catalytic metal ions in human disease: an overview, p. 1-85. *In* A. J. Parker and A. N. Glazer (ed.), Oxygen radicals in biological system. Academic Press, New York, N.Y.).

ROI, including superoxide (O_2^-), hydrogen peroxide (H_2O_2), and hydroxyl radical ($OH\cdot$), can cause oxidative damage to DNA, RNA, proteins, and lipids. Virtually all organisms possess mechanisms to counter these potentially toxic ROI generated during aerobic growth. The primary cellular antioxidant defense in prokaryotes and eukaryotes is the metalloenzyme family of superoxide dismutases (SODs), which dismutate O_2^- to molecular oxygen (O_2) and hydrogen peroxide (H_2O_2) at rates nearly sufficient to limit diffusion. H_2O_2 then is detoxified by catalase and/or members of the peroxidase family of enzymes. SODs are classified into three types depending on their prosthetic metal cofactors—manganese (MnSOD), iron (FeSOD), and copper-zinc (CuZnSOD)—encoded by the *sodA*, *sodB*, and *sodC* genes, respectively. In addition, nickel- and iron-zinc-containing isozymes have been identified in bacteria.

In addition to their detoxifying function during aerobic growth, **bacterial SODs have been shown to be important virulence factors. SODs protect *Salmonella enterica* serovar Choleraesuis, *Staphylococcus aureus*, and *Mycobacterium tuberculosis* from the bactericidal effects of the host macrophages and polymorphonuclear leukocytes.** The present report addresses the role of a recently reported FeSOD in *Francisella tularensis* in the aerobic survival of the organism and the pathogenesis of tularemia.

F. tularensis, the etiological agent of tularemia, is a facultative intracellular pathogen that primarily infects macrophages. ***F. tularensis* requires oxygen for growth and has been shown to possess ROI-scavenging enzymes such as SODs, peroxidases, and catalases.** *F. tularensis*, like many gram-negative bacteria, contains two SODs: an FeSOD and a CuZnSOD.

In accordance with the recent definition of a virulence factor, FeSOD meets the criteria for inclusion as such since it promotes *F. tularensis* survival, which in turn results in greater host damage and higher mortality than is observed with mice infected with wild-type *F. tularensis* LVS. FeSOD may have a dual role in protecting *F. tularensis* from oxidative stress. First, FeSOD binds iron with high affinity and limits the availability of iron that is needed for production of the highly lethal OH ·. Second, dismutation of O_2^- prevents cellular damage of DNA, proteins, and lipids associated with O_2^- toxicity. FeSOD dismutation activity can also protect bacteria from peroxynitrite ($ONOO^-$) toxicity by minimizing the interaction of O_2^- with nitric oxide (NO). Indeed, $ONOO^-$ has been shown to have a major role in the gamma-interferon-induced killing of *F. tularensis* LVS by murine macrophages. Superoxide-dependent $ONOO^-$ toxicity may be an important factor in defective invasion and colonization and in rapid clearance of the $sodB_{Ft}$ mutant by C57BL/6 and BALB/c mice.

The increased survival of mice infected with the $sodB_{Ft}$ mutant supports the hypothesis that FeSOD plays a role in virulence; however, linking virulence to one gene is simplistic.

(Superoxide Dismutase B Gene (sodB)-Deficient Mutants of Francisella tularensis Demonstrate Hypersensitivity to Oxidative Stress and Attenuated Virulence. Chandra Shekhar Bakshi et al. Journal of Bacteriology, September 2006, p. 6443-6448, Vol. 188, No. 17). **I believe that study says that a deficiency of the antioxidant enzyme, SOD, makes the tularensis more vulnerable to oxidative death.**

2.1.3.7 SOD deficiency may cause AMD (adult-onset macular degeneration)

Mice deficient in superoxide dismutase 1 (Sod1(-/-) mice) develop many features seen in patients with age-related macular degeneration (AMD) including choroidal neovascularization (NV). (RMH Note: this means that these mice are not making hydrogen peroxide and they are EMOD deficient.) Investigators sought to determine if the absence of SOD1 contributes to the pro-angiogenic environment in the subretinal space or whether it is completely secondary to other changes in Bruch's membrane and the retinal pigmented epithelium (RPE) that precede the development of choroidal NV. In an ischemic retinopathy model or a transgenic model in which the rhodopsin promoter drives expression of vascular endothelial growth factor (VEGF) in photoreceptor there was significantly more NV in Sod1(-/-) compared to Sod1(+/+) mice. **The compromised antioxidant defense system in Sod1(-/-) mice contributes to the pro-angiogenic environment, because treatment of Sod1(-/-)**

mice with a mixture of antioxidants caused a significant reduction in ischemia-induced retinal NV. Wild-type mice treated with the same antioxidants also showed reduced ischemia-induced retinal NV, reduced VEGF-induced subretinal NV, and reduced choroidal NV at Bruch's membrane rupture sites. **These data suggest that reactive oxygen species contribute to several types of ocular NV.** This could explain why in the Age-Related Eye Disease Trial, antioxidant treatment reduced conversion from non-neovascular to neovascular AMD and severe vision loss, and suggest that potent antioxidants should be considered for other diseases complicated by ocular NV. (J. Cell. Physiol. 219: 544-552, 2009). **I believe that they have confused SOD as being an antioxidant and it is a prooxidant. This will markedly affect the interpretation of their data.**

2.1.3.8 SOD produced H2O2 and Gpx1 regulate cerebral vascular tone

Although arachidonic acid (AA) has diverse vascular effects, the mechanisms that mediate these effects are incompletely defined. The goal of our study was to use genetic approaches to examine the role of hydrogen peroxide (H2O2), glutathione peroxidase (Gpx1, which degrades H2O2), and CuZn-superoxide dismutase (SOD1, which produces H2O2 from superoxide) in mediating and in determining vascular responses to AA. In basilar arteries in vitro, AA produced dilation in nontransgenic mice, and this response was reduced markedly in transgenic mice overexpressing Gpx1 (Gpx1 Tg) or in those genetically deficient in SOD1. For example, AA (1 nmol/L to 1 mumol/L) dilated the basilar artery and this response was reduced by approximately 90% in Gpx1 Tg mice ($P<0.01$), although responses to acetylcholine were not altered. Dilation of cerebral arterioles in vivo in response to AA was inhibited by approximately 50% by treatment with catalase (300 U/mL) ($P<0.05$) and reduced by as much as 90% in Gpx1 Tg mice compared with that in controls ($P<0.05$). These results provide the first evidence that **Gpx1 has functional effects in the cerebral circulation, and that AA-induced vascular effects are mediated by H2O2 produced by SOD1.** In contrast, cerebral vascular responses to the endothelium-dependent agonist acetylcholine are not mediated by H2O2. **I believe that this emphasizes the crucial role of SOD for the production of H2O2 in the brain vasculature.** (Modrick M. et al. Role of hydrogen peroxide and the impact of glutathione peroxidase-1 in regulation of cerebral vascular tone. Journal of cerebral blood flow and metabolism. 2009-Jun; vol 29 (issue 6) : pp 1130-7).

2.1.3.9 Life long SOD deficiency has negative effect on heart function

The mitochondrially expressed manganese-dependent superoxide dismutase (MnSOD, SOD2) is an essential antioxidative enzyme that is necessary for normal heart function. In this study, we investigated the heart function of mice that were exposed to increased oxidative stress for time periods of up to 6 months due to decreased MnSOD activity caused by heterozygous deletion of the MnSOD gene. METHODS AND RESULTS: We generated a mouse strain in which the gene encoding MnSOD was exchanged against a cassette containing the SOD cDNA under the control of the tetracycline response element. After breeding with mice carrying the tetracycline receptor, compound mice express MnSOD depending on the presence of tetracycline. Without tetracycline receptor the MnSOD gene is fully inactivated, and animals show an MnSOD-deficient phenotype. Using echo-cardiographic recordings, we found an impairment of left ventricular functions: MnSOD+/- mice displayed a decrease in fraction shortening and ejection fraction and an increase in left ventricular internal diameter in systole. Furthermore, MnSOD+/- mice developed heart hypertrophy with accompanying fibrosis and necrosis revealed by immunhistochemical analysis. Although we did not find an increase in apoptosis in MnSOD+/- hearts under normal conditions, we observed an increase of the number of apoptotic cells and vascular senescence after treatment with doxorubicin. CONCLUSION: Our study demonstrates **that lifelong reduction of MnSOD activity has a negative effect on normal heart function.** This animal model presents a valuable tool to investigate the mechanism of heart pathology reported in patients bearing different polymorphic variants of the MnSOD gene and to develop new therapeutic strategies through manipulation of the antioxidative defence system (Loch T. et al. Different extent of cardiac malfunction and resistance to oxidative stress in heterozygous and homozygous manganese-dependent superoxide dismutase-mutant mice. 2009-Jun; vol 82 (issue 3) : pp 448-57).

2.1.3.10 SOD over expression protects cancer cell exposed to hyperthermia ==

It has been hypothesized that **exposure of cells to hyperthermia results in an increased flux of reactive oxygen species (ROS), primarily superoxide anion radicals**, and that increasing antioxidant enzyme levels will result in protection of cells from the toxicity of these ROS. In this study, the prostate cancer cell line, PC-3, and its manganese superoxide dismutase (MnSOD)-overexpressing clones were subjected to hyperthermia (43 degrees C, 1 h). Increased expression of MnSOD increased the mitochondrial membrane potential (MMP). Hyperthermic exposure of PC-3 cells resulted in increased ROS production, as determined by aconitase inactivation, lipid peroxidation, and H2O2 formation with a reduction in cell survival. In contrast, PC-3 cells overexpressing MnSOD had less ROS production, less lipid peroxidation, and greater cell survival compared to PC-3 Wt cells. **Since MnSOD removes superoxide, these results suggest that superoxide free radical or its reaction products are responsible for part of the cytotoxicity associated with hyperthermia and that MnSOD can reduce cellular injury and thereby enhance heat tolerance** (Venkataraman Sujatha; Wagner Brett A; Jiang Xiaohong; Wang Hong P; Schafer Freya Q; Ritchie Justine M; Patrick Burns C; Oberley Larry W; Buettner Garry R. **Overexpression of manganese superoxide dismutase promotes the survival of prostate cancer cells exposed to hyperthermia.** Free radical research 2004;38(10):1119-32). **In light of their data showing that SOD increases peroxide formation in the ETC, this study shows that increased EMODs increase tumoricidal activity and cancer kill and that reduced EMODs reduces an apoptotic response.**

2.1.4.0 Hydrogen peroxide

2.1.4.1 Hydrogen peroxide in the human body (Halliwell)

(Halliwell, B et al. *FEBS Letters, 486(1), 2000)* (Federation of European Biochemical Societies).

Because hydrogen peroxide (H2O2) is widely regarded as a cytotoxic agent, levels must be minimized by the action of antioxidant defence enzymes. **In fact, H2O2 is poorly reactive in the absence of transition metal ions.** Exposure of certain human tissues to H2O2 may be greater than is commonly supposed. Levels of H2O2 in the body may be controlled not only by catabolism, but also by excretion, and H2O2 could play a role in the regulation of renal function and as an antibacterial agent in the urine. Urinary H2O2 levels are influenced by diet, but under certain conditions might be a valuable biomarker of `oxidative stress'.

2.1.4.2 Introduction

Hydrogen peroxide is freely miscible with water and is apparently able to cross cell membranes readily, **high (usually 50+ micro-M) levels being cytotoxic**.

It is therefore widely thought that H_2O_2 is very toxic in vivo and must be rapidly eliminated, employing enzymes such as catalases, peroxidases (especially glutathione peroxidases) and thioredoxin-linked systems.

Paradoxically, however, in chemical terms, **H_2O_2 is poorly reactive: it can act as a mild oxidizing or as a mild reducing agent, but it does not oxidize most biological molecules readily, including lipids, DNA and proteins** (unless the latter have hyper-reactive thiol groups or methionine residues). The danger of H_2O_2 largely comes from its ready conversion to the indiscriminately reactive **hydroxyl radical, either by exposure to ultraviolet light or by interaction with a range of transition metal ions,** of which the most important is probably iron.

Living organisms have evolved mechanisms to sequester transition metal ions into protein-bound forms that cannot catalyze hydroxyl radical formation and other free radical reactions in vivo. These mechanisms are especially important in such extracellular fluids as the blood plasma. Nevertheless, H_2O_2 can contribute to Fenton chemistry not only by being one of the substrates but also by providing the other, e.g. by liberating iron from heme proteins. **Addition of H_2O_2 to cells in culture can lead to transition metal ion-dependent hydroxyl radical-mediated oxidative DNA damage**, although this damage appears to be rapidly repaired provided that the cells are not rendered non-viable by an excess of H_2O_2. *(Spencer J, et al, Biochem. Biophys. Res. Commun, 224, 1996)*

However, **levels of H_2O_2 at or below about 20-50 micro-M seem to have limited cytotoxicity to many cell types**. Indeed, there is a growing literature showing that H_2O_2 can be used as an inter- and intra-cellular signalling molecule. **At sites of inflammation, H_2O_2 generated by activated phagocytes appears to modulate the inflammatory process,** e.g. by up-regulating expression of adhesion molecules, controlling cell proliferation or apoptosis and modulating platelet aggregation.

2.1.4.3 Exposure of human tissues to H_2O_2

Hydrogen peroxide is generated in vivo by the dismutation of superoxide radical both non-enzymatically and catalyzed by superoxide dismutase enzymes. **Hydrogen peroxide is also directly produced by a range of oxidase enzymes including glycollate and monoamine oxidases as well as by the peroxisomal pathway for beta-oxidation of fatty acids.** With the apparent **exception of cardiac muscle, mitochondria in most tissues appear to have limited capacity to remove H_2O_2**, in that they readily generate substantial amounts of H_2O_2 in vitro and probably in vivo. Although mitochondria contain glutathione peroxidase and thioredoxin-linked peroxidase activities, the efficiency of these enzymes in removing H_2O_2 is uncertain given the **ease with which mitochondria release H_2O_2**. It thus seems likely that **most or all human cells are exposed to some level of H_2O_2**, with the mitochondria being an important source. However, certain tissues may be exposed to higher H_2O_2 concentrations.

2.1.4.4 The oral cavity, oesophagus and stomach

Several beverages commonly drunk by humans can contain **H_2O_2** at concentrations **above 100 micro-M, including green and black tea and especially instant coffee.** When such beverages are ingested, the H_2O_2 they contain presumably rapidly diffuses into the cells of the oral cavity and upper part of the gastrointestinal tract. **Oral bacteria also produce H_2O_2**, although the resulting levels of exposure of the oral tissues are uncertain. It is often suggested that H_2O_2 released into saliva is used by salivary peroxidase to oxidize thiocyanate into products toxic to certain bacterial strains.

2.1.4.5 The respiratory system

The cells lining the respiratory system, in common with the oral and oesophageal epithelium, are exposed to high O2 concentrations (21%) as compared with most other body tissues. **Hydrogen peroxide is present in exhaled air of humans from phagocytes (e.g. alveolar macrophages, neutrophils in the oral cavity, or neutrophils recruited to the lungs in inflammatory lung diseases) or other lung cells.** Amounts of exhaled H_2O_2 appear greater in subjects with inflammatory lung diseases.

2.1.4.6 The kidney, urinary tract and bladder

Substantial quantities of H_2O_2, at concentrations sometimes exceeding 100 micro-M can be detected in freshly voided human urine, even in babies. The H_2O_2 detected in human urine appears to arise, at least in part, by superoxide radical-dependent auto-oxidation of urinary molecules, some of which originate from diet. Traces of superoxide dismutase are present in urine: this enzyme, as well as the acidic pH of urine, should facilitate both enzymic and non-enzymic dismutation of superoxide radicals to H_2O_2. The high levels of H_2O_2 that can be detected in some urine samples, strongly suggest that **at least some H_2O_2 generation occurs within the bladder.** Hydrogen peroxide has an antibacterial effect and it may be that its presence at high levels in urine could be advantageous in diminishing infections of the bladder and urinary tract. Indeed, there are suggestions that H_2O_2 is involved in modulation of renal function. Excretion of H_2O_2 may also represent a metabolic mechanism for controlling its levels in the human body, a valuable tool for assessment of `oxidative stress'.

2.1.4.7 Vascular endothelial and circulating blood cells

Some studies have claimed substantial levels of H_2O_2 (up to ~35 micro-M) in human blood plasma, but others have claimed levels to be very low. In part, it is degraded by the traces of catalase present, but H_2O_2 can also react with heme proteins, ascorbate, and protein-SH groups. In vivo, H_2O_2 generated in plasma could also diffuse into erythrocytes, white cells, endothelial cells and platelets for metabolism. **Human plasma may be continuously generating H_2O_2,** at least under pathological conditions.

2.1.4.8 Ocular tissues

The presence of H_2O_2, at widely varying levels (in some cases, 100 micro-M or more), has been reported in human and other animal aqueous and vitreous humors. Any impairment in the capacity of the lens epithelium, retina or other ocular tissues to dispose of H_2O_2 would then result in its accumulation. The origin of this H_2O_2 is uncertain, but oxidation of glutathione or ascorbate is one possibility.

2.1.4.9 Conclusion

Hydrogen peroxide appears to be a ubiquitous molecule. We exhale it, excrete it and take it in from diet. It can be detected in drinking water, rain-water and sea water *(Willey J et al, Eco. Prog Ser. 178, 1999; Fujiwara K, Nippon Bunseki Kagakkai 9, 1999.)* These data emphasize the importance of metal ion sequestration in preventing the toxicity of H_2O_2 in vivo by decreasing the occurrence of Fenton chemistry.

CAUTION: Hydrogen peroxide is an irritant of the eyes, mucous membranes, and skin. Inhalation of high concentrations of the vapor or mist may cause extreme irritation of the nose and throat. Severe systemic poisoning may cause headache, dizziness, vomiting, diarrhea, tremors, numbness, convulsions, pulmonary edema, unconsciousness, and shock. Exposure for a short period of time to the mist or spray may cause stinging and tearing of the eyes. Skin contact with liquid hydrogen peroxide causes a temporary whitening or bleaching of the skin; if the skin is not washed promptly, redness and blisters may develop. Ingestion of hydrogen peroxide may cause irritation of the upper gastrointestinal tract and severe damage to the esophagus and stomach. *(Hathaway G et al. Proctor and Hughes' chemical hazards of the workplace. Van Nostrand Reinhold. 1991)* Splashes of high concentrations of hydrogen peroxide in the eyes may cause severe corneal damage. At very low concentrations (1 to 3 percent), instillation of hydrogen peroxide into the eye causes severe pain that later subsides. *(Grant W, Toxicology of the eye. Charles C Thomas, 1986)*

2.1.5.0 T-cells contain 10-100 μM peroxide

T cells are exposed to ROS at sites of inflammation where activated macrophages and neutrophils produce large amounts of superoxide and its derivatives via the phagocytic isoform of NADPH oxidase. It is estimated that **during this oxidative burst the local H2O2 concentration may reach 10-100 μM in the vicinity of T cells** (Nathan & Root, 1977) (Nathan CF, Root RK. Hydrogen peroxide release from mouse peritoneal macrophages: dependence on sequential activation and triggering. J Exp med 146:1648-1662, 1977).

A growing body of evidence demonstrates that T lymphocytes are strongly regulated in their activities by ROS such as H2O2.

2.1.5.1 Hydrogen peroxide bactericidal activity is increased by blue light

Investigators evaluated the possibility of **enhancing the phototoxic effect on *Streptococcus mutans* using a potentially antibacterial synergic effect between blue light and hydrogen peroxide (H_2O_2),** and to investigate the antibacterial mechanism involved.

Methods: Growth of *S. mutans* samples was determined after exposure to light in the presence and absence of H_2O_2. The effect of such light on H_2O_2 degradation, on reactive oxygen species (ROS) generation and on the exposed-medium temperature was examined.

Results: **The combination of light exposure for 20 s (~23 J/cm^2) and a concentration of 0.3 mM H_2O_2 yielded 96% growth inhibition, whereas, when applied separately, light exposure decreased bacterial growth by 3% and H_2O_2 by 30% compared with the control.** The results showed no direct effect of the light on H_2O_2 degradation, a partial protective effect of ROS scavengers on *S. mutans* and a non-lethal increase in the medium temperature after light exposure.

Conclusions: **An antibacterial synergic effect between blue light and H_2O_2 was observed.** The mechanism of the phototoxic effect on *S. mutans* was basically a photochemical process, in which **ROS were involved.** Application of such light in combination with H_2O_2 to an infected tooth could be an alternative to or serve as an additional minimally invasive antibacterial treatment.

Blue non-coherent light sources, such as the plasma-arc curing (PAC) light, the halogen lamp and the light emitting diode, are often used in dentistry for photocuring resin composites. Previous studies have shown that visible light at **wavelengths of 400–500 nm (blue light)** induced an oxygen-dependent phototoxic effect on the periopathogenic bacteria Porphyromonas gingivalis and Fusobacterium nucleatum, in which reactive oxygen species (ROS) such as hydroxyl radicals (OH ·) were involved. These ROS have been shown to cause damage to proteins, lipids and nucleic acids. Indeed, although nonionizing, visible light (wavelengths 408–750 nm) causes mutagenic and metabolic damage to Escherichia coli cells.

Light source

A xenon lamp with a combined filter for transmission of blue light (450–490 nm) (MSq, Caesarea, Israel), the dental PAC light, was applied. The distance between the light source tip and the exposed sample was fixed to obtain a constant power density. An average light power of 440 mW was measured using a power meter (Ophir, Jerusalem, Israel) over a spot of 0.7 cm diameter. To calculate power density, the average power was divided by the area of the light spot.

The results of the present study show a synergic antibacterial effect between blue light and H_2O_2. The combination of light exposure for 20 s (_23 J/cm2) and a concentration of 0.3 mM H_2O_2 yielded 96% growth inhibition, whereas, when they were applied separately, bacterial growth was decreased by 3% when exposed to light and by 30% in the presence of H_2O_2 as compared with the control. (Synergic antibacterial effect between visible light and hydrogen peroxide on *Streptococcus mutans*. Osnat Feuerstein, Daniel Moreinos and Doron Steinberg. Journal of Antimicrobial chemotherapy. Vol. 57, No. 5, pp. 872-876).

I believe that this study was likely generating singlet oxygen, which accounted for the increased bacterial kill.

2.1.5.2 Hydrogen peroxide plus blue light kills germs in oral biofilms

Oral biofilms are associated with the most common infections of the oral cavity. Bacteria embedded in the biofilms are less sensitive to antibacterial agents than planktonic bacteria are. Recently, an antibacterial synergic effect of noncoherent blue light and hydrogen peroxide (H_2O_2) on planktonic *Streptococcus mutans* was demonstrated. In this study, we tested the effect of a combination of light and H_2O_2 on the vitality and gene expression of *S. mutans* embedded in biofilm. Biofilms of *S. mutans* were exposed to visible light (**wavelengths, 400 to 500 nm**) for 30 or 60 s (equivalent to 34 or 68 J/cm^2) in the presence of 3 to 300 mM H_2O_2. The antibacterial effect was assessed by microbial counts of each treated sample compared with that of the control. The effect of light combined with H_2O_2 on the different layers of the biofilm was evaluated by confocal laser scanning microscopy. Gene expression was determined by real-time reverse transcription-PCR. Our results show that **noncoherent light, in combination with H_2O_2, has a synergistic antibacterial effect through all of the layers of the biofilm**. Furthermore, this treatment was more effective against bacteria in biofilm than against planktonic bacteria. The combined light and H_2O_2 treatment up-regulated the expression of several genes such as *gtfB*, *brp*, *smu630*, and *comDE* but did not affect *relA* and *ftf*. The ability of noncoherent visible light in combination with H_2O_2 to affect bacteria in deep layers of the biofilm suggests that this treatment may be applied in biofilm-related diseases as a minimally invasive antibacterial procedure (Genetic and Physiological Effects of Noncoherent Visible Light Combined with Hydrogen Peroxide on Streptococcus mutans in Biofilm. Doron Steinberg, Daniel Moreinos, John Featherstone, Moshe Shemesh, and Osnat Feuerstein. Antimicrobial Agents and Chemotherapy, July 2008, p. 2626-2631, Vol. 52, No. 7).

2.1.6.0 Myeloperoxidase is involved in H_2O_2-induced apoptosis of HL-60 human leukemia cells ==

Investigators examined the mechanism of H_2O_2-induced cytotoxicity and its relationship to oxidation in human leukemia cells. The HL-60 promyelocytic leukemia cell line was sensitive to H_2O_2, and at concentrations up to about 20-25 micrometer, the killing was mediated by apoptosis. There was limited evidence of lipid peroxidation, suggesting that the effects of H_2O_2 do not involve hydroxyl radical. When HL-60 cells were exposed to H_2O_2 in the presence of the spin trap alpha-(4-pyridyl-1-oxide)-N-tert-butylnitrone (POBN), we detected a 12-line electron paramagnetic resonance spectrum assigned to the POBN/POBN(.) N-centered spin adduct previously described in peroxidase-containing cell-free systems. Generation of this radical by HL-60 cells had the same H_2O_2 concentration dependence as initiation of apoptosis. In contrast, studies with the K562 human erythroleukemia cell line, which is often used for comparison with the HL-60, and with high passaged HL-60 cells (spent HL-60) studied under the same conditions failed to generate POBN(.). Cellular levels of antioxidant enzymes superoxide dismutase, glutathione peroxidase, and catalase did not explain the differences between these cell lines. **Interestingly, the K562 and spent HL-60 cells, which did not generate the radical, also failed to undergo H_2O_2-induced apoptosis.** Based on this we reasoned that the difference in H_2O_2-induced apoptosis might be due to the enzyme myeloperoxidase. Only the apoptosis-manifesting HL-60 cells contained appreciable immunoreactive protein or enzymatic activity of this cellular enzyme. **When HL-60 cells were incubated with methimazole or 4-aminobenzoic acid hydrazide, which are inhibitors of myeloperoxidase, they no longer underwent H_2O_2-induced apoptosis. Hypochlorous acid stimulated apoptosis in both HL-60 and spent HL-60 cells, indicating that another oxidant generated by myeloperoxidase induces apoptosis and that it may be the direct mediator of H_2O_2-induced apoptosis.** Taken together these observations indicate that H_2O_2-induced apoptosis in the HL-60 human leukemia cell is mediated by myeloperoxidase and is linked to a non-Fenton oxidative event marked by POBN(.) (Wagner B A; Buettner G R; Oberley L W; Darby C J; Burns C P. **Myeloperoxidase is involved in H_2O_2-induced apoptosis of HL-60 human leukemia cells.** The Journal of biological chemistry 2000;275(29):22461-9). **This emphasizes the role of EMOD-induced apoptosis in cancer cell kill. I have seen this over and over.**

2.1.7.0 Hydrogen peroxide and melanogenesis

(May 2008, Soap, Cosmetics and Perfumery) RMH Note: I do not put much credence in this paper but will include it as general information of questionable reliability. I included it to show another extreme.

By **Ratan Chaudhuri**

Hydrogen peroxide and its impact on the production of melanin

Ever wondered why hydrogen peroxide bubbles when you put it on an abrasion? The answer is simple. The hydrogen peroxide decomposes into water and oxygen and the bubbles you see are oxygen bubbles. Hydrogen peroxide should really be called hydrogen dioxide as its chemical formula is H_2O_2. Hydrogen peroxide is odourless and almost colourless, but not tasteless, and is slightly more viscous than water.

It is a weak acid and its strong oxidising property makes it a powerful bleaching agent. **H_2O_2 is one of the most powerful oxidisers known and is stronger than chlorine, chlorine dioxide and potassium permanganate**. It is used in a number of household products and it is a component of some tooth whitening products. **(RMH Note: I do not believe that this is true in physiological systems. In fact, it is a weak oxidizer.)**

Surprisingly, **H_2O_2 therapy, as well as other oxygen-based treatments, is rapidly gaining in popularity within the alternative medicine community**. Newer research indicates that **we need hydrogen peroxide for a multitude of chemical reactions that take place throughout the body**.

2.1.7.1 The role of melanin in skin

The skin is the main barrier to the external environment and relies on melanocytes to provide, among other things, photoprotection and thermoregulation by producing melanin. In addition to carotenoids and hemoglobulin, complexion colouration in humans is primarily regulated by the amount and type of melanin synthesised by the epidermal melanocytes. Human skin colour is variable around the world and no-one has truly black, white or yellow skin.

Skin lightening products in the European market tend to be used to treat age spots and freckles or to obtain even toning effects, whereas in Asia and Africa it is used to change or modify skin colour.

Although human beings generally possess a similar concentration of melanocytes in their skin, the melanocytes in some individuals and ethnic groups more frequently or less frequently express the melanin-producing genes, thereby conferring a greater or lesser concentration of skin melanin.

There are two types of melanins: eumelanin and pheomelanin. Both are found in human skin and hair, but eumelanin is the most abundant melanin in humans. Of these, eumelanin is presumed photoprotective and pheomelanin phototoxic. Pheomelanin is widely thought to be causally related to susceptibility to the harmful effects of ultraviolet radiation; epidemiological studies show that those with a higher ratio of pheomelanin to eumelanin in hair have higher rates of melanoma. Eumelanin and pheomelanin in human skin, before and following irradiation, are positively related to skin colour and inversely with cancer susceptibility. The ratio of melanin classes is similar in people with widely different cancer rates and ultra violet radiation (UVR) sensitivity.

2.1.7.2 Hydrogen peroxide & melanin

So what's the connection between the two? Well, **hydrogen peroxide does have a major role to play in melanogenesis.** Melanogenesis is the process of production of melanin by melanocytes within the skin follicles. Melanocytes have specialised organelles, termed melanosomes, which contain several enzymes that catalyse the production of melanin. The copper-containing enzyme tyrosinase (a tyrosinase hydroxylase) catalyses the oxidation of the amino acid tyrosine into DOPA and dopamine, which on auto-oxidation produces DOPAquinone and dopaminoquinone, electrophilic molecules that rapidly cyclise to form DOPAchrome and dopaminochrome respectively.

Subsequent reaction generates dihydroxyindole-2-carboxylic acid (DHIC) and dihydroxy indole (DHI) that polymerise to form brown-black pigment termed eumelanin. At least two additional melanosomal enzymes are involved in the eumelanogenesis pathway that produces brown and black pigments, tyrosine-related protein-1 (TRP-1, DHIC oxidase) and tyrosine-related protein-2 (TRP-2, DOPA chrome tautomerase). Depending on the incorporation of a sulphur-containing reactant (such as cystein or glutathione) into the products, the melanogenesis pathway diverges, producing eumelanins or pheomelanins (red-yellow pigments) or both. **H_2O_2 does have a key role to play in melanogenesis.** The steps involving H_2O_2 can be summarised in the diagram: Hydrogen peroxide and melanogenesis.

2.1.7.3 Dealing with the problem

Tyrosinase inhibitory activity is not a prerequisite for a skin lightening effect. Inhibition of alternate oxidative pathways – namely peroxidase/ **H_2O_2**, Fe2+/ **H_2O_2** or nitric oxide (NO) – can also provide the desired skin lightening effect. **Phenolic antioxidants do play a role in inhibiting melanin synthesis mediated by H_2O_2.** Some skin lighteners, such as **standardised fruit extract of Phyllanthus emblica (Emblica), highly purified hexylresorcinol**

(Synovea HR) and resveratrol have all been shown to act as skin lighteners by inhibiting tyrosinase and peroxidase/ H_2O_2 pathways. Both resveratrol and hexylresorcinol also inhibit H_2O_2-induced DNA damage, thereby not only inhibiting DNA-fragment induced melanin synthesis but also giving additional skin protection against sun-induced damage. Skin lighteners that work by inhibiting multiple pathways are a better choice because **H_2O_2-induced skin damage and hyperpigmentation are intertwined** (see Hydrogen peroxide & skin ageing, SPC, p21, January 2008).

2.1.8.0 Hydrogen peroxide and melanogenesis

2.1.8.1 Hydrogen peroxide & skin aging

(SPC January 2008)

By **Ratan Chaudhuri**

Ratan Chaudhuri looks for protection from hydrogen peroxide induced ageing

Hydrogen peroxide (H_2O_2) was first isolated in 1818 by Louis Jacqueous Thenard by reacting barium peroxide with nitric acid. It is a pale blue liquid which appears colourless in a dilute solution. It is a weak acid and has a strong oxidizing property and is therefore a powerful bleaching agent. It is one of the most powerful oxidisers known and is stronger than chlorine, chlorine dioxide and potassium permanganate. It is used in a number of products, including hair dyes, and it is a component of some tooth whitening products.

Well, it has a major role to play in chronological as well as in photoageing. Hydrogen peroxide plays a pivotal role **because it is generated from nearly all sources of oxidative stress and oxygen radicals.** Mitochondria are the major sources of production of hydrogen peroxide. Mitochondria are sometimes described as cellular powerhouses because they generate most of the cell's supply of adenosine triphosphate (ATP), used as a source of chemical energy. The reactive oxygen species that are generated by mitochondrial respiration, including hydrogen peroxide, are potent inducers of oxidative damage and mediators of ageing. **(RMH Note: This is highly debatable.)**

It is not clear, however, whether oxidative stress is the result of a genetic programme or the byproduct of physiological processes. Recent findings demonstrate that a fraction of mitochondrial H2O2, produced by a specialised enzyme as a signalling molecule in the pathway of apoptosis, induces intracellular oxidative stress and accelerates ageing. **It is quite conceivable to assume that the genes that control H_2O_2 production are selected determinants of lifespan. I have reported on the essential nature of the role of peroxide in apoptosis, especially for prooxidant pathogen and neoplasia protection.**

2.1.8.2 How does hydrogen peroxide cause chronological ageing?

Hydrogen peroxide and superoxide anion (O2-) are **normal metabolites** in aerobic cells. For example, H_2O_2 is formed from O2+ in the presence of superoxide dismutase (SOD) and then converted to H2O and O2 by the enzymes catalase or glutathione peroxidase. **Glucose oxidase produces H_2O_2 directly whereas xanthine oxidase produces O2-, which then gets converted to H_2O_2 by SOD, which can react with free iron or copper to form the hydroxyl radical (HO).**

In addition to these **toxic electron transport chain reactions** of the inner mitochondrial membrane, **the mitochondrial outer membrane enzyme monoamine oxidase catalyses the oxidative deamination of biogenic amines resulting in a large production of H_2O_2** that contributes to an increase in the steady state concentrations of reactive oxygen species within both the mitochondrial matrix and cytosol. Reactive oxygen species generated by mitochondria, or from other sites in or outside the cell, cause damage to mitochondrial components and initiate degradation. **I believe that this is an incorrect model in the living/breathing cell and it has been shown by Halliwell and Singapore investigators that mitochondrial DNA does not suffer any more damage than does nuclear DNA.**

H_2O_2 can be increased in inflammatory states and can also be formed by exposure to radiation. It has also been shown that **light driven formation of hydrogen peroxide is responsible for advanced glycation end products (AGE) phototoxicity**, supporting the general hypothesis that extracellular matrix (ECM)-bound chromophores are endogenous sensitisers of UV phototoxicity in human skin. **I have reported on the beneficial effects of EMODs generated by photodynamic and sonodynamic therapy.**

Hydrogen peroxide is able to cross cell membranes easily and, in conjunction with Fe2+, generates highly toxic hydroxyl radical. Both singlet oxygen and hydroxyl radical can initiate lipid peroxidation. **It has been shown that H_2O_2 can induce cell death in normal human keratinocytes.**

Both prokaryotic and eukaryotic cells have inducible and adaptive defences to counter oxidative damage. To counteract the harmful effects of reactive oxygen species (ROS), the skin is equipped with antioxidant defence systems consisting of a variety of low molecular weight antioxidants (eg vitamins C and E) and antioxidant defence enzymes (eg superoxide dismutase, glutathione peroxidase, catalase) forming an **antioxidant network.** The antioxidant network is responsible for maintaining the equilibrium between pro-oxidants and antioxidants. However, the antioxidant defence can be overwhelmed by increased exposure to exogenous sources of ROS. **I believe that this is based on the erroneous concept of oxidative stress.**

The molecular mechanisms by which hydrogen peroxide is sensed and the increasing evidence that antioxidant enzymes play multiple, key roles as sensors and regulators of signal transduction in response to hydrogen peroxide. **Hydrogen peroxide has been shown to act as a second messenger mediating intracellular redox-sensitive signal transduction**. Hydrogen peroxide is also able to transmit pro-inflammatory signals from one cell to the other and this action can be inhibited by endogenous produced glutathione peroxidase or catalase.

Signalling functions of superoxide and hydrogen peroxide in enzymatic phosphorylation/dephosphorylation reactions are now well documented. Hydrogen peroxide signalling in the dephosphorylation reactions by protein phosphatases and in the activation of protein kinases is actually mediated by superoxide formed during the conversion of H_2O_2 into superoxide by the oxidised superoxide dismutase. There are at least three options for skin protection:

1. Quenching superoxide anion radicals: A wide variety of polyphenolics are very effective superoxide anion quenchers. For example, standardised extracts of green tea, Phyllanthus emblica (Emblica) etc or well-defined natural polyphenolics like epigallo catechin 3-gallate.

2. Inhibiting the activity of glucose oxidase or monoamine oxidase enzymes: For example, **resveratrol is an efficient inhibitor of glucose oxidase**. It is wise to stay away from **monoamine oxidase inhibitors for skin protection purposes as they are used as anti-depressants**.

3. Converting hydrogen peroxide to water and oxygen: This can be achieved by inducing synthesis of glutathione peroxidase or catalase. For example, **hexylresorcinol (Synovea HR) and resveratrol are very effective stimulators**

of glutathione peoxidase whereas Emblica is a good stimulator for catalase.

Topical formulations using compounds capable of reducing hydrogen peroxide-induced skin damage are likely to lead to further improvements in the way we protect our skin from overexposure to the sun. **That is the opinion of Mr. Chaudhuri.**

2.1.9.0 Hydrogen peroxide said to be causative of gray hair

Gray or white hair develops with advancing age in **an entirely natural aging process** which results in the generation of less and less color pigments. Researchers of the Johannes Gutenberg University Mainz in Germany und the University of Bradford in Great Britain have now unlocked the secret of hair turning white or gray in old age. According to them, **free oxygen radicals are significantly involved in the loss of hair color. "The originator of the entire process is hydrogen peroxide**, which we also know as a bleaching agent," explains Professor Heinz Decker of the Institute of Biophysics at Mainz University.

"With advancing age, hydrogen peroxide builds up in larger amounts in the hair follicle and ultimately inhibits the synthesis of the color pigment melanin." The biophysicists in Mainz together with dermatologists from Bradford have revealed the molecular mechanisms of this process for the first time, and they published their findings in the Feb. 2009 professional journal, The FASEB Journal.

Hydrogen peroxide - or H_2O_2 by its the chemical formula - is a by-product of metabolism, and as such it is generated in small amounts throughout the human body, consequently also in hair follicles. With increasing age, the quantity builds up, because the human body can no longer keep up neutralizing the hydrogen peroxide using the enzyme catalyse, which breaks down hydrogen peroxide into its two components water and oxygen. In their work, the **scientists showed that in aging cells catalase is still present but in very limited concentration.** This has dramatic consequences. **Hydrogen peroxide attacks the enzyme tyrosinase by oxidizing an amino acid, methionine, at the active site. As a consequence, this key enzyme, which normally starts the synthesizing pathway of the coloring pigment melanin, does not function anymore.**

"We now know the specific molecular dynamic that underlies this process," elucidates Decker. The scientists at the Institute of Biophysics at Mainz University have been working for about ten years already on research concerning tyrosinases, which are enzymes present in all organisms and performing a variety of functions. In computer simulations that helped to reveal the molecular mechanisms, the biophysicists were supported by the newly established research focus on "Computer-based Research Methods in the Natural Sciences" at Johannes Gutenberg University Mainz.

Oxidation by hydrogen peroxide not only interferes with the production of melanin, but also inhibits other enzymes that are needed for the repair of damaged proteins. As a result, a cascade of events is set off, at the end of which stands the gradual loss of pigments in the entire hair from its root to its tip. With this research work, the scientists from Mainz and Bradford not only solved - on a molecular level - the age-old riddle of why hair turns gray in old age, but also have pointed out approaches for future therapy of vitiligo, a skin pigment disorder. For **melanin is not only the pigment in hair, but it is also responsible for color in skin and eyes. Thus, I ask, "Why doesn't the eye pigment bleach out? The eye has one of the highest oxygen utilization rates in the entire body and it is exposed to photooxidation as long as the eyelid is open."**

The researchers in Mainz were supported by the Collaborative Research Center 490 "Mechanisms of Invasion and Persistence of Infectious Agents," and the Research Training Group 1043 "Antigen-specific Immunotherapy", both funded by the German Research Foundation (DFG).

(J. M. Wood, H. Decker, H. Hartmann, B. Chavan, H. Rokos, J. D. Spencer, S. Hasse, M. J. Thornton, M. Shalbaf, R. Paus, and K. U. Schallreuter. Senile hair graying: H2O2-mediated oxidative stress affects human hair color by blunt-ing methionine sulfoxide repair. The FASEB Journal, online published on 23 February 2009, doi: 10.1096/fj.08-125435) (T. Schweikardt, C. Olivares, F. Solano, E. Jaenicke, J.C. Garcia-Borron and H. Decker. A three-dimensional model of mammalian tyrosinase active site accounting for loss of function mutations. Pigment Cell Research (2007) 20:394-401).

The generation of H_2O_2 in the melanin biosynthesis pathway is of great importance because of its **"alleged" great cytotoxic capacity**.

2.2.0.0 Human body glows in the dark

7-22-09 **The human body literally glows, emitting a visible light in extremely small quantities at levels that rise and fall with the day, scientists now reveal.**

Past research has shown that the body emits visible light, 1,000 times less intense than the levels to which our naked eyes are sensitive. In fact, **virtually all living creatures emit very weak light, which is thought to be a byproduct of biochemical reactions involving free radicals.**

(This visible light differs from the infrared radiation - an invisible form of light - that comes from body heat.)

To learn more about this faint visible light, scientists in Japan employed extraordinarily sensitive cameras capable of detecting single photons. Five healthy male volunteers in their 20s were placed bare-chested in front of the cameras in complete darkness in light-tight rooms for 20 minutes every three hours from 10 a.m. to 10 p.m. for three days.

The researchers found the body glow rose and fell over the day, with its lowest point at 10 a.m. and its peak at 4 p.m., dropping gradually after that. These findings suggest there is light emission linked to our body clocks, most likely due to how our metabolic rhythms fluctuate over the course of the day. **I believe that this is in agreement with my theory on sleep, peak EMOD emission and rejuvenation.**

Faces glowed more than the rest of the body. This might be because faces are more tanned than the rest of the body, since they get more exposure to sunlight - the pigment behind skin color, **melanin, has fluorescent components that could enhance the body's miniscule light production**.

Since **this faint light is linked with the body's metabolism**, this finding suggests cameras that can spot the weak emissions could help spot medical conditions, said researcher Hitoshi Okamura, a circadian biologist at Kyoto University in Japan.

"If you can see the glimmer from the body's surface, you could see the whole body condition," said researcher Masaki Kobayashi, a biomedical photonics specialist at the Tohoku Institute of Technology in Sendai, Japan.

Schematic illustration of experimental setup that found the human body, especially the face, emits visible light in small quantities that vary during the day. B is one fo the test subjects. The other images show the weak emissions of visible light during totally dark conditions. The chart corresponds to the images and shows how the emissions varied during the day. The last image (I) is an infrared image of the subject showing heat emissions. Credit: Kyoto University; Tohoku Institute of Technology

2.2.1.0 Iron and ascorbate increase PDT effect

Photofrin, a photosensitizer used in the photodynamic therapy of cancer, selectively localizes in cellular membranes. Upon exposure to visible light, **Photofrin produces singlet oxygen (1O2), which reacts with membrane polyunsaturated fatty acids forming lipid hydroperoxides. Transition metals, such as Fe2+, catalyze the production of cytotoxic free radicals from lipid hydroperoxides.** Ascorbate reduces ferric to ferrous iron, further augmenting lipid peroxidation. Therefore, to increase the efficacy of Photofrin photosensitization, we added 20 microM ferrous sulfate and 100 microM ascorbic acid, in an aqueous layer over SCC-25 oral squamous cell carcinoma cells during in vitro illumination. In electron paramagnetic resonance spin trapping experiments, using POBN (alpha-(4-pyridyl-1-oxide)-N-tert-butylnitrone), we observed that **the presence of this pro-oxidant combination greatly increases the production of membrane-derived lipid free radicals.** The effect was time dependent but only partially concentration dependent. Trypan blue dye exclusion demonstrated that this increase in lipid radical formation correlated with cytotoxicity. These observations support the hypothesis that **Photofrin photosensitization leads to lipid hydroperoxide formation, which increases the cell's susceptibility to iron-induced Fenton chemistry. The resulting free radical-mediated lipid peroxidation results in cell death**. From these data we hypothesize that the efficacy of photodynamic therapy of superficial cancer might be increased by the topical application of the pro-oxidant combination of iron and ascorbate. Furthermore, their use will probably allow lower doses of Photofrin without compromising antitumor effect. (Kelley E E; Domann F E; Buettner G R; Oberley L W; Burns C P. **Increased efficacy of in vitro Photofrin photosensitization of human oral squamous cell carcinoma by iron and ascorbate.** Journal of photochemistry and photobiology. B, Biology 1997;40(3):273-7).

2.2.1.1 Ascorbate as a prooxidant

Trace levels of transition metals can participate in the metal-catalyzed Haber-Weiss reaction (superoxide-driven Fenton reaction) as well as catalyze the oxidation of ascorbate. Generally ascorbate is thought of as an excellent reducing agent; it is able to serve as a donor antioxidant in free radical-mediated oxidation processes. However, **as a reducing agent it is also able to reduce redox-active metals such as copper and iron, thereby increasing the pro-oxidant chemistry of these metals.** Thus **ascorbate can serve as both a pro-oxidant and an antioxidant. In general, at low ascorbate concentrations, ascorbate is prone to be a pro-oxidant, and at high**

concentrations, it will tend to be an antioxidant. Hence there is a **crossover effect.** We propose that the "position" of this crossover effect is a function of the catalytic metal concentration. In this presentation, we discuss: (1) the role of catalytic metals in free radical-mediated oxidations; (2) ascorbate as both a pro-oxidant and an antioxidant; (3) catalytic metal catalysis of ascorbate oxidation; (4) use of ascorbate to determine adventitious catalytic metal concentrations; (5) use of ascorbate radical as a marker of oxidative stress; and (6) use of ascorbate and iron as free radical pro-oxidants in photodynamic therapy of cancer (Buettner G R; Jurkiewicz B A. **Catalytic metals, ascorbate and free radicals: combinations to avoid.** Radiation research 1996;145(5):532-41). **Actually, I believe that this is a good way to increase the overall oxidative capacity and fight cancer.**

2.2.2.0 Effect of topically applied tocopherol on ultraviolet radiation-mediated free radical damage in skin

Previously, we demonstrated by electron paramagnetic resonance (EPR) spectroscopy that ultraviolet radiation induces free-radical formation in Skh-1 hairless mouse skin. Because free-radical oxidative stress is thought to play a principal role in skin photoaging and cancer, oxidative stress and subsequent photodamage should be decreased by supplementation of skin with antioxidants. Using both the ascorbate free radical and an EPR spin-trapping system to detect short-lived radicals, we evaluated the effect of the topically applied antioxidants tocopherol sorbate, alpha-tocopherol, and tocopherol acetate on ultraviolet radiation-induced free-radical formation. We show that tocopherol sorbate significantly decreases the ultraviolet radiation-induced radical flux in skin. With our chronically exposed mouse model, tocopherol sorbate was also found to be significantly more protective against skin photoaging than alpha-tocopherol and tocopherol acetate. These results extend our previous observations of ultraviolet radiation-induced free-radical generation in skin and indicate the utility of tocopherol sorbate as an antioxidant in providing significant protection against ultraviolet radiation-induced oxidative damage (Jurkiewicz B A; Bissett D L; Buettner G R. **Effect of topically applied tocopherol on ultraviolet radiation-mediated free radical damage in skin.** The Journal of investigative dermatology 1995;104(4):484-8).

2.2.2.1 Vitamin E slows the rate of free radical-mediated lipid peroxidation in cells ==

Much of what is known about the antioxidant mechanism of vitamin E has been learned from studies of lipid dispersions, solutions, or subcellular organelles. We have investigated the effect of vitamin E supplementation on intact live eucaryotic cells. L1210 murine leukemia cells were exposed to an oxidative stress induced by 20 microM Fe2+ and 100 microM ascorbic acid introduced immediately before oxidative measurements were begun, and the kinetics of the generation of lipid-derived free radicals, as measured by EPR spin trapping (a product) and O2 consumption (a reactant) were measured. Cells grown for 24 h with supplemental (5-100 microM) vitamin E in their media had a slower rate of lipid radical generation compared to cells grown without vitamin E supplementation; this inhibition in the rate of oxidation was generally dependent upon the amount of vitamin E supplementation. In complementary studies measuring O2 consumption, 5-100 microM vitamin E slowed the rate of oxidation (10-fold with 100 microM supplemental vitamin E) consistent with the EPR studies. The membrane active drug edelfosine accentuated the vitamin E effects; vitamin E introduced a discernible lag phase (time delay) in both lipid radical generation and O2 consumption that was not seen in the absence of edelfosine. Vitamin E supplementation of cells also altered the kinetics of ascorbate free radical formation. We conclude that vitamin E inhibits lipid peroxidation in cells by slowing the rate of lipid peroxidation; but with iron/ascorbate as the initiating system, vitamin E does not delay the onset of peroxidation. Of special interest is that these free radical peroxidation events parallel cell membrane damage as detected using trypan blue exclusion. These observations are consistent with the free radical events preceding and causing the observed membrane damage (Wagner B A; Buettner G R; Burns C P. **Vitamin E slows the rate of free radical-mediated lipid peroxidation in cells.** Archives of biochemistry and biophysics 1996;334(2):261-7). **I believe that this argues that vitamin E will block EMOD-induced apoptosis.**

2.2.3.0 EMODs and CVD

Fundamental problems remain with implicating oxidative modification as a (requisite) pathophysiologically important cause for atherosclerosis. These include the poor performance of antioxidant strategies in limiting either atherosclerosis or cardiovascular events from atherosclerosis, and observations in animals that suggest dissociation between atherosclerosis and lipoprotein oxidation. Indeed**, it remains to be established that oxidative events are a cause rather than an injurious response to atherogenesis.** (Role of oxidative modifications in atherosclerosis. Stocker R, Keaney JF Jr. Physiol Rev. 2004 Oct;84(4):1381-478).

Direct evidence that oxidative stress in general, and the oxidative modification of low-density lipoprotein in particular, is both necessary and sufficient for atherosclerosis has been difficult to find. There are many potential reasons for this difficulty, not the least of which is our lack of sufficient knowledge delineating the precise molecular events that beget oxidative stress in the vessel wall, and the precise mediators involved. (New insights on oxidative stress in the artery wall. Stocker R, Keaney JF Jr. J Thromb Haemost. 2005 Aug;3(8):1825-34)

2.2.3.1 Multiple sclerosis not cured by antioxidants or vitamins B12 or D

Antioxidants. Some patients use anti-oxidant vitamins or supplements (A, E, C, Q10, pycnogenol, OPC, grape seed extract), since the destruction in the MS disease process may be partly due to oxidation (chemical damage from particles called oxygen free radicals). Theoretically, however, **antioxidants can trigger T-cells and macrophages (inflammatory components of the immune system) and, therefore, may pose some danger to MS patients.**

Small studies to date have not found any worsening of the disease from taking vitamin supplements, but patients should wait for more research. **No vitamins studied for MS, including carotenoids, vitamin C, vitamin E, B12 injections or vitamin D, have been proven to be beneficial to date.**

About.com accessed 10-24-08

2.2.4.0 Anthocyanins have unknown bioavailabity

Scientist are creating purple tomatoes to increase antioxidants and prevent cancer.

Anthocyanins also act as powerful antioxidants. However, it is not clear whether anthocyanins can significantly contribute to scavenging of free-radicals produced through metabolic processes in leaves, since they are located in the vacuole, and thus, spatially separated from metabolic reactive oxygen species.

Anthocyanins are the largest group of water-soluble pigments in the plant kingdom and belong to the family of compounds known as flavonoids. Major sources of anthocyanins are blue-berries, cherries, raspberries, strawberries, black currants, purple grapes and red wine. In recent years several studies have shown that anthocyanins display a wide range of biological activities including antioxidant, anti-inflammatory, antimicrobial and anti-carcinogenic activities. In addition they display a variety of effects on blood vessels, platelets and lipoproteins able to reduce the risk of coronary heart diseases. However, until the absorption and metabolic fate of anthocyanins *in vivo* is unravelled, **it would be unwise to conclude that a high consumption of them will reduce the risk of chronic diseases.** Long-term intervention trials must be properly designed and carried out to provide definite proof. In the meantime a more complete knowledge of the identity of anthocyanin metabolites and their tissue distribution should be reached. (Ann Ist Super Sanità 2007 | Vol. 43, No. 4: 369-374 Anthocyanins and heart health. **Giuseppe (Joe) Mazza)**

2.2.4.1 Antioxidant and prooxidant activities of elderberry

Antioxidant and prooxidant activities of elderberry (Sambucus nigra) extract in low-density lipoprotein oxidation

Auteur(s) / Author(s)

ABUJA P. M. [1] ; MURKOVIC M. [2] ; PFANNHAUSER W. [2] ;

Affiliation(s) du ou des auteurs / Author(s) Affiliation(s)

[1] Institute of Biochemistry, SFB Biomembrane Research Center, Karl-Franzens University, Schubertstrasse 1, 8010 Graz, AUTRICHE

[2] Institute of Biochemistry and Food Chemistry, Graz University of Technology, Petersgasse 12, 8010 Graz, AUTRICHE

Résumé / Abstract

Spray-dried elderberry juice, containing high amounts of anthocyanin glucosides, was investigated for its antioxidant and prooxidant potentials and mechanisms. A strong, concentration-dependent prolongation of the lag phase of copper-induced oxidation of human low-density lipoprotein (LDL) was found, but the maximum oxidation rate was unchanged. Peroxyl-radical-driven LDL oxidation showed both prolongation of lag time and reduction of maximum oxidation rate. In the case of copper-mediated oxidation, **the anthocyanins were able to reduce α-tocopheroxyl radical to α-tocopherol. Clear prooxidant activity in copper-mediated oxidation was observed,** depending on the time of addition of extract: whenever the extract was present from the beginning or added within the first 10 min, the antioxidant effect prevailed. Addition at later times led to a considerable reduction of lag phase and increase of maximum oxidation rate. No such effect was found in peroxyl-radical-mediated LDL oxidation; on the contrary, the extract was even able to reduce the propagation rate considerably.

Revue / Journal Title

Journal of agricultural and food chemistry **ISSN** 0021-8561 **CODEN** JAFCAU

Source / Source

1998, vol. 46, n°10, pp. 4091-4096

(Antioxidant and prooxidant activities of elderberry (Sambucus nigra) extract in low-density lipoprotein oxidation. Abuja P. M., Murkovic M., Pfannhauser W. Journal of agricultural and food chemistry. 1998, vol. 46, n°10, pp. 4091-4096)

2.2.4.2 Anthocyanin induces apoptosis in human leukemia cells via EMODs ==

Delphinidin 3-sambubioside, a Hibiscus anthocyanin, induces apoptosis in human leukemia cells through reactive oxygen species-mediated mitochondrial pathway. Hou,-D-X; Tong,-X; Terahara,-N; Luo,-D; Fujii,-M. Arch-Biochem-Biophys. 2005 Aug 1; 440(1): 101-9.

Delphinidin 3-sambubioside (Dp3-Sam), a Hibiscus anthocyanin, was isolated from the dried calices of Hibiscus sabdariffa L. Dp3-Sam could induce a dose-dependent apoptosis in human leukemia cells (HL-60) as characterized by cell morphology, DNA fragmentation, activation of caspase-3, -8, and -9, and inactivation of poly(ADP)ribose polymerase (PARP). Molecular data showed that Dp3-Sam induced Bid truncation, mitochondrial membrane potential (DeltaPsi(m)) loss, and cytochrome c release from mitochondria to cytosol. Moreover, **Dp3-Sam caused a time- and dose-dependent elevation of intracellular reactive oxygen species (ROS) level in HL-60 cells, and antioxidants such as N-acetyl-L-cysteine (NAC) and catalase could effectively block Dp3-Sam-induced ROS generation, caspase-3 activity, and DNA fragmentation.** These data indicate that Dp3-Sam might induce apoptosis in HL-60 cells through a ROS-mediated mitochondrial dysfunction pathway. These findings enhance our understanding for anticancer function of Hibiscus anthocyanins in herbal medicine (**Delphinidin 3-sambubioside, a Hibiscus anthocyanin, induces apoptosis in human leukemia cells through reactive oxygen species-mediated mitochondrial pathway.** Hou,-D-X; Tong,-X;

Terahara,-N; Luo,-D; Fujii,-M. Arch-Biochem-Biophys. 2005 Aug 1; 440(1): 101-9). **I believe that this confirms the prooxidant activity of anthocyanins.**

2.2.4.3 Anthocyanins block colon cancer cells ==

Nutr Cancer. 2003 ;46 (2):186-96 14690795 (P,S,G,E,B)

Anthocyanin-Rich Extract From Aronia meloncarpa E. Induces a Cell Cycle Block in Colon Cancer but Not Normal Colonic Cells.

Minnie Malik, Cuiwei Zhao, Norberta Schoene, M Monica Guisti, Mary P Moyer, Bernadene A Magnuson

Department of Nutrition and Food Science, University of Maryland, College Park, MD.

Anthocyanin-rich extracts, potent antioxidants and commercially available food coloring agents, have been reported to inhibit growth of various cancer cell lines. We investigated the effect of semipurified anthocyanin-rich extract from fruits of Aronia meloncarpa, on normal colon and colon cancer cell lines. A 24-h exposure to 50 mg monomeric anthocyanin/ml of Aronia extract resulted in 60% growth inhibition of human HT-29 colon cancer cells. The treated cells showed a blockage at G1/G0 and G2/M phases of the cell cycle. The cell cycle arrest coincided with an increased expression of the p21WAF1 and p27KIP1 genes and decreased expression of cyclin A and B genes. Prolonged exposure to the extract resulted in no further change in the cell number, indicating a cytostatic inhibition of cell growth. NCM460 normal colon cells demonstrated <10% growth inhibition at the highest concentration of 50 mg/ml extract. A 35% decrease in the cyclooxygenase-2 gene expression was observed within 24 h of exposure of HT-29 cells but did not translate into decreased protein levels or protein activity. These results support the need for further research to identify the specific component(s) in this extract that suppress cancer cell growth and the genes affected by these natural compounds.

2.2.4.4 Anthocyanins prevent cellular malignant transformation ==

Prevention of malignant transformation: Anthocyanins prevent cellular malignant transformation. Moreover, anthocyanins have been probed to induce apoptosis in some malignant cells. This characteristic is extremely important since, as was shown above, anthocyanins are protective for normal cells. A recent publication from Feng et al (Feng 2007) brings light over this apparent contradiction and reinforces the selectivity of anthocyanins anti-tumorous activity. **Feng found that Cyanidin-3-rutenoside selectively kills leukemic cells (HL-60 cells) by induction of oxidative stress. Anthocyanins induce peroxide accumulation and apoptosis in HL-60 cells.** In addition, cyanidin-3-rutinoside treatment resulted in reactive oxygen species (ROS)-dependent activation of p38 MAPK and c-jun NH2-terminal kinase (JNK), which contributed to cell death by activating the mitochondrial pathway mediated by Bim. Notably, cyanidin-3-rutinoside treatment did not lead to Increased ROS accumulation in normal human peripheral blood mononuclear cells and had no cytotoxic effects on these cells (Feng 2007). Molecular mechanisms behind the chemoprotective effects of anthocyanins can be inferred from all the biological effects already mentioned. Hou et al (Hou 2004) proposed similar mechanisms including modulation of MAPK pathway, AP-1 factor, NF-kB pathway, Cyclooxigenase-2 gene and JNK-mediated caspase activation. Though more information is available every day; the current information should be enough to support the use of anthocyanines.

(Feng R., Ni H., Wang S.Y., Tourkova I. L., Shurin M. R., Harada H. and Yin X. **Cyanidin-3-rutinoside, a Natural Polyphenol Antioxidant, Selectively Kills Leukemic Cells by Induction of Oxidative Stress.** *The journal of biological chemistry.* 2007; 282(18): 13468–13476).

Block et al (Block 2007) performed a systematic review of the literature in order to compile results from randomized trials that evaluate concurrent use of antioxidants with chemotherapy.

Still, Block et al. concluded that the review "provides suggestive evidence that antioxidant supplementation helps reduce some adverse reactions including neurotoxicity, thrombocytopenia, diarrhea, thus enabling increased or uninterrupted dosing in patients who otherwise may discontinue treatment due to side effects". The review did not detect diminished chemotherapeutic efficacy in patients receiving antioxidant supplementation in randomized trials and suggest that "the clinical application of antioxidant supplementation during chemotherapy should be further explored" (Block 2007). Block K. I., Koch M. C., Mead M. N., M. N., Tothy P. K.,

Newman R.A., Gyllenhaal C. **Impact of antioxidant supplementation on chemotherapeutic efficacy: A systematic review of the evidence from randomized controlled trials.** *Cancer Treat Rev.* 2007 doi:10.1016/j.ctrv.2007.01.005

2.2.5.0 Down Syndrome: The fallacy of the big vitamin deficiency.

By way of an update on Down Syndrome vitamins, a prestigious number of people in between 2006 and 2008, including several research fellows, a professor of clinical epidemiology, a professor of biochemistry, a senior lecturer in statistics, a senior lecturer in community child health, a consultant developmental paediatrician, a professor of paediatric epidemiology and several others of note, undertook a major research project into the effect of vitamins, antioxidants and folinic acid on the development of infants with Down Syndrome.

The infants with Down Syndrome were started on the vitamins etc prior age 7 months and continued taking the vitamins etc to age 18 months. **The findings were categorically negative - the vitamins etc did not help improve language nor psychomotor development of infants with Down Syndrome.**

Further, they pointed out that using these vitamins etc could prove dangerous in the long term and that as there was no value demonstrated in taking the vitamins etc for those with Down Syndrome, that the selling of such to those with Down Syndrome was **based on commercial interests of those selling them.**

So the bottom line appears to be the one I came to several years ago, that Downs Syndrome vitamins don't work.

Source: http://www.cdadc.com/ds/vitamins.htm

2.2.6.0 Pau d'Arco

This treatment modality is used in place of conventional therapies to treat cancer. Seek advice from a qualified physician before replacing standard cancer therapy with pau d'arco therapy.

What does pau d'arco therapy involve? Pau d'arco is a tree found in the rainforests of Central and South America. Its common names include lapacho, taheebo and trumpet tree. The inner bark of pau d'arco is used by native tribes to treat cancer, lupus, infectious diseases, wounds, backache, toothache and sexually transmitted diseases. Pau d'arco is available in health food stores as capsules, tablets, alcohol solutions, dried bark and tea. However, **pau d'arco must be boiled**

for at least eight minutes to release the active ingredients, making a tea from the bark ineffective unless properly prepared.

How is pau d'arco thought to treat cancer? The medicinal value of pau d'arco is thought to reside in certain compounds, called naphthaquinones, in the inner bark. Proponents claim that naphthaquinones enhance the immune system, cleanse the body and stimulate the production of red blood cells, which can increase the amount of oxygen the blood can carry contributing to healing.

What has been proven about the benefit of pau d'arco? Naphthaquinones, the active commons in pau d'arco bark, have shown potent antifungal properties in laboratory tests. These same compounds also have anticancer properties. Pau d'arco has killed lung cancer cells grown in the laboratory and reduced the rate of lung tumor growth in mice. Unfortunately, it must be taken in very toxic doses for any effects to occur. **Because of the toxic effects, the National Cancer Institute did not seek approval to use pau d'arco as an anticancer drug** and research has, for the most part, ceased. The **American Cancer Society urges patients to avoid pau d'arco** as an alternative treatment for cancer until more evidence is available.

What is the potential risk or harm of pau d'arco? The whole bark has no known side effects. The unrefined bark is much safer than taking extracts of the active ingredients. High doses of **naphthaquinones** can cause uncontrolled bleeding, nausea and vomiting.

How much does pau d'arco cost? Costs will vary depending on the health food store where it is purchased. Because health food products are not regulated for quality and purity, the amount of pau d'arco in different products varies. Some may only contain trace amounts of the active ingredients.

Source: University of California, San Diego

Pau d'arco

source: ACS website

common name(s): lapachol, lapacho, lapacho morado, lapacho Colorado, ipe roxo, ipes, taheebo, tahuari, trumpet bush, trumpet tree

Scientific/medical name(s): *Tabebuia impetiginosa* or *Tabebuia avellanedae*; other species include *Tabebuia heptaphylla, Tabebuia ipé*

Description

Pau d'arco is a large tree that grows in the rainforests of Central and South America, although it may be cultivated in southern Florida. There are about 100 species of the tree, which produces large flowers and can grow to 150 feet tall and 6 feet in diameter. *Tebebuia impetiginosa* produces purple or pink flowers, while other varieties produce yellow or white. The inner bark of the tree is used in herbal remedies.

Overview

Laboratory and animal studies suggest that lapachol and other compounds extracted from or made from pau d'arco may have some effects against certain illnesses, but available evidence from well-designed, controlled studies has not supported this substance as an effective treatment for cancer in humans. Pau d'arco also has potentially dangerous side effects. (See the section "Are there any possible problems or complications?" below.)

How is it promoted for use?

Pau d'arco is promoted as a cure for dozens of illnesses and medical conditions, including arthritis, ulcers, diabetes, and cancer. Proponents also claim that when taken internally it relieves infections, reduces inflammation, promotes digestion, strengthens the immune system, flushes toxins from the body, and protects against cardiovascular disease and high blood pressure. They also use it to treat lupus, osteomyelitis, Parkinson's disease, psoriasis, and to relieve pain. Some use boiled bark externally as a poultice, or the strained liquid as a skin wash to treat skin inflammation, fungal infections, hemorrhoids, eczema, and wounds. The consensus of available scientific evidence does not support claims that pau d'arco can prevent or cure disease.

What does it involve?

Pau d'arco is available in capsules, tablets, salves, liquid extracts, powder, and teas from health food stores and over the Internet. Recommended dosage varies by manufacturer. When making tea, practitioners say the bark must be boiled or simmered for at least 8 minutes to release the active ingredients, which do not dissolve easily in water.

What is the history behind it?

A tea made from pau d'arco is thought to have been a popular herb among the **ancient Incas** and natives of the South American rain forests, who used it to cure disease and as a tonic to strengthen the body and improve overall health. Caribbean folk healers reportedly use the leaf and the bark to treat backaches, toothaches, and sexually transmitted diseases. The native tribes of Brazil used the tree to make bows for hunting. When the Portuguese colonized Brazil, they named the tree **pau d'arco, which means "bow stick**." The herb remains a popular Brazilian folk remedy.

New interest in pau d'arco arose in the mid-1960s when a Brazilian physician claimed that the substance relieved pain, increased the number of red blood cells, and cured numerous illnesses, including cancer. Since the early 1980s, the herb has been sold in health food stores in the United States, where it is promoted as a treatment for virtually every kind of medical complaint.

What is the evidence?

One of the active ingredients in pau d'arco that has been studied is called lapachol. In laboratory animals, lapachol was found to be effective against malaria and certain kinds of animal tumor cells, such as sarcoma, but it did not have an effect against other kinds of cancer, including leukemia and adenocarcinoma. Even though animal and laboratory studies may show promise, further studies are required to find out if the results apply to humans.

There have only been a few studies on lapachol in humans. An uncontrolled study sponsored by the National Cancer Institute in the early 1970s found no toxic effects on liver or kidney tissue, although **it did prevent blood from clotting. Doses that were thought to be high enough to affect tumors posed a serious risk of bleeding.** Clotting times returned to normal when the drug was stopped. Based on these results, approval was not sought for lapachol as a new anti-cancer drug, research in the area was discontinued, and **Canada banned the substance in 1985**.

Pau d'arco contains at least 20 other active compounds, including naphthaquinones (such as lapachol), anthraquinones, alkaloids, and quercetin and other flavonoids whose effects are not fully known. Unconfirmed tests showed that crude extracts of the tree bark stimulated activity of certain immune system cells (macrophages). The substance also killed lung cancer and liver cancer cells grown in test tubes and reduced the rate of lung cancer spread in mice after they had surgery to remove the initial tumor. The bark extract also may kill bacteria or fungi. In a 2004 study, two compounds made from naphthaquinones **showed promise in animal studies for malaria treatment.** It is also important to note that extracted compounds are not the same as the raw bark, and study results are not likely to show the same effects.

2.2.7.0 EMOD generation in thyroid cells by naphthaquinone

Investigators examined whether superoxide (O_2^-) is produced as a precursor of hydrogen peroxide (H_2O_2) in cultured thyroid cells using the cytochrome c method and the electron paramagnetic resonance (EPR) method. No O_2^- or its related radicals was detected in thyroid cells under the physiological condition. The presence of quinone, 2,3-dimethoxy-l-naphthoquinone (DMNQ), or 2-methyl-1, 4-naphthoquinone (menadione), in the medium produced O_2^- and hydroxyl radicals (OH•); the amount of H_2O_2 generation was also increased. Incubation of follicles with DMNQ or menadione inhibited iodine organification (a step of thyroid hormone formation) and its catalytic enzyme, thyroid peroxidase (TPO). **This inhibition should be caused by reactive oxygen species because the two quinones, particularly DMNQ, exert their effect through the generation of reactive oxygen species.** It is speculated that the site-specific inactivation of TPO might have occurred at the heme-linked histidine residue of the TPO molecule, a critical amino acid for enzyme activity because OH• (vicious free radicals) can be formed at the iron-linked amino acid. TPO mRNA level and electrophoretic mobility of TPO were not inhibited by quinones. Our study suggests **that thyroid H_2O_2 is produced by divalent reduction of oxygen without O_2^- generation.** If thyroid cells happen to be exposed to significant amount of reactive oxygen species, TPO and subsequent thyroid hormone formation are inhibited.

The thyroid gland produces H_2O_2 by the NADPH oxidase system of the apical membrane and it utilizes H_2O_2 as a substrate of thyroid peroxidase (TPO) for thyroid hormone formation. The thyroid gland contains superoxide dismutase (SOD), which converts O_2^- to H_2O_2. However, whether the thyroid cell actually produces O_2^- has been controversial; conflicting results have been published. In a simplified cell-free experiment, incubation of lactperoxidase (an analog of TPO) with excess H_2O_2 in the presence of iodide has been shown to produce O_2^- and hydroxyl radicals (OH•).

(Generation of Oxygen Free Radicals in Thyroid Cells and Inhibition of Thyroid Peroxidase. Masahiro Sugawara, Yoshinobu Sugawar, Katherine Wen and Cecilia Giulivi. *Experimental Biology and Medicine* 227:141-146 (2002).

2.2.8.0 Lapacho (naphthoquinone) generates tumoricidal EMODs ==

The highly active, quinone-containing anticancer drugs, Adriamycin, daunorubicin, carminomycin, rubidazone, nogalamycin, aclacinomycin A, and steffimycin (benzanthraquinones); mitomycin C and streptonigrin (/V-heterocyclic quiÃ±ones); and lapacho (naphthoquinone) interact with mammalian microsomes and function as free radical carriers. These quinone drugs augment the flow of electrons from reduced nicotinamide adenine dinucleotide phosphate to molecular oxygen as measured by enhanced reduced nicotinamide adenine dinucleotide phosphate oxidation and oxygen consumption. This reaction is catalyzed by microsomal protein and **produces a free radical intermediate form of the drugs** as determined by electron paramagnetic resonance spectroscopy. Microsomes from mouse and rat liver, heart, lung, and spleen and mouse L1210 and P388 tumors all catalyze the augmented oxygen consumption. Apparent Km values determined with normal rat liver microsomes range from 0.49 x 10~ "Mfor steffimycin to 13.4 x 10~" M for lapacho. Since SKF 525A and carbon monoxide have little effect on this reaction, cytochrome P-450 is probably not involved. Several nonquinone anticancer agents were tested and were found inactive in the system. Since quinone anticancer drugs are associated with chromosomal damage that appears to be dependent on metabolic activation of these drugs, we propose that the intracellular activation of these drugs to a free radical state may be primary to their cytotoxic activity. As free radicals, these drugs, because of their high affinity and selective binding to nucleic acids, have the potential to be "site-specific free radicals" that bind to DNA or RNA and either react directly or **generate oxygen-dependent free radicals such as Superoxide radical or hydroxyl radical to cause the damage associated with their cytotoxic actions.** (A General Mechanism for Microsomal Activation of Quinone Anticancer Agents to Free Radicals. Nicholas R. Bachur, Sandra L. Gordon, and Malcolm V. Gee. CANCER RESEARCH 38, 1745-1750, June 1978).

2.2.9.0 Oysters contain EMOD-apoptosis-inducing ceramides (blocked by antioxidants)

Ceramide is one of the major sphingosine-based lipid second messengers that is generated in response to various extracellular agents. However, while widespread attention has focused on ceramide as a second messenger involved in the induction of apoptosis, important issues with regard to the mechanisms of ceramide formation and mode of action remain to be addressed. Several lines of evidence suggest that ceramide and oxidative stress are intimately related in cell death induction. This review focuses on the putative relationships between oxidative stress and sphingolipid metabolism in the apoptotic process and discusses the potential mechanisms that connect and regulate the two phenomena (Ceramide in apoptosis signaling: relationship with oxidative stress. Nathalie Andrieu-Abadie et al. Free Radical Biology and Medicine. Volume 31, Issue 6, 15 September 2001, Pages 717-728).

Anthracyclines such as daunorubicin (DNR) generate radical oxygen species (ROS), which account, at least in part, for their cytotoxic effect. We observed that early ceramide generation (within 6–10 min) through neutral sphingomyelinase stimulation was **inhibitable by the antioxidants *N*-acetylcysteine and pyrrolidine dithiocarbamate, which led to a decrease in apoptosis** (.95% decrease in DNA fragmentation after 6 h). Furthermore, we observed that DNR triggers the c-Jun N-terminal kinase (JNK) and the transcription factor activated protein-1 through an antioxidant-inhibitable mechanism. **Treatment of U937 cells with cell-permeant ceramides induced both an increase in ROS generation and JNK activation, and apoptosis, all of which were antioxidant-sensitive.** In conclusion, DNR-triggered apoptosis implicates a ceramide-mediated, ROS-dependent JNK and activated protein-1 activation. (Implication of Radical Oxygen Species in Ceramide Generation, c-Jun N-Terminal Kinase Activation and Apoptosis Induced by Daunorubicin. Ve´ Ronique Mansat-De Mas et al. Molecular Pharmacology, 56:867–874 (1999).

2.2.9.1 Onion oil EMOD-induced apoptosis blocked by NAC and glutathione ==

Protective effects of Allium vegetables against cancers have been shown extensively in experimental animals and epidemiologic studies. We investigated cell proliferation and the induction of apoptosis by **onion oil** extracted from Allium cepa, a widely consumed Allium vegetable, in **human lung cancer A549 cells**. GC/MS analysis suggested that propyl sulfides but not allyl sulfides are major sulfur-containing constituents of onion oil. Onion oil at 12.5 mg/L significantly induced apoptosis (13% increase of apoptotic cells) as indicated by sub-G1 DNA content. It also caused cell cycle arrest at the G2/M phase; 25 mg/L onion oil increased the percentage of G2/M cells almost 6-fold compared with the dimethyl sulfoxide control. The action of onion oil may occur via a reactive oxygen species–dependent pathway because **cell cycle arrest and apoptosis were blocked by the antioxidants N-acetylcysteine and exogenous glutathione.** Marked collapse of the mitochondrial membrane potential suggested that **dysfunction of the mitochondria may be involved in the oxidative burst and apoptosis induced by onion oil.** Expression of phospho-cdc2 and phospho-cyclin B1 were downregulated by onion oil, perhaps accounting for the G2/M arrest. Overall, these results suggest that onion oil may exert chemopreventive action by inducing cell cycle arrest and apoptosis in tumor cells (The Production of Reactive Oxygen Species and the Mitochondrial Membrane Potential Are Modulated during Onion Oil–Induced Cell Cycle Arrest and Apoptosis in A549 Cells. Xin-jiang Wu et al. American Society for Nutrition J. Nutr. 136:608-613, March 2006).

2.3.0.0 EMODs control apoptosis ==

Reactive oxygen species are widely generated in biological systems. Consequently humans have evolved antioxidant defence systems that limit their production. **Intracellular production of active oxygen species such as –√OH, O_2– and H_2O_2 is associated with the arrest of cell proliferation. Similarly, generation of oxidative stress in response to various external stimuli has been implicated in the activation of transcription factors and to the triggering of apoptosis.** Investigators reviewed how free radicals induce DNA sequence changes in the form of mutations, deletions, gene amplification and rearrangements. **These alterations may result in the initiation of apoptosis signalling leading to cell death, or to the activation of several proto-oncogenes and/or the inactivation of some tumour suppressor genes.** The regulation of gene expression by means of oxidants, antioxidants and the redox state remains as a promising therapeutic approach. **Several anticarcinogenic agents have been shown to inhibit reactive oxygen species production and oxidative DNA damage, inhibiting tumour promotion. (RMH Note: this is merely showing that a low level of EMODs allows for the development of neoplasia and not that EMODs are causing cancer.).** In addition, **recombinant vectors expressing radical-scavenging enzymes reduce apoptosis.** In conclusion, oxidative stress has been implicated in both apoptosis and the pathogenesis of cancer providing contrived support for two notions: free radical reactions may be increased in malignant cells and oxidant scavenging systems may be useful in cancer therapy (Role of reactive oxygen species in apoptosis: implications for cancer therapy. José M. Matés and Francisca M. Sánchez-Jiménez. The International Journal of Biochemistry & Cell Biology. Volume 32, Issue 2, February 2000, Pages 157-170).

2.3.1.0 EMODs cause spontaneous regression of cancer (melanoma)

Investigators described before that **oxidative burst of granulocytes is cytotoxic for melanoma B16F10 and for Walker 256 carcinoma (W256)**. Therefore, we assumed that granulocytes could also be important mechanism of the host defence against tumour. In current study we report **massive granulocyte infiltration at the site of W256 transplanted in the hind limb of Sprague–Dawley associated with spontaneous tumour regression observed for 22/25 rats (87%). Peripheral blood granulocytes of these animals were highly cytotoxic for W256 cells cultured in vitro.** After the tumour disappearance the inflammatory oxidative burst of the granulocytes ended. Distraction of granulocytes from the tumour by s.c. Sephadex injection decreased the incidence of the W256 regression to only 7/25 animals (30%). These results suggest that **innate immunity based on immune competent granulocytes may be the cause of well known phenomenon of spontaneous regression of W256 carcinoma** (The involvement of granulocytes in spontaneous regression of Walker 256 carcinoma. M. Jaganjac, M. Poljak-Blazi, K. Zarkovic, R. Schaur, N. Zarkovic. *Cancer Letters*, Volume 260, Issue 1, 18 February 2008, Pages 180-186).

2.3.1.1 Lipid coated viruses and bacteria

Lipid coated viruses:

Human immunodeficiency virus HIV-1 or HIV+
Measles virus
Herpes simplex virus-1 (HSV-1)
Herpes simplex virus-2 (HSV-2)
Herpes viridae (all)
Human lymphotropic viruses (type 1)
Vesicular stomatitis virus (VSV)
Vienna virus
Cytomegalovirus
Epstein-Barr virus
Influenza virus
Leukemia virus
Pneumonovirus
Sarcoma virus
Synctial virus
Rubeola virus

Lipid coated Bacteria
Listeria monocytogenes
Heliobacter pylori (gram negative)
Hemophilus influenzae (gram positive)
Staphylococcus agalactiae
Groups A, B, F and G streptococci
Gramm-positive organisms
Gram-negative organisms if pretreated with chelator
Source: http://www.lauric.org/lcv.html

I believe that all of the above organisms can be treated by increasing oxidative levels, such that the lipid coats are destroyed and the organism is inactivated and rendered harmless. Prevention can be effected by sustaining an EMOD sufficiency.

2.3.2.0 Spontaneous Cancer Regression in Melanoma Pigs

Incomplete spontaneous regression of melanoma is common. However, complete melanoma regression is still a very rare phenomenon. Because **melanoma is the most immunogenic human malignancy**, the mechanisms leading to regression, based on accumulative evidence, are the host's immune responses. Unfortunately, therapies aiming to enhance the patient's natural immunity against melanoma have yet to meet their expectations. Reasons for failure include various immune escape mechanisms, induced by the tumor, that subsequently lead to tolerance. Here, we performed time-dependent gene expression profiling to unravel molecular changes involved in the transition of progressive melanoma to complete tumor regression using a porcine model. **The melanoblastoma-bearing Libechov minipigs are highly suitable for this study because these animals exhibit naturally occurring and regressing melanomas.** We were able to identify a molecular signature of the melanoma regression process. Genes regulated in this signature were associated with 1) cell cycle, 2) immune response, and 3) melanocyte differentiation. These genes may shed light on molecular mechanisms involved in complete melanoma regression and indicate what improvements are needed for successful antimelanoma therapy (Gene Expression Signature for Spontaneous Cancer Regression in Melanoma Pigs. Florian Rambow et al. Neoplasia. 2008 July; 10(7): 714–726).

2.3.3.0 Hyperthermia inhibits tumor growth ==

Also, we must remember that hyperthermia has tumoricidal properties, which is in part due to increased EMODs.

Tumour cells are selectively inhibited by hyperthermia (41–42.5°C) in the same conditions where normal cells are not damaged. At higher temperature, also normal cells are injured. In spite of the large number of reports on the cytotoxic effect of hyperthermia the mechanisms of heat cytotoxicity are yet unclear. It appears plausible that concomitant phenomena, triggered by heat and related each other, may be involved. The major points on this subject are the following:

Heat appears to increase the flux of oxygen free radicals mediating in part the cytotoxicity.

(On the Biochemical Basis of Tumour amage by Hypothermia. Paola Pietrangeli and Bruno Mondovì. Book: Hyperthermia in Cancer Treatment: A Primer. SpringerLink May 8, 2008**).**

2.3.4.0 Hyperoxia increases spontaneous regression

Pulmonary neuroendocrine cell (PNEC) hyperplasia is associated with chronic lung diseases in humans, where it is thought to play a role in reparative responses to lung injury. To investigate the kinetics of strongly induced PNEC hyperplasia in an animal model, we exposed hamsters to a combination of **hyperoxia (60% O2)** and diethylnitrosamine (DEN) for up to 20 weeks. We thus demonstrate not only **the induction but also spontaneous regression of intense PNEC differentiation and growth, which are much more intense than those observed with DEN alone**. (Induction and Spontaneous Regression of Intense Pulmonary Neuroendocrine Cell Differentiation in a Model of Preneoplastic Lung Injury. Mary E. Sunday2 and Christopher G. Willett. (CANCER RESEARCH (SUPPL.) 52. 2677s-2686s. May l. 1992). **I believe that this illustrates the positive impact of hyperoxia on spontaneous regression.**

2.3.5.0 Spontaneous regression of cancer

Because most cancers that are detected are also treated**, there are only a few reports documenting spontaneous regression of breast cancer** (Dussan C, Zubor P, Fernandez M, Yabar A, Szunyogh N, Visnovsky J. Spontaneous regression of a breast carcinoma: a case report. *Gynecol Obstet*

Invest. 2008;65(3):206-211) (Krutchik AN, Buzdar AU, Blumenschein GR, Lukeman JM. Spontaneous regression of breast carcinoma. *Arch Intern Med.* 1978;138(11):1734-1735).

However, **spontaneous regression of advanced cancer has long been recognized in metastatic melanoma and metastatic renal cell carcinoma**, and, in fact, such observations have motivated the interest in immunotherapy in these settings (Printz C. Spontaneous regression of melanoma may offer insight into cancer immunology. *J Natl Cancer Inst.* 2001;93(14):1047-1048) (Gleave ME, Elhilali M, Fradet Y; et al, Canadian Urologic Oncology Group. Interferon gamma-1b compared with placebo in metastatic renal-cell carcinoma. *N Engl J Med.* 1998;338(18):1265-1271) (de Gast GC, Klümpen HJ, Vyth-Dreese FA; et al. Phase I trial of combined immunotherapy with subcutaneous granulocyte macrophage colony-stimulating factor, low-dose interleukin 2, and interferon alpha in progressive metastatic melanoma and renal cell carcinoma. *Clin Cancer Res.* 2000;6(4):1267-1272).

Furthermore, **more systematic investigations of spontaneous regression are beginning to be reported in the context of screen-detected abnormalities.** There are data suggesting that **regression routinely occurs in colonic adenomas** (both from the National Polyp Study and others) (Loeve F, Boer R, Zauber AG; et al. National Polyp Study data: evidence for regression of adenomas. *Int J Cancer.* 2004;111(4):633-639) (Hofstad B, Vatn MH, Andersen SN; et al. Growth of colorectal polyps: redetection and evaluation of unresected polyps for a period of three years. *Gut.* 1996;39(3):449-456).

There is a growing literature **documenting regression in precancerous lesions of the cervix** (Schlecht NF, Platt RW, Duarte-Franco E; et al. Human papillomavirus infection and time to progression and regression of cervical intraepithelial neoplasia. *J Natl Cancer Inst.* 2003;95(17):1336-1343) (Moscicki AB, Shiboski S, Hills NK; et al. Regression of low-grade squamous intra-epithelial lesions in young women. *Lancet.* 2004;364(9446):1678-1683).

Documentation of regression in screen-detected cancer is limited to neuroblastoma, for which investigators have found that screening detects far more cancer than will ever become clinically apparent and that a substantial proportion regress (Schilling FH, Spix C, Berthold F; et al. Neuroblastoma screening at one year of age. *N Engl J Med.* 2002;346(14):1047-1053) (Yamamoto K, Hanada R, Kikuchi A; et al. Spontaneous regression of localized neuroblastoma detected by mass screening. *J Clin Oncol.* 1998;16(4):1265-1269).

Spontaneous regression has been seen in:

- **metastatic melanoma**
- **metastatic renal cell carcinoma**
- **precancerous lesions of the cervix**
- **neuroblastoma**
- **some prostate**
- **some lungs**

2.3.5.1 Spontaneous regression of malignant breast cancer

Spontaneous regression of malignant tumors is a rare event. It is defined as partial or total disappearance of a proven malignant tumor without adequate medical treatment. The causes of this phenomenon are various. Nevertheless, **malignant tumors do regress occasionally for no apparent reason,** as evidenced by many clinical observations. We report a case of a 68-year-old woman, who was presented with a several-month history of a painless firm lump, initially of 1 cm in diameter and growing to a large solid regular tumor of 2.5 × 2.5 cm in size, in the upper outer quadrant of her right breast. Preoperative histopathological diagnosis revealed ductal invasive carcinoma. Later on, while awaiting surgical treatment, she suffered an arm injury requiring a 1-month delay of surgery. After recovery, on the date of surgery the tumor disappeared, and, in addition, it was not found in tissue specimens obtained from quadrantectomy. After 78 months of follow-up there was no evidence of relapse. In this report, we discuss clinical and histopathological findings, patient management and possible mechanisms of cancer regression (Spontaneous Regression of a Breast Carcinoma: A Case Report. Carlos Dussan, Pavol Zubor, Manuel Fernandez, Alejandro Yabar, Norbert Szunyogh, Jozef Visnovsky. *Gynecol Obstet Invest* 2008;65:206-211). **I believe that the "trauma" of the biopsy could have stimulated a strong oxidative WBC response, which produced EMODs and caused the apoptosis.**

2.3.5.2 Some breast cancers may resolve without treatment

Provided by: Canadian Press

Written by: Helen Branswell, THE CANADIAN PRESS

Nov. 24, 2008

A significant portion of invasive breast cancers may regress on their own without treatment, a new study that is bound to provoke controversy suggests.

The study, published 11/24/08 in the journal Archives of Internal Medicine, suggested **breast cancer screening may be leading to over diagnosis of cancer**, with upwards of 22 per cent of cases likely to resolve themselves without treatment.

Once a breast cancer is found, however, it wouldn't currently be considered ethical not to treat. So - **if the theory is correct - large numbers of women may be having surgeries, radiation, chemotherapy and other treatments that would never have been needed if their cancers hadn't been detected**.

"If we are right, then this is a kind of paradigm shift," said lead author Dr. Per-Henrik Zahl, a senior statistician with the Norwegian Institute of Public Health. Zahl, who admitted he has been trying to get the study published for about four years, said the risks of over diagnosis of breast cancer are real.

Radiation can do significant and permanent damage to the heart and coronary arteries. Chemotherapy can cause cognitive confusion. And surgery that involves the removal of lymph nodes can cause lymphedema, the painful swelling of the arm closest to the involved breast.

Dr. Patrick Remington has been studying the idea of self-limiting breast cancers since the early 1990s, when the introduction of breast screening programs showed a sharp and sustained increase in the incidence of the disease in the United States. **He is convinced some invasive breast cancers do regress**; they have become known as **LMPs or cancers of "limited malignant potential."**

"I would say a very good guess would be about one out of three women have cancers detected today that would not have progressed otherwise," said Remington, a professor of population health sciences at the University of Wisconsin. Remington was not involved in this study. He notes **some other types of cancers - prostate and recently lung - have been shown to spontaneously regress in some patients**.

In the case of prostate cancer, some physicians urge an approach known as watchful waiting, where patients are monitored to see if their disease is progressing; only then is it treated. That approach is not currently an option with breast cancer.

Zahl's findings are likely to spark heated debate. In fact, he acknowledged several journals refused to publish the study before it was accepted by Archives of Internal Medicine, a journal published by the American Medical Association.

But an editorial in the journal stressed that **the findings are consistent with several observations about breast cancer that have troubled investigators for years**.

And the editorial's authors, Dr. Robert Kaplan of the UCLA School of Public Health and Dr. Franz Porzsolt of Germany's Clinical Economics University of Ulm, said **the hypothesis of breast cancer regression, while counterintuitive, is "difficult to rule out**."

"We know from autopsy studies that a significant number of women die (from other causes) without knowing that they had breast cancer," they noted.

Dr. Steven Narod, a leading breast cancer researcher at Toronto's Sunnybrook Health Sciences Centre, agreed the findings are persuasive. "I do agree with them that the best explanation of the findings is that about 10 to 20 per cent of the breast cancers ... disappeared on their own," he said. "I'm still a bit skeptical and there's alternative explanations, but I think this one is worth paying attention to."

In what Narod described as an "elegant" study design, Zahl and his colleagues used the introduction of a breast cancer screening program in Norway to explore the question.

They compared breast cancer rates among nearly **120,000 women** who had three rounds of mammography between 1996 and 2001 to those among nearly 110,000 women of the same age range (50 to 64) in the five-year period preceding the start of the breast cancer screening program. Those women, known as the controls, had one mammogram.

In statistical terms, the two groups of women were identical. Their educational profile was closely matched, they had roughly the same average family income and the same average number of children. So the rates of cancers in the two groups should have been equal.

In fact, **the women who hadn't been regularly screened had 22 per cent fewer breast cancers.**

The authors explore a number of arguments about why that might be. They noted for instance that use of hormone replacement therapy in the part of Norway where the women lived increased substantially between 1996 and 2001, the period when the screened women were undergoing regular mammograms. **HRT use is linked to increased risk of breast cancer.**

But the authors conclude none of the potential other explanations could account for such a large difference between the two groups.

"All the caveats that could be explored have been explored in terms of accounting for the things that people would call ... weaknesses" of the study, agreed Dr. Cornelia Baines, a professor in the University of Toronto's school of public health and co-principal investigator of a landmark study into mammography, the Canadian National Breast Screening Study.

Baines, who has been diagnosed with breast cancer which was earlier missed in a mammogram, said the findings are important. But she added that even if Zahl and his co-authors are correct, there's no way currently to put the findings into application. "The incontrovertible truth is that once you've screened a woman and you find an abnormality, you have to biopsy," she said.

"If you biopsy, you have to follow through with surgery if the biopsy reveals malignant tissue. You can't stop that. You can't say: 'Well, I've been screened and there is a chance that this is over diagnosis.' You can't do that."

Finding ways to answer the questions raised by the study will be difficult, experts said. And Remington noted even if doctors could differentiate, women and-or their health-care professionals might still opt for treatment to play it safe.

He suggested, though, **studying women whose cancers regress on their own could teach scientists how to trigger the same response in women whose cancers aren't self-limiting**, and maybe even to prevent breast cancer from developing.

And in the meantime, Baines said, this study may serve as an important reminder to women and the medical community.

"What is important and it seems to me it's been ignored for a long, long time is that ... screening doesn't only have upsides. It has downsides," she said.

"And if women want to accept the downsides and proceed with screening, then that's great. But I personally believe that they should only make that choice when they are fully informed. And a lot of them have not been fully informed about the over diagnosis scenario."

Abstract: November 24, 2008 edition of the *Archives of Internal Medicine*

Prof Randolph M. Howes MD, PhD

The Natural History of Invasive Breast Cancers Detected by Screening Mammography

Per-Henrik Zahl, MD, PhD; Jan Moehlen, MD, PhD; H. Gilbert Welch, MD, MPH

Background: The introduction of screening mammography has been associated with sustained increases in breast cancer incidence. The natural history of these screen-detected cancers is not well understood.

Methods: We compared cumulative breast cancer incidence in age-matched cohorts of women residing in 4 Norwegian counties before and after the initiation of biennial mammography. The screened group included all women who were invited for all 3 rounds of screening during the period 1996 through 2001 (age range in 1996, 50-64 years). The control group included all women who would have been invited for screening had there been a screening program during the period 1992 through 1997 (age range in 1992, 50-64 years). All women in the control group were invited to undergo a 1-time prevalence screen at the end of their observation period. Screening attendance was similar in both groups (screened, 78.3%, and controls, 79.5%). Counts of incident invasive breast cancers were obtained from the Norwegian Cancer Registry (in situ cancers were excluded).

Results: As expected, before the age-matched controls were invited to be screened at the end of their observation period, the cumulative incidence of invasive breast cancer was significantly higher in the screened group than in the controls (4-year cumulative incidence:1268vs810per100 000 population; relative rate, 1.57;95%confidenceinterval,1.44-1.70). Even after prevalence screening in controls, however, the cumulative incidence of invasive breast cancer remained 22% higher in the screened group (6-year cumulative incidence: 1909vs1564per100 000population; relative rate, 1.22;95%confidence interval, 1.16-1.30). Higher incidence was observed in screened women at each year of age.

Conclusions: Because the cumulative incidence among controls never reached that of the screened group, **it appears that some breast cancers detected by repeated mammographic screening would not persist to be detectable by a single mammogram at the end of 6 years.** This raises the possibility that **the natural course of some screen-detected invasive breast cancers is to spontaneously regress**.

2.3.6.0 Two paths for apoptosis death ==

Apoptosis occurs primarily through two well-recognized pathways in cells, including the intrinsic, or mitochondrial-mediated, effector mechanism and the extrinsic, or death receptor–mediated, effector mechanism.

However, death not only can follow the well-characterized type I apoptotic pathway but also can proceed by nonapoptotic modes such as type II (macroautophagy-related) and type III (necrosis) or combinations thereof. In contrast to apoptosis, the induction of macroautophagy may contribute to either the survival or death of cells in response to a stressor.

2.3.7.0 Resveratrol

2.3.7.1 Resveratrol blocks EMOD-induced apoptosis ==

Epidemiological studies suggest that **Mediterranean diets rich in resveratrol are associated with reduced risk of coronary artery disease**. However, the mechanisms by which resveratrol exerts its vasculoprotective effects are not completely understood. Because oxidative stress and endothelial cell injury play a critical role in vascular aging and atherogenesis, we evaluated whether resveratrol inhibits oxidative stress-induced endothelial apoptosis. We found that oxidized LDL and TNF-α elicited significant increases in caspase-3/7 activity in endothelial cells and cultured rat aortas, which were prevented by resveratrol pretreatment (10^{-6}–10^{-4} mol/l). The protective effect of resveratrol was attenuated by inhibition of glutathione peroxidase and heme oxygenase-1, suggesting a role for antioxidant systems in the antiapoptotic action of resveratrol. Indeed, **resveratrol treatment protected cultured aortic segments and/or endothelial cells against increases in intracellular H_2O_2 levels and H_2O_2-mediated apoptotic cell death induced by oxidative stressors (exogenous H_2O_2, paraquat, and UV light)**. Resveratrol treatment also attenuated UV-induced DNA damage (comet assay). Resveratrol treatment upregulated the expression of glutathione peroxidase, catalase, and heme oxygenase-1 in cultured arteries, whereas it had no significant effect on the expression of SOD isoforms. Resveratrol also effectively scavenged H_2O_2 in vitro. Thus **resveratrol seems to increase vascular oxidative stress resistance by scavenging H_2O_2 and preventing oxidative stress-induced endothelial cell death**. We propose that the antioxidant and antiapoptotic effects of resveratrol, together with its previously described anti-inflammatory actions, are responsible, at least in part, for its cardioprotective effects (Resveratrol increases vascular oxidative stress resistance. Zoltan Ungvari. Am J Physiol Heart Circ Physiol 292: H2417-H2424, 2007).

2.3.7.2 Resveratrol prooxidant activity ==

Investigators recently showed that efficient apoptotic signaling is a function of a permissive intracellular milieu created by a decrease in the ratio of superoxide to hydrogen peroxide and cytosolic acidification. **Resveratrol, a phytoalexin found in grapes and wines, triggers apoptosis in some systems and inhibits the death signal in others**. In this regard, **the reported inhibitory effect on hydrogen peroxide-induced apoptosis has been attributed to its antioxidant property**. Here, we provide evidence that exposure of human leukemia cells to low concentrations of resveratrol (4-8 micro M**) inhibits** caspase activation and DNA fragmentation induced by incubation with hydrogen peroxide or upon triggering apoptosis with a novel compound **that kills via intracellular hydrogen peroxide production.** At these concentrations, **resveratrol elicits pro-oxidant properties as evidenced by an increase in intracellular superoxide concentration.** This pro-oxidant effect is further supported by our observations that the drop in intracellular superoxide and cytosolic acidification induced by hydrogen peroxide is completely blocked in cells preincubated with resveratrol. Thus, **the inhibitory effect of resveratrol on hydrogen peroxide-induced apoptosis is not due to its antioxidant activity, but contrarily via a pro-oxidant effect that creates an intracellular environment nonconducive for apoptotic execution** (Pro-oxidant activity of low doses of resveratrol inhibits hydrogen peroxide-induced apoptosis. Ahmad KA, Clement MV, Pervaiz S. Ann N Y Acad Sci. 2003 Dec;1010:365-73). **The prooxidant activity is well documented but not well known. I believe that its benefits are due to this prooxidant activity, including those with anti-aging. However, the above study is conflicted regarding the mechanism of action of resveratrol.**

2.3.7.3 Resveratrol increases vascular oxidative stress resistance ==

Epidemiological studies suggest that Mediterranean diets rich in resveratrol are associated with reduced risk of coronary artery disease. However, the mechanisms by which resveratrol exerts its vasculoprotective effects are not completely understood. Because oxidative stress and endothelial cell injury play a critical role in vascular aging and atherogenesis, we evaluated whether resveratrol inhibits oxidative stress-induced endothelial apoptosis. We found that oxidized LDL and TNF-α elicited significant increases in caspase-3/7 activity in endothelial cells and cultured rat aortas, which were prevented by resveratrol pretreatment (10^{-6}–10^{-4} mol/l). The protective effect of resveratrol was attenuated by inhibition of glutathione peroxidase and heme oxygenase-1, suggesting a role for antioxidant systems in the antiapoptotic action of resveratrol. Resveratrol treatment protected cultured aortic segments and/or endothelial cells against increases in intracellular H_2O_2 levels and H_2O_2-mediated apoptotic cell death induced by **oxidative stressors (exogenous H_2O_2, paraquat, and UV light)**. Resveratrol treatment also attenuated UV-induced DNA damage (comet assay). Resveratrol treatment upregulated the expression of glutathione peroxidase, catalase, and heme oxygenase-1 in cultured arteries, whereas it had no significant effect on the expression of SOD isoforms. Resveratrol also effectively scavenged H_2O_2 in vitro. Thus resveratrol seems to increase vascular oxidative stress resistance by scavenging H_2O_2 and preventing oxidative stress-induced endothelial cell death. We propose that the antioxidant and antiapoptotic effects of resveratrol, together with its previously described anti-inflammatory actions, are responsible, at least in part, for its cardioprotective effects (Resveratrol increases vascular oxidative stress resistance. Zoltan Ungvari et al. Am J Physiol Heart Circ Physiol 292: H2417-H2424, 2007). **Basically, this tells you that resveratrol in low levels blocks EMOD induced apoptosis.**

2.3.8.0 Catalase over-expression blocks apoptosis and increases tumor growth ==

Glucocorticoids are used for the treatment of lymphoid neoplasms, taking advantage of the well-known ability of these compounds to cause apoptosis in lymphoid tissues. Previously, we have shown that **dexamethasone, a synthetic glucocorticoid, causes a down-regulation of several antioxidant defense enzymes and proteins, including catalase and thioredoxin, concomitant with the induction of apoptosis in WEHI7.2 mouse thymoma cells.** To test whether this down-regulation plays a critical role in the mechanism of steroid-induced apoptosis, WEHI7.2 cells were transfected with rat catalase. Two clones, expressing 1.4-fold and 2.0-fold higher catalase specific activity, respectively, when compared with vector-only transfectants were selected for further study. An increase to 1.4-fold parental cell catalase activity delayed cell loss after dexamethasone treatment, whereas a 2.0-fold parental catalase activity prevented dexamethasone-induced cell loss for 48 h after treatment. Dexamethasone treatment of the WEHI7.2 cells stimulated a release of cytochrome *c* into the cytosol. **Catalase-overexpressing cells showed a delay or lack of cytochrome c release from the mitochondria, which correlated temporally with**

the delay or prevention of cell loss in the culture after dexamethasone treatment. A decreased amount of cell death from WEHI7.2 cells overexpressing catalase was also seen in tumor xenografts in severe combined immunodeficient mice when compared with tumors from vector-only transfected cells. Similarly, thioredoxin-overexpressing WEHI7.2 cells, shown previously to be apoptosis resistant, showed decreased cell death in tumor xenografts. This resulted in larger tumors from cells overexpressing these proteins. Cell death in control transfectant tumor xenografts was primarily attributable to apoptosis. In contrast, the cell death we observed in tumors from thioredoxin- or catalase-overexpressing cells had a higher frequency of a nonapoptotic, nonnecrotic type of cell death termed **para-apoptosis.** These data suggest that: (*a*) **oxidative stress plays a critical role in steroid-induced apoptosis prior to the commitment of the cells to undergo apoptosis; and (*b*) resistance to oxidative stress can contribute to tumor growth** (Catalase-overexpressing Thymocytes Are Resistant to Glucocorticoid-induced Apoptosis and Exhibit Increased Net Tumor Growth. Margaret E. Tome, Amanda F. Baker, Garth Powis, Claire M. Payne and Margaret M. Briehl. *Cancer Research* 61, 2766-2773, March 15, 2001). **I believe that again this emphasizes the true nature of EMOD induced apoptosis in tumor cells.**

2.3.9.0 A Polyphenol antioxidant kills by increasing EMODs ==

Anthocyanins are a group of naturally occurring phenolic compounds widely available in fruits and vegetables in human diets. **They have broad biological activities including anti-mutagenesis and anticarcinogenesis, which are generally attributed to their antioxidant activities.** We studied the effects and the mechanisms of the most common type of anthocyanins, cyanidin-3-rutinoside, in several leukemia and lymphoma cell lines. We found that cyanidin-3-rutinoside extracted and purified from the black raspberry cultivar Jewel **induced apoptosis** in HL-60 cells in a dose- and time-dependent manner. **Paradoxically, this compound induced the accumulation of peroxides, which are involved in the induction of apoptosis in HL-60 cells**. In addition, cyanidin-3-rutinoside treatment resulted in reactive oxygen species (ROS)-dependent activation of p38 MAPK and JNK, which contributed to cell death by activating the mitochondrial pathway mediated by Bim. Down-regulation of Bim or overexpression of Bcl-2 or Bcl-x_L considerably blocked apoptosis. Notably, **cyanidin-3-rutinoside treatment did not lead to increased ROS accumulation in normal human peripheral blood**

mononuclear cells and had no cytotoxic effects on these cells. These results indicate that cyanidin-3-rutinoside has the potential to be used in leukemia therapy with the advantages of being widely available and selective against tumors (Cyanidin-3-rutinoside, a Natural Polyphenol Antioxidant, Selectively Kills Leukemic Cells by Induction of Oxidative Stress. Rentian Feng, Hong-Min Ni, Shiow Y. Wang, Irina L. Tourkova, Michael R. Shurin, Hisashi Harada and Xiao-Ming Yin. J. Biol. Chem., Vol. 282, Issue 18, 13468-13476, May 4, 2007.). **This is the pattern which I see over and over again. EMODs kill cancer cells selectively and do not harm normal cells.**

2.4.0.0 Lung cancer patients have higher GPx and lower SOD levels

The present study aimed to determine the alterations of antioxidant activities in erythrocytes from patients with nonsmall cell lung carcinoma (NSCLC).

A comparative study of the systemic antioxidant activities in red blood cell lysate from subjects with NSCLC and healthy control subjects was conducted. The antioxidants catalase, superoxide dismutase (SOD) and glutathione peroxidase (GPx) were measured using chemical kinetic reactions under spectrophotometry.

In total, 189 cases of mostly advanced-stage IIIB or stage IV NSCLC and 202 healthy controls were studied. In subjects with lung cancer, there was similar catalase activity, **lower SOD activity** (median (interquartile range) 13.4 (9.0–27.2) *versus* 48.7 (27.0–64.3) U ·(ghaemoglobulin(Hb)$^{-1}$), and **higher GPx activity** (175.2 (126.6–288.3) *versus* 49.2 (39.5–59.2) mU ·(gHb)$^{-1}$) compared with controls. The antioxidant activities in lung cancer subjects were not associated with age, sex, smoking status, or tumour cell types. However, **more advanced disease (stage IV compared with stage IIIB) was associated with lower SOD activity**. Using multivariable analysis, the presence of lung cancer independently predicted SOD and GPx activities.

In conclusion, nonsmall cell lung carcinoma in Chinese subjects is associated with alterations in systemic antioxidant activities, which may play an important role in carcinogenesis (Disturbance of systemic antioxidant profile in nonsmall cell lung carcinoma. J. C. Ho et al. Eur Respir J 2007; 29:273-278). **I predicted that lung cancer patients would have higher GPx levels and lower SOD levels. The GPx would lead to an EMOD insufficiency and the low SOD would**

produce lowered amounts of tumoricidal peroxide. Both situations are conducive to allowing tumor growth.

2.4.1.0 Photodynamic therapy for Barrett's esophagus

Photodynamic therapy (PDT) has been used to palliate advanced, obstructing, or bleeding esophageal cancers (ECs) and Barrett's high-grade dysplasia (HGD). Few investigators, though, have described using PDT to cure either disease.

Methods: We performed a retrospective review from 1997–2005 of **50 patients** with HGD or EC. All patients refused surgical resection or were physiologically unfit. They were instead **treated using PDT with curative intent**. Clinical follow-up, long-term survival, complications, and recurrence were evaluated.

Results: Thirteen patients (26%) had Barrett's HGD, 6 (12%) had small, intramural carcinomas, 16 (32%) had T1 N0 tumors, 14 (28%) had T2 N0 tumors, and 1 (2%) had a small, polypoid T3 lesion. The mean length of follow-up was 28.1 months. Sixteen patients (32%) are alive without recurrence, 15 (30%) are living with residual or recurrent disease and have received additional PDT, and the remainder (38%) died of recurrent EC or other causes and had known recurrence. Sixteen (32%) patients received adjuvant chemotherapy, radiation, or both. Esophageal stricture occurred in 21 (42%) patients. There was no procedure-related mortality.

Conclusions: PDT may represent a reasonable alternate to esophagectomy for high-risk patients with HGD or superficial esophageal cancer. Due to superior survival and local control, we still favor esophagectomy for patients without physiologic impairment. However, **PDT appears to potentially cure approximately one-third of superficial esophageal cancers and provide local control of high-grade dysplasia in a similar subset of patients** (Photodynamic Therapy with Curative Intent for Barrett's Esophagus with High Grade Dysplasia and Superficial Esophageal Cancer. Samuel B. Keeley et al. Annals of Surgical Oncology 14:2406-2410 (2007). **PDT generates EMODs, which are tumoricidal.**

2.4.2.0 Lung Cancer Chemoprevention: Evidence-Based Clinical Practice Guidelines (2nd Edition) 2007

American College of Chest Physicians (ACCP) Evidence-Based Clinical Practice Guidelines (2nd Edition) Jhanelle Gray, MD; Jenny T. Mao, MD, FCCP;

Eva Szabo, MD; Michael Kelley, MD; Jonathan Kurie, MD and Gerold Bepler, MD, PhD. *Chest*. **2007; 132:56S-68.**

Lung cancer is the most common cause of cancer death in the United States. Cigarette smoking is the main risk factor. Former smokers are at a substantially increased risk for lung cancer compared with lifetime never-smokers. Chemoprevention is the use of specific agents to reverse, suppress, or prevent the process of carcinogenesis. This article reviews the major agents that have been studied for chemoprevention.

Methods: Articles of primary, secondary, and tertiary prevention trials were reviewed and summarized to obtain recommendations.

Results: **None of the phase III trials with the agents beta carotene, retinol, 13-cis-retinoic acid, α-tocopherol, N-acetylcysteine, or acetylsalicylic acid has demonstrated beneficial, reproducible results.**

2.4.3.0 No effect of vitamin C, E, or beta carotene on cardiovascular events among women at high risk for CVD

Randomized trials have largely failed to support an effect of antioxidant vitamins on the risk of cardiovascular disease (CVD). Few trials have examined interactions among antioxidants, and, to our knowledge, no previous trial has examined the individual effect of ascorbic acid (vitamin C) on CVD.

Methods The Women's Antioxidant Cardiovascular Study tested the effects of ascorbic acid (500 mg/d), vitamin E (600 IU every other day), and beta carotene (50 mg every other day) on the combined outcome of myocardial infarction, stroke, coronary revascularization, or CVD death among **8171 female health professionals** at increased risk in a 2 x 2 x 2 factorial design. Participants were 40 years or older with a history of CVD or 3 or more CVD risk factors and were followed up for a mean duration of 9.4 years, from 1995-1996 to 2005.

Results A total of 1450 women experienced 1 or more CVD outcomes. There was no overall effect of ascorbic acid (relative risk [RR], 1.02; 95% CI, 0.92-1.13 [*P* = .71]), vitamin E (RR, 0.94; 95% CI, 0.85-1.04 [*P* = .23]), or beta carotene (RR, 1.02; 95% CI, 0.92-1.13 [*P* = .71]) on the primary combined end point or on the individual secondary outcomes of myocardial infarction, stroke, coronary revascularization, or CVD death. A marginally significant reduction in the primary outcome with active vitamin E was observed among the prespecified subgroup of women with prior CVD (RR, 0.89; 95% CI, 0.79-1.00 [P = .04]; P value for interaction, .07). There were no significant interactions between agents for the primary end point, but those randomized to both active ascorbic acid and vitamin E experienced fewer strokes (P value for interaction, .03).

Conclusion There were no overall effects of ascorbic acid, vitamin E, or beta carotene on cardiovascular events among women at high risk for CVD (**A Randomized Factorial Trial of Vitamins C and E and Beta Carotene in the Secondary Prevention of Cardiovascular Events in Women. Results From the Women's Antioxidant Cardiovascular Study.** Nancy R. Cook, ScD; Christine M. Albert, MD; J. Michael Gaziano, MD; Elaine Zaharris, BA; Jean MacFadyen, BA; Eleanor Danielson, MIA; Julie E. Buring, ScD; JoAnn E. Manson, MD, DrPH. *Arch Intern Med.* 2007;167(15):1610-1618).

2.4.4.0 Supplemental vitamin E does not protect against prostate cancer

Supplemental vitamin E (α-tocopherol) has been linked to lower prostate cancer incidence in one randomized trial and several, although not all, observational studies. The evidence regarding dietary intake of individual vitamin E isoforms and prostate cancer is **limited and inconclusive**, however. We prospectively examined the relations of supplemental vitamin E and dietary intakes of α-, β-, γ-, and δ- tocopherols to prostate cancer risk among 295,344 men, ages 50 to 71 years and cancer-free at enrollment in 1995 to 1996, in the NIH-AARP Diet and Health Study. At baseline, participants completed a questionnaire that captured information on diet, supplement use, and other factors. Proportional hazards models were used to estimate relative risks (RR) and 95% confidence intervals (95% CI) of prostate cancer. During 5 years of follow-up, 10,241 incident prostate cancers were identified. Supplemental vitamin E intake was not related to prostate cancer risk (for >0-99, 100-199, 200-399, 400-799, and ≥800 IU/d versus never use: RR, 0.97, 0.89, 1.03, 0.99, and 0.97 (95% CI, 0.87-1.07) respectively; P_{trend} = 0.90). However, dietary γ-tocopherol, the most commonly consumed form of vitamin E in the United States, was significantly inversely related to the risk of advanced prostate cancer (for highest versus lowest quintile: RR, 0.68; 95% CI, 0.56-0.84; P_{trend} = 0.001). These results suggest that **supplemental vitamin E does not protect against prostate cancer,** but that increased consumption of γ-tocopherol from foods is associated with a reduced risk of clinically relevant disease. The potential benefit of γ-tocopherol for prostate cancer prevention deserves further attention. (Supplemental and Dietary Vitamin E Intakes and Risk of Prostate Cancer in a Large Prospective

Study. Margaret E. Wright, Stephanie J. Weinstein, Karla A. Lawson, Demetrius Albanes, Amy F. Subar, L. Beth Dixon, Traci Mouw, Arthur Schatzkin and Michael F. Leitzmann. Cancer Epidemiol Biomarkers Prev 2007;16(6):1128–35).

2.4.5.0 AHA Scientific Statement-2007. Do not recommend C or E

Drug Therapy of High-Risk Lipid Abnormalities in Children and Adolescents

A Scientific Statement From the American Heart Association Atherosclerosis, Hypertension, and Obesity in Youth Committee, Council of Cardiovascular Disease in the Young, With the Council on Cardiovascular Nursing. Brian W. McCrindle, MD, MPH, Chair; Elaine M. Urbina, MD; Barbara A. Dennison, MD, FAHA; Marc S. Jacobson, MD, FAHA; Julia Steinberger, MD, MS; Albert P. Rocchini, MD, FAHA; Laura L. Hayman, PhD, RN, FAHA; Stephen R. Daniels, MD, PhD, FAHA. *Circulation.* 2007;115:1948-1967

The impact of adjuvant therapies on vascular structure and function also has been explored. Engler and colleagues performed a **double-blind randomized crossover trial** in **15 children** with familial or familial combined hypercholesterolemia, comparing placebo with **500 mg/d vitamin C and 400 U vitamin E** given over a 6-week period. Although flow-mediated dilatation as assessed by vascular ultrasound of the brachial artery was similarly reduced at baseline in the diet-only phase and in the placebo phase, it returned toward near normal with intake of the antioxidant vitamins (Engler MM, Engler MB, Malloy MJ, Chiu EY, Schloetter MC, Paul SM, Stuehlinger M, Lin KY, Cooke JP, Morrow JD, Ridker PM, Rifai N, Miller E, Witztum JL, Mietus-Snyder M. Antioxidant vitamins C and E improve endothelial function in children with hyperlipidemia: Endothelial Assessment of Risk from Lipids in Youth (EARLY) Trial. *Circulation.* 2003; 108: 1059–1063).

Nonetheless, **it is difficult to make a recommendation for their use because long-term efficacy trials in adults, often with cardiovascular disease or other medical conditions, have not shown benefit** (Lonn E, Bosch J, Yusuf S, Sheridan P, Pogue J, Arnold JM, Ross C, Arnold A, Sleight P, Probstfield J, Dagenais GR, for the HOPE and HOPE-TOO Trial Investigators. Effects of long-term vitamin E supplementation on cardiovascular events and cancer: a randomized controlled trial. JAMA. 2005; 293: 1338–1347) (Lee IM, Cook NR, Gaziano JM, Gordon D, Ridker PM, Manson JE, Hennekens CH, Buring JE. Vitamin E in the primary prevention of cardiovascular disease and cancer: the Women's Health Study:

a randomized controlled trial. JAMA. 2005; 294: 56–65) (Yusuf S, Dagenais G, Pogue J, Bosch J, Sleight P. Vitamin E supplementation and cardiovascular events in high-risk patients: the Heart Outcomes Prevention Evaluation Study Investigators. N Engl J Med. 2000; 342: 154–160) (Rapola JM, Virtamo J, Ripatti S, Huttunen JK, Albanes D, Taylor PR, Heinonen OP. Randomised trial of alpha-tocopherol and beta-carotene supplements on incidence of major coronary events in men with previous myocardial infarction. Lancet. 1997; 349: *1715–1720)*. **Accessed 12-1-08 http://circ.ahajournals.org/cgi/content/full/115/14/1948#BIBL**

2.4.6.0 Thioredoxin blocks EMOD-induced apoptosis for human neuroblastoma ==

Human neuroblastoma cells, SH-SY5Y, contain relatively low levels of thioredoxin (Trx); thus, they serve favorably as a model for studying oxidative stress-induced apoptosis. Interestingly, **thioredoxin is upregulated by cGMP/protein kinase G in human neuroblastoma cells, protecting cells from oxidative stress–induced apoptosis** (Andoh T, Chiueh CC, Chock PB. Cyclic GMP-dependent protein kinase regulates the expression of thioredoxin and thioredoxin peroxidase-1 during hormesis in response to oxidative stress-induced apoptosis. *J Biol Chem*. 2003; 278: 885–890).

2.4.7.0. Summary of American Heart Association Diet and Lifestyle Recommendations Revision 2006: supplements not recommended

Antioxidant Supplements

Antioxidant vitamin supplements or other supplements such as selenium to prevent CVD are not recommended (Kris-Etherton PM, Lichtenstein AH, Howard BV, Steinberg D, Witztum JL. Nutrition Committee of the American Heart Association Council on Nutrition, Physical Activity, and Metabolism. Antioxidant vitamin supplements and cardiovascular disease. *Circulation*. 2004; 110: 637–641) (Lee IM, Cook NR, Gaziano JM, Gordon D, Ridker PM, Manson JE, Hennekens CH, Buring JE. Vitamin E in the primary prevention of cardiovascular disease and cancer: the Women's Health Study: a randomized controlled trial. *J Am Med Assoc*. 2005; 294: 56–65) (Lonn E, Bosch J, Yusuf S, Sheridan P, Pogue J, Arnold JM, Ross C, Arnold A, Sleight P, Probstfield J, Dagenais GR. HOPE and HOPE-TOO Trial Investigators. Effects of long-term vitamin E supplementation on cardiovascular events and cancer: a randomized controlled trial. *J Am Med Assoc*. 2005; 293: 1338–1347) (Miller ER 3rd, Pastor-Barriuso R, Dalal D, Riemersma RA, Appel LJ,

Guallar E. Meta-analysis: high-dosage vitamin E supplementation may increase all-cause mortality. *Ann Intern Med.* 2005; 142: 37–46).

Nevertheless, food sources of antioxidant nutrients, principally from a variety of plant-derived foods such as fruits, vegetables, whole grains, and vegetable oils are recommended. (Summary of American Heart Association Diet and Lifestyle Recommendations Revision 2006. Alice H. Lichtenstein; Lawrence J. Appel; Michael Brands; Mercedes Carnethon; Stephen Daniels; Harold A. Franch; Barry Franklin; Penny Kris-Etherton; William S. Harris; Barbara Howard; Njeri Karanja; Michael Lefevre; Lawrence Rudel; Frank Sacks; Linda Van Horn; Mary Winston; Judith Wylie-Rosett. *Arteriosclerosis, Thrombosis, and Vascular Biology.* 2006;26:2186).

2.4.8.0 American Cancer Society Guidelines on Nutrition and Physical Activity for Cancer Prevention 2006

Vitamin A

Does vitamin A lower cancer risk? Vitamin A (retinol) is obtained from foods in two ways: preformed from animal food sources, and derived from beta carotene in plant-based foods. Vitamin A is needed to maintain healthy tissues. **Vitamin A supplements, whether in the form of beta carotene or retinol, have not been shown to lower cancer risk, and high-dose supplements may, in fact, increase the risk for lung cancer in current and former smokers** (The effect of vitamin E and beta carotene on the incidence of lung cancer and other cancers in male smokers. The Alpha-Tocopherol, Beta Carotene Cancer Prevention Study Group. N Engl J Med 1994;330:1029–1035) (Omenn GS, Goodman GE, Thornquist MD, et al. Effects of a combination of beta carotene and vitamin A on lung cancer and cardiovascular disease. N Engl J Med 1996;334:1150–1155).

Vitamin C

Does vitamin C lower cancer risk? Vitamin C is found in many vegetables and fruits, particularly oranges, grapefruit, and peppers. Many studies have linked consumption of vitamin C–rich foods with a reduced risk for cancer (Fruits and Vegetables, vol. 8. Lyon, France: International Agency for Research on Cancer, World Health Organization; 2003).

The few studies in which vitamin C has been given as a supplement, however, have not shown a reduced risk for cancer.

Vitamin D

Does vitamin D lower cancer risk? There is a growing body of evidence from epidemiologic studies (not yet tested in RCTs) that **vitamin D may have beneficial effects on some types of cancer, including cancers of the colon, prostate, and breast** (Giovannucci E. The epidemiology of vitamin D and cancer incidence and mortality: a review (United States). Cancer Causes Control 2005;16:83–95).

Vitamin D is obtained through skin exposure to ultraviolet (UV) radiation, and through diet, particularly products fortified with vitamin D such as milk and cereals, and supplements. Many Americans, however, do not consume sufficient amounts of vitamin D (Whiting SJ, Calvo MS. Dietary recommendations to meet both endocrine and autocrine needs of Vitamin D. J Steroid Biochem Mol Biol 2005;97:7–12).

The current national recommended levels of intake of vitamin D of 200 to 600 IU may be inadequate to meet needs, especially among those with little sun exposure, the elderly, individuals with dark skin, and exclusively breast-fed babies. More research is needed to define optimal blood and intake levels for cancer risk reduction, but recommended intake is likely to fall between 200 and 2000 IU, depending on age and other factors that modify vitamin D status. To minimize the health risks associated with UVB radiation exposure while maximizing the potential benefits of optimum vitamin D levels, a balanced diet, supplementation, and limiting sun exposure to small amounts are the preferred methods of obtaining vitamin D.

Vitamin E

Does vitamin E lower cancer risk? Alpha-tocopherol is recognized as the most active form of **vitamin E in humans and is a powerful biological antioxidant**. A reduction in prostate cancer incidence was observed among men randomly assigned to receive alpha-tocopherol in the Alpha-Tocopherol Beta Carotene (ATBC) trial, a study that included only male smokers.[76]

However, this **association was not observed in the HOPE-TOO trial** (Lonn E, Bosch J, Yusuf S, et al. Effects of long-term vitamin E supplementation on cardiovascular events and cancer: a randomized controlled trial. JAMA 2005;293:1338–1347), **in postintervention follow up of the ATBC trial** (Virtamo J, Pietinen P, Huttunen JK, et al. Incidence of cancer and mortality following alpha-tocopherol and beta-carotene supplementation:

a postintervention follow-up. JAMA 2003;290:476–485), **or in two large prospective observational studies** (Chan JM, Stampfer MJ, Ma J, et al. Supplemental vitamin E intake and prostate cancer risk in a large cohort of men in the United States. Cancer Epidemiol Biomarkers Prev 1999;8:893–899) (Rodriguez C, Jacobs EJ, Mondul AM, et al. Vitamin E supplements and risk of prostate cancer in US men. Cancer Epidemiol Biomarkers Prev 2004;13:378–382), and may have been a result of chance. While ongoing randomized trials will eventually provide further information, **the promise of alpha-tocopherol as a cancer prevention agent appears to be dimming.** (American Cancer Society Guidelines on Nutrition and Physical Activity for Cancer Prevention-2006. Reducing the Risk of Cancer With Healthy Food Choices and Physical Activity*. Lawrence H. Kushi, ScD, Tim Byers, MD, MPH, Colleen Doyle, MS, RD, Elisa V. Bandera, MD, PhD, Marji McCullough, ScD, RD, Ted Gansler, MD, MBA, Kimberly S. Andrews, Michael J. Thun, MD, MS and The American Cancer Society 2006 Nutrition and Physical Activity Guidelines Advisory Committee. CA Cancer J Clin 2006; 56:254-281).

2.4.9.0 AHA Scientific Statement. Diet and Lifestyle Recommendations Revision 2006: supplements not recommended for CVD

Antioxidant Supplements

Antioxidant vitamin supplements or other supplements such as selenium to prevent CVD are not recommended (Kris-Etherton PM, Lichtenstein AH, Howard BV, Steinberg D, Witztum JL; Nutrition Committee of the American Heart Association Council on Nutrition, Physical Activity, and Metabolism. Antioxidant vitamin supplements and cardiovascular disease. *Circulation.* 2004; 110: 637–641) (Lee IM, Cook NR, Gaziano JM, Gordon D, Ridker PM, Manson JE, Hennekens CH, Buring JE. Vitamin E in the primary prevention of cardiovascular disease and cancer: the Women's Health Study: a randomized controlled trial. *JAMA.* 2005; 294: 56–65).

Although observational studies have suggested that high intakes of antioxidant vitamins from food and supplements are associated with a lower risk of CVD, **clinical trials of antioxidant vitamin supplements have not confirmed benefit. Some trials, in fact, have documented potential harm, including an increased risk of lung cancer from beta-carotene supplements in smokers and an increased risk of heart failure and the possibility of increased total mortality from high-dose vitamin E supplements.** Although antioxidant supplements are not recommended, food sources of antioxidant nutrients, principally from a variety of plant-derived foods such as fruits, vegetables, whole grains, and vegetable oils are recommended (AHA Scientific Statement. Diet and Lifestyle Recommendations Revision 2006. A Scientific Statement From the American Heart Association Nutrition Committee. Alice H. Lichtenstein, DSc, FAHA, Chair; Lawrence J. Appel, MD, FAHA, Vice-Chair; Michael Brands, PhD, FAHA; Mercedes Carnethon, PhD; Stephen Daniels, MD, PhD, FAHA; Harold A. Franch, MD, FAHA; Barry Franklin, PhD, FAHA; Penny Kris-Etherton, RD, PhD, FAHA; William S. Harris, PhD, FAHA; Barbara Howard, PhD, FAHA; Njeri Karanja, PhD; Michael Lefevre, PhD, FAHA; Lawrence Rudel, MD, PhD, FAHA; Frank Sacks, MD, FAHA; Linda Van Horn, PhD, RD, FAHA; Mary Winston, EdD; Judith Wylie-Rosett, EdD, RD. *Circulation.* 2006;114:82-96).

2.5.0.0 Vitamins C and E not recommended to treat or prevent cancer

Investigators evaluated the evidence of the supplements vitamin C and vitamin E for treatment and prevention of cancer.

Thirty-eight studies showed scant (inadequate) evidence that vitamin C or vitamin E beneficially affects survival. In the ATBC Cancer Prevention Study Group, no statistically significant effect of treatment was seen for any cancer individually, and our pooled relative risk (regardless of tumor type) for α-tocopherol alone was 0.91 (95% confidence interval [CI]: 0.74, 1.12). All cause mortality was not significant. In the Linxian General Population Trial, the relative risks for cancer death for vitamin C (combined with molybdenum) was 1.06 (95% CI: 0.92, 1.21) and for vitamin E (combined with β-carotene and selenium) was 0.87 (95% CI: 0.76, 1.00). We identified only 3 studies that reported statistically significant beneficial results: vitamin C (in combination with BCG) was found to be beneficial in a single trial of bladder cancer and vitamin E (in combination with ω-3 fatty acid) increased survival in patients with advanced cancer. In the ATBC trial, in analyses of 6 individual cancers, the prevention of prostate cancer in subjects treated with α-tocopherol was statistically significant (RR = 0.64, 95% CI: 0.44, 0.94).

CONCLUSIONS

The **systematic review of the literature does not support the hypothesis that the use of supplements of vitamin C or vitamin E in the doses tested helps prevent and/or treat cancer in the populations tested.** There were isolated findings of benefit, which require confirmation (Antioxidants

Vitamin C and Vitamin E for the Prevention and Treatment of Cancer. Ian D Coulter et al. J Gen Intern Med. 2006 July; 21(7): 735–744).

2.5.1.0 How household bleach works to kill bacteria

Nov 13 , General Science

Despite the fact that household bleach is commonly used as a disinfectant, exactly how it works to fight bacteria remained an open question. Now, a report in the November 14, 2008 issue of the journal **Cell**, a Cell Press publication, provides an answer. The researchers found that **hypochlorous acid, the active ingredient in bleach, causes the unfolding of proteins in bacteria in much the same was that heat stress or fever does.** Those denatured proteins then clump together irreversibly into a mass in living cells, similar to what happens to proteins when you boil an egg, according to the researchers.

The bacteria aren't totally defenseless, however. Under those circumstances, **a protein chaperone called heat shock protein Hsp33 springs to action, protecting proteins from the aggregation effect and increasing the bacteria's bleach resistance. Protein chaperones are generally defined as proteins whose function is to help other proteins.**

"We found both in vitro and in vivo that bleach attacks proteins," said Ursula Jakob of the University of Michigan, Ann Arbor. "They lose structure much like they would under high temperature. Under those circumstances, the [Hsp33] protein is specifically activated to increase resistance." Jakob emphasized that **this newly discovered mechanism is clearly one way bleach kills bacteria, but it may not be the only way.**

Why would bacteria have a system specifically designed to deal with bleach?

"Hypochlorous acid is an important part of host defense," Jakob said. **"It's not just something we use on our countertops."**

In fact, **the innate immune systems of mammals, and specifically immune cells known as neutrophils, release high concentrations of hypochlorous acid (aka bleach) upon recognizing microbial invaders.** In addition, Jakob said, some evidence suggests that **enzymes that produce bleach may help keep the bacteria in our guts in check.**

The specific effects of hypochlorous acid on proteins help to explain why hydrogen peroxide is an inferior antimicrobial agent even though both chemicals are expected to act as strong oxidants, Jakob said. **Hydrogen peroxide doesn't do much for your countertops, she said, because it doesn't provoke these effects on proteins.**

Hsp33 also represents another example of an emerging concept in protein biology: that some proteins actually become activated through the act of partial unfolding. Indeed, chaperones react to stress by unfolding in the same way that other proteins do. Far from leaving them useless, however, that change in conformation is exactly what turns them on. "Usually, we think proteins need structure to be active, but here they must lose structure to be active," Jakob said.

As for whether the findings will have any practical implications, Jakob said she isn't yet sure. For instance, **she has doubts that bleach could be made to work any more effectively than it does, particularly given that it works so rapidly and so well as it is even at low concentrations.**

The findings in bacteria could perhaps offer new insight into the damaging effects of bleach on our own proteins, she added, noting that **hypochlorous acid produced by the immune system has been suspected to play a role in chronic inflammation.** The protein unfolding seen in bacteria might explain what the chemical agent is doing, perhaps yielding clues about what might be done to stop it.

Source: Cell Press

2.5.2.0 Baths with Bleach Help Kids' Eczema

4-27-09

When treating children for chronic eczema, pediatricians may want **to look in the laundry room,** according to a new study published this week in the journal *Pediatrics*. The study reports that adding a small amount of household bleach to a child's bathwater can **dramatically reduce the itching, rashes and discomfort caused by eczema.**

The treatment sounds harsh, but the findings confirm what many pediatric dermatologists have seen anecdotally for years. The theory is that **the antimicrobial properties of bleach** help relieve symptoms of eczema not by acting directly on that skin condition, but by improving children's skin infections of staph bacteria — a common co-occurrence that exacerbates the irritating symptoms of eczema.

In the new study, researchers followed 31 children between the ages of 6 months and 17 years, who had both conditions: atopic dermatitis, the most common form of childhood eczema, which affects 17% of the school-aged population, as well as a co-infection of *Staphylococcus aureus*. Although antibiotics are typically used successfully to combat such staph infections, the emergence of drug-resistant MRSA (or methicillin-resistant *Staphylococcus aureus*) has physicians increasingly wary of overusing the medicines.

"The bottom line is that the more antibiotics we use, the higher the risk for something becoming resistant to them," says Dr. Amy Paller, a study author, specialist in pediatric dermatology and chair of the dermatology department at Northwestern University's Feinberg School of Medicine. **"The beauty of something like dilute bleach is that one doesn't get resistance to it."**

Each study participant was given an identically labeled bleach bottle, but only half of the bottles actually contained bleach. (Although patients, or at least their parents, could easily distinguish whether they were in the bleach group or the placebo group by smelling the contents of their bottle, they were instructed not to tell the researchers which group they were in.) Those who received real bleach were instructed to draw a bath twice a week with a heavily diluted bleach solution — **a half-cup of bleach per 40 gallons of water** — and immerse their limbs and torsos, leaving the neck and head above water, for five to 10 minutes each time. They were told to pat dry afterward and apply a heavy slathering of moisturizer. The placebo group was not given restrictions about the frequency of baths. Both groups of patients were also treated with oral antibiotics and the nasal ointment muciprocin to control staph infections, which often exist in the nostrils.

After three months, the group using bleach baths reported improvement of symptoms in the areas of the body that had been submerged, with 67% of those using bleach baths benefiting, compared with just 15% of those who bathed in normal water. "This is so simple, and it's really working." Paller says.

Dr. Nanette Silverberg, director of pediatric and adolescent dermatology at Beth Israel Medical Center in New York, has been using bleach baths with her patients for years. (She first learned of the treatment during her fellowship in pediatric dermatology studying under Paller.) She says parents and patients are usually dumbfounded when she first suggests the remedy. "They call in relatives from the waiting room to witness the insanity," Silverberg laughs. "Many patients look at me like I've lost my marbles."

But in her practice, when combined with other treatments, the baths have been a valuable and successful technique, Silverberg says. **"The bleach baths do work,"** she says. "I'm a big believer in using them."

If bleach baths work, then perhaps children with chronic eczema and persistent staph infections could be treated with fewer courses of antibiotics. Continuous antibiotic treatment is not a viable option, especially given the emergence of MRSA, say Silverberg and Paller. "We have been looking for agents that are antibacterial but would not have the problems that we see with antibiotics, where you can and will develop resistance over time," Silverberg says. "With the bleach bath, you reduce the chances of getting grossly infected and needing to go on the antibiotics, and it has benefits in the general community — you're not walking around with staph [lesions]."

Paller and Silverberg underscore that bleach baths should be used as one component of a larger treatment strategy for chronic eczema, always in consultation with a doctor, and that **bleach should never be applied directly to the skin**. For patients with severe skin damage such as cracking, baths of any kind — including dilute bleach — may initially be too painful, and should be introduced later in treatment only after the skin has begun to improve.

When used correctly, Paller says the baths are extremely safe for patients with eczema. What's more, she adds light-heartedly, "It keeps the tub clean too."

I believe that the bleach, hypochlorite, generates EMODs which kill the bacteria.

2.5.3.0 Lung airway cells activate vitamin D and increase immune response

Nov 04 , Medicine & Health

Vitamin D is essential to good health but needs to be activated to function properly in the human body. Until recently, this activation was thought to happen primarily in the kidneys, but a new University of Iowa study finds that the activation step can also occur in lung airway cells. The study also links the vitamin D locally produced in the lung airway cells to activation of two genes that help fight infection. The study results appear in the **Nov. 15, 2008 issue of the *Journal of Immunology***, now online.

In addition to contributing to calcium absorption and bone health, vitamin D is increasingly recognized for its beneficial effects on the immune system. **Vitamin D deficiency has been recently linked to increased risk of some infections, autoimmune diseases such as multiple sclerosis and type 1 diabetes, and some cancers.**

"The more scientists have been studying vitamin D, the more we learn about new roles it plays in the human body," said the study's lead author Sif Hansdottir, M.D., fellow in internal medicine in the University of Iowa Carver College of Medicine. "**The active form of vitamin D is known to affect the expression of more than 200 genes**, so we were interested both in the possible lung-specific production of active vitamin D and in vitamin D-dependent production of proteins that fight infections."

The first step in vitamin D activation takes place in the liver, where an enzyme called 25-hydroxylase converts vitamin D into a "storage" form. **The next step takes place typically in the kidneys, but in recent years, tissue and organs such as skin, intestines, breast and prostate have been found also to express the enzyme that completes vitamin D conversion.**

The University of Iowa team, based in the laboratory of Gary Hunninghake, M.D., professor of internal medicine and the study's senior author, used cells from deceased human donors to demonstrate that the presence of the enzyme 1 alpha-hydroxylase in the airway cells helps convert the storage form of vitamin D into its active form.

"When we put the storage form of vitamin D on the lung airway cells, we saw them convert it to the active form," Hansdottir said. "The next step was to investigate whether this active form could affect the expression of genes."

The team then showed that vitamin D activated by airway cells affects two genes involved in immune defense. One gene expresses a protein called cathelicidin that can kill bacteria. The second gene, called CD14, produces a protein that helps cells recognize different kinds of pathogens that could be a threat.

"Vitamin D converted by the kidneys circulates in the bloodstream, but vitamin D converted by other organs appears to stay within those

organs and protect them from infection," Hansdottir said. "We were able to see this happen in cells lining the trachea and main bronchi."

The team also found that when lung airway cells are infected by a virus, they express more of the enzyme that activates vitamin D. Hansdottir said the team is very interested in pursuing studies on the role of viral infections in vitamin D production and subsequent effects on lung infections.

"Vitamin D not only increases proteins involved in bacterial killing but also can dampen inflammation," Hansdottir said. "Controlling inflammation through vitamin D is good because too much inflammation can cause problems such as sepsis and seems to contribute to autoimmune disease." **I believe that this is a great example of a prooxidant acting as an anti-inflammatory.**

Hansdottir noted that vitamin D insufficiencies and deficiencies (which are more severe) are fairly common, particularly for people living in northern latitudes. While vitamin D can be generated through sun exposure, such exposure is generally not recommended as a remedy because of skin cancer risks. Instead, supplements can be used.

The American Academy of Pediatrics recently recommended that the vitamin D dosage for children be increased to 400 IU (international units) per day. Optimal daily intake for adults is still being studied but may be as high as 800 to 1,000 IU.

Source: University of Iowa

2.5.4.0 HOCl vs H_2O_2

Some of the following was excerpted or modified from: (Contrasting Effects of Hypochlorous Acid and Hydrogen Peroxide on Endothelial Permeability. Prevention with cAMP Drugs. LUIS OCHOA, GREGORY WAYPA, JOHN R. MAHONEY Jr., LUIS RODRIGUEZ, and FRED L. MINNEAR. Am. J. Respir. Crit. Care Med., Volume 156, Number 4, October 1997, 1247-1255).

An increase in vascular endothelial permeability to protein and the development of pulmonary edema are characteristic features of the lung pathophysiology associated with inflammation, embolism, sepsis, and trauma. Polymorphonuclear leukocytes have been implicated in the pathogenesis as these cells when activated produce toxic, reactive oxygen metabolites and proteases that can increase the pulmonary vascular permeability to the movement of water and protein leading to pulmonary edema and the onset of acute respiratory distress syndrome. **Upon activation, these cells assemble a nicotinamide adenine dinucleotide phosphate (NADPH) oxidase on the cell surface and generate a cascade of reactive oxygen metabolites that include superoxide radical (O^-_2), hydrogen peroxide (H_2O_2), hypochlorous acid (HOCl), hydroxyl radical ($^{\cdot}OH$), and peroxynitrite radical ($ONOO^-$).** The first four of these oxidants have been reported to increase endothelial permeability.

H_2O_2, produced by the spontaneous or enzymatic dismutation of O^-_2, is lipid soluble and readily diffuses into endothelial cells, where it can react with ferrous iron to produce the extremely toxic $^{\cdot}OH$. **Approximately 40% of the H_2O_2 formed by activated polymorphonuclear leukocytes can be oxidized by myeloperoxidase (MPO) in the presence of Cl^-, the most abundant halide in plasma, to HOCl** (Weiss, S. J., R. Klein, A. Slivka, and M. Wei. 1982. Chlorination of taurine by human neutrophils: evidence for hypochlorous acid generation. *J. Clin. Invest* 70: 598-607), which is highly reactive and does not accumulate in biologic systems).

HOCl is a powerful oxidant that is ~ 100-fold more potent as an antimicrobial compound than H_2O_2 (Chesney, J., J. W. Eaton, and J. R. Mahoney Jr.. 1996. Bacterial glutathione: a sacrificial defense against chlorine oxidants. *J. Bacteriol* 178: 2131-2135) **and that can degrade structural proteins and inactivate enzymes** (Schraufstatter, I. U., K. Browne, A. Harris, P. A. Hyslop, J. H. Jackson, O. Quehenberger, and C. G. Cochrane. 1990. Mechanisms of hypochlorite injury of target cells. *J. Clin. Invest* 85: 554-562).

Although the effects of H_2O_2 on vascular endothelial permeability have been studied extensively, the effects of HOCl are represented by only one study (Tatsumi, T., and H. Fliss. 1994. Hypochlorous acid and chloramines increase endothelial permeability: possible involvement of cellular zinc. *Am. J. Physiol* 267: H1597-H1607).

The purpose of the present study was to compare and contrast the effects of H_2O_2 and HOCl on the permeability of the vascular endothelium.

(Contrasting Effects of Hypochlorous Acid and Hydrogen Peroxide on Endothelial Permeability. Prevention with cAMP Drugs. LUIS OCHOA, GREGORY WAYPA, JOHN R. MAHONEY Jr., LUIS RODRIGUEZ, and FRED L. MINNEAR. Am. J. Respir. Crit. Care Med., Volume 156, Number 4, October 1997, 1247-1255).

HOCl caused rapid, within 1 to 3 min, changes in cell shape and electrical resistance, whereas H_2O_2 required ~ 30 min to induce these changes. HOCl produced greater increases in endothelial protein permeability and decreases in electrical resistance and more extensive cell retraction at much lower concentrations than H_2O_2.

Generation of HOCl by the conversion of H_2O_2 with MPO produced results similar to the direct administration of HOCl.

The increase in endothelial protein permeability induced by H_2O_2 was prevented by isoproterenol and 8-bromo-cAMP, but the increased permeability induced by HOCl was prevented only by 8-bromo-cAMP. These findings demonstrate that HOCl is a more potent oxidant than H_2O_2 in altering endothelial cell shape and permeability and that an elevation in the intracellular level of cAMP can prevent the increase in endothelial protein permeability induced by either oxidant.

Previous studies have shown that both H_2O_2 and HOCl increase endothelial protein permeability *in vitro* and that cAMP-enhancing agents can prevent the increased permeability induced by H_2O_2. **H_2O_2 has been reported to increase permeability in a dose range from 50 to 100 μM, with doses > 100 μM causing cellular damage** as assessed by release of lactate dehydrogenase or ^{51}Cr (Bhat, G. B., S. B. Tinsley, J. K. Tolson, J. M. Patel, and E. R. Block. 1992. Hypoxia increases the susceptibility of pulmonary artery endothelial cells to hydrogen peroxide injury. *J. Cell. Physiol* 151: 228-238).

HOCl was found to increase permeability at doses equal to and greater than 25 μM (Tatsumi, T., and H. Fliss. 1994. Hypochlorous acid and chloramines increase endothelial permeability: possible involvement of cellular zinc. *Am. J. Physiol* 267: H1597-H1607).

The present study confirms these findings and, in addition, directly compares the potency and temporal response of these two oxidants using four different methodologies. First, the potency of these two oxidants was compared by the measurement of endothelial protein permeability. **The direct administration of HOCl produced a variable increase in permeability at 10 μM and consistent increases at 25, 50, and 100 μM, whereas H_2O_2 produced consistent increases at 50 and 100 μM.**

Secondly, **HOCl produced by conversion of H_2O_2 with MPO significantly increased endothelial protein permeability at doses of 25, 50, and 100 μM compared directly to the same doses of H_2O_2 administered**

alone as the control groups. At 50 and 100 μM, HOCl doubled the protein permeability of the H_2O_2 control groups.

Thirdly, the potency and time course of changes in endothelial electrical resistance were compared directly using the ECIS apparatus. HOCl caused almost an immediate decrease in electrical resistance, whereas H_2O_2 required ~ 30 min to induce a significant change in resistance. Furthermore, HOCl decreased endothelial electrical resistance to a twofold greater extent than H_2O_2.

Fourthly, HOCl caused a more rapid (within 3 min) and extensive alteration in cell shape than H_2O_2 (~ 30 min), as depicted by a greater number of and wider intercellular gaps and more extensive formation of intercellular strands. **The dose of HOCl (10 μM) that readily produced cell retraction was much lower than that required for H_2O_2 (400 μM).** These four comparisons demonstrate that HOCl induces a more rapid and potent change in electrical resistance, protein permeability, and shape change of endothelial cell monolayers than H_2O_2.

Similar findings with regard to the time course leading to cellular damage and potency of these two oxidants have been reported for murine macrophage-like tumor cells (P388D1) exposed to HOCl and H_2O_2. Low concentrations (10 to 20 μM) of HOCl caused oxidation of plasma membrane sulfhydryls and disturbances of plasma membrane functions such as inactivation of glucose uptake, loss of cellular K^+, and an increase in cell volume. Higher concentrations led to generalized oxidation of sulfhydryl, methionine, and tryptophan residues, ATP depletion, and cell lysis. H_2O_2 on the other hand, induced sulfhydryl oxidation of glyceraldehyde-3-phosphate dehydrogenase, depletion of ATP, degradation of NAD, and strand breaks in DNA.

Compared with H_2O_2, which caused cell death after several hours, HOCl induced cell lysis within an hour at one-tenth of the molar concentration (Schraufstatter, I. U., K. Browne, A. Harris, P. A. Hyslop, J. H. Jackson, O. Quehenberger, and C. G. Cochrane. 1990. Mechanisms of hypochlorite injury of target cells. *J. Clin. Invest* 85: 554-562).

HOCl increased endothelial protein permeability when administered either directly or by conversion of H_2O_2 with MPO. Enzymatic production of HOCl was used to mimic the *in vivo* production of HOCl by polymorphonuclear leukocytes. A similar protocol has been used to induce glomerular injury in rats. MPO was shown by electron microscopy to localize, presumably by electrostatic interactions, to the glomerular capillary wall. Subsequent administration of H_2O_2 produced a greater than threefold increase in urine protein excretion from the MPO and H_2O_2 control groups. These investigators concluded that **HOCl produced by the conversion of H_2O_2 by MPO and Cl^- may be important in polymorphonuclear leukocyte-mediated glomerulonephritis.**

Under ideal conditions, the conversion of H_2O_2 to HOCl catalyzed by MPO in the presence of Cl^- should be one-to-one. Under physiologic conditions and in the present study, probably not all of the H_2O_2 was converted to HOCl. Some of the H_2O_2 was inaccessible to MPO because it had already diffused into the cell. Furthermore, **HOCl interferes with its own production by inhibiting the reduction of H_2O_2 by MPO.** Although the added H_2O_2 was not detectable, using the xylenol orange assay, after conversion by MPO to HOCl, most likely all of the H_2O_2 was not converted to HOCl. Thus, the comparisons of potency and temporal changes between H_2O_2 and HOCl produced indirectly are probably limited by the fact that not all of the H_2O_2 was converted by MPO to HOCl. However, this indirect method of production of HOCl is probably required for studies involving intact animals or isolated lungs perfused with protein, since **proteins scavenge HOCl**. Furthermore, this indirect production of HOCl simulates the *in vivo* condition whereby polymorphonuclear leukocytes produce HOCl via the release of MPO, which binds electrostatically to endothelial cells, and H_2O_2.

They noted that the **doses of H_2O_2 from 10 to 200 μM did not always produce consistent increases in protein permeability.** Both H_2O_2 and HOCl have been shown by other investigators to produce reversible changes in endothelial cell shape. For H_2O_2, changes in cell shape were maximal within 4 to 6 h and reversible by 24 h. HOCl caused changes in cell shape that were noticeable within 2 to 6 min and reversible by 4 h. The reversible response of HOCl was observed with noncytotoxic concentrations of 10 and 25 μM and when the HOCl was incubated with the cells for 2 min but not when incubated for 6 min.

With both oxidants, the changes in endothelial cell shape have been reported to include cell retraction, the formation of thin intercellular strands connecting the separated cells early in the retraction process, and the reorganization of actin microfilaments. Although both oxidants caused cell retraction, the differences in time of onset and the extent of intercellular strand formation would suggest that these two oxidants function by different mechanisms. Schraufstatter and associates have demonstrated that HOCl and H_2O_2 interact with similar and different cellular targets. For example, HOCl reacts with the closest targets, often components of the plasma membrane, whereas H_2O_2 diffuses freely into cells and causes site-directed damage presumably due to the formation of metal-dependent $^{\cdot}OH$.

A variety of cAMP-enhancing agents have been used to attenuate the H_2O_2-induced increase in endothelial permeability *in vitro*. **Pretreatment with prostaglandin E_1, forskolin, type III and IV phosphodiesterase inhibitors, and β_2-adrenergic agonists have been effective in the prevention of the H_2O_2-induced increase in endothelial permeability.** There are a number of mechanisms whereby an increase in the intracellular level of cAMP might protect against the H_2O_2 response. **H_2O_2 has been shown to reduce intracellular levels of ATP, NAD, and glutathione and activate the inositol phosphate pathway which increases intracellular Ca^{2+} and activates protein kinase C.**

8-Bromo-cAMP prevented the increased protein permeability induced by either oxidant, whereas isoproterenol failed to modify the HOCl response. Administered as a co-treatment, HOCl as well as H_2O_2 could directly alter the structure of isoproterenol and/or oxidize the sulfhydryl groups in the β-adrenergic receptor and subsequently depress the function of the receptor. That HOCl may react directly with isoproterenol and is a more potent oxidant than H_2O_2 might explain why isoproterenol was protective against H_2O_2 but not HOCl.

I believe that this entire paper merely re-emphasizes the point that HOCl is a much more potent oxidant than is peroxide.

2.5.5.0 Oxidant stress and endothelial cell dysfunction

Reactive oxygen species (ROS) are generated at sites of inflammation and injury, and **at low levels, ROS can function as signaling molecules participating as signaling intermediates in regulation of fundamental cell activities such as cell growth and cell adaptation responses, whereas at higher concentrations, ROS can cause cellular injury and death.** The vascular endothelium, which regulates the passage of macromolecules and circulating cells from blood to tissues, is a major target of oxidant stress, playing a critical role in the pathophysiology of several vascular diseases and disorders. Specifically, oxidant stress increases vascular endothelial permeability and promotes leukocyte adhesion, which are coupled with alterations in endothelial signal transduction and redox-regulated transcription factors such as activator protein-1 and nuclear factor-κB. This review discusses recent findings on the cellular and molecular mechanisms by which ROS signal events leading to impairment of endothelial barrier function and promotion of leukocyte adhesion. Particular emphasis is placed on the regulation of cell-cell and cell-surface adhesion molecules, the actin cytoskeleton, key protein kinases, and signal transduction events (Oxidant stress and endothelial cell dysfunction. H. Lum and K.A. Roebuck. Am J Physiol Cell Physiol, April 1, 2001; 280(4): C719 - C741).

2.5.6.0 Exercise

2.5.6.1 Exercise and sleep drastically reduce cancer risk

Get your exercise, but be sure to get a good night's sleep, too, if you want to lower your risk of getting cancer.

A new study suggests that **regular physical activity can lower a woman's risk of developing cancer, but only if she sleeps more than seven hours a night**.

The study found that **women who measured in the upper 50 per cent for physical activity levels had an 80 per cent drop in overall cancer risk and a 75 per cent reduction in breast cancer risk.**

However, the study also showed that women under the age of 65 who measured in the upper 50 per cent for physical activity levels but slept less than seven hours a night had a **1.5-fold increase in risk for developing cancer**.

Researchers have long known that exercise can reduce overall cancer risk, but lack of sleep can have the opposite effect.

While the researchers can't say for sure how exercise lowers cancer risk, they speculated that physical activity has an impact on body functions that are linked to cancer development, such as hormone levels, immune function and body weight.

"Greater participation in **physical activity has consistently been associated with reduced risk of cancer incidence at several sites, including breast and colon cancers**," lead study author James McClain, cancer prevention fellow at the National Cancer Institute, said in a statement. "Short duration sleep appears to have opposing effects of physical activity on several key hormonal and metabolic parameters, which is why we looked at how it affected the exercise/cancer risk relationship."

McClain presented his study, which included data from nearly **6,000 women**, at the **American Association for Cancer Research's International Conference on Frontiers in Cancer Prevention Research.**

The findings must be confirmed by other studies, McClain cautioned. But the study suggests that research must be done on how exactly sleep and exercise impact the development of cancer. **I have written for years that exercise increases EMOD levels and stage 4 sleep increases EMODs. Both will help keep cancer cells in abeyance. On the other hand, an EMOD insufficiency allows for cancer (and a plethora of other diseases) to manifest themselves.**

2.5.6.2 Total antioxidant capacity tended to be lower in athletes

Exercise has been shown to increase the production of reactive oxygen species to a point that can exceed antioxidant defenses to cause oxidative stress. Dietary intake of antioxidants, physical activity levels, various antioxidants and oxidative stress markers were examined in 20 exercise-trained "athletes" and 20 age- and sex-matched sedentary "controls." Plasma F-2-isoprostanes, antioxidant enzyme activities, and uric acid levels were similar in athletes and sedentary controls. **Plasma alpha-tocopherol and beta-carotene were higher in athletes compared with sedentary controls. Total antioxidant capacity tended to be lower in athletes,** with a significant difference between male athletes and male controls. Dietary intakes of antioxidants were also similar between groups and well above recommended dietary intakes for Australians. These findings suggest that athletes who consume a diet rich in antioxidants have elevated plasma alpha-tocopherol and beta-carotene that were likely to be brought about by adaptive processes resulting from regular exercise (Oxidative stress and antioxidants in athletes undertaking regular exercise training. Watson, Trent A. University of Newcastle, MacDonald-Wicks, Lesley K. University of Newcastle, Garg, Manohar Lal. University of Newcastle; The University of Newcastle. 2005; journal article). **The question for the followers of the FRT is, "If exercise increases EMODs drastically, why doesn't the body react by increasing total antioxidant capacity?" I believe that is because the body needs the additional beneficial disease fighting effects of EMODs.**

2.5.6.3 Antioxidants not recommended during strenuous exercise

Investigators determined the effect of dietary antioxidant restriction on oxidative stress, antioxidant defenses, and exercise performance in athletes. **Oxidative stress has been shown to increase during exercise.** To alleviate oxidative stress, a high intake of antioxidant rich foods or supplements may be required in trained athletes. Methods: Plasma oxidative stress and antioxidant defenses were examined in 17 trained athletes who underwent two separate exercise tests. Before the initial exercise test participants followed their habitual (high) antioxidant (H-AO) diets. Then they followed a 2-wk restricted-antioxidant (R-AO) diet before the second exercise test. Blood was taken at rest, after submaximal and high-intensity exhaustive exercise, and after 1 h of recovery. Results: The R-AO diet induced a threefold reduction in antioxidant intake when compared with habitual-antioxidant (H-AO) diets. F-2-isoprostane concentration (marker of oxidative stress) was significantly higher after submaximal exercise (38%), exhaustion (45%), and 1 h of recovery (31%) when following the R-AO diet compared with the H-AO diet. Rate of perceived exertion was increased on the R-AO diet whilst **exercise time to exhaustion was not affected.** Total antioxidant capacity and circulating antioxidant concentrations, although not significantly different, tended to be lower when following the R-AO diet. Conclusion: Athletes regularly participating in up to 40 min of acute high-intensity exercise may require higher intakes of exogenous antioxidants to defend against increased oxidative stress during exercise, which can be met through an adequate intake of high-antioxidant foods. Thus, **there seems no valid reason to recommend antioxidant supplements to athletes participating in acute high-intensity exercise events up to 40 min in duration**, except in those known to be consuming a low-antioxidant diet for prolonged periods (Watson TA, et al. (2005) Med Sci Sports Exerc. 37:63-71).

2.5.6.4 "Exercise, Good; Antioxidants, Bad"

The following is an editorial I (RMH) published on 5-13-09:

Exercise is consistently seen as being good for overall health, as has eating a diet of fresh fruits and vegetables. Unfortunately, the diet data has been misinterpreted to suggest that the antioxidants contained in fruits and vegetables are the specific agents responsible for their good effects, but that is not the case. Being made aware of facts that contradict decades of erroneous teaching is at the least disturbing, if not "stunning." One must have an open mind to consider the strength of the current scientific data on commonly marketed antioxidants, such as vitamins A, C and E. Years of intense study on oxygen metabolism presented me with reliable data which questioned the accuracy of a preponderance of non-scientific publications praising dietary supplements, especially the antioxidant vitamins. Please remember that dietary supplements are a $23 billion business and their advertising influence is demonstrably powerful. German scientists from the University of Jena have found that the antioxidant vitamins C and E can undo some of the most important health benefits of exercise and that taking vitamins C and E after a workout appears to prevent physical exercise improvement of the body's energy regulation. These vitamins appear to block the good effect that exercise has on insulin sensitivity, which could lead to Type 2 diabetes and insulin resistance. The findings add to the growing evidence that antioxidants, including vitamins A, C and E, have complex effects on the body which can do harm as well as good. Also, the much derided oxygen free radicals have been shown to have crucial beneficial effects, including energy production, immunity and protection from cancer and pathogens. In fact, these often maligned oxygen free radicals are essential for our well being. I have presented a world literature review (free of charge) to document these facts at www.thepundit.com and www.medi.philica.com or www.iwillfindthecure.org. Presenting unsupported health care advice and perpetuation of medical misinformation is truly dangerous and irresponsible. There should be legal culpability for giving medical advice which does not have patient safety as its number one priority.

In the America that I love, we will put away misleading medical mythology, get our health information from the most reliable sources available and realize that as our database changes, so should our conclusions. Medical recommendations from only a few years ago may seem foolhardy today. We can not let a dogmatic, arrogant tendency deny our current state of ignorance. **RMH**

2.5.6.5 Habitual exercise and arterial aging

Aging affects the function and structure of arteries and increases the risk of cardiovascular diseases (CVD). In healthy sedentary adults, **aging is associated with increased stiffness (reduced compliance) of large elastic arteries; impaired vascular endothelial function, including reductions in endothelium-dependent dilation (EDD), release of tissue-type plasminogen activator (fibrinolytic capacity) and endothelial progenitor cell number and function; increased intima-media wall thickness (IMT); and peripheral vasoconstriction (decreased basal leg blood flow).**

Habitual physical activity/increased aerobic exercise capacity is associated with reduced risk of CVD. Compared with their sedentary peers, adults who regularly perform aerobic exercise demonstrate smaller or no age-associated increases in large elastic artery stiffness, reductions in vascular endothelial function, and increases in femoral artery IMT. A short-term, moderate-intensity aerobic exercise intervention (**brisk daily walking for 12 wk**) improves carotid artery compliance and can restore vascular endothelial function in previously sedentary middle-aged and older adults. **Reduced oxidative stress may be an important mechanism contributing to these effects.** Habitual resistance exercise increases (high-intensity) or does not affect (moderate-intensity) large elastic artery stiffness, and prevents/restores the age-associated reduction in basal leg blood flow independent of changes in leg fat-free mass. Habitual exercise favorably modulates several expressions of arterial aging, thus preserving vascular function and possibly reducing the risk of CVD (Habitual exercise and arterial aging. Habitual exercise and arterial aging. Douglas R. Seals et al. *J Appl Physiol* 105: 1323-1332, 2008). **Actually, it appears to be logical that habitual exercise is associated with increased EMOD production.**

2.5.7.0 Oxidative stress in development of cardiovascular complications in diabetes mellitus

Diabetes represents a serious risk factor for the development of cardiovascular problems such as coronary heart disease, peripheral arterial disease, hypertension, stroke, cardiomyopathy, nephropathy and retinopathy. Identifying the pathogenesis of this increased risk provides a basis for secondary intervention to reduce morbidity and mortality in diabetic patients. Hyperglycemia and protein glycation, increased inflammation, a prothrombotic state and endothelial dysfunction have all been implicated as possible mechanisms for such complications. A linking element between many of these phenomena could possibly be, among other factors, increased production of reactive oxygen species. Vascular endothelial cells have several physiological actions that are essential for the normal function of the cardiovascular system. These include the production of nitric oxide (NO), which regulates vasodilatation, anticoagulation, leukocyte adhesion, smooth muscle proliferation and the antioxidative capacity of endothelial cells. However, **under conditions of hyperglycemia, excessive amounts of superoxide radicals are produced inside vascular cells** and this can interfere with NO production leading to the possible complications (Role of oxidative stress in development of cardiovascular complications in diabetes mellitus. Haidara MA, Yassin HZ, Rateb M, Ammar H, Zorkani MA. Curr Vasc Pharmacol. 2006 Jul;4(3):215-27). **Actually, hyperglycemia decreases EMOD levels.**

In Watson's study, vitamin E actually increased oxidative stress in the body.

2.5.7.1 Endothelial dysfunction in diabetes mellitus

Diabetes mellitus is associated with an increased risk of cardiovascular disease, even in the presence of intensive glycemic control. Substantial clinical and experimental evidence suggest that both diabetes and insulin resistance cause a combination of endothelial dysfunctions, which may diminish the anti-atherogenic role of the vascular endothelium. **Both insulin resistance and endothelial dysfunction appear to precede the development of overt hyperglycemia in patients with type 2 diabetes.** Therefore, in patients with diabetes or insulin resistance, endothelial dysfunction may be a critical early target for preventing atherosclerosis and cardiovascular disease. Microalbuminuria is now considered to be an atherosclerotic risk factor and predicts future cardiovascular disease risk in diabetic patients, in elderly patients, as well as in the general population. It has been implicated as an independent risk factor for cardiovascular disease and premature cardiovascular mortality for patients with type I and type 2 diabetes mellitus, as well as for patients with essential hypertension. A complete biochemical understanding of the mechanisms by which hyperglycemia causes vascular functional and structural changes associated with the diabetic milieu still eludes us. In recent years, the numerous biochemical and metabolic pathways postulated to have a causal role in the pathogenesis of diabetic vascular disease have been distilled into several unifying hypotheses. The role of chronic hyperglycemia in the development of diabetic microvascular complications and in neuropathy has been clearly established. However, the biochemical or cellular links between elevated blood glucose levels, and the vascular lesions remain incompletely understood. A number of trials have demonstrated that statins therapy as well as angiotensin converting enzyme inhibitors is associated with improvements in endothelial function in diabetes. **Although antioxidants provide short-term improvement of endothelial function in humans, all studies of the effectiveness of preventive antioxidant therapy have been disappointing (failed).** Control of hyperglycemia thus remains the best way to improve endothelial function and to prevent atherosclerosis and other cardiovascular complications of diabetes. In the present review we provide the up to date details on this subject (Endothelial dysfunction in diabetes mellitus. Hadi HA, Suwaidi JA. Vasc Health Risk Manag. 2007;3(6):853-76). **This argues strongly that EMODs are not responsible for diabetes.**

2.5.8.0 High Blood Glucose Levels in Early Pregnancy May Deprive Embryo of Oxygen and Lead to Birth Defects

Oct. 4 /PRNewswire/ -- **The babies of women with diabetes are two to five times more likely to develop birth defects than offspring of women without the disease.** A recent study in animals by scientists at **Joslin Diabetes Center in Boston** helps explain why. The research, appearing in the **October 2005 issue of the American Journal of Physiology: Endocrinology and Metabolism**, suggests that **high blood glucose levels early in pregnancy deprive the embryo of oxygen, interfering with its development.**

"Until recently, it was not understood how diabetic pregnancy could cause birth defects. My laboratory wanted to explore this research because the more we know about the effects of the mother's diabetes on the embryo, the more tools we have to identify therapies that may prevent birth defects in diabetic pregnancy," says the study's lead investigator, Mary R. Loeken, Ph.D., an investigator in Joslin's Section on Developmental and Stem Cell Biology and Assistant Professor of Medicine at Harvard Medical School.

Women with both type 1 and type 2 diabetes run a high risk of having babies with birth defects, especially of the heart and spinal cord. Because **these organs form during the first few weeks of pregnancy,** coinciding with the time that a woman may first learn she is pregnant, aggressive control of blood glucose levels just before and after conception is critical. "Women with diabetes should be consulting with their healthcare team to be sure they have good glycemic control before becoming pregnant," says Dr. Loeken. Maintaining blood glucose control continues to be important throughout the pregnancy, but it is particularly important during the first eight weeks, when an embryo's organs are forming.

In addition to recommending that women with diabetes have good control of their glucose levels before becoming pregnant, Dr. Loeken recommends that obese women who don't know if they have diabetes but who are planning to become pregnant be tested for diabetes. **There have been several recent reports of increased birth defects in the pregnancies of obese women**. **"Many obese individuals have type 2 diabetes and do not know it,** so it is a good idea to bring glucose levels to within the normal range before becoming pregnant, and to monitor women with pre-diabetes closely during pregnancy to make sure that they don't develop diabetes," Dr. Loeken says.

In the new study, Dr. Loeken and her colleagues examined embryos of pregnant mice injected with glucose (the sugar that is elevated in the blood during diabetes) to mimic diabetic pregnancy. The researchers knew that **oxygen is needed by cells to break down glucose and produce energy, and that normally, when oxygen is consumed, more oxygen is delivered to tissues by increasing blood flow to those tissues**. However, at the stage of embryonic development in which birth defects in women with diabetes frequently are believed to occur, the embryo does not yet have a heart or blood supply, and so the scientists theorized it might not be possible to replace oxygen as rapidly as it is consumed. This has the potential to cause hypoxic stress, or damage to cells caused by low oxygen (hypoxia).

Working in collaboration with Peter Smith, Ph.D., Director of the BioCurrents Research Center at the Marine Biological Laboratory at Woods Hole, Mass., Dr. Loeken found that **the oxygen concentrations in embryos of mice injected with glucose were significantly lower than in control embryos.** This demonstrated that breaking down higher amounts of glucose caused oxygen to be used up faster than it could be delivered.

The researchers then injected pregnant mice with glucose, or exposed them to varying levels of oxygen to see if raising and lowering oxygen delivery to the embryos had the same effect as raising and lowering glucose. The scientists' goal was to see whether oxygen deprivation is what mediates the effects of high glucose on the embryo in pregnant diabetic mice. Dr. Loeken's lab had previously found that **inducing high blood glucose levels in pregnant mice suppressed Pax3 expression in embryos. Pax3 is a gene required for healthy formation of the brain and spinal cord.**

In the new study, the researchers found that **restricting oxygen delivery** (by housing pregnant mice for one day in cages containing 12 percent oxygen -- a concentration that did not cause any stress to the mothers, but which might significantly reduce the amount of oxygen delivered to the uterus – instead of 20 percent oxygen contained in room air at sea level) **had the same effect as high glucose.** In fact, **embryos from pregnant mice with high blood glucose levels, or oxygen-restricted mice, had five-fold decreases in Pax3 expression and eight-fold increases in a severe type of birth defect called neural tube defects.** Conversely, **increasing the oxygen delivery to pregnant diabetic mice (by housing them in cages containing 30 percent oxygen) blocked the decrease in Pax3 expression and neural tube defects in their embryos.**

Neural tube defects occur when parts of the brain, spinal cord, or their protective coverings fail to develop properly. For example, spina bifida -- the most common neural tube defect in humans -- results from the incomplete closure of the spinal cord. **Neural tube defects and heart abnormalities are the most common birth defects affecting babies born to women with diabetes.**

Previous research by Dr. Loeken and others has shown **that in pregnant mice, high blood glucose levels boost an embryo's production of free radicals** -- products of metabolism that cause oxidative stress, and that oxidative stress leads to birth defects. These new experiments showed that glucose also caused hypoxic stress in embryos. However, what Dr. Loeken and her colleagues did not know was whether glucose caused two different disturbances, hypoxic stress and oxidative stress, each having separate effects on Pax3 expression, or whether the two disturbances were linked. **To their surprise**, when they investigated the production of free radicals, they found that **embryos of oxygen-restricted mice showed the same three- to five-fold changes in markers of oxidative stress as did embryos of glucose-injected mice**. Conversely, **the markers of oxidative stress were suppressed in embryos of oxygen-supplemented diabetic mice.**

These results suggest that the lack of oxygen caused by increased glucose consumption triggers the production of free radicals, which then causes birth defects, Dr. Loeken explains.

The researchers also found that **administration of high levels of antioxidants** -- which keep free radicals from wreaking cellular havoc -- **prevented the decrease in Pax3 expression and birth defects in embryos of diabetic mice.** This lends weight to the theory that lack of oxygen and the accompanying increase in free radical production that occurs in mice with high blood glucose levels are what ultimately increase risk of birth defects.

"We're trying to pinpoint all the steps that occur between oxygen deprivation and gene expression, and to identify the signals and molecules that regulate Pax3," Dr. Loeken says. (Am J Physiol Endocrinol Metab 289:E591-E599, 2005 (October).

2.5.8.1 Iron in Pregnancy: Free Radical Generation

Jul 16, 2007

Transitional metals, specifically iron, are important in the production of free radicals. Free radical damage is not uncommon and can be detrimental to the fetus.

Iron in pregnancy and its effect on the fetus is one of the most common studies and has led to **an intense focus on free radical generation**. From early pregnancy the human placenta influences maternal homeostasis. **When fully developed the placenta is rich in mitochondria and consumes approximately 1% of the basal metabolic rate of the pregnant woman.**

Pregnancy favors oxidative stress. Oxidative stress can be defined as the disturbance in the pro-oxidant-antioxidant balance, which can lead to potential damage due to free radical generation. **Oxidative stress peaks by the second trimester** of pregnancy and is a vulnerable period for health and gestational progress.

Transitional metals, especially iron, are important in the production of free radicals and are particularly abundant in the placenta. **Free radical damage indications include conditions such as gestational hypertension, insulin resistance and diabetes, which are conditions restricted to pregnancy**. One way of ameliorating early fetal damage is by avoiding excess of iron. It is known that there is an increase in free iron liberation as the placenta starts to develop and mature. **As the placenta's vascularization develops, it changes from a hypoxic environment to an oxygen-rich environment and favours the production of reactive oxygen species (ROS).** These reactive oxygen species allows iron to be liberated from iron-sulphur clusters. Together with the production of ROS is the production of **nitric oxide, which is locally produced by the placenta.**

Nitric oxide and other reactive nitrogen species in the presence of transitional metals can contribute to potential oxidative stress by damaging cellular DNA, proteins and lipids. **There is little data that strongly suggests that the fetus is protected from placental ROS, particularly during the last few weeks of pregnancy**. However, there is special concern about conditions that can induce ROS during organogenesis phases. ROS damage has been observed and explained in many of the effects secondary to temporary iron excess such as acute iron intoxication and hemolytic episodes. The role of vitamin C and E in preventing free radical damage is well known and their nutritional adequacy is important in pregnancy. Vitamin C and vitamin E are known as non-enzymatic free radical protectors and scavengers. A vitamin C deficiency will have a major impact on placental structure and ROS and possibly facilitate placental infections resulting in an increased risk of premature rupture of placental membranes and premature birth (Sadzadeh SM, Saffori Y. Iron and Brain Disorders. Am J Clin Pathol. 2004;121:564-70) (Bucnocore G, Perrane S, Bracci R. Free Radicals and Brain Damage in the Newborn. Biol Neonate. 2001;79:180-6) (Casaneuva E, Viteri FE. Nutrition as a Preventive Strategy Against Adverse Pregnancy Outcomes. Iron and Oxidative stress. J Nutr. 2003;133:1700).

2.5.8.2 Vitamin C, oxidative stress in pregnancy

L-Ascorbic Acid Status Of Pregnant Women And Its Potential Role In Pregnancy-Induced Stress

The increased metabolic activity during pregnancy leads to an increased oxygen requirement. This in turn leads to an increased intake

and utilization of oxygen resulting in elevated levels of oxidative stress via the production of reactive oxygen species. Thus, I believe that increased EMODs appear to be 'Normal" for pregnancy, in order to protect the developing fetus from infections or neoplastic changes.

The concentration of serum L-ascorbic acid was assayed in **90 pregnant women** (age range 20-35 years) and a control group of 30 age-matched women with the aim of assessing the variation in L-ascorbic acid levels and its availability for scavenging reactive oxygen species and controlling oxidative stress during pregnancy.

Results: Serum L-ascorbate was found to generally decrease during the entire period of pregnancy. Inter-trimester mean L-ascorbic acid concentrations in serum were all lower than the control serum L-ascorbic acid concentration. The lowest serum concentration of L-ascorbic acid was found in the first trimester, 1.10 ± 0.01 mg/dl, $p < 0.05$ relative to the control serum L-ascorbic acid concentration of 3.05 ± 0.13 mg/dl. Within trimester L-ascorbate was lowest in the 1-2 months of pregnancy, 0.84 ± 0.01 mg/dl vs. 3.05 ± 0.13 mg/dl (control), $p < 0.05$. **I believe that the decrease in the antioxidant vitamin C appears to be the "normal" response during pregnancy to reduce harmful antioxidant levels.**

Conclusion: These results indicate a compromised ability to scavenge reactive oxygen species, significant perturbation of other L-ascorbate-requiring metabolic/physiological activities during pregnancy and the need for vitamin C supplementation for pregnant women (I. H. Garba, G.A. Ubom, D. Gatsing, R. Aliyu, C. D. Onyeagwa: L-Ascorbic Acid Status Of Pregnant Women And Its Potential Role In Pregnancy-Induced Stress. *The Internet Journal of Nutrition and Wellness*. 2005. Volume 1 Number 2).

Oxygen free radicals

The following is taken from the above Garba paper: **Many free radicals are produced in the body as a result of the myriad of biochemical processes taking place in normal metabolism** (Skaper SD, Fabris M, Ferrari V, Carbonare MD, Leon A. Quercetin protects cutaneous tissue-associated cell types from oxidative stress induced by glutathione depletion: cooperative effects of ascorbic acid. *Free Rad Biol Med* 1997; 22: 669-678). **Please remember that both quercetin and ascorbate can act as prooxidants.**

Oxygen-derived free radicals account for 95 % of such radicals (Du WD, Yuan ZR, Sun J, Tang JX, Cheng AQ, Shen DM, Song XH, Yu XF, Zheng SB. Therapeutic efficacy of high dose vitamin C on acute pancreatitis and its potential mechanisms. *World J Gastroenterol* 2003; 11: 2565-2569).

These **free radicals perform some physiologic function** to some degree in the body such as, **participating in xenobiotics metabolism, biosynthesis and clearance of microorganisms** (Braganza JM, Scott P, Bilton G, Schofield D, Chaloner C, Shiel N, Hunt LP, Bottiglieri T. Evidence for early oxidative stress in acute pancreatitis. Clues for correction. *Int J Pancreatol* 1995; 17: 69-81) (Wereszczynska S, Dabrowski A, Jedynak M, Gabryelewicz A. Oxidative stress as an early prognostic factor in acute pancreatitis (AP): its correlation with serum phospholipase A2 (pla2) and plasma polymorphonuclear elastase (PMN-E) in different severity forms of human AP. *Pancreas* 1998; 17: 163-168) (Fentone JC, Ward PA. Role of oxygen derived free radicals and metabolites in leukocyte-dependent inflammatory reactions. *Am J Pathol* 1982; 107: 397-418).

The normal homeostasis of these free radicals is maintained by anti-oxidants and anti-oxidases, leading to a dynamic balance between production and clearance (Sudha K, Rao AV, Rao S, Rao A. Free radical toxicity and antioxidants in Parkinson's disease. *Neurol India* 2003; 51: 60-61).

An imbalance between reactive oxygen species and anti-oxidant defense mechanisms of a cell leads to an excessive production of oxygen metabolites, creating a condition known as 'oxidative stress' (Sudha K, Rao AV, Rao A. Oxidative stress and antioxidants in epilepsy. *Clin Chim Acta* 2001; 303: 19-24).

Such free radicals can attack polyunsaturated fatty acids of membranes, leading to lipid peroxidation and disruption of intracellular calcium homeostasis and consequent cellular **apoptosis** (Buttke TM, Sandsrom PA. Oxidative stress as mediator of apoptosis. *Immunol Today* 1994; 15: 7-10).

Free radicals can also destroy key intracellular enzymes, including free radical scavenger enzymes, disrupt DNA replication and initiate the process of carcinogenesis (Wiseman H, Halliwell B. Damage to DNA by reactive oxygen and nitrogen species: Role in inflammatory disease and progression to cancer. *Biochem J* 1996; 313: 17-29) (Sundstrom H, Korpela H, Viinikka L, Kauppila A. Serum selenium and GP and plasma lipid peroxides in uterine, ovarian and vulvar cancer, and their responses to antioxidants in patients with ovarian cancer. *Cancer Lett* 1984; 24: 1-10).

Free radical-induced oxidative injury have been reported to have a role in the pathogenesis of a number of diseases, including cancer, atherosclerosis, diabetes mellitus, epilepsy, radiation damage, cellular aging, reperfusion damage, inflammatory diseases and Parkinsonism (Sundstrom H, Korpela H, Viinikka L, Kauppila A. Serum selenium and GP and plasma lipid peroxides in uterine, ovarian and vulvar cancer, and their responses to antioxidants in patients with ovarian cancer. *Cancer Lett* 1984; 24: 1-10) (Plachta H, Bartkowska E, Obara A. Lipid peroxides in blood from patients with atherosclerosis of coronary and peripheral arteries. *Clin Chim Acta* 1992; 211: 101-102) (Oberley LW. Free radicals and diabetes. *Free Rad Biol Med* 1988; 5: 113-124) (Bowling AC, Beal MF. Bioenergetics and oxidative stress in neurodegenerative diseases. *Life Sci* 1995; 56: 1151-1) (Ames BN, Shigenaga MK, Hagen TM. Antioxidants and the degenerative diseases of aging. *Proc Natl Acad Sci USA* 1993; 90: 7915-7922) (Yondim MB, Riederer P. Understanding Parkinson's disease. *Sci Am* 1997; 1: 38-45).

Free radical defenses in the body consist of a complex anti-oxidant system comprising of vitamins A, C, E, glutathione and anti-oxidant enzymes (Halliwell B, Gutteridge JMC. The antioxidants of human extracellular fluids. *Arch Biochim Biophys* 1990; 280: 1-8) (Bravenboer B, Kapelle AC, Hamers EPT, Van Buren DW, Erkelens DW, Gispen WH. Potential use of glutathione for the prevention and treatment of diabetic neuropathy in the streptozocin-induced diabetic rat. *Diabetologia* 1992; 35: 813-817).

These enzymes include glutathione reductase, glutathione peroxidase, superoxide dismutase and catalase (Halliwell B, Gutteridge JMC. The antioxidants of human extracellular fluids. *Arch Biochim Biophys* 1990; 280: 1-8).

Pregnancy is a developmental crisis in a woman's life. It places a great demand on her body and requires adaptation. Changes in many of the body's biochemical function during pregnancy leads to a high demand for energy and an increased oxygen requirement (Bray JJ, Cragg PA, Macknight ADC, Mills RG. Lecture notes on human physiology, 4th ed. Blackwell Scientific Publications, USA. 1999).

This leads to intake and utilization of oxygen, resulting in increased levels of oxidative stress and the consequent acceleration in the production of reactive oxygen species (Renata G, Miroslow K, Wlodizimierz K, Ryszard K, Ewa S. Changes in antioxidant components in blood of mares during pregnancy and after foaling. *Bull Vet Inst Pulaway* 2002; 46: 301-305).

In this study, the serum concentration of L-ascorbic acid which makes up over 80% of the vitamin C activity was assessed in pregnant women in three different trimesters of pregnancy with the aim of determining the effect of pregnancy on serum L-ascorbic acid concentration and its availability for the scavenging of reactive oxygen species produced as a result of pregnancy-induced oxidative stress. **There is a significant reduction in the serum L-ascorbic acid concentration throughout the period of pregnancy with the highest decrease in the first trimester.** As reported by Renata et al.**changes in the physiological state during pregnancy necessitates an increase oxygen intake and utilization.This leads to an increased level of oxidative stress.**

I believe that Darwinian evolution would argue that EMOD increases during pregnancy is a good and necessary event, especially considering the vulnerability of a developing fetus and embryo.The EMODs are protect of disease and neoplasia.

Considering the catalytic role of ascorbic acid in enhancing iron absorption, the low serum ascorbate can lead to a decrease in the absorption and subsequent utilization of iron which is required for the proper maintenance of pregnancy and fetal growth. In addition, **during pregnancy resistance to infection is generally decreased. Similarly fetal and neonatal immunity is low.**

Low serum L-ascorbic acid will further complicate this delicate immune status since L-ascorbic acid is known to play a significant role in boosting immunity. Since earlier reports have confirmed the importance of vitamin C in safe delivery and the prevention of premature abortions, we conclude from these results that pregnant women should be placed on daily supplemental doses of vitamin C to boost maternal antioxidant defenses and help improve maternal and fetal immune status. **I believe that this is an erroneous recommendation, based on old, out-dated data.**

2.5.9.0 Vitamin Deaths

2.5.9.1 Fifteen infant deaths in India may be due vitamin A

Newscientist.com 24 November 2001 Magazine issue 2318

Fifteen infants have died and over 3000 are severely ill in Assam in north-east India after receiving vitamin A supplements as part of a drive to combat night blindness in under-fives.The joint UNICEF-Assam government campaign has now been stopped and an enquiry ordered. Indian health officials fear that either the children's doses were too high, or the supplements were contaminated. They also say that the campaign is unnecessary. "Vitamin A overdose increases brain pressure in babies. Besides, its deficiency is no longer a public health problem here," says Coluthur Gopalan, president of the Nutritional Foundation of India.

Wikipedia Death by vitamin poisoning appears to be quite uncommon in the US, typically none in a given year. Before 1998, several deaths per year were associated with pharmaceutical iron-containing supplements, especially brightly-colored, sugar-coated, high-potency iron supplements, and most deaths were children.[2] Unit packaging restrictions on supplements with more than 30 mg of iron have since reduced deaths to 0 or 1 per year. (Tenenbein M (2005). "Unit-dose packaging of iron supplements and reduction of iron poisoning in young children". *Arch Pediatr Adolesc Med* 159 (6): 557–60).

2.5.9.2 Vitamin death-link hard pill to swallow (*Bjelakovic*)

Vitamin supplements might make you die sooner, say researchers.

Goran Bjelakovic and his colleagues, from the University of Copenhagen, looked at the results from 230,000 people who had taken part in 67 previously published placebo-controlled trials of anti-oxidant vitamins and their effects on health and disease.

Combining the data together in this way can make a study much more powerful because bias and error can be reduced, and subtle, possibly previously-invisible trends are easier to spot.

What emerged from this analysis, which included both healthy volunteers and patients with a range of diseases, was that taking anti-oxidants such as vitamin A or vitamin E are not linked to a lower death rate. In fact, when the researchers focused on the results of the 46 trials with the least risk of bias, a worrying statistic emerged. **There was a 16% higher death rate amongst the users of vitamin A, patients given beta-carotene had a roughly 7% higher mortality rate, and those on vitamin E had a 4% rise in mortality.** Vitamin C and selenium didn't seem to increase nor decrease mortality rates, but the team stress that more data is needed to form firm conclusions about these agents.

The use of vitamin supplements, and **anti-oxidants in particular, is based on sound science,** since researchers think that most of the effects of ageing and diseases linked to it like heart disease are caused by damage done to cells by reactive chemicals called free radicals. Antioxidants are thought shield cells from the damaging effects of free radicals, and therefore taking them as supplements might help to fend off disease and the effects of the ageing process.

Whilst that may be true, what this study shows is that obtaining anti-oxidants from a packet is not beneficial to your health and may even **paradoxically increase mortality**. Instead the only proven way to cut cancer and heart disease deaths is to eat five or more portions of fruit and veg daily, which has consistently emerged in trials as the best predictor of living to a ripe old age.

2.5.9.3 Orthomolecular News report *20th Apr 2008*

A 23-year review of US poison control center annual reports confirms the true and largely ignored story: **vitamins are extraordinarily safe**. The American Association of Poison Control Centers (AAPCC), which maintains the USA's national database of information from 61 poison control centers, provides data showing that even including intentional and accidental misuse, **the number of alleged vitamin fatalities is strikingly low, averaging less than one death per year for more than two decades**. In 16 of those 23 years, AAPCC reports that there was not one single death due to vitamins. These statistics specifically include vitamin A, niacin (B-3), pyridoxine (B-6), other B-complex, C, D, E, and "other" vitamin(s), such as vitamin K. (Annual Reports of the American Association of Poison Control Centers' National Poisoning and Exposure Database (formerly known as the Toxic Exposure Surveillance System). AAPCC, 3201 New Mexico Avenue, Ste. 330, Washington, DC 20016).

Michael Janson, MD, said, "In decades of people taking a wide variety of dietary supplements, few adverse effects have been noted, and zero deaths as a result of the dietary supplements. **There is far more risk to public health from people stopping their vitamin supplements than from people taking them."**

2.5.9.4 E-Ferol

http://www.cdc.gov/mmwr/preview/mmwrhtml/00000319.htm MMWR weekly. April 13, 1984 / 33(14);198-9.

2.5.9.5 Unusual Syndrome with Fatalities among Premature Infants: Association with a New Intravenous Vitamin E Product

Since March 9, 1984, CDC has received reports from two hospitals of clusters of an unusual illness occurring among low-birthweight (less than 1,500 grams), premature infants in neonatal intensive-care units. Thirteen affected infants in these two hospitals developed clinically significant ascites, in addition to some or all of the following abnormalities: hepatomegaly, splenomegaly, cholestatic jaundice, azotemia, and thrombocytopenia. **Eight infants have died.** All affected infants had received parenteral nutrition therapy, in addition to other supportive measures and therapeutic interventions common to the care of low-birthweight infants. An intravenous vitamin E preparation, containing 25 mg/ml vitamin E, 9% polysorbate 80 and 1% polysorbate 20 in 2-ml vials (**E-Ferol Aqueous SolutionR**, distributed by O'Neal, Jones & Feldman, St. Louis, Missouri), was introduced in each hospital for addition to parenteral nutrition solutions approximately 1 month before the onset of illness in the first infant in both clusters. All affected infants received E-Ferol; some affected infants received up to 1 ml or more daily. Both outbreaks ceased shortly after use of E-Ferol was discontinued.

In collaboration with the state health departments, CDC is conducting ongoing epidemiologic investigations at both institutions. Although the etiology and pathophysiology of this syndrome are presently unclear, the U.S. Food and Drug Administration (FDA) and CDC recommend that E-Ferol not be used. FDA and the distributor have initiated a voluntary recall of the product. The product, which has been marketed since December 1983, is not the subject of an Approved New Drug Application by FDA. Reported by V Lorch, MD, MD Murphy, MD, University of Tennessee Research Center and Hospital, Knoxville, RH Hutcheson, MD, State Epidemiologist, Tennessee Dept of Health and Environment; N Kosmetatos, MD, D Frank, MD, Good Samaritan Hospital, Cincinnati, TJ Halpin, MD, State Epidemiologist, Ohio State Dept of Health; Center for Drugs and Biologics, US Food and Drug Administration; Hospital Infections Program, Div of Viral Diseases, Center for Infectious Diseases, Center for Environmental Health, CDC.

Editorial Note

Editorial Note: Premature neonates are reported to have a relative deficiency of vitamin E at birth, which has been associated with hemolytic anemia in premature infants (1). Although vitamin E is reported to have a therapeutic benefit in treating this form of hemolytic disease in premature infants and may have a role in preventing the development of retrolental fibroplasia and bronchopulmonary dysplasia in infants requiring oxygen therapy, the benefit, risk, and dosage relationships are, at present, uncertain (Ehrenkranz RA. Vitamin E and the neonate. Am J Dis Child 1980;134:1157-66) (Hittner HM, Godio LB, Rudolph AJ, et al. Retrolental fibroplasia: efficacy of vitamin E in a double blind clinical study of preterm infants. N Eng J Med 1981;305:1365-71).

Other vitamin E preparations are available for enteral, subcutaneous, and intramuscular administration. Vitamin E is a component, at lower concentrations, of multivitamin preparations for intravenous use. Use of these alternative vitamin E preparations has not been temporally associated with the severe clinical syndrome described above. However, other complications, such as cholestatic jaundice, have been associated with total parenteral nutrition therapy (Bernstein J, Chang CH, Brough AJ, Heidelberger KP. Conjugated hyperbilirubinemia in infancy associated with parenteral alimentation. J Pediatr 1977;90;361-7), and thrombocytopenia with lipid emulsion therapy (Lipson AH, Pritchard J, Thomas G. Thrombocytopenia after intralipid infusion in a neonate. Lancet 1974;I:1462-3).

Additional reports of similar severe illness should be reported through appropriate state health officials to the Epidemiology Development Branch, Division of Drug and Biologic Experience, FDA (301) 443-6410 or the Hospital Infections Program, Center for Infectious Diseases, CDC (404) 329-3406.

2.5.9.6 Supplements have quality problems

6-9-09 The following was taken from: http://news.yahoo.com/s/ap/20090609/ap_on_bi_ge/us_med_unproven_remedies_safety

Lead in ginkgo pills. Arsenic in herbals. Bugs in a baby's colic and teething syrup. Toxic metals and parasites are part of nature, and all of these have been found in "natural" products and dietary supplements in recent years. Set aside the issue of whether vitamin and herbal supplements do any good.

Are they safe? Is what's on the label really what's in the bottle? Tests by researchers and private labs suggest the answer sometimes is no.

One quarter of supplements tested by an independent company over the last decade have had some sort of problem. Some contained contaminants. Others had contents that did not match label claims. Some had ingredients that exceeded safe limits. Some contained real drugs masquerading as natural supplements.

"We buy it just as the consumer buys it" from stores, said Dr. Tod Cooperman, president of **ConsumerLab.com.** The company tests pills for makers that want its seal of approval, and publishes ratings for subscribers, much as Consumer Reports does with household goods.

Other tests, reported in scientific journals, found prenatal vitamins lacking claimed amounts of iodine, and supplements short on ginseng and hoodia — an African plant sparking the latest diet craze.

"There's at least 10 times more hoodia sold in this country than made in the world, so people are not getting hoodia," said Dr. Mehmet Oz, a heart surgeon and frequent Oprah Winfrey guest who occasionally has touted the stuff.

Industry groups say that quality problems are the exception rather than the rule.

"I believe that the problem is narrow, that the well-established and reputable brands deserve their reputations," said Michael McGuffin, president of the American Herbal Products Association.

Of course, prescription drugs have had problems, too. Dozens of deaths were linked last year to tainted heparin, a blood thinner produced in China, for example. However, **pharmaceutical drugs must show evidence to the government of safety and effectiveness before they go on sale. Not so for dietary supplements**.

Fifteen years ago, Congress passed a law that treats supplements like food and allows them to go straight to market without federal Food and Drug Administration approval. The FDA can act only after consumers get sick or a safety issue comes to light.

"We called it 'the body rule,'" said William Obermeyer, a chemist who left the FDA to found ConsumerLab.com with Cooperman. If a supplement was harmful, "we had to have so many adverse events before we could make a move on it. It was really like closing the barn door after all the animals left."

The law said the FDA could write quality control rules for products sold in the U.S. It took the FDA 13 years to adopt these, and they are just now taking effect. But the rules do not say what tests companies must do to prove what is in their products, and some tests can be fooled by subbing other ingredients. The rules also set no limits on toxins such as lead; nor do they change the fundamental way these products are sold to the public.

"It leaves the level of quality up to the manufacturer," Cooperman said.

In a written statement, FDA spokeswoman Susan Cruzan said the new rules contain what is "needed to ensure quality," and that products that contain contaminants or whose labels do not honestly describe their contents, are considered adulterated and subject to further action by the agency. But she conceded that the agency is spread thin.

"In that FDA has limited resources to analyze the composition of food products, including dietary supplements, it focuses these resources first on public health emergencies and products that may have caused injury or illness," she wrote.

Millions of Americans take vitamin, herbal or other dietary supplements. Annual sales exceed $23 billion, and more than 40,000 products are on the market.

Tens of thousands of supplement-related health problems are handled by U.S. poison control centers each year, according to a report in the New England Journal of Medicine in 2002.

Until last year, supplement makers were not required to report problems to the FDA, and even now they must report only serious ones. The agency estimates that more than 50,000 safety problems a year are related to supplement use.

The Institute of Medicine, an independent science panel that advises the government, studied the situation in 2005. "The committee is concerned about the quality of dietary supplements in the United States. **Product reliability is low**," says its report, which urged amending the 1994 law to tighten consumer protections.

Trade associations say the FDA's new rules do that.

"We are FDA-regulated products," though not in the same way as prescription or over-the-counter drugs, said Steven Mister, president of the Council for Responsible Nutrition.

The FDA can ask law enforcement to act against any company selling an adulterated product, said McGuffin of the herbal products association. "You can go to jail, you can have your company seized," he said.

"We represent companies that we consider the responsible center of the industry," who are working to comply with the new rules, he said. But **his group only represents 250 of the 1,500 companies selling such products.** And even though millions of people take supplements with no apparent ill effects, there have been many quality problems that a consumer might never realize because they don't always produce symptoms:

_CONTAMINANTS

ConsumerLab.com found lead in at least one brand each of zinc, black cohosh and ginkgo products tested in recent years. Lead can accumulate and cause many health problems, and the testing company wants a national limit of 0.5 micrograms per day — a level that in California requires a warning on the label.

A fungal toxin was found in four red yeast rice products in March 2008. And in 2007, federal officials warned about **a liquid herbal supplement sold for colic and teething pain after finding cryptosporidium**, a waterborne parasite that causes severe diarrhea.

Ayurvedics — popular herbals used in traditional medicines from India — often contain hazardous metals, studies in medical journals report. In 2004, researchers tested 70 ayurvedic remedies in the Boston area and found that one in five had potentially harmful levels of lead, mercury or arsenic. Tests in Houston, Chicago, San Francisco and New York City turned up similar results.

Metals naturally accumulate in certain herbs and come from the soil they are grown in. Many supplement ingredients come from Europe, India and China. "We don't know how much of the ingredients are imported — whether they're coming from across town or across the world," Mister of the trade association conceded. But even manufacturers get duped, said Jana Hildreth of the Analytical Research Collective, a group of scientists advocating better supplement testing.

"Companies started going to China and demanding lower prices," and unscrupulous suppliers sometimes spiked products with cheap ingredients that can trick lab tests, she said. An example: a buckwheat derivative, rutin, in place of pricier ginkgo.

_POTENCY PROBLEMS

In ConsumerLab.com testing last November, four out of seven supplements contained less ginkgo than claimed on their labels, and one failed to break apart properly to release its ingredients. Seven out of nine failed in tests in 2003, as did six out of 13 in 2005.

"It is now believed that **ginkgo is among the most adulterated herbs**," the company reports. Tests by California scientists of two dozen ginseng supplements, reported in a nutrition journal in 2001, found that many differed from their labels. The concentrations of some ginseng compounds varied by up to 200-fold from product to product.

In ConsumerLab.com tests, six out of nine chondroitin supplements failed testing in April 2007. One had only 8 percent of what it claimed to contain, and one "maximum strength" product had none.

Vitamins and minerals had problems, too. A "high potency" iron supplement contained less than half the amount claimed. Of 23 top-selling vitamin C pills, one provided less than half the amount promised; the suggested dosages of some others were beyond recommended safe levels. Of 10 vitamin A supplements, one provided twice its stated amount, raising concern about toxic side effects.

Last year, nearly 200 people were sickened by supplements containing up to 200 times the amount of selenium stated on the label. Symptoms included hair loss, discolored and painful fingernails, muscle cramps, joint pain, diarrhea and fatigue.

_HIDDEN PRESCRIPTION DRUGS

The FDA has repeatedly warned about herbal pills found to contain versions of Viagra and similar drugs to help men get an erection. These can pose a heart hazard, especially when taken with certain medications.

In December, the FDA expanded warnings about dozens of brands of weight loss pills. Though the labels did not say so, some contained sibutramine, a controlled substance that poses heart risks; rimonabant, a drug not approved in the United States; a seizure medicine, and a diuretic.

Red yeast rice, a traditional Chinese medicine, has compounds that may block cholesterol in a way similar to statin drugs. Some red yeast rice products have been found to contain lovastatin, the active ingredient in the drug Mevacor. Problems can occur at high doses or with other medicines.

_OTHER RISKS

Even "safe" supplements can be harmful. Beta-carotene takers still had increased rates of lung cancer six years after one study was stopped. These supplements "appear to increase rates of the disease, particularly among smokers," the National Cancer Institute warns.

In another study, men taking vitamin E were slightly more likely to get prostate cancer, and those taking selenium were a little more likely to develop diabetes. The results could have been due to chance, but federal officials were taking no chances and stopped the study last October.

Other studies suggest that **high doses of vitamin C may help shield cancer cells from treatments designed to kill the cancer**.

"Antioxidants are not the magic bullets that the supplement industry would like consumers to believe," said David Schardt, a nutrition expert with the consumer advocacy group, the Center for Science in the Public Interest. **"They're not even necessarily benign."**

Herbal sex pills containing the African tree bark extract yohimbe have landed men in hospitals with heart rhythm problems. This herb can cause high blood pressure, increased heart rate and other symptoms, the government warns.

The most serious side effects occurred with diet pills containing ephedra — heart problems, seizures and even deaths. The FDA banned it in 2004. The battle started in 1997, when the agency wanted strong warnings on labels, and it became a test case of FDA authority that went all the way to the U.S. Supreme Court, where the FDA ultimately prevailed.

_DRUG INTERACTIONS

Ginkgo, vitamin K, garlic, ginseng and other herbals can cause bleeding or clotting problems if taken with certain medications or before surgery. St. John's wort, promoted for depression, affects metabolism of more than half of all prescription drugs and can undermine birth control pills. Other supplements that can interfere with medicines include glucosamine, saw palmetto, soy and valerian.

_OVERSTATED HEALTH CLAIMS

Makers can say a supplement addresses a nutrient deficiency, supports health, or reduces the risk of developing a problem, but then must say the product "is not intended to diagnose, treat, cure, or prevent any disease."

So consumers will see vague claims, such as "promotes healthy immune system function." The immune system has dozens of parts, and modifying one can be helpful or harmful, so "it's a quack concept," said Dr. Stephen Barrett, a retired physician who runs Quackwatch, a Web site on medical scams.

The Federal Trade Commission has stepped up actions against deceptive ads, said commission lawyer Rich Cleland. "It is a little like playing Whack-A-Mole," because each time one problem is resolved, more seem to pop up, he said.

Last year, his agency reached a settlement against the makers of Airborne, a supplement aimed at people in crowded places such as airplanes, offices and schools. Company founders "made false claims that Airborne products are clinically proven to treat colds," and there is also no evidence the products can prevent colds, the FTC complaint says.

Airborne's makers agreed to add $6.5 million to the $23.5 million they had already agreed to pay to settle a related private class-action lawsuit, bringing the total settlement fund to $30 million.

Industry also has stepped up self-policing. The Council for Responsible Nutrition gave money to the Council of Better Business Bureaus so it could hire a lawyer to investigate some supplement sellers' sketchy claims.

"There were cancer cures and 'blast off 29 pounds in 39 days' — really **the Wild West of advertising. It was totally out of control,"** said the BBB's advertising division director, Andrea Levine.

The BBB council targets the worst claims in popular categories, such as diet, cold and flu, menopause, joint problems and sleep aids. "We can't do them all," but want to send a broad signal about what kinds of claims are over the line for each type of product, she said.

On the Net:

FDA: http://www.fda.gov/consumer/updates/supplements080408.html

Government supplement advice: http://tinyurl.com/alpr98

2.6.0.0 Hyperuricemia Deaths

Uric acid general information (source: eMedicine.com accessed 11/20/08).

Uric acid is the final product of purine metabolism in human beings. Despite the fact that uric acid was first identified approximately 2 centuries ago, certain pathophysiologic aspects of hyperuricemia are still not clearly understood. For years, hyperuricemia has been identified with or thought to be the same as gout, but uric acid has now been identified as a marker for a number of metabolic and hemodynamic abnormalities.

Unlike allantoin, the more soluble end product found in lower animals, uric acid is a poorly soluble end product of purine metabolism in humans. Human beings have higher levels of uric acid, in part, because of a deficiency of the hepatic enzyme, uricase, and a lower fractional excretion of uric acid. **Approximately two thirds of total body urate is produced endogenously, while the remaining one third is accounted for by dietary purines.** Approximately 70% of the urate produced daily is excreted by the kidneys, while the rest is eliminated by the intestines. However, during renal failure, the intestinal contribution of urate excretion increases to compensate for the decreased elimination by the kidneys.

The blood levels of uric acid are a function of the balance between the breakdown of purines and the rate of uric acid excretion. Theoretically, alterations in this balance may account for hyperuricemia, although clinically defective elimination accounts for most cases of hyperuricemia. (source: eMedicine.com accessed 11/20/08).

Hyperuricemia has been associated with increased morbidity in patients with hypertension and is associated with increased mortality in women and elderly persons. The cause for this is unknown, but hyperuricemia is probably a marker for comorbid risk factors rather than a causative factor, per se.

A high prevalence of hyperuricemia exists in indigenous races of the Pacific, which appears to be associated with a low fractional excretion of uric acid. **African American persons develop hyperuricemia more commonly than white persons.**

Hyperuricemia, and particularly gouty arthritis, are far more common in men than in women. Only 5% of patients with gout are female, but **uric acid levels increase in women after menopause.**

The normal serum uric acid level is lower in children than in adults. The upper limit of the reference range for children is 5 mg/dL (0.30 mmol/L). The upper limit of the reference range for men is 7 mg/dL (0.42 mmol/L) and for women is 6 mg/dL (0.36 mmol/L). **The tendency to develop hyperuricemia increases with age.**

2.6.0.1 Antioxidant uric acid increases death risk

Hyperuricemia is clearly a powerful predictive factor for ischemic cardiovascular disease (CVD; and poor outcomes in these conditions), as recently reviewed. But **hyperuricemia and gout are commonly associated with hypertension, metabolic syndrome, and dyslipidemia**, and the role of serum urate as an independent risk factor has remained controversial despite many decades of study. Substantial differences in patient populations and study design have been proposed as explanations for discrepancies of results for this question, including assessment of subjects with existing cardiovascular and metabolic disorders. For example, **the recently published National Health and Nutrition Examination Survey I (NHANES I) study of 5926 subjects concluded that increased uric acid is independently and significantly associated with cardiovascular mortality.**

Death because of ischemic heart disease in men and women increased when serum urate levels were in their highest quartile compared with the lowest quartile (men, risk ratio 1.77 [95% confidence interval (CI) 1.08–3.98]; women, risk ratio 3.00 [95% CI 1.45–6.28]). In contrast, earlier results from the Framingham database [3] suggested that the apparent association of serum urate with cardiovascular events was probably because of confounding by other cardiovascular risk factors, particularly by diuretic use. These discrepancies, and lack of direct attention to metabolic syndrome in the NHANES study, prompted Niskanen *et al.* to further examine this clinical association.

This population-based prospective cohort study was conducted on **1423 healthy middle-aged Finnish males** (*ie*, subjects who were initially without CVD, cancer, or diabetes). Baseline uric acid levels were obtained as well as other potentially confounding variables (*ie*, waist circumference, hypertension, smoking history, serum cholesterol levels, and so on). Patients were stratified by uric acid into thirds (tertile limits, 5.04 and 5.88 mg/dL) and **followed-up for a mean of**

11.9 years. The primary outcome measure was death from CVD. The associations of serum urate tertiles with cardiovascular mortality were analyzed with forced Cox proportional hazard models and multivariate adjustment.

Results: There were 157 deaths during the 11.9 years follow-up and of these, 55 were CVD deaths. **In univariate Cox proportional hazard analyses, serum urate concentration was associated with CVD mortality. Uric acid levels also tended to be associated with death from any cause during follow-up** ($P = .06$). Multivariate analysis was performed using three different models: age-adjusted, age adjusted plus cardiovascular risk factors (smoking, low density lipoprotein cholesterol level, family history for cardiac disease, systolic blood pressure, use of diuretics, use of blood pressure medications, body mass index, alcohol intake, serum creatinine level, and adult socioeconomic level), and age adjusted plus cardiovascular risk factors and metabolic syndrome variables (fasting serum insulin, triglyceride, and high-density lipoprotein cholesterol concentrations, fasting blood glucose levels, conditioning exercise, and cardiorespiratory fitness). **In all three models, serum urate in the second and third tertiles was associated with a higher relative risk of death from CVD than the lowest third tertile.** Taking into account cardiovascular as well as metabolic syndrome risk factors, **serum urate levels in the upper thirds were associated with a 4.77 greater risk from cardiac death than the lower third**. Interestingly, in this same model of analysis, the middle uric acid tertile had an (approximately) equally high risk from cardiac death (4.98) relative to the highest tertile.

This was a well-conducted study that, unlike some of its predecessors, adjusted for key components of the metabolic syndrome (*ie*, waist circumference and levels of glucose, insulin, high-density lipoprotein cholesterol and triglycerides). The study also adjusted for physical conditioning, an important variable given that muscle and tissue ischemia increase uric acid production. Serum urate levels are a sensitive surrogate marker of metabolic syndrome, which is also associated with cardiovascular mortality.

(Niskanen L, Laaksonen D, Nyyssonen K, *et al.*: **Uric acid level as a risk factor for cardiovascular and all-cause mortality in middle-aged men.** *Arch Intern Med* 2004, **164:**1546–1551).

2.6.0.2 Hyperuricemia increases risk of death in all causes

A positive association between hyperuricemia and cardiovascular disease has been reported, but no study has evidenced yet the precise role of serum uric acid in the development of cardiovascular disease. In addition, **no epidemiological studies have so far documented a decreased risk of cancer among people**

with hyperuricemia, even though **the antioxidant action of uric acid has recently been stressed to inhibit DNA damage.** The present prospective cohort study investigates the relationship between hyperuricemia and health hazards in a Japanese working population. The subjects were 49,413 Japanese male railroad workers, aged 25-60 years at enrollment. Serum uric acid and other baseline data were provided by annual health-survey records from 1975 to 1982. The vital status of the subjects was traced until the end of 1985 for those who remained alive. During an average 5.4-year study period, 984 deaths were recorded. Those with serum uric acid over 8.5 mg/dl showed elevated relative risks (RRs) of death in all causes (RR 1.62, $p<0.01$), coronary heart disease (RR 1.52), stroke (RR 2.33, $p<0.01$), hepatic disease (RR 3.58, $p<0.01$), and renal failure (RR 8.52, $p<0.01$), as compared with those with serum uric acid levels of 5.0-6.4mg/dl. The RR of death in all causes still remains statistically significant when adjusted by age and serum total cholesterol (2.00, $p<0.01$), age and alcohol intake (1.85, $p<0.001$), age and smoking (1.69, $p<0.001$), age and gout treatment (1.61, $p<0.05$), and also age and BMI (1.50, $p< 0.05$). On the other hand, the RR of all causes decreased but was still above 1.0 when adjusted by age and blood glucose (1.62), age and systolic blood pressure (1.32), age and GOT (1.23), and also age and history of cardiovascular disease (1.17). These results showed that **hyperuricemia has a strong association with the RRs of death in all causes, coronary heart disease, stroke, hepatic disease and renal failure, and indicated that serum uric acid seems to be a considerable risk factor for reduced life expectancy** (Does hyperuricemia affect mortality? A prospective cohort study of Japanese male workers. Tomita M. et al. J Epidemiol. 2000 Nov;10(6):403-9).

I must ask, "How can a great antioxidant, like uric acid, cause such bad effects and death?" To do so is counter to the free radical theory.

2.6.0.3 Men with gout have increased all cause mortality

Although gout and hyperuricemia are related to several conditions that are associated with reduced survival, no prospective data are available on the independent impact of gout on mortality. Furthermore, although many studies have suggested that hyperuricemia is associated with cardiovascular disease (CVD), limited data are available on the impact of gout on CVD. METHODS AND RESULTS: Over a 12-year period, we prospectively examined the relation between a history of gout and the risk of death and myocardial infarction in 51,297 male participants of the Health Professionals Follow-Up Study. During the 12 years of follow-up, we documented 5825 deaths from all causes, which included 2132 deaths from CVD and 1576 deaths from coronary heart disease (CHD). Compared with men without history of gout and CHD at baseline, the multivariate relative risks among men with history of gout were 1.28 (95% confidence interval [CI], 1.15 to 1.41) for total mortality, 1.38 (95% CI, 1.15 to 1.66) for CVD deaths, and 1.55 (95% CI, 1.24 to 1.93) for fatal CHD. The corresponding relative risks among men with preexisting CHD were 1.25 (95% CI, 1.09 to 1.45), 1.26 (95% CI, 1.07 to 1.50), and 1.24 (95% CI, 1.04 to 1.49), respectively. In addition, men with gout had a higher risk of nonfatal myocardial infarction than men without gout (multivariate relative risk, 1.59; 95% CI, 1.04 to 2.41). CONCLUSIONS: These prospective data indicate that **men with gout have a higher risk of death from all causes.** Among men without preexisting CHD, the increased mortality risk is primarily a result of an elevated risk of CVD death, particularly from CHD (Independent impact of gout on mortality and risk for coronary heart disease. Choi HK, Curhan G. Circulation. 2007 Aug 21;116(8):894-900).

2.6.0.4 Framingham study: Uric acid not causal in deaths

Hyperuricemia is associated with risk for cardiovascular disease and death. However, the role of uric acid independent of established risk factors is uncertain. OBJECTIVE: To examine the relation of serum uric acid level to incident coronary heart disease, death from cardiovascular disease, and death from all causes. DESIGN: Community-based, prospective observational study. SETTING: Framingham, Massachusetts. PATIENTS: **6763 Framingham Heart Study participants** (mean age, 47 years). MEASUREMENTS: Serum uricacid level at baseline (1971 to 1976); event rates per 1000 person-years by sex-specific uric acid quintile. RESULTS: During 117,376 person-years of follow-up, 617 coronary heart disease events, 429 cardiovascular disease deaths, and 1460 deaths from all causes occurred. In men, after adjustment for age, elevated serum uric acid level was not associated with increased risk for an adverse outcome. In women, after adjustment for age, uric acid level was predictive of coronary heart disease (P = 0.002), death from cardiovascular disease (P = 0.009), and death from all causes (P = 0.03). After additional adjustment for cardiovascular disease risk factors, uric acid level was no longer associated with coronary heart disease, death from cardiovascular disease, or death from all causes. In a stepwise Cox model, diuretic use was identified as the covariate responsible for rendering serum uric acid a statistically nonsignificant predictor of outcomes. CONCLUSIONS: These findings indicate that **uric acid does not have a causal role in the development of coronary heart disease, death from cardiovascular disease, or death from all causes.** Any apparent association with these outcomes is probably due to the association of uric acid level with other risk factors (Serum uric acid and risk for cardiovascular disease and death: the Framingham Heart Study. Culleton BF, Larson MG, Kannel WB, Levy D. Ann Intern Med. 1999 Jul 6;131(1):7-13).

2.6.0.5 Confusion: hyperuricemia induces oxidative stress

Endothelial dysfunction is a characteristic feature during the renal damage induced by mild hyperuricemia. The mechanism by which uric acid reduces the bioavailability of intrarenal nitric oxide is not known. We tested the hypothesis that oxidative stress might contribute to the endothelial dysfunction and glomerular hemodynamic changes that occur with hyperuricemia. Hyperuricemia was induced in Sprague-Dawley rats by administration of the uricase inhibitor, oxonic acid (750 mg/kg per day). The **superoxide scavenger, tempol** (15 mg/kg per day), or placebo was administered simultaneously with the oxonic acid. All groups were evaluated throughout a 5-wk period. Kidneys were fixed by perfusion and afferent arteriole morphology, and tubulointerstitial 3-nitrotyrosine, 4-hydroxynonenal, NOX-4 subunit of renal NADPH-oxidase, and angiotensin II were quantified. Hyperuricemia induced intrarenal oxidative stress, increased expression of NOX-4 and angiotensin II, and decreased nitric oxide bioavailability, systemic hypertension, renal vasoconstriction, and afferent arteriolopathy. **Tempol treatment reversed the systemic and renal alterations induced by hyperuricemia despite equivalent hyperuricemia.** Moreover, because tempol prevented the development of preglomerular damage and decreased blood pressure, glomerular pressure was maintained at normal values as well. **Mild hyperuricemia induced by uricase inhibition causes intrarenal oxidative stress, which contributes to the development of the systemic hypertension and the renal abnormalities induced by increased uric acid**. Scavenging of the superoxide anion in this setting attenuates the adverse effects induced by hyperuricemia (Role of oxidative stress in the renal abnormalities induced by experimental hyperuricemia. Laura G. Sánchez-Lozada et al. Am J Physiol Renal Physiol 295: F1134-F1141, 2008).

2.6.0.6 Hyperuricemic Syndromes in Cancer Patients

Tumor lysis syndrome is a challenging complication of cancer therapy. This review focuses on the risk factors and pathologies of patients at risk for hyperuricemic complications. Methods: A review of the literature was performed that included original articles and related reviews from MEDLINE (PubMed) and published abstracts of meeting presentations. Results: **Both host-related and tumor-related factors predispose cancer patients to hyperuricemic syndromes**. Host-related factors include low urinary flow, pre-existing hyperuricemia, renal failure, dehydration, acidic urine, and suppressed renal uric acid excretion. Tumor-related risk factors include a high tumor cell proliferation rate, large tumor burden, and tumor chemosensitivity. Acute renal failure may occur after cytoreductive chemotherapy in patients with active disease and a high tumor burden. **Patients with advanced Burkitt's leukemia/lymphoma, high-grade lymphoma, or acute leukemia with elevated leukocyte counts are at high risk for complications of hyperuricemia.** The use of nonrecombinant (uricozyme) or recombinant urate oxidase to prevent or treat urate nephropathy may improve the outcome of patients. Conclusion: Early recognition of metabolic abnormalities in cancer patients at risk for hyperuricemia is essential for proper therapy (Ronco C, Rodeghiero F (eds): Hyperuricemic Syndromes: Pathophysiology and Therapy. Contrib Nephrol. Basel, Karger, 2005, vol 147, pp 47-60 (DOI: 10.1159/000082541).

2.6.0 7 Hyperuricemia may cause chronic disease

Fructose-induced hyperuricemia might have a causal role in metabolic syndrome, hypertension, and other chronic disease. However, no study has investigated whether sugar added to foods or sugar-sweetened beverages, which are major sources of fructose, are associated with serum uric acid concentration in free-living populations. We examined the relationship between the intakes of added sugars and sugar-sweetened beverages and serum uric acid concentrations in the National Health and Nutrition Examination Survey 2001–2002, a nationally representative sample of men and women. We included 4073 subjects (1988 men and 2085 women) >18 years of age in the current study. Dietary intake was assessed by a single 24-hour recall. We used multivariate linear regression to adjust for age, gender, intake of energy and alcohol, body mass index, use of diuretics, ß-blockers, and other covariates. Male subjects in the highest intake quartile of estimated intake of added sugars or sugar-sweetened drinks had higher plasma uric acid concentrations than those in the lowest intake quartiles ($P<0.001$ for both) after adjusting for potential confounders, whereas we did not observe significant associations for females (P for trend>0.2; P for interaction <0.01). Further research is needed to confirm causality of these associations and the observed difference by gender (Intake of Added Sugar and Sugar-Sweetened Drink and Serum Uric Acid Concentration in US Men and Women. Xiang Gao et al. *Hypertension.* 2007;50:306)

2.6.1.0 Hyperbilirubinemia deaths

Hyperbilirubinemia is a condition of mammals, specifically humans, in which there are excessive amounts of bilirubin in the blood. Bilirubin is the chief pigment in human bile. It is derived from hemoglobin which is the red pigment of the red corpuscles. The main site of bilirubin is the liver. It is also made in the bone marrow, the spleen and the lymph glands.

Free bilirubin is the most toxic substance produced by the human body. In normal adults, however, the bilirubin is conjugated in the liver, i.e. converted to a nontoxic form known as bilirubin-glucuronide. Conjugation of bilirubin in the liver is catalyzed by the enzyme UDP-glucuronyl transferase. The conjugated form of bilirubin is water-soluble and can be excreted into the bile. While bile is passed into the intestines and the gall bladder, part of the bilirubin is converted into sterco-bilin and excreted in the feces. The remainder is reabsorbed in the bloodstream and of this portion the bulk returns to the liver to be reexcreted into the bile.

Hyperbilirubinemia frequently occurs in the first five days of life of a newborn baby and may clear up within seven to fourteen days. This condition known as "physiological jaundice of newborns" or "neonatal jaundice" is due to incomplete development of certain mechanisms of the body resulting in a decreased ability to conjugate bilirubin with glucronic acid. Specifically, the key enzyme, UDP-glucuronyl transferase, is not present in the newborn, requiring several weeks to be fully induced. As a result, the bilirubin cannot be conjugated and is retained in the body for some time. The condition is usually mild and self-limiting, though in premature infants, the hyperbilirubinemia may be more severe, last longer, and more frequently result in kernicterus. Kernicterus may result in severe neurological deficits, mental retardation, loss of IQ and even death.

It is estimated that as many as twenty-five percent of newborns are afflicted with this malady. **In adults, hyperbilirubinemia, commonly referred to as "Gilbert's Disease", frequently results in death.**

Neonatal jaundice has been successfully treated by complete blood transfusion, administration of phenobarbital and total body irradiation by visible light (phototherapy). Blood transfusion is quite inconvenient for babies. **The most popular treatment is phototherapy.**

Jaundice, or yellowing of the skin, is common in newborns. The condition results from an accumulation of bilirubin, a yellowish substance produced when red blood cells are broken down. Ordinarily, bilirubin is removed from the body by the liver.

For most infants with jaundice, the yellow skin color will fade after a few days and the infant won't suffer any ill effects. In some infants, however, the liver fails to remove bilirubin rapidly enough, and potentially toxic levels accumulate. The condition is known as hyperbilirubinemia. Untreated, hyperbilirubinemia may cause severe brain injury, which could result in cerebral palsy, profound intellectual and developmental disability, blindness, and severe hearing loss.

The first line of treatment for newborn hyperbilirubinemia is phototherapy — exposure to high intensity light. The light penetrates the skin and converts bilirubin to a less toxic substance, which is eliminated through the urine.

2.6.2.0 Earlier Jaundice Treatment Decreases Brain Injury In Preemies

A study from a National Institutes of Health research network found that an early treatment to prevent severe newborn jaundice in extremely early preterm infants reduced the infants' rate of brain injury, a serious complication of severe jaundice.

The study also found that the smallest, most frail infants in the study were more likely to die than were the larger infants, regardless of whether they received the early or the conventional treatment. Moreover, the study found a trend toward a higher proportion of deaths among the smaller infants in the early treatment group, when compared to the smaller infants receiving the conventional treatment. However, this trend was within the statistical margin of error.

The study, appearing in the Oct. 30, 2008 *New England Journal of Medicine*, was conducted by researchers in the Neonatal Research Network of NIH's Eunice Kennedy Shriver National Institute of Child Health and Human Development (NICHD). The study's first author was Brenda H. Morris, M.D., a researcher at the University of Texas Medical School at Houston when the study was conducted.

Bilirubin can be very toxic and it is also an antioxidant.

2.6.3.0 Heart Disease Deaths Fall as Obesity and Diabetes Increase

12 Jul 2007. Epidemiologists at the University of Liverpool and the Heart of Mersey have found that **approximately half the recent fall in coronary heart disease deaths in the US is due to positive life style changes and a further half to medical therapies.**

The team found that a decrease in smoking, cholesterol, blood pressure and physical inactivity contributed to the fall in deaths from coronary heart disease, yet this decrease could have been substantially more had it not been for the increases in obesity and diabetes cases.

Coronary heart disease (CHD) death rates in the US almost halved between 1980 and 2000. To understand how this fall occurred scientists combined information on medical treatments with national changes in the levels of major risk factors, such as smoking and high cholesterol. The UK has seen similar falls in heart disease, but **this fall is mainly attributed to healthier diets rather than medication.**

From 1980 to 2000, the US death rates for CHD fell from 543 to 267 per 100,000 population among men and from 263 to 134 per 100,000 population among women. Overall there were 341, 745 fewer CHD deaths in 2000 than in 1980.

The team found that this decrease was attributed to reductions in risk factors such as total cholesterol, systolic blood pressure, smoking and physical inactivity. However, they found that this reduction could have been 15% more had it not been for an increase in obesity and diabetes. Approximately half the fall in CHD deaths was also attributed to medical treatments, including medications for heart failure and emergency treatments for heart attacks and angina.

Professor Simon Capewell, from the University of Liverpool's Division of Public Health and Trustee at CHD prevention charity, Heart of Mersey, said: "Using a sophisticated computer model called IMPACT we were able to combine and analyze data on the uptake and effectiveness of specific cardiac treatments and changes in risk factors among adults aged 25 to 84 years in the US. Data included results from trials, official statistics and national surveys. We found that CHD death rates halved, and 47% of the fall was attributed to medical treatments and approximately 44% to changes in risk factors. Prevalence of smoking, for example had fallen by 12%. Decreases in physical inactivity however, were offset by increases in body mass index and diabetes."

Robin Ireland, Chief Executive at Heart of Mersey, added: "We have recently seen similar falls in heart disease here in the UK. **These changes mainly reflect healthier diets, not tablets.** However the increase in obesity and diabetes are a wakeup call. They reflect the increasing consumption of large helpings of junk food. We need legislation to encourage food manufacturers and supermarkets to provide healthier food options."

The research is published in the *New England Journal of Medicine.*

(Source: *New England Journal of Medicine*: University of Liverpool: July 2007).

2.6.4.0 Ginkgo Biloba and Cell Phone Free Radical Damage

Ginkgo Biloba has previously been shown to improve blood flow to the brain and lower extremities, boost visual acuity, and enhance memory in those diagnosed with Alzheimer's. (RMH Note: This is wrong.) Now, researchers in Turkey have found that Ginkgo Biloba can prevent the free radical damage that occurs in the brains of rats after exposure to electromagnetic radiation from cell phones. The increasing use of cell phones has led to the emergence of research to determine the consequences of exposure to the low-intensity electromagnetic radiation emitted by mobile phones. Several experimental studies have **suggested that reactive oxygen species**—in other words, free radicals—play a role in electromagnetic radiation damage in tissues. In the current study, researchers investigated the effect of Ginkgo Biloba on cell-phone-induced oxidative damage in brain tissue of rats.

Researchers exposed rats to **900 MHz electromagnetic radiation** from mobile phones, one hour per day for seven days.

2.6.5.0 Ginkgo Biloba Preserves Brain's Antioxidant Enzyme Activity, SOD & GPx

One group of rats was pretreated with Ginkgo Biloba prior to being exposed to the electromagnetic radiation. Another group served as untreated controls. Oxidative stress markers and pathological changes in brain tissue were examined for each group.

In the group of rats that did not receive Ginkgo but were exposed to the cell phone radiation, researchers noted a number of changes that indicated oxidative damage. One of these changes included a decrease in the activities of brain **superoxide dismutase and glutathione peroxidase,** two antioxidant enzymes that play a key role in neutralizing oxidative damage caused by free radicals. **Please remember that SOD is a prooxidant enzyme.**

In the rats treated with Ginkgo Biloba, however, the researchers did not notice any of the changes associated with free radical damage. Furthermore, **Ginkgo Biloba prevented the cell-phone-induced cellular injury in brain tissue.**

The researchers concluded that **Ginkgo can preserve antioxidant enzyme activity in brain tissue exposed to radiation from mobile phones, thereby reducing oxidative stress in brains exposed to cell phones.** (Ilhan A, Gurel A, Armutcu F, Kamisli S, Iraz M, Akyol O, Ozen S. Ginkgo biloba prevents mobile phone-induced oxidative stress in rat brain. Clin Chim Acta 2004 Feb;340(1-2):153-62).

2.6.6.0 Cell phones can affect sperm quality

Keeping a cell phone on talk mode in a pocket can decrease sperm quality, according to new research from the Cleveland Clinic. 11/24/08

http://www.cnn.com/2008/HEALTH/conditions/09/18/cellphone.sperm/index.html

"We believe that these devices are used because we consider them very safe, but it could cause harmful effects due to the proximity of the phones and the exposure that they are causing to the gonads," says lead researcher Ashok Agarwal, the Director of the Center for Reproductive Medicine.

In the small study, Agarwal's team took semen samples from **32 men** and brought them to the lab. Each man's sample was placed into small, conical tubes and divided into two parts: a test group and a control group. The control group was unexposed to cell phone emissions, but kept under the same conditions and temperature as the test group.

The semen in the test group was placed 2.5 centimeters from an **850 MHz cell phone** in talk mode for 1 hour. Researchers say that **850 MHz is the most commonly used frequency.**

They used the measurement of **2.5 centimeters to mimic the distance between the trouser pocket and the testes. What?** Agarwal reasoned that many men keep their active cell phones in their pants pocket while talking on their headsets.

Overall, **researchers found an increase in oxidative stress such as a significant increase in free radicals and oxidants and a decrease in antioxidants.** Agarwal says that equals a decrease in sperm's quality, including motility and viability. Evidence of oxidative stress can appear under other conditions, including exposure to certain environmental pollutants or infections in the urinary genital tract.

"On average, **there was an 85 percent increase in the amount of free radicals for all the subjects in the study**. Free radicals have been linked to a variety of diseases in humans including cancer," said Agarwal. **Free radicals have been linked to decreased sperm quality in previous studies.**

However, the study does have major limitations, he acknowledged, such as the small sample size. It also was conducted in a lab and so cannot account for the protection a human body might offer, such as layers of skin, bone and tissue. Agarwal is in the early stages of further research that can model the human body's role in protecting from radio-frequency electromagnetic waves emitted from cell phones.

Agarwal also admits that there is no clear explanation of this demonstrated effect, but he shared some of his theories. "Perhaps the cell phone radiation is able to affect the gonads through a thermal effect thereby increasing the temperature of the testes and causing damaging effects in the sperm cell."

In a previous study, **Agarwal and his team found that men who used their cell phones more than four hours a day had significantly lower sperm quality than those who used their cell phones for less time.** Those findings were based on self-reported data from 361 subjects.

While representatives from the cell phone industry had not yet reviewed the latest study, they were careful not to give this study much merit. "The weight of the published scientific evidence, in addition to the opinion of global health organizations, shows that **there is no link between wireless usage and adverse health effects**," said Joe Farren, a spokesman for the CTIA-the Wireless Association.

"We support good science and always have," he said. "It's important to look at studies that are peer-reviewed and published in leading journals and to listen to the experts."

Agarwal emphasized that it is far too early for men to start changing cell phone carrying habits, noting that his own cell phone was in his pocket as he talked to CNN.

"**Our study has not provided proof that you should stop putting cell phones in your pocket.** There are many things that need to be proven before we get to that stage," he said.

2.6.7.0 Ginkgo proves ineffective in preventing dementia, Alzheimer's disease

One of the most widely used herbal supplements for improving memory and cognition has **no impact on the development of dementia or Alzheimer's disease**, according to new results from a $30 million, multi-center study.

The Ginkgo biloba for the Evaluation of Memory (GEM) Study was the largest clinical trial ever to evaluate the effects of the dietary supplement ginkgo biloba (ginkgo) on the occurrence of dementia. The study tested the effectiveness of 120 milligrams (mg) of ginkgo twice daily versus placebo in lowering the incidence of dementia and Alzheimer's in normal, elderly people and those with mild cognitive impairment.

Results from the study show that 240 mg of ginkgo daily has no effect on the onset of dementia or development of Alzheimer's. The study appears in this week's issue of the *Journal of the American Medical Association*.

Many people today use ginkgo leaf extracts hoping to improve memory, to treat or help prevent Alzheimer's and other types of dementia, to decrease intermittent claudication (leg pain caused by narrowing arteries) and to treat sexual dysfunction, multiple sclerosis, tinnitus, and other health conditions. **In Europe and the United States, ginkgo supplements are among the best-selling herbal medications and it consistently ranks as a top medicine prescribed in France and Germany.**

"Alzheimer's disease is a devastating disease affecting large numbers of older adults," said Gregory Burke, M.D., M.Sc., the lead investigator for the Wake Forest University Baptist Medical Center clinical site. "Our best strategy is to prevent dementia before it begins."

The study was conducted primarily to determine if ginkgo would decrease the incidence of all types of dementia and, more specifically, reduce the incidence of Alzheimer's. The study also aimed to evaluate ginkgo for its effects on overall cognitive decline, functional disability, incidence of cardiovascular disease and stroke, and total mortality.

The results were disappointing and surprising, said Burke and Jeff Williamson, M.D., M.H.S., principal investigator for the GEM Study Clinical Coordinating Center at Wake Forest Baptist.

"In addition to its widespread use based on the belief that it helps memory function," Williamson said, "Ginkgo biloba had enough promising circumstantial evidence from laboratory and animal studies and enough safety information to warrant a full-scale test in humans."

Dementia is a form of brain disease that can seriously affect a person's ability to carry out daily activities. It is caused by many conditions, some of which are reversible. **Alzheimer's is one of the most common forms of dementia in older people, affecting nearly 4.5 million Americans**, according to the National Institute on Aging. It is an incurable disease with a slow progression beginning with mild memory loss and ending with severe brain damage and death.

The GEM Study was conducted at four clinical sites: Wake Forest Baptist, the University of Pittsburgh, Johns Hopkins University, and the University of California-Davis.

Investigators followed a total of **3,069 participants** age 75 or older, who had either normal cognition or mild cognitive impairment. Participants were randomized to receive twice-daily doses of either 120 mg of ginkgo extract or placebo. The dose of ginkgo was selected based on prior clinical study results that found 120 mg twice daily to be the most effective dose. The gingko product used in the study was supplied by Schwabe Pharmaceuticals and is sold in the United States as Ginkgold MaxTM, under the Nature's Way label.

Patients were followed for an average of about six years**, with a maximum of just over seven years. During the study, 523 participants were diagnosed with dementia, 246 in the placebo group and 277 in the ginkgo group, leading researchers to declare that ginkgo showed no overall effect for reducing all types of dementia or Alzheimer's.**

"It is very unlikely that ginkgo biloba is effective at any dose over a five-year period and in anyone over 75 years old," Williamson said. "It is also ineffective in people with signs of early memory loss. What is not known yet is whether the effect of ginkgo biloba might require taking the drug for many, many years, say 15 years, before there is even a sign of memory loss."

For the millions of people spending their money on over-the-counter ginkgo for the perceived promise of protection from dementia and Alzheimer's, Williamson suggests they spend their money elsewhere, while remaining mentally and physically active.

And though ginkgo failed to perform as hoped, Williamson explained that the trial was valuable in many ways to the scientific community. The study experience itself demonstrates the feasibility of conducting large dementia prevention trials in older adults, the researchers said.

"One of the most important findings from this study is that we can recruit and follow adequate numbers of volunteers for this purpose, even in the rapidly growing population of people over age 75," he said. "This will be critical for the most cost-effective use of scarce Medicare dollars in the future.

"Secondly, we are already learning a lot of new information from the GEMS volunteers about how dementia develops and how not all memory change is a sign of impending dementia," Williamson added.

Source: Wake Forest University Baptist Medical Center

The dietary supplement ginkgo, long promoted as an aid to memory, didn't help prevent dementia and Alzheimer's disease in the longest and largest test of the extract in older Americans.

"We don't think it has a future as a powerful anti-dementia drug," said Dr. Steven DeKosky of the University of Virginia School of Medicine, who led the federally funded study.

Extracts from ginkgo tree leaves have antioxidant and anti-inflammatory effects, but earlier research on ginkgo and memory showed mixed results. Annual U.S. sales of the supplement reached $107 million in 2007, according to **Nutrition** Business Journal estimates.

Ginkgo has been believed to protect the brain by preventing the build-up of an Alzheimer's-related protein or by preventing cell-damaging oxidative stress. It's been used for leg pain, ringing in the ears and sexual dysfunction. For the new study, appearing in Wednesday's Journal of the American Medical Association, researchers recruited more than 3,000 people, ages 75 and older, from voter and mailing lists in Maryland, Pennsylvania, California and North Carolina.

Half were randomly assigned to take 120 milligrams of ginkgo biloba twice a day, a typical dose taken by people who think it may help memory. The others took identical dummy pills. Participants were screened for dementia every six months.

After six years, dementia had been diagnosed at a similar rate in both groups; 277 in the ginkgo group and 246 in the group taking the dummy tablets. When the researchers looked only at Alzheimer's disease, that rate too was similar.

At the start, some people showed mild difficulties with thinking; ginkgo didn't work to prevent dementia in those people either. Ginkgo appears relatively safe, DeKosky said. There was no difference in the rate of adverse events such as heart attacks and gastrointestinal bleeding between the groups. There were 16 strokes from bleeding in the brain in the ginkgo group versus eight in the placebo group, a difference that wasn't statistically significant, he said, because the number of strokes was too small.

A new role?

Would ginkgo work better to prevent dementia if people started taking it earlier, say, in middle age? The study didn't look at that, DeKosky acknowledged, adding that following people for 25 years from middle age to old age would be expensive research. The study also didn't test whether ginkgo improves thinking and memory in the short term. "It would have been terrific if this worked. It's inexpensive, available and relatively safe," said Paul Solomon, professor of neuroscience at Williams College in Williamstown, Mass., who wasn't involved in the new study but has studied ginko. "Now with this kind of evidence, you can confidently tell people it didn't show benefit in more than 3,000 people in six years of research," Solomon said.

There may still be a role for ginkgo in treating, rather than preventing, Alzheimer's disease, said Michael McGuffin, president of the American Herbal Products Association, a trade association. Some previous ginkgo trials have shown no benefit in Alzheimer's symptom treatment, while others have found it comparable to prescription drugs such as Aricept, also known as donepezil.

A four-month supply of ginkgo can cost less than $10. But not all brands contain what their labels claim. ConsumerLab.com, which tests the ingredients in supplements, reported Tuesday that of seven ginkgo products it reviewed, five failed to pass its tests. An eighth ginkgo product also passed the group's test in a voluntary certification program. The dementia study was funded by a grant from the National Institutes of Health's National Center for Complementary and Alternative Medicine, which is undertaking large, scientific tests of a number of commonly used dietary supplements. The agency said it's the largest-ever randomized trial of a botanical medicine. There have been larger studies of vitamins and minerals.

DeKosky reported receiving grants from and acting as a consultant for several drug companies, including some that make dementia drugs. Schwabe Pharmaceuticals of Karlsruhe, Germany, provided the ginkgo tablets and identical placebos.

People on the blood thinner warfarin shouldn't take ginkgo because of the risk of increased bleeding.

Once again, the antioxidant, i.e., ginkgo, failed miserably.

2.6.8.0 Fact or Fiction?: Cell Phones Can Cause Brain Cancer

By Melinda Wenner

This summer, Ronald Herberman, director of the University of Pittsburgh Cancer Institute, sent a memo to staffers warning them to limit their cell phone use and to use hands-free sets in the wake of "growing evidence that we should reduce exposure" to cell phone radiation. Among the possible consequences: an increased risk of brain cancer.

Five months later, a top official at the National Cancer Institute (NCI) told a congressional panel that published scientific data indicates cell phones are safe.

So what's the deal? Do cell phones cause cancer—or not?

It depends on whom you ask: Herberman, Robert Hoover, director of NCI's Epidemiology and Biostatistics Program, and other health officials recently clashed during a hearing before the House Subcommittee on Domestic Policy held to determine whether mobile phones are safe.

"**Long term and frequent use of cell phones which receive and emit radio frequency may be associated with an increased risk of brain tumors**," Herberman told lawmakers. "I find the old adage 'better to be safe than sorry' to be very apt to this situation."

Hoover, **on the other hand, insisted that the pervasive technology was safe, testifying that "its effect on the body appears to be insufficient to cause genetic damage**."

The debate became so heated at one point that Rep. Dennis Kucinich (D–Ohio), who called the hearing, snapped at Hoover for interrupting David Carpenter, director of the Institute for Health and the Environment at the University at Albany, State University of New York, as he argued there was enough evidence to warrant more scrutiny and a government warning of potential damage.

Cell phones use non-ionizing radiation, which differs from the ionizing radiation of x-rays and radioactive material in that it does not have enough energy to knock around—or ionize—electrons or particles in atoms. Cell phone radiation falls into the same band of nonionizing radio frequency as microwaves used to heat or cook food. But Jorn Olsen, chair of epidemiology at the University of California, Los Angeles, School of Public Health says that **unlike microwaves, cell phones do not release enough radiation or energy to damage DNA or genetic material, which can lead to cancer.**

Recent research suggests, however, that although short-term exposure is harmless, long-term cell phone use may be a different story. **Three studies since 1999 indicate that people who have used cell phones for more than a decade may have as much as three times greater risk of developing brain tumors on the side of the head against which they most often hold their phone**—an argument for, at the least, shifting ears regularly or, even better, using an earpiece or the speakerphone feature while chatting.

For people who've used their cell phones for more than 10 years and who use their phone on the same side as the tumor, it appears there's an association," Lawrie Challis, emeritus physics professor at the University of Nottingham in England and former chairman of the U.K.'s Mobile Telecommunications and Health Research program, told ScientificAmerican.com during a recent interview.

Worldwide, one in 29,000 men and one in 38,000 women on average develop brain tumors each year, with people in industrial nations twice as likely as those in developing countries to be diagnosed with one, according to the World Health Organization's International Agency for Research on Cancer (IARC) in Lyon, France. If cell phone use does, in fact, triple the odds of getting cancer, these stats would suggest that over 60 years a man's risk of developing a brain tumor from cell phone use increases from 0.206 percent to 0.621 percent, and a woman's from 0.156 percent to 0.468 percent.

IARC in 2000 launched a study called Interphone, funded by the European Union, the International Union against Cancer and other national and local funding bodies. Interphone compared surveyed cell phone use in 6,420 people with brain tumors to that of 7,658 healthy people in 13 developed countries—Australia, Canada, Denmark, Finland, France, Germany, Israel, Italy, Japan, New Zealand, Norway, Sweden and the U.K.—to try to determine whether people with brain tumors had used their cell phones more than healthy people, an association that might suggest that cell phones caused the tumors.

The results are expected by the end of this year. "The interpretation of the results is not simple because of a number of potential biases which can affect the results," says project leader Elisabeth Cardis, a professor at the Center for Research in Environmental Epidemiology at the Barcelona Biomedical Research Park. "These analyses are complex and have, unfortunately, taken much time." Among factors that might skew the results: failure of participants—especially those with tumors—to accurately recall exactly how long and often they talk on their cell phones.

According to the U.S. Centers for Disease Control and Prevention (CDC), the average time between first exposure to a cancer-causing agent and clinical recognition of the disease is 15 to 20 years or longer—and cell phone use in the U.S. has only been popular for about a decade. (In 1996 there were 34 million U.S. cell phone users compared with more than 200 million today, according to CTIA–The Wireless Association, a Washington, D.C.–based cell phone industry group.)

Carpenter told the congressional panel that most of the studies that have shown an increased risk are from Scandinavia, where cell phones have been popular since the early 1990s. Herberman added that most of the research showing cell phones are safe is based on surveys of consumers who have used them for less than 10 years.

Despite a dearth of human studies, more than 400 experiments have been done since the early 1970s to determine how cell phone radiation affects animals, cells and DNA. They, too, have produced conflicting results. Some suggest that cell phone radiation damages DNA and/or nerve cells, others do not. At the hearing, Carpenter suggested that **cell phones may increase the brain's production of reactive forms of oxygen called free radicals**, which can interact with and damage DNA.

Contradictory findings could be a sign of poor study quality, according to NCI expert Hoover. But Jerry Phillips, a biochemist who performed cell phone research at U.S. Department of Veterans Affairs's Pettis VA Medical Center in Loma

Linda, Calif., in the 1990s, believes that conflicting results are to be expected given the nature of the radiation being scrutinized.

Phillips says, for instance, that sometimes the body will respond to radiation by initiating a series of intrinsic repair mechanisms designed to fix the harmful effects. In other words, the effects from radiation exposure may be different in different people. And these varied responses may help explain the contradictory results, says Phillips, who is now director of the Science/Health Science Learning Center at the University of Colorado at Colorado Springs.

There is plenty of anecdotal evidence out there claiming a link between cell phone use and cancer: Keith Black, chairman of neurosurgery at Cedars-Sinai Medical Center in Los Angeles, says that **the brain cancer (malignant glioma) that killed O. J. Simpson's attorney, Johnnie Cochran, was the result of frequent cell phone use, based on the fact that the tumor developed on the side of the head against which he held his phone.** And in May, a week after Massachusetts Sen. Edward Kennedy was diagnosed with a glioma, The EMR Policy Institute, a Marshfield, Vt.–based nonprofit organization that supports research on the effects of electromagnetic radiation, released a statement linking his tumor to heavy cell phone use. But the **NCI maintains that there is no definitive evidence that cell phones increase cancer risk.**

In other words, the verdict is still out. "We can't rule out the possibility of risk," Nottingham's Challis says. "There hadn't been as much work in this area as is now demanded." http://www.sciam.com/article.cfm?id=fact-or-fiction-cell-phones-can-cause-brain-cancer. Accessed 11-24-08.

2.6.9 0 Metals, Fenton chemistry and antioxidants

Attention is focused on structural, chemical and biochemical aspects of free radicals, the endogenous and exogenous sources of their generation, **the metal (iron, copper, chromium, cobalt, vanadium, cadmium, arsenic, nickel)-mediated formation of free radicals (e.g. Fenton chemistry),** the DNA damage (both mitochondrial and nuclear), the damage to lipids and proteins by free radicals, the phenomenon of oxidative stress, cancer and the redox environment of a cell, the mechanisms of carcinogenesis and the role of signalling cascades by ROS; in particular, ROS activation of AP-1 (activator protein) and NF-kappaB (nuclear factor kappa B) signal transduction pathways, which in turn lead to the transcription of genes involved in cell growth regulatory pathways. The role of) in the process of carcinogenesis as well as the antioxidant interactions with various regulatory factors, including Ref-1, NF-kappaB,

AP-1 are also reviewed. (Chem Biol Interact. 2006 Mar 10;160(1):1-40. Epub 2006 Jan 23).

2.7.0.0 Aging/anti-aging

2.7.1.0 Antioxidants can not extend normal life span

FREE RADICALS AND THE THEORY OF AGING: Severe oxidative stress progressively leads to cell dysfunction and ultimately cell death. Oxidative stress is defined as an imbalance between pro-oxidants and/or free radicals on the one hand, and anti-oxidizing systems on the other. The oxygen required for living may indirectly be responsible for negative effects; these deleterious effects are due to the production of free radicals, which are toxic for the cells (superoxide anions, hydroxyl radicals, peroxyl radicals, hydrogen peroxide, hydroperoxides and peroxinitrite anions). Free radical attacks are responsible for cell damage and the targeted cells are represented by the cell membranes, which are particularly rich in unsaturated fatty acids, sensitive to oxidation reactions; DNA is also the target of severe attacks by these reactive oxygen species (ROS). THE DEFENCE SYSTEMS: These are represented by the enzymes and free radical captors. The latter are readily oxidizable composites. **The free radical captor or neutralization systems of these ROS use a collection of mechanisms**, vitamins (E and C), enzymes [superoxide dismutase (SOD), glutathion peroxidase (GPx) and others], and glutathion reductase (GSH), capable of neutralizing peroxinitrite. The efficacy of this system is dependent on the genome for the enzymatic defence systems, and on nutrition for the vitamins. Some strategies aimed at reducing oxidative stress-related alterations have been performed in animals. However, only a few can be used and are efficient in humans, such as avoidance of unfavourable environmental conditions (radiation, dietary carcinogens, smoking...) and antioxidant dietary supplementation. DIETARY SUPPLEMENTATION: Epidemiological data suggest that antioxidants may have a beneficial effect on many age-related diseases: atherosclerosis, cancer, some neurodegenerative and ocular diseases. However, **the widespread use of supplements is hampered by several factors: the lack of prospective and controlled studies; insufficient knowledge on the pro-oxidant, oxidant and ant-oxidant properties of the various supplements; growing evidence that free radicals are not only by-products, but also play an important role in cell signal transduction, apoptosis and infection control**.

RECOMMENDATIONS: Although **current data indicate that antioxidants cannot prolong maximal life span,** the beneficial impact of antioxidants on various age-related degenerative diseases may forecast an improvement in life span and enhance quality of life. **The current lack of sufficient data does not permit the systematic recommendation of anti-oxidants.** Nevertheless, antioxidant-rich diets with fruit and vegetables should be recommended (Antioxidants to slow aging, facts and perspectives. Bonnefoy M, Drai J, Kostka T. Presse Med. 2002 Jul 27;31(25):1174-84).

2.7.2.0 Support for antioxidants in aging is scarce and equivocal

The free radical theory of aging **hypothesizes** that oxygen-derived free radicals are responsible for the age-related damage at the cellular and tissue levels. In a normal situation, a balanced-equilibrium exists among oxidants, antioxidants and biomolecules. Excess generation of free radicals may overwhelm natural cellular antioxidant defences leading to oxidation and further contributing to cellular functional impairment. **The identification of free radical reactions as promoters of the aging process implies that interventions aimed at limiting or inhibiting them should be able to reduce the rate of formation of aging changes with a consequent reduction of the aging rate and disease pathogenesis.** Even if antioxidant supplementation is receiving growing attention and is increasingly adopted in Western countries, **supporting evidence is still scarce and equivocal.** Major limitations in literature are still needed to be addressed to better evaluate the potential benefits from antioxidant supplementation: 1) an improved understanding of oxidation mechanisms possibly at the basis of the aging process, 2) the determination of reliable markers of oxidative damage and antioxidant status, 3) the identification of a therapeutic window in which an eventual antioxidant supplementation may be beneficial, 4) a deeper knowledge of the antioxidant molecules which in several conditions act as pro-oxidants. In the present paper, after a preliminary introduction to the free radical theory of aging and the rationale of antioxidant supplementation as an anti-aging intervention, we will present an overview of evidence relating antioxidant supplementations with clinical conditions typical of older age (ie, cardiovascular disease, Alzheimer's disease, cancer). Given the large amount of data available on the antioxidant supplementation topic, this overview is **not intended to be exhaustive.** The aim of this paper is to provide the main basis from which future studies should start and indicate which the main limitations that need to be addressed are. (Effects of antioxidant supplementation on the aging process. Fusco D, Colloca G, Lo Monaco MR, Cesari M. Clin Interv Aging. 2007;2(3):377-87)

2.7.3.0 Aging studies inconsistent on antioxidant defenses

Age-related increase in ROS generation/oxidative stress may also be a consequence of a decline of antioxidant defence systems. However, **the pattern of age-related changes in antioxidants in many tissues and species has been inconsistent**.

On one hand, some studies supported the notion that **a decline in antioxidant defence systems occurs with aging** (Hagen TM. Oxidative stress, redox imbalance, and the aging process. Antioxid. Redox Signal (2003) 5:503–506), but substantial data also exist indicating that **there is no generalized decrease in antioxidant defence enzymes** (Hatao H, Oh-ishi S, Itoh M, Leeuwenburgh C, Ohno H, Ookawara T, Kishi K, Yagyu H, Nakamura H, et al. Effects of acute exercise on lung antioxidant enzymes in young and old rats. Mech. Ageing Dev (2006) 127:384–390) (Gomi F, Matsuo M. Effects of aging and food restriction on the antioxidant enzyme activity of rat livers. J. Gerontol. A Biol. Sci. Med. Sci (1998) 53:B161–B167) (Sohal RS, Mockett RJ, Orr WC. Mechanisms of aging: an appraisal of the oxidative stress hypothesis. Free Radic. Biol. Med (2002) 33:575–586) (Andziak B, O'Connor TP, Buffenstein R. Antioxidants do not explain the disparate longevity between mice and the longest-living rodent, the naked mole-rat. Mech. Ageing Dev (2005) 126:1206–1212) **with some studies even showing an age-associated increase in antioxidant enzyme activities** (Judge S, Jang YM, Smith A, Hagen T, Leeuwenburgh C. Age-associated increases in oxidative stress and antioxidant enzyme activities in cardiac interfibrillar mitochondria: implications for the mitochondrial theory of aging. FASEB J (2005) 19:419–421) (Ji LL. Antioxidant signaling in skeletal muscle: a brief review. Exp. Gerontol (2007) 42:582–593). **I would have predicted either that the antioxidant enzymes would have been either unchanged or increased with aging, to account for the concomitant EMOD insufficiency and the increase in disease.**

Thus **the correlation between antioxidant enzymes and aging is, at best, weak and sometimes contradictory, suggesting that antioxidant enzymes may not necessarily be a limiting factor governing the degree of cellular oxidative damage with aging** (DNA damage, cellular senescence and organismal ageing: causal or correlative? Jian-Hua Chen, C. Nicholes Hales and Susan E. Ozanne. Nucleic Acids Research 2007 35(22):7417-7428).

At present, the correlative relationship between DNA damage and ageing is strong and a causative role of compromised DNA maintenance or accelerated mtDNA mutations in premature ageing is convincing. However, **whether DNA damage plays a causative role in normal aging still remains to be established.** Hayflick, who first described cellular senescence over four decades ago, recently keenly declared that 'Biological ageing is no longer an unsolved problem' (Hayflick L. Biological aging is no longer an unsolved problem. Ann. NY Acad. Sci (2007) 1100:1–13).

2.7.4.0 Antioxidants 'cannot slow aging' (Nematode worms)

1 December 2008. **Diets and creams claiming their antioxidant properties could cheat aging may be worthless, a study says.** Using Nematode worms, scientists found even those given enhanced antioxidant powers to deal with tissue damaging "free radicals" did not live longer.

The team from University College London said, in the **Genes and Development journal**, there was "no clear evidence" they could slow ageing.

Antioxidants are a staple of the beauty and health industries.

This has been based on a 50-year-old theory.

***"The free radical theory has filled a knowledge vacuum for over 50 years now, but it doesn't stand up to the evidence."* Dr David Gems, University College London**

In 1956, it was suggested that aging was caused by a build-up of molecular damage caused by reactive forms of oxygen, called superoxides or free radicals, circulating in the body. This is known as oxidative stress. Antioxidants supposedly worked to mop up these free radicals, minimising their damage. This week's study, however, could explain why **many studies aimed at proving the theory have been inconclusive.**

Nematode worms

The tiny Nematode worm, despite appearing to be far-removed from the human species, is a useful tool for scientists who want to explore how our bodies work. They share many genes with humans, and, crucially, have a lifespan measured in days, which allows scientists to get clues about long-term changes.

The UCL team, led by Dr David Gems, genetically manipulated nematodes so that their bodies were able to "mop up" surplus free radicals. This, in theory, should give them an advantage over normal nematodes in terms of ageing and lifespan. However, these worms lived just as long as the others, suggesting that **"oxidative stress" is less of a factor in the ageing of our cells and tissues as some have suggested**.

Dr Gems said: "The fact is that we don't understand much about the fundamental mechanisms of aging - the free radical theory has filled a knowledge vacuum for over 50 years now, but it doesn't stand up to the evidence.

"It is clear that if superoxide is involved, it plays only a small part in the story - oxidative damage is clearly not a universal, major driver of the aging process."

He said a healthy, balanced diet was important for reducing the risk of many "old age" diseases, such as cancer, diabetes and osteoporosis, but **there was no clear evidence that eating antioxidants could slow or prevent aging, and even less evidence to support the claims made by antioxidant pills and creams.**

'No magic bullet'

The research was supported by the Wellcome Trust, and Dr Alan Schafer, its head of molecular and physiological sciences, said: "Research such as this points to how much we have to learn about ageing, and the importance of understanding the mechanisms behind this process."

A spokesman for the British Dietetic Association said that it had been hard to find the evidence to support antioxidants from previous studies.

She said: "All the evidence has come from epidemiological studies looking at the whole diet - where there was some sign of benefit to people who ate diets with antioxidants, but also who ate lots of other good things." **What this shows is that there is likely to be no one 'magic bullet' in terms of diet and health** -the important thing is still achieving a healthy balance."

A spokesman for the Cosmetic Toiletry and Perfumery Association said cosmetic companies carry out extensive research and rigorous scientific studies to ensure claims are supported by robust evidence. "Findings on the genetics of a particular nematode worm may not be directly relevant to the complex process of ageing as it happens in higher animals such as the human," the association added.

Pamela Mason, of the Health Supplements Information Service, said: "Antioxidant vitamins, like any other vitamins were never intended for the prevention of chronic disease and mortality. They are not magic bullets.

"They are intended for health maintenance on the basis of their various physiological roles in the body and in the case of the antioxidant vitamins, this does, in appropriate amounts, include a protective antioxidant effect in the body's tissues."

This paper supports my UTOPIA theory and my assertions of the failures of antioxidants for over the past half decade. This also directly supports my Philica.com paper on the failures of antioxidants. Hallelujah, Brother!

2.7.5.0 Aging Not Slowed By Antioxidants, Study Rejects 50 Year Old Theory

Research led by scientists in the UK has upturned a 50-year old theory that maintains antioxidants stop or slow aging by counteracting the oxidative stress on cells caused by free radicals, **a finding that will undermine claims made by beauty and diet products that promote the antiaging properties of antioxidants**.

The research which was funded by the Wellcome Trust, was led by Dr David Gems of the Institute of Healthy Ageing at University College, London, and is published in the **30 November 2008 issue of the journal *Genes & Development*.**

Superoxide free radicals are a natural byproduct of metabolism. They are essentially unstable oxygen molecules with too many electrons that go in search of compounds they can bond with that are happy to accept their extra electrons. This process is similar to when iron becomes rusty and turns into iron oxide, except that in the human body, biological mechanisms exist that can stop or reverse it.

In 1956 the biogerontologist **Denham Harman proposed** that aging was the result of an accumulation of "oxidative stress" such as that inflicted on cells by free radicals. Gems and colleagues now suggest **this theory is not correct and that superoxide is not a major cause of aging.**

Gems said **the free radical theory of aging, which has dominated the field for over 50 years, "just doesn't stand up to the evidence."**

For this study, he and his team studied the way genes controlled the removal of superoxide from the bodies of *Caenorhabditis elegans*, a type of nematode worm often used in aging research. They were able to switch the genes on and off and influence the extent to which the worms' bodies were able to get rid of surplus superoxide and thus reduce the potential damage it could cause through oxidation.

According to the free radical theory, Gems and colleagues expected to see a significant link between the worms' lifespan and the extent to which their bodies were able to mop up excess superoxide, but this is not what they observed. **Another study on mice led by researchers at the University of Texas came to similar conclusions, supporting the idea that the 50-year old free radical theory is not correct,** said Gems and his team.

If superoxide is involved in the accumulation of molecular damage that characterizes the aging process, it only plays a small part, said Gems.

"Oxidative damage is clearly not a universal, major driver of the ageing process. Other factors, such as chemical reactions involving sugars in our body, clearly play a role," he added.

On the strength of these findings, Gems suggested that anti-aging products that claim to have anti-oxidant effects are unlikely to be as effective as they say. He said that while a healthy and balanced diet reduced the risk of developing diseases of aging such as cancer, diabetes and osteoporosis, there was:

"No clear evidence that dietary antioxidants can slow or prevent ageing. There is even less evidence to support the claims of most anti-ageing products," he said.

Dr Alan Schafer, Head of Molecular and Physiological Sciences at the Wellcome Trust, said this new study should encourage researchers to explore new areas of aging research:

"Research such as this points to how much we have to learn about ageing, and the importance of understanding the mechanisms behind this process," added Schafer.

(*"Against the oxidative damage theory of aging: superoxide dismutases protect against oxidative stress but have little or no effect on life span in Caenorhabditis elegans.*

Doonan, R. et al. *Genes and Development*, Published online 30 Nov 2008).

2.7.6.0 Survival Mode That Protects Cells When Oxygen Is Low (HIF) Also Slows Aging

4-16-09 **A biochemical pathway that helps keep cells alive when oxygen is low also plays a role in longevity and resistance against some diseases of old age**, according to a report to be published April 16, 2009 in the journal *Science*.

A cell's protective reaction to a drop in oxygen is called the **hypoxic response**. Researchers at the University of Washington (UW) have found that **nematode worms live longer if their genetic make-up permits their cells to turn on the hypoxic response under normal oxygen conditions.**

Not only do these worms live longer, the researchers noted, their cells are relatively free from the toxic proteins that accumulate and clump together as an animal ages. I believe that this is support for my contention that oxidation can break up or destroy microaggregates, such as plaque or amyloid.

Dr. Matt Kaeberlein, UW assistant professor of pathology and the senior author on the study, said that defining cellular mechanisms that prevent accumulation of these proteins may point to new therapeutic targets for devastating diseases that often accompany old age in people. **Toxic protein aggregations, he explained, are seen in the brain cells of those with Alzheimer's disease, Huntington's disease, and several other degenerative conditions that afflict the elderly**.

The co-lead authors, Dr. Ranjana Mehta and Dr. Katy Steinkraus, uncovered the life-extending role of the hypoxic response while studying the mechanism by which dietary restriction slows aging in nematodes. **Dietary restriction has been shown to increase life span in many different organisms, including worms, flies and mice**. Kaeberlein's group had previously found that **dietary restriction also protects against toxic protein aggregation in nematode models of Huntington's and Alzheimer's diseases. To their surprise,** however, genetic experiments mapped the hypoxic response to a previously unknown longevity pathway, different from dietary restriction.

"The research findings suggest that **the hypoxic response promotes longevity and reduces the accumulation of toxic proteins by a mechanism that is distinct from both dietary restriction and insulin-like signaling**. It appears to be an alternative pathway," Kaeberlein said. "However, we don't know if future studies might reveal that all of these different genetic pathways converge somewhere down the line into a common mechanism for delaying the effects of age."

The key factor that controls the hypoxic response is called **HIF**. HIF is regulated by another protein called VHL-1, which tags HIF to be destroyed by a cellular machine called the proteasome. Destruction of HIF by VHL-1 keeps the hypoxic response "off" when oxygen is present. The UW researchers bred worms that could not produce VHL-1, leading to persistence of HIF even in the presence of high oxygen levels. They found that **these worms, which were able to turn on the hypoxic response under normal oxygen conditions, lived about 30 percent longer than worms whose cells made VHL-1**.

Thus, I believe that HIF increases EMOD production, which breaks up aggregates and promotes longevity by not allowing the appearance of other harmful diseases.

They also found that **animals lacking VHL-1 were resistant to the toxic proteins known to cause Alzheimer's and Huntington's diseases, and that their cells accumulated less of an age-pigment called lipofuscin**. Lipofuscin is thought to be one indicator of an animal's health during aging. According to Kaeberlein, "These observations may suggest that **the hypoxic response not only increases life span, but also lengthens health span and protects against the molecular processes that lead to neurodegenerative diseases in people**." Health span refers to the period of an organism's life that is relatively free of disease.

The authors note that the hypoxic response, including HIF and VHL-1, is very well conserved in organisms from nematodes to humans, raising the possibility that modulating HIF activity may be useful for treating some age-associated diseases, and perhaps even slowing aging, in people. Kaeberlein cautions, however, that **"mutation of VHL-1 is associated with a variety**

of tumors, and any therapies targeted toward activation of HIF would most likely need to be specific for cells that are not rapidly dividing, such as brain cells or muscle cells."

"What we're focused on now," says Mehta, "is figuring out how HIF is protecting the animals from aging." In both worms and people, HIF regulates the activity of several factors involved in growth and resistance to stress. "One or more of these factors must be the key." **(I believe that the key factor is that HIF creates an EMOD sufficiency.)**

Kaeberlein agrees. "This is a completely new pathway for aging and age-associated disease. If we can understand at a very detailed level how HIF is slowing aging, we may be able to use that information to develop effective therapies for treating age-associated diseases in people."

The researchers on the study entitled "Proteasomal Regulation of the Hypoxic Response Modulates Aging in C. elegans," in addition to Kaeberlein, Mehta, and Steinkraus, were George Sutphin, Fresnida J. Ramos, Lara S. Shmieh, Alexander Huh, Christina Davis, and Devon Chandler-Brown, all from the UW Department of Pathology or the UW Molecular and Cellular Biology Program.

2.7.7.0 Anti-aging creams don't work

A new study, conducted by researchers at University College London, has revealed that diets and creams claiming their antioxidant properties could slow ageing, have little or no effect.

London, Dec 1, 2008: A new study, conducted by researchers at University College London, has revealed that **diets and creams claiming their antioxidant properties could slow ageing, have little or no effect.**

While conducting a study with Nematode worms, the researchers found that **even those given enhanced antioxidant powers to deal with tissue damaging "free radicals" did not live longer.** The researchers said that **there was "no clear evidence" they could slow ageing.**

Antioxidants are a staple of the beauty and health industries. This has been based on a 50-year-old theory. In 1956, it was suggested that ageing was caused by a build-up of molecular damage caused by reactive forms of oxygen, called superoxides or free radicals, circulating in the body. This is known as oxidative stress. Antioxidants supposedly worked to mop up these free radicals, minimising their damage.

However, the new data could help explain why **many studies aimed at proving the theory have been inconclusive.** The research team, led by Dr David Gems, genetically manipulated nematodes so that their bodies were able to "mop up" surplus free radicals. However, **these worms lived just as long as the others**, suggesting that "oxidative stress" is less of a factor in the ageing of our cells and tissues as some have suggested.

"The fact is that we don't understand much about the fundamental mechanisms of ageing - **the free radical theory has filled a knowledge vacuum for over 50 years now, but it doesn't stand up to the evidence**," BBC quoted Gems, as saying.

"It is clear that if superoxide is involved, it plays only a small part in the story - **oxidative damage is clearly not a universal, major driver of the ageing process,"** Gems added.

He said a healthy, balanced diet was important for reducing the risk of many "old age" diseases, such as cancer, diabetes and osteoporosis, but **there was no clear evidence that eating antioxidants could slow or prevent ageing, and even less evidence to support the claims made by antioxidant pills and creams.**

The study is published in the **Genes and Development journal**.

2.7.8.0 Mice with increased catalase live longer

Seattle Times 5/05/2008

In a study that **bolsters the free-radical theory of aging**, University of Washington scientists have genetically engineered mice to live 20 percent longer than normal. The **Methuselah mice produce large amounts of an antioxidant enzyme that protects their cells from damage and also staves off the cataracts and heart damage that usually come with age. Don't go rushing for the Vitamin E and other antioxidant supplements**, cautions lead researcher Peter Rabinovitch, a UW pathologist.

While the experiment shows a specific antioxidant can slow the aging process in mice, it also demonstrates how difficult it will be to translate that into a pill for people.

To get a significant increase in life span, the researchers not only had to insert a souped-up gene into the mice, they had to target the gene to cell structures called mitochondria. That suggests where and how antioxidants are delivered to tissues and cells may be key to any life-extending benefits, Rabinovitch said.

This may help explain why **scientists have not been able to find clear improvements in the health or life span of people who take antioxidants - despite the mega-million-dollar industry's claims.**

"There is more and more evidence that antioxidant supplements are not beneficial, and there have been a few examples where they might have been harmful," Rabinovitch said.

A study this year hinted that **high doses ofVitamin E may raise the risk of heart disease**. Earlier research has found **beta carotene, another popular antioxidant, puts smokers at higher risk of lung cancer**.Yet it's clear health improves when people eat antioxidant-rich fruits and vegetables, Rabinovitch said."We don't know yet how to deliver the health benefits of fruit and vegetable antioxidants in a pill form."

The free-radical theory of aging blames highly reactive byproducts of metabolism, like hydrogen peroxide, for cell damage that builds up over a lifetime. The mitochondria, where cells "burn" glucose for energy, churn out high levels of these oxidizing free-radicals.

Working with colleagues from the University of California and the University of Texas, the UW researchers focused on **catalase, an enzyme in mice and people that neutralizes hydrogen peroxide. Mice with higher levels of catalase in their mitochondria lived 5.5 months longer than the controls**, whose average life span is about two years. **Mice with high catalase in other cell structures, including the nucleus, showed only modest life extension.**

The oldest of nearly 1,000 experimental mice lived to the ripe age of three years and four months - watched closely by scientists who couldn't start their analysis until all the mice had died. "Waiting those last few months for the experiment to be done was like waiting until the day finally arrives to open a present," Rabinovitch said. In addition to living longer, **the genetically engineered mice had less heart damage and fewer cataracts than normally aging mice.**

"It's a pretty strong case that several different aspects of aging, including terminal disease, have been delayed or decelerated," said pathologist Richard Miller, of the University of Michigan Geriatrics Center. Miller, who was not involved in the UW study, analyzed its significance for Science Express, the online version of Science magazine that published the study yesterday.

Miller and several other scientists have extended mouse, worm and fruit-fly life spans by genetically tampering with growth hormones. The resulting **dwarf mice can live 50 percent longer, though most are infertile.**

Small dogs, which produce low levels of growth hormone, live longer than big breeds. And mice and rats fed near-starvation diets also have life spans up to 50 percent longer than animals that eat normally.

The UW study is the first to extend mouse life spans by reducing free-radical damage, Miller said. The big question researchers are trying to answer now is how all these bits of evidence fit together to explain the underlying causes of aging - and whether the process can be slowed.

"The only way to increase maximum life span to a major extent is by fiddling around with the aging process itself," Miller said. It's possible antioxidants may be tied in with growth hormones, diet and cell structures called telomeres, which break down with age, blocking cell division. Or there could be several separate mechanisms responsible for different aspects of aging.

"That's the 64,000 dollar question," Rabinovitch said. **"Now that we know antioxidants can extend life spans,** we want to know whether they work through similar or different mechanisms than caloric restriction or dwarfism."

He and his co-workers are raising a new generation of genetically engineered mice, hoping to boost life spans further by targeting antioxidants to more types of tissue throughout the animals' bodies. "We propose this is just the tip of the iceberg."

2.7.9.0 Superoxide is not a major determinant of aging in C. elegans: Against the oxidative damage theory of aging

The superoxide radical (O(2)(-)) has long been considered a major cause of aging. O(2)(-) in cytosolic, extracellular, and mitochondrial pools is detoxified by dedicated superoxide dismutase (SOD) isoforms. **We tested the impact of each SOD isoform in Caenorhabditis elegans by manipulating its five sod genes and saw no major effects on life span**. sod genes are not required for daf-2 insulin/IGF-1 receptor mutant longevity. However, loss of the extracellular Cu/ZnSOD sod-4 enhances daf-2 longevity and constitutive diapause, suggesting a signaling role for sod-4. Overall, these findings imply that **O(2)(-) is not a major determinant of aging in C. elegans (Against the oxidative damage theory of aging**: superoxide dismutases protect against oxidative stress but have little or no effect on life span in Caenorhabditis elegans. R Doonan, JJ e, F Matthijssens, GA Walker, K Houthoofd, P Back, A Matscheski, JR Vanfleteren, D Gems. Genes Dev (2008) 22: 3236-3241).

2.8.0.0 Xanthine oxidase produces superoxide in route to making antioxidant, uric acid

Superoxide is produced by several other enzymes (steps I and iii in the electron transport system), an example of which is xanthine oxidase (involved in the formation of uric acid).

When cellular superoxide dismutase comes into contact with superoxide, the SOD a reaction takes place, which results in the production of hydrogen peroxide. For each two superoxides that are encountered by the SOD, one hydrogen peroxide (H2O2) is created. Hydrogen peroxide does however pose a great danger to the cell as it transforms easily into the highly reactive hydroxyl radical. **I believe that this predicts that patients without catalase (acatalasemia) would have disastrous consequences and be a fatal genetic flaw. However, acatalasemic patients live basically normal lives, troubled only by gum infections. This fact, alone, discounts the doom and gloom predictions of the free radi-crap theory.**

A process involving the Fenton chemistry (described previously). Luckily, there does exist an efficient mechanism for dealing with the hydrogen peroxide. The enzyme **catalase is produced by the rough endoplasmic reticulum and is concentrated in peroxisomes surrounding the mitochondria** (as well as being present in lower concentrations throughout the cell). The catalase reacts with the hydrogen peroxide to produce water and oxygen. As stated before, **acatalasemics live basically normal lives and have a normal life span.**

Over 90% of the dioxygen used by an organism is processed in the mitochondria (B Chance, H Sies and A Boveris, Physiol Rev, 59, 527±605(1979).

2.8.1.0 A Fountain of Youth?

The canny world of advertising has caught on to the free radical theory of aging, **marketing a whole array of antioxidants for preventing anything from wrinkles to dry hair to reducing the risk of heart disease — promising to help slow the hands of time.**

Nevertheless, numerous studies of people taking antioxidant pills have failed to show a benefit, and the supplements may even be harmful. A study earlier this year hinted that high doses of the antioxidant vitamin E may raise the risk of heart disease, while earlier research has found that beta carotene, another popular antioxidant, puts smokers at higher risk of lung cancer (Role of Oxidants and Antioxidants in Atherosclerosis: Results of In Vitro and In Vivo Investigations. Siekmeier et al. *J CARDIOVASC PHARMACOL THER* 2007;12:265-282).

2.8.2.0 Hydrogen peroxide induces senescence in human fibrobsasts

Premature senescence of human fibroblasts is established after exposure to an acute sublethal concentration of H_2O_2. Overexpression of transforming growth factor-beta1 (TGF-beta1) was shown to be responsible for the appearance of the biomarkers of senescence in these conditions. Other studies have shown that incubation of human fibroblasts with TGF-beta1 leads to overexpression of H_2O_2. In this work, **we show an increased production of H_2O_2 by human fibroblasts as premature senescence is established after an initial exposure to H_2O_2.** (Establishment of H_2O_2-induced premature senescence in human fibroblasts concomitant with increased cellular production of H_2O_2. Zdanov S, Remacle J, Toussaint O. Ann N Y Acad Sci. 2006 May;1067:210-6).

2.8.3.0 Hydrogen peroxide increase senescence in Werner fibroblasts

Normal human diploid fibroblasts (HDFs) exposed to a single H_2O_2 subcytotoxic stress display features of premature senescence, termed stress-induced premature senescence (SIPS). In this work, our aim was to study SIPS in Werner syndrome (WS) fibroblasts, derived from a patient with WS, a disease resembling accelerated aging.

The subcytotoxic dose for WS fibroblasts was found to be inferior to that of normal HDFs, indicating WS fibroblasts are more sensitive to hydrogen peroxide than normal HDFs. SA beta-gal activity has been shown to occur both in vitro and in vivo, and we studied the proportion of WS cells positive for SA beta-gal. **Intriguingly, the percentage of positive cells did not increase with the dose of H_2O_2 used. Contrary to other HDFs, the DNA-binding activity of p53 in WS fibroblasts did not increase in SIPS.** We found, based on our results, that WS fibroblasts feature an altered stress response and **do not reach SIPS from H_2O_2.** We suggest that the proportion of cells that in normal HDFs would enter SIPS instead die in WS fibroblasts. Last, we propose that aging derives from a loss of integrity of the chromatin structure, which occurs faster in WS patients (No increase in senescence-associated beta-galactosidase activity in Werner syndrome fibroblasts after exposure to H_2O_2. de Magalhães JP, et al. Ann N Y Acad Sci. 2004 Jun;1019:375-8). **I suggest that this indicates that peroxide is not the cause of aging.**

2.8.4.0 Werner syndrome

Werner syndrome (WS) is a premature aging disorder used as a model of normal human aging. **WS individuals have several characteristics of normal aging, such as cataracts, hair graying, and skin aging, but manifest these at an early age.** Additionally, **WS individuals have high levels of inflammatory diseases, such as atherosclerosis and type 2 diabetes.** The in vivo aging in WS is associated with accelerated aging of fibroblasts in culture. **The cause of the accelerated senescence is not understood,** but may be due to the genomic instability that is a hallmark of WS. Genome instability results in activation of stress kinases, such as p38, and the p38-specific inhibitor SB203580, prevents the accelerated senescence seen in WS fibroblasts. However, **oxidative damage plays a role, as low oxygen conditions and antioxidant treatment revert some of the accelerated senescence phenotype.** The effects of oxidative stress appear to be suppressible by SB203580; however, it does not appear to be transduced by p38. As SB203580 is known to inhibit other kinases in addition to p38, this suggests that more than one kinase pathway is involved. The recent development of p38 inhibitors with different binding properties, specificities, and oral bioavailability, and of new potent and selective inhibitors of JNK and MK2, will make it possible to dissect the roles of various kinase pathways in the accelerated senescence of WS cells. If this accelerated senescence is reflective of WS aging in vivo, these kinase inhibitors may well form the basis of antiaging therapies for individuals with WS (The role of cellular senescence in Werner syndrome: toward therapeutic intervention in human premature aging. Davis T, Wyllie FS, Rokicki MJ, Bagley MC, Kipling D. Ann N Y Acad Sci. 2007 Apr;1100:455-69).

As I have said before, even anaerobes age and progeria patients do not utilize oxygen at 8X normal rates (oxygen consumption is normal), even though they age 8X faster than normal.

2.8.6.0 Cytochrome produced EMODs do not contribute to aging

Oxidative stress impairs endothelium-dependent dilation (EDD) with aging in healthy sedentary adults. **Increased cytochrome P-450 2C9 (CYP 2C9) signaling can contribute to oxidative stress-mediated suppression of EDD, but its role in aging is unknown.** We hypothesized that inhibition of CYP 2C9 signaling with sulfaphenazole would improve EDD in older, but not young, healthy sedentary adults. At baseline, increases in forearm blood flow (FBF; venous occlusion plethysmography) in response to brachial artery infusions of ACh (1, 2, 4, and 8 μg ·100 ml forearm volume^{-1} ·min^{-1}), an endothelium-dependent dilator, were smaller in older [n = 14, 63 ± 1 (SE) yr] than in young (n = 11, 23 ± 2 yr) adults ($P < 0.05$), with a reduction in peak FBF of 32% (11.8 ± 1.7 vs. 17.3 ± 2.3 ml ·100 ml tissue^{-1} ·min^{-1}). Infusion of sulfaphenazole at doses that block CYP 2C9 signaling in humans did not affect the FBF responses to ACh in the older (peak FBF = 13.0 ± 4.3 ml ·100 ml tissue^{-1} ·min^{-1}, P = 0.41) or the young (peak FBF = 17.1 ± 1.9 ml ·100 ml tissue^{-1} ·min^{-1}, P = 0.55) adults. Coadministration of the nitric oxide inhibitor L-NMMA and sulfaphenazole decreased the FBF response to ACh in young and older subjects ($P < 0.05$); the effect was smaller in the older subjects, but group differences in EDD remained ($P < 0.05$). Endothelium-independent dilation assessed with sodium nitroprusside was not different in the young and older subjects. These results provide the first support for the concept that **increased CYP 2C9 signaling does not contribute to impairments in EDD with aging in healthy adults** (Cytochrome P-450 2C9 signaling does not contribute to age-associated vascular endothelial dysfunction in humans. Anthony J. Donato et al. J Appl Physiol 105: 1359-1363, 2008). **I believe that we see more and more evidence that the entire free radical theory has been nullified.**

2.9.0.0 Hydrogen peroxide linked to longer life

The following was taken from: http://www.scientificblogging.com/news_articles/oxidative_stress_linked_aging_cancer_and_now_longer_life

Oxidative stress has been linked to aging, cancer and other diseases in humans. **Paradoxically, researchers have suggested that small exposure to oxidative conditions may actually offer protection from acute doses.** Now, scientists at the University of California, San Diego, have discovered the gene responsible for this effect. Their study, published in *PLoS Genetics* on May 29, 2009 explains the underlying mechanism of the process that prevents cellular damage by reactive oxygen species (ROS).

"We may drink pomegranate juice to protect our bodies from so-called 'free radicals' or look at restricting calorie intake to extend our lifespan," said **Trey Ideker, PhD, chief of the Division of Genetics in the Department of Medicine at UC San Diego's School of Medicine and professor of bioengineering at the Jacobs School of Engineering.** "But our study suggests why **humans may actually be able to prolong the aging process by regularly exposing our bodies to minimal amounts of oxidants.**"

Reactive oxygen species (ROS), ions that form as a natural byproduct of the metabolism of oxygen, play important roles in cell signaling. These very small molecules include oxygen ions, free radicals and peroxides. However, during times of environmental stress (for example, **ultraviolet radiation or heat or chemical exposure), ROS levels can increase dramatically.** This can result in significant damage to cellular damage to DNA, RNA and proteins – cumulating in an effect called oxidative stress.

One major contributor to oxidative stress is **hydrogen peroxide**, converted from a type of free radical that leaks from the mitochondria as it produces energy. While the cell has ways to help minimize the damaging effects of hydrogen peroxide by converting it to oxygen and water, this conversion isn't 100 percent successful. **RMH Note: It would be tragic for all peroxide to be instantaneously converted to oxygen and water. It is crucially needed for many normal activities within the cell and for prooxidant pathogen and neoplasia protection.**

Ideker and first author Ryan Kelley used the rich functional genomics toolbox of yeast to identify pathways involved in the cell's adaption to hydrogen peroxide. **Adaption (or hormesis) is an effect where a toxic substance acts like a stimulant in small doses, but is an inhibitor in large doses.**

To shed light on the molecular mechanisms of adaptation, Ideker and Kelley designed a way to identify genes involved in adaptation to hydrogen peroxide. **They elicited adaptation by pre-treating cells with a mild dose of hydrogen**

peroxide, followed by a high dose. They observed that the cells undergoing this adaptation protocol exhibited a smaller reduction in viability than cells exposed to only an acute treatment protocol (in which about half of the cells died.) **In other words, I believe that the exposure to peroxide resulted in greater viability, in a preconditioning type reaction.**

To figure out which genes might control this adaptation mechanism, Kelley and Ideker ran a series of experiments in which cells were forced to adapt while each gene in the genome was removed, one by one – covering a total of nearly **5,000 genes**. By systematically removing genes, they identified a novel factor called **Mga2** – and discovered that this transcription factor is essential for adaptation.

"This was a surprise, because Mga2 is found at the control point of a completely different pathway than those which respond to acute exposure of oxidative agents," said Ideker. "This second pathway is only active at lower doses of oxidation."

2.9.1.0 Caloric restriction may raise ROS

This finding may explain **recent studies suggesting that eating less may, in fact, raise ROS levels** – and, in doing so, provide protection from acute doses of oxidants. **This is counter to the hypothesis that caloric restriction extends lifespan in some species because it reduces ROS** produced as a by-product of the energy regenerated by mitochondria. **I have been saying this for years!**

"It may be that adaption to oxidative stress is the main factor responsible for the lifespan-expanding effects of caloric restriction," said Ideker. "Our next step is to figure out how Mga2 works to create a separate pathway – to discover the upstream mechanism that senses low doses of oxidation and triggers a protective mechanism downstream." Further efforts to understand this process may have broad implications on models of aging and disease. (Kelley R, Ideker T (2009) Genome-Wide Fitness and Expression Profiling Implicate Mga2 in Adaptation to Hydrogen Peroxide. PLoS Genet 5(5): e1000488. doi:10.1371/journal.pgen.1000488).

-the following is taken from the original Plos article:

Caloric restriction extends lifespan, an effect once thought to involve attenuation of reactive oxygen species (ROS) generated by aerobic metabolism. However, recent evidence suggests that caloric restriction may in fact raise ROS levels, which in turn provides protection from acute doses of oxidant through a process called adaptation. To shed light on the molecular mechanisms of adaptation, we designed a series of genome-wide deletion fitness and mRNA expression screens to identify genes involved in adaptation to hydrogen peroxide. Combined with known transcriptional interactions, the integrated data **implicate Yap1 and Skn7 as central transcription factors of both the adaptive and acute oxidative responses. They also identify the transcription factors Mga2 and Rox1** as active exclusively in the adaptive response and show that Mga2 is essential for adaptation. These **findings are striking** because Mga2 and Rox1 have been thought to control the response to hypoxic, not oxidative, conditions. Expression profiling of *mga2Δ* and *rox1Δ* knockouts shows that these factors most strongly regulate targets in ergosterol, fatty-acid, and zinc metabolic pathways. Direct quantitation of ergosterol reveals that its basal concentration indeed depends on Mga2, but that Mga2 is not required for the decrease in ergosterol observed during adaptation.

Reactive oxygen species (ROS) damage a variety of structures within the cell, resulting in disease and aging. **RMH Note: I vehemently disagree with this statement.**

In a seemingly **paradoxical** effect termed adaptation, it is possible to prevent damage caused by ROS by pre-treating the cell with a small amount of oxidant. We studied this process in order to identify the mechanisms that provide this protection. Our study identified a number of genes and processes with previously unappreciated roles in adaptation. **The mechanisms we identified are remarkable because they are distinct from those previously known to protect the cell from ROS.** Although this study is conducted in yeast, the wide conservation of adaptation among many organisms suggests that the results from this study may be widely applicable.

2.9.1.1 Introduction

Oxidative stress is caused by a number of reactive oxygen species (ROS) generated as a result of aerobic metabolism or chemical exposure. These compounds damage a variety of cellular products, including DNA, proteins, and lipid membranes, and are associated with a number of human pathologies (**associated with but not proven causative**). For example, **in cardiovascular disease, oxidation of low-density lipoprotein causes an inflammatory response** (Lusis AJ (2000) Atherosclerosis. Nature 407: 233–241).

The sensitivity of neurons to oxidative stress implicates ROS in neurodegenerative diseases, such as Parkinson's and Alzheimer's (Jenner

P (2003) Oxidative stress in Parkinson's disease. Ann Neurol 53: Suppl 3S26–36. discussion S36–28) (Markesbery WR (1997) Oxidative stress hypothesis in Alzheimer's disease. Free Radic Biol Med 23: 134–147) (Christen Y (2000) Oxidative stress and Alzheimer disease. Am J Clin Nutr 71: 621S–629S).

A continuing source of controversy is the role of oxidative stress in aging. Caloric restriction has been shown to extend lifespan in a number of species (Weindruch R, Naylor PH, Goldstein AL, Walford RL (1988) Influences of aging and dietary restriction on serum thymosin alpha 1 levels in mice. J Gerontol 43: B40–42).

Initially, **it was hypothesized that the effect on lifespan occurs primarily because caloric restriction reduces the level of aerobic respiration, a major source of ROS** (Harman D (1956) Aging: a theory based on free radical and radiation chemistry. J Gerontol 11: 298–300). **I believe that this proved to be wrong because it was based on the flawed free radical theory of Harman.**

Newer evidence is challenging this hypothesis, since caloric restriction paradoxically increases respiration (Lin SJ, Kaeberlein M, Andalis AA, Sturtz LA, Defossez PA, et al. (2002) Calorie restriction extends Saccharomyces cerevisiae lifespan by increasing respiration. Nature 418: 344–348). **I believe that this is a very important observation and is consistent with my UTOPIA theory.**

Increased respiration, in turn, can generate mild levels of ROS which protect against high doses of oxidant (Schulz TJ, Zarse K, Voigt A, Urban N, Birringer M, et al. (2007) Glucose restriction extends Caenorhabditis elegans life span by inducing mitochondrial respiration and increasing oxidative stress. Cell Metab 6: 280–293).

2.9.1.2 Hormesis and caloric restriction

This process is known as adaptation or **hormesis** (Jamieson DJ (1992) Saccharomyces cerevisiae has distinct adaptive responses to both hydrogen peroxide and menadione. J Bacteriol 174: 6678–6681) and is widely conserved among eukaryotes.

One hypothesis is that adaptation to oxidative stress is the basis for the lifespan-extending effect of caloric restriction (Masoro EJ (2000) Caloric restriction and aging: an update. Exp Gerontol 35: 299–305) (Masoro EJ (2005) Overview of caloric restriction and ageing. Mech Ageing Dev 126: 913–922).

Thus, further efforts to understand the process of adaptation may have broad implications on models of aging and disease.

In one model of adaptation, the cell increases the activity of the enzymes and pathways required to rid the cells of ROS, leaving it better equipped to process acute dosages of oxidant when they arise. Under this model, genes involved in the adaptive response are expected to be a subset of those that become active in the acute response. Many such candidates have been identified, including a variety of biosynthetic enzymes which produce small molecular compounds or proteins with reduction potential, such as **glutathione (GSH), thioredoxin, NADPH, and trehalose**. Different enzymes facilitate this process for different ROS, including catalases and peroxidases (which deal with peroxide radicals) and superoxide dismutases (which deal with superoxide radicals). Additional proteins serve to repair the damage caused by oxidative stress. Heat shock proteins act as chaperones within the cell, allowing damaged proteins to fold properly or preparing them for disposal. DNA repair genes are also vital, as oxidative stress can damage both nucleotides and the phosphodiester DNA backbone. Several studies have implicated classical oxidative stress proteins and pathways in adaptation, including the transcription factor Yap1 and glutathione synthesis.

In contrast to this model, a second body of evidence suggests that **adaptation may be governed by novel pathways not directly involved in the response to acute oxidation**. In a study of adaptation to the oxidant linoleic acid, Alic *et al.* found that adaptation can occur without induction of oxidative or general stress response genes following pretreatment. Instead, various metabolic processes were activated and protein synthesis was inhibited. Moreover, machinery with a central role in the acute response, such as the mitochondria or the Msn2/4 environmental stress response factors, are not required for adaptation.

Nonetheless, expression studies of acute oxidative damage have helped to identify a set of genes involved in the common environmental stress response (ESR) and implicated the Msn2/4 transcription factors in control of this gene set. In fitness studies of yeast deletion strains, Thorpe *et al.* identified a set of genes required for the response to **hydrogen peroxide,** mainly dealing with the proper functioning of the mitochondria. However, to-date these genome-scale approaches have focused on the acute, rather than the adaptive, response. One study to date that has screened for adaptive genes focused on a set of 268 genes selected based on previous literature.

Here, we use the rich functional genomics toolbox of yeast to identify pathways involved in adaptation to **hydrogen peroxide**. To accomplish this goal, we use barcode arrays to screen the *Saccharomyces cerevisiae* gene deletion collection for genes required in the acute and adaptive responses, and we couple these data with genome-wide mRNA expression profiles to build a system-wide model of adaptation.

They elicited adaptation using a protocol consisting of a **mild pretreatment of hydrogen peroxide (0.1 mM H_2O_2 for 45 min**) followed by a later **high dose (0.4 mM H_2O_2 for 1 hr)**. For purposes of comparison, we also conducted an acute protocol which exposed cells to the high dose only (0.4 mM H_2O_2 for 1 hr). Consistent with previous findings, we observed that **yeast cells undergoing the adaptation protocol exhibited a smaller reduction in viability compared to cells exposed to the acute treatment protocol**.

2.9.2.0 Some pathogens have catalase to protect against peroxide

Hydrogen peroxide is used as a potent antimicrobial agent when cells are infected with a pathogen. Pathogens that are catalase-positive, such as *Mycobacterium tuberculosis, Legionella pneumophila*, and *Campylobacter jejuni*, make catalase in order to deactivate the peroxide radicals, thus allowing them to survive unharmed within the host (Srinivasa Rao PS, Yamada Y, Leung KY (September 2003). "A major catalase (KatB) that is required for resistance to H_2O_2 and phagocyte-mediated killing in Edwardsiella tarda". *Microbiology (Reading, Engl.)* 149 (Pt 9): 2635–44).

Very few aerobic microorganisms are known that do not use catalase. *Streptococcus* species are an example of aerobic bacteria that do not possess catalase. Catalase has also been observed in some anaerobic microorganisms, such as *Methanosarcina barkeri* (Brioukhanov AL, Netrusov AI, Eggen RI (June 2006). "The catalase and superoxide dismutase genes are transcriptionally up-regulated upon oxidative stress in the strictly anaerobic archaeon Methanosarcina barkeri". *Microbiology (Reading, Engl.)* 152 (Pt 6): 1671–7**)**.

I find it incredible that peroxide is such an effective cidal agent that certain bacteria have evolved the synthesis of catalase as a defense.

2.9.3.0 Hydrogen peroxide important signaling clue in cancer cells

A significant breakthrough in understanding the communication system within the body's cells could aid research into cancer. Scientists

have found that the chemical hydrogen peroxide - better known as a form of bleach - plays a central role in this communication process. It appears to be one of the ways to tell cells when they should divide and when they die.

However, **if the signalling system goes awry, then it may lead to cancer.**

Hydrogen peroxide is a by-product of the energy-creating process in cells. **Usually it is toxic to cells** and is broken down by an enzyme called peroxiredoxin. **RMH Note: this is not true.**

But researchers from Oregon State University and Wake Forest University in the US found **peroxiredoxin is only effective when levels of hydrogen peroxide are low.** When levels of the chemical rise it appears to neutralise the enzyme which is then unable to break it down.

The evolution of this complex system suggests that **at certain special times the body, rather than needing to get rid of hydrogen peroxide, actually requires the chemical to perform a specialised function.**

The researchers believe **these special times can include moments when a cell is ordered to divide, or when it is ordered to die - and that the sudden increase in hydrogen peroxide levels stimulates these processes. Under normal circumstances, they believe, the enzyme keeps hydrogen peroxide levels in check so that no accidental signals are sent within the body's cells.**

But when hydrogen peroxide is needed to stimulate the signalling process, **the cells produce a sudden burst of hydrogen peroxide**, which overwhelms the enzyme, switching it off and permitting the signal. The scientists believe **cancer may be linked to the over-production of peroxiredoxin. I believe that cancer is "allowed" to manifest itself due to an EMOD/peroxide insufficiency.**

In this case there is so much of the enzyme that it is not switched off by a burst of hydrogen peroxide production. Thus it is able to break down peroxide and prevent it from signalling to cells that they should commit suicide in the normal way. Thus the cancer cells don't die off, but instead begin to divide in a controlled way. **This is the effect of adding antioxidants, in that they allow the cancer cells to continue to divide and negate the apoptotic action of peroxide.**

Researcher **Professor Andrew Karplus told BBC News Online**: "What we have discovered is a remarkable and unexpected way that **cells can protect themselves from the negative effects of hydrogen peroxide,** yet still use it as a signalling molecule. "Our work shows that the enzyme peroxiredoxin is the key to sorting out these two roles. "Given that in many cases the peroxide signalling pathways have gone awry in diseases like cancer (**this is not true**), this opens up novel possibilities for future medical applications."

Dr Zac Wood, who also worked on the study, said: "Hydrogen peroxide is an effective signalling molecule because it is rapidly produced, is reactive and is easily controlled by enzymes."

Nicola O'Connor, from the charity Cancer Research UK, told BBC News Online that the **peroxiredoxins had been linked to wide range of biological activities that implicate them in fundamental processes that control cell growth and death.**

"There is increasing evidence that **some cancers have abnormal levels of peoxiredoxins, suggesting that an imbalance of these enzymes could be involved in tumour development."** The research is published in the journal Science in June, 2009.

http://news.bbc.co.uk/2/hi/health/2973555.stm

2.9.4.0 Stem Cells

2.9.4.1 ROS required for signaling cascades initiating cardiovascular differentiation

Growing stem cells are subjected to mechanical forces, which may initiate differentiation programs. Mechanical strain stimulated cardiovascular differentiation of mouse embryonic stem (ES) cells as evaluated by quantification of contracting cardiac foci and capillary areas, respectively. **Mechanical strain rapidly elevated intracellular reactive oxygen species (ROS).** After 24 h up-regulation of NADPH oxidase subunits p22-phox, p47-phox, p67-phox, and Nox-4 as well as *Nox-1* and *Nox-4* mRNA was observed. In parallel, mechanical strain increased hypoxia-inducible factor-1 (HIF-1α) and vascular endothelial growth factor (VEGF) mRNA and protein as well as *MEF2C* and *GATA-4* mRNA, which are involved in cardiovascular development. Furthermore, phosphorylation of extracellular-regulated kinase 1,2 (ERK1,2), p38, and c-jun N-terminal kinase (c-Jun NH2-terminal kinase (JNK)) was observed. Stimulation of cardiovascular commitment,

HIF-1α, VEGF, and *MEF2C* expression as well as MAPK activation were **abolished by free radical scavengers**, whereas *GATA-4* expression was increased. Cardiomyogenesis was inhibited by the p38 inhibitor SB203580, the ERK1,2 inhibitor UO126, and the JNK inhibitor SP600125. Vasculogenesis/angiogenesis was blunted following inhibition of ERK1,2 and JNK, whereas p38 inhibition was ineffective. Our data outline a role of ROS as mechanotransducing molecules in mechanical strain-stimulated cardiovascular differentiation of ES cells, and point toward **a microenvironment of elevated ROS required for signaling cascades initiating cardiovascular differentiation programs.** (Schmelter, M., Ateghang, B., Helmig, S., Wartenberg, M., Sauer, H. Embryonic stem cells utilize reactive oxygen species as transducers of mechanical strain-induced cardiovascular differentiation. *The FASEB Journal.* 2006;20:1182-1184).

2.9.5.0 Pro-vasculogenic stem cell effects are mediated by Ca^{2+}-induced ROS generation

Platelet-derived growth factor BB (PDGF-BB) has been assigned a critical role in vascular growth and recruitment of perivascular mural cells. The purpose of the present study is to investigate the signalling events underlying the stimulation of vasculogenesis of mouse embryonic stem (ES) cells by PDGF-BB.

Methods and results: PDGF-BB increased vascular sprouting and branching of capillary-like structures in embryoid bodies as evaluated by computer-assisted analysis of CD31-positive cell structures. It also activated extracellular-regulated kinase 1,2 (ERK1,2) and c-Jun N-terminal kinase but not p38 mitogen-activated protein kinase or PI 3-kinase. Microfluorometric analysis of fluo-4 fluorescence revealed that treatment with PDGF-BB raised intracellular Ca^{2+} levels in differentiating ES cells expressing the PDGF receptor β, an effect that was abolished in the presence of the intracellular Ca^{2+} chelator BAPTA. Furthermore, **PDGF-BB raised reactive oxygen species (ROS) levels in embryoid bodies** as evaluated using the redox-sensitive dye H_2DCF-DA. ROS generation was blunted in the presence of the NADPH oxidase inhibitors diphenylen iodonium (DPI) and apocynin as well as in the presence of BAPTA, suggesting that **ROS generation is regulated by intracellular Ca^{2+} transients.** The stimulation of vasculogenesis of ES cells upon treatment with PDGF-BB was significantly inhibited by the ERK1,2 inhibitor U0126, the NADPH oxidase inhibitors DPI, apocynin, 4-(2-aminoethyl)benzenesulfonylfluoride and VAS2870, the free radical scavengers vitamin E, and N-(2-mercaptopropionyl)glycin as well as by BAPTA.

Conclusion: Our data demonstrate that **the pro-vasculogenic effects of PDGF-BB are mediated by Ca^{2+}-induced ROS generation, resulting**

in the activation of an ERK1,2-mediated signal transduction cascade (Platelet-derived growth factor BB stimulates vasculogenesis of embryonic stem cell-derived endothelial cells by calcium-mediated generation of reactive oxygen species. Sabine Lange et al. Cardiovascular Research Advance Access first published online on September 20, 2008

This version [Corrected Proof] published online on October 22, 2008

Cardiovascular Research, doi:10.1093/cvr/cvn258).

2.9.6.0 Reactive Oxygen Species and Genomic Stability in Hematopoietic Stem Cells

Hematopoietic stem cells (HSCs) are defined by their ability both to self-renew and to give rise to fresh blood cells throughout the lifetime of an animal. The failure of HSCs to self-renew during aging is believed to depend on several intrinsic (cell-autonomous) and extrinsic (non–cell-autonomous) factors. In this review, we focus on how **dysregulation of reactive oxygen species (ROS) and disruptions of genomic stability can impair HSC functions.** Recently, it was shown that **long-term self-renewing HSCs normally possess low levels of intracellular ROS**. However, **when intracellular ROS levels become excessive, they cause senescence or apoptosis, resulting in a failure of HSC self-renewal.**

Repression of intracellular ROS levels in HSCs by **treatment with an antioxidant that scavenges ROS can rescue HSC functions,** indicating that excess ROS levels are at the root of HSC failure. Products of numerous genes that are involved in either DNA-damage responses or longevity related signaling contribute to the maintenance of the HSC self-renewal capacity. Further investigations on the molecular mechanisms of ROS regulation and on the manipulation of excess ROS levels could lead to the development of novel therapeutics for hematopoietic diseases, regenerative medicine, and the prevention of leukemia (Kazuhito Naka, Teruyuki Muraguchi, Takayuki Hoshii, Atsushi Hirao. Antioxidants & Redox Signaling. November 1, 2008, 10(11): 1883-1894).

2.9.7.0 ROS control hematolymphopoiesis

Reactive oxygen species (ROS) have been shown to stimulate proliferation and growth responses in a variety of mammalian cell types and to act as important mediators in many cellular processes, including hematolymphopoiesis. We examined the effect on primitive murine hematopoietic progenitor cells (HPC) of ROS generated by xanthine plus xanthine oxidase (xanthine/XO) and various antioxidants. Pretreatment of murine HPC (C57BL/6) with xanthine/XO produced a dose-dependent enhancement of clonogenic response to granulocyte/macrophage colony- stimulating factor (GM-CSF) but not to interleukin-3 or granulocyte colony-stimulating factor. Stem cell factor (SCF), a potent comitogen for many hematopoietic growth factors, also synergized with GM-CSF. However, the synergistic enhancement of GM-CSF with xanthine/XO and SCF was not additive, indicating that xanthine/XO and SCF may target the same subpopulation of HPC. These findings indicate that **xanthine/XO mimics SCF in stimulating a subpopulation of murine HPC to proliferate and that SCF synergy with GM-CSF in this population is sensitive to antioxidant inhibition**. (Reactive oxygen species mediate stem cell factor synergy with granulocyte/macrophage colony-stimulating factor in a subpopulation of primitive murine hematopoietic progenitor cells. DW Pyatt, WS Stillman and RD Irons. Molecular Pharmacology. Volume 49, Issue 6, pp. 1097-1103, 06/01/1996).

3.0.0.0 Hypoxia

3.0.0.1 Intermittent Hypoxia: Cause of or Therapy for Systemic Hypertension?

During acute episodes of hypoxia, chemoreceptor-mediated sympathetic activity increases heart rate, cardiac output, peripheral resistance and systemic arterial pressure. However, **different intermittent hypoxia paradigms produce remarkably divergent effects on systemic arterial pressure in the post-hypoxic steady state.** The hypertensive effects of **obstructive sleep apnea (OSA)** *vs.* the depressor effects of therapeutic hypoxia exemplify this divergence. **OSA, a condition afflicting 15–25% of American men and 5–10% of women,** has been implicated in the pathogenesis of systemic hypertension and is a major risk factor for heart disease and stroke. OSA imposes a series of brief, intense episodes of hypoxia and hypercapnia, leading to persistent, maladaptive chemoreflex-mediated activation of the sympathetic nervous system which culminates in hypertension. Conversely, **extensive evidence in animals and humans has shown controlled intermittent hypoxia conditioning programs to be safe, efficacious modalities for prevention and treatment of hypertension.** This article reviews the pertinent literature in an attempt to reconcile the divergent effects of intermittent hypoxia therapy and obstructive sleep apnea on hypertension. Special emphasis is placed on research conducted in the nations of the former Soviet Union, where intermittent hypoxia conditioning programs are being applied therapeutically to treat hypertension in patients. Also reviewed is evidence regarding mechanisms of the pro- and anti-hypertensive effects of intermittent hypoxia (Intermittent Hypoxia: Cause of or Therapy for Systemic Hypertension? Tatiana V. Serebrovskaya et al. *Experimental Biology and Medicine* 233:627-650 (2008).

3.0.1.0 Intermittent hypoxia has salutary effect

Intermittent hypoxia (IH) has been found to protect brain from ischemic injury. We investigated whether IH mitigates brain oxidative stress and behavioral deficits in rats subjected to ethanol intoxication and abrupt ethanol withdrawal (EW). The effects of IH on overt EW behavioral signs, superoxide generation, protein oxidation, and mitochondrial permeability transition pore (PTP) opening were examined. Male rats consumed dextrin or 6.5% (wt/vol) ethanol for 35 days. During the last 20 days, rats were treated with repetitive (5–8 per day), brief (5–10 min) cycles of hypoxia (9.5–10% inspired O_2) separated by 4-min normoxia exposures. Cerebellum, cortex, and hippocampus were biopsied on *day 35* of the diet or at 24 h of EW. Superoxide and protein carbonyl contents in tissue homogenates and absorbance decline at 540 nm in mitochondrial suspensions served as indicators of oxidative stress, protein oxidation, and PTP opening, respectively. Although IH altered neither ethanol consumption nor blood ethanol concentration, it sharply lowered the severity of EW signs including tremor, tail rigidity, and startle response. Compared with dextrin and ethanol per se, in the three brain regions, EW increased superoxide and protein carbonyl contents and accelerated PTP opening in a manner ameliorated by IH. **Administration of antioxidant *N*-acetylcysteine throughout the IH program abrogated the reductions in EW signs and superoxide content**, implicating **IH-induced ROS as mediators of the salutary adaptations.** We conclude that **IH conditioning during chronic ethanol consumption attenuates oxidative damage to the brain and mitigates behavioral abnormalities during subsequent EW. IH-induced ROS may evoke this powerful protection** (Intermittent hypoxia conditioning prevents behavioral deficit and brain oxidative stress in ethanol-withdrawn rats. Marianna E. Jung et al. J Appl Physiol 105: 510-517, 2008).

RMH observation: Chronic hypoxia is cardioprotective and is a valid treatment for hypertension. Chronic hypoxia increases EMODs. Ergo, EMODs are not causative of hypertension or of cardiac failure.

3.0.2.0 EMOD cardioprotection is blocked by NAC

Reactive oxygen species (ROS) play a crucial role in the pathophysiology of ischemic heart disease by causing cardiac dysfunction and cell death. Several redox-sensitive anti- and pro-apoptotic transcription factors including NFkappaB and AP-1 progressively and steadily increase in the heart as a function of the duration of ischemia and reperfusion. When the heart is preconditioned to ischemic stress by repeated short-term ischemia and reperfusion, NFkappaB remains high while AP-1 is lowered to almost baseline value. **The anti-apoptotic gene Bcl-2 is downregulated in the ischemic/reperfused heart, while it is upregulated in the adapted myocardium. Cardioprotective abilities of the preconditioning are abolished when heart is pre-perfused with N-acetyl cysteine, a scavenger for ROS, suggesting the role of ROS in redox signaling.** Mammalian heart is protected by several defense systems which include among others, redox-regulated protein, thioredoxin. Reperfusion of ischemic myocardium results in the downregulation of thioredoxin 1 (Trx 1) expression, which was upregulated in the preconditioned myocardium. The increased expression of Trx 1 is completely blocked with an inhibitor of Trx 1, CDDP, which also abolished cardioprotection afforded by ischemic adaptation. The cardioprotective role of Trx 1 is confirmed further with transgenic mouse hearts overexpressing Trx 1. The Trx 1 mouse hearts displayed significantly improved post-ischemic ventricular recovery and reduced myocardial infarct size and apoptosis as compared to the corresponding wild-type mouse hearts. Taken together, preconditioning appears to potentiate redox signaling, which converts the "death signal" into "survival signal." (Preconditioning potentiates redox signaling and converts death signal into survival signal. Das DK, Maulik N. Arch Biochem Biophys. 2003 Dec 15;420(2):305-11).

3.0.3.0 Ischemic preconditioning

ISCHEMIC PRECONDITIONING describes the phenomenon whereby sublethal ischemia reduces subsequent lethal ischemic injury (Murry CE, Jennings RB, and Reimer KA. Preconditioning with ischemia: a delay of lethal cell injury in ischemic myocardium. *Circulation* 74: 1124–1136, 1986).

The phenomenon is highly reproducible and has been shown in many species, probably including humans (Lambiase PD, Edwards RJ, Cusack MR, Bucknall CA, Redwood SR, and Marber MS. Exercise-induced ischemia initiates the second window of protection in humans independent of collateral recruitment. *J Am Coll Cardiol* 41: 1174–1182, 2003) (Marber M, Walker D, and Yellon D. Ischaemic preconditioning. *BMJ* 308: 1–2, 1994).

Preconditioning has a number of identifiable triggers, including reactive oxygen species (ROS) (Das DK, Engelman RM, and Maulik N. Oxygen free radical signaling in ischemic preconditioning. *Ann NY Acad Sci* 874: 49–65, 1999).

It has been shown that ischemic preconditioning can be blocked by ROS scavengers (Tanaka M, Fujiwara H, Yamasaki K, and Sasayama S. Superoxide dismutase and N-2-mercaptopropionyl glycine attenuate infarct size limitation effect of ischaemic preconditioning in the rabbit. *Cardiovasc Res* 28: 980–986, 1994).

Moreover, it has been suggested that **ROS contribute to the threshold necessary for the activation of signals leading to cardioprotection** (Baines CP, Goto M, and Downey JM. Oxygen radicals released during ischemic preconditioning contribute to cardioprotection in the rabbit myocardium. *J Mol Cell Cardiol* 29: 207–216, 1997).

Furthermore, it has been shown that **ROS are generated during preconditioning cycles in cardiomyocytes** (vanden Hoek TL, Becker LB, Shao Z, Li C, and Schumacker PT. Reactive oxygen species released from mitochondria during brief hypoxia induce preconditioning in cardiomyocytes. *J Biol Chem* 273: 18092–18098, 1998).

In whole organ and whole animal models there is remaining controversy as to the effect of ROS scavengers on cardioprotection (Becker LB. New concepts in reactive oxygen species and cardiovascular reperfusion physiology. *Cardiovasc Res* 61: 461–470, 2004).

Although at high concentrations ROS are detrimental, there is increasing evidence that at lower concentrations they may play a subtle role in initiating protective cell signaling pathways (Droge W. Free radicals in the physiological control of cell function. *Physiol Rev* 82: 47–95, 2002).

Antimycin A is thought to generate mitochondrial ROS through an action on site III of the electron transport chain. At this site it blocks the conversion of ubisemiquinone to ubiquinol, thereby causing accumulation of superoxide ROS. In support of this action being of relevance to protection is **evidence that other mitochondrial ROS generators, such as menadione, also initiate cardioprotection** (Yue Y, Krenz M, Cohen MV, Downey JM, and Critz SD. Menadione mimics the infarct-limiting effect of preconditioning in isolated rat hearts. *Am J Physiol Heart Circ Physiol* 281: H590–H595, 2001).

Although in studies using anesthetic as a protective agent, a number of groups have demonstrated that ROS can trigger cardioprotection through activation of PKC; the specific isoform involved is unclear.

Antimycin A initiates cardioprotection that is blocked by MPG, suggesting a role for ROS in the mechanism of protection. Yue et al. have shown previously that another mitochondrial ROS generator menadione can cause cardioprotection through a pathway involving p38 mitogen-activated protein kinase (MAPK) activation (Yue Y, Krenz M, Cohen MV, Downey JM, and Critz SD. Menadione mimics the infarct-limiting effect of preconditioning in isolated rat hearts. *Am J Physiol Heart Circ Physiol* 281: H590–H595, 2001).

At high concentrations, ROS are detrimental to cells. However, there is increasing evidence that at lower concentrations they have a role to play in the signaling mechanisms of preconditioning (**Tritto I and Ambrosio G.** Role of oxidants in the signaling pathway of preconditioning. *Antioxid Redox Signal* 3: 3–10, 2001).

3.0.4.0 Controversial role of antioxidants

Increasingly complex behavior of free radicals and reactive oxygen species (ROS) are noted within biological systems. Classically free radicals and ROS were considered injurious, however current mechanisms describe both protective and deleterious effects. A burst of ROS has been well described with the first moments of reperfusion and is associated with injury. However ROS can also be protective as signal preconditioning protection and induce stress responses that lead to survival. ROS generation is appreciated to occur during ischemia despite the low oxygen tension, from a likely mitochondria source, and ROS-induced ROS release may amplify its signal. The burst of ROS seen during reperfusion may originate from a different cellular source than during ischemia and is not yet fully identified. **ROS and cellular redox conditions regulate a large number of vital pathways (energy metabolism, survival/stress responses, apoptosis, inflammatory response, oxygen sensing, etc).**

While cellular systems may demonstrate reperfusion injury, whole organ and animal models continue to report contradictory results on reperfusion injury and the role of antioxidants as a therapy. Collectively, these data may offer insight into why **clinical trials of antioxidants have had such mixed and mostly negative results.**

Future antioxidant therapies are likely to be effective but they must become: more specific for site of action, not have deleterious effects on other signaling pathways, be targeted to a specific reactive oxygen species or cellular compartment, and be "time sensitive" so they deliver the correct therapy at precisely the correct time in ischemia and reperfusion (New concepts in reactive oxygen species and cardiovascular reperfusion physiology. Lance B Becker. Cardiovascular Research 2004 61(3):461-470).

Aerobic organisms utilize molecular oxygen as a terminal electron acceptor to enable metabolism of organic carbon for providing energy. In this respiratory process, oxygen is consumed along with metabolic substrates while ATP, water, and carbon dioxide are generated. While the energetic payoffs of this process (38 moles of ATP per mole of glucose) are critical to the existence of most multi-cellular life, the risk we oxygen consumers must adapt to is the production of some toxic intermediates as this process occasionally goes astray leading to production of ROS (Droge W. Free radicals in the physiological control of cell function. Physiol. Rev. (2002 (January)) 82(1):47–95).

Under normal conditions, oxygen is reduced to H_2O in the myocardium via two paths. Mitochondrial electron transport reduces 95% of O_2

by tetravalent reduction to H_2O without any free radical intermediates. However, **the remaining 5% of oxygen is reduced via the univalent pathway in which free radicals are produced.** When oxygen accepts an electron the superoxide (O_2^-) anion is formed. Superoxide is in equilibrium with its protonated form, $^{\bullet}HO_2$. **During acidosis, as occurs in ischemia, the protonated form $^{\bullet}HO_2$ is favored and more reactive. $^{\bullet}HO_2$ is capable of oxidative injury to fatty acids and cell membranes, which is prevented within the cell by dismutation (primarily by superoxide dismutase) to H_2O_2.**

H_2O_2 is only directly toxic at high concentrations not thought to occur under normal conditions in cells. Cells have a well-adapted method to continue the reduction of H_2O_2 to H_2O via catalase or the glutathione system. In this manner superoxide, a byproduct of respiration, is safely metabolized to water. **Our tissues have substantial ability to tolerate ROS under normal conditions.** However, the setting of ischemia and then reperfusion alters this carefully orchestrated homeostasis. With ischemia antioxidant defenses are eroded and a new danger exists as elevated H_2O_2 becomes increasingly capable of generating the destructive hydroxyl radical ($^{\bullet}OH$) (Hess M.L., Manson N.H. Molecular oxygen: friend and foe. The role of the oxygen free radical system in the calcium paradox, the oxygen paradox and ischemia/reperfusion injury. J. Mol. Cell. Cardiol. (1984 (November)) 16(11):969–985).

Metal ions, particularly iron, may play a role in generating hydroxyl radicals, hence the rationale for metal chelation during oxidative stress. Hydroxyl radicals are extremely reactive and may cause direct cell membrane damage, lipid peroxidation, and damage to proteins and sulfhydryl bonds. Additional oxygen-related free radicals (nitric oxide, peroxynitrate, etc.) can also be produced and have important biological effects that can be likewise destructive or protective.

Despite the very sensible notion that ROS are produced primarily with the reintroduction of oxygen following ischemia, several investigators began to also observe ROS generation during ischemia. While seeming paradoxical at first, there is much literature to support this observation (Hess M.L., Manson N.H. Molecular oxygen: friend and foe. The role of the oxygen free radical system in the calcium paradox, the oxygen paradox and ischemia/reperfusion injury. J. Mol. Cell. Cardiol. (1984 (November)) 16(11):969–985).

While a 90% reduction in oxygen delivery would render the heart ischemic (i.e. insufficient oxygen delivery to meet metabolic demands), considerable molecular O_2 would still be present. Total anoxia is unlikely to exist even with clinically important ischemia. With ischemia the respiratory cytochromes become redox-reduced allowing them to directly transfer (i.e. "leak") electrons to oxygen. **A redox-reduced cell in the presence of molecular oxygen appears capable of producing large amounts of superoxide anions** (Nohl H., Jordan W. The mitochondrial site of superoxide formation. Biochem. Biophys. Res. Commun. (1986) 138:533–539).

The concept that ischemia causes generation of ROS is of major importance because these ischemia-generated ROS appear to play an important signaling role, may contribute to direct cellular oxidant damage, and are likely to be the same source of ROS that has been reported to trigger preconditioning.

The site of ROS generation along the electron transport chain is suggested by these results with mitchondrial inhibitors and would suggest that oxidant generation must be distal to site I but proximal to site IV. All these **inhibitors (amytal, rotenone, myxothiazol, and cyanide) block mitochondrial electron transport**, but only those acting upstream of the ubisemiquinone site were able to attenuate the oxidant signal, indicating that the response is not a non-specific response to a blockage of mitochondrial phosphorylation or electron transport. Collectively the findings suggest that mitochondrial ubisemiquinone functions as the primary source of ROS generation during ischemia in this model.

An important additional concept is the notion of ROS-induced ROS release described by Zorov et al.. Working with isolated adult rat cardiomyctes, they created "triggering" or "inducing" ROS (likely to be singlet oxygen or superoxide anions) via intracellular photoactivation of tetramethylrhodamine compounds. Thus triggering ROS leads to electron transport inhibition which redox reduces the respiratory electron transport complexes which then pass electrons to molecular oxygen resulting in superoxide formation (Zorov D.B., Filburn C.R., Klotz L.O., Zweier J.L., Sollott S.J. Reactive oxygen species (ROS)-induced ROS release: a new phenomenon accompanying induction of the mitochondrial permeability transition in cardiac myocytes. J. Exp. Med. (2000 (October 2)) 192(7):1001–1014).

Additional work also suggests the very important role in protection that oxidant signaling may also play within the cell. With these studies comes the current concept that oxidants can also be protective—not simply injurious. Much insight into this came out of work in preconditioning. In the late 1980s Murry et al. described ischemic preconditioning wherein a brief non-lethal episode of ischemia conferred both short and longer-term protection to tissues against an ensuing lethal ischemic insult. Preconditioning pathways have been the subject of many studies, and still offers hope that by understanding this natural adaptive protective mechanism new therapies for ischemia will be developed. However, another important lesson is contained (and was almost overlooked) within this seminal description of preconditioning, that **antioxidants abolished the preconditioning protection.** In other words, **treatment with antioxidants interfered with preconditioning protection and made the injury worse.**

Vanden Hoek et al. demonstrates the loss of preconditioning protection with antioxidants clearly in cardiomyocytes (Vanden Hoek T.L., Becker L.B., Shao Z., Li C., Schumacker P.T. Reactive oxygen species released from mitochondria during brief hypoxia induce preconditioning in cardiomyocytes. J. Biol. Chem. (1998) 273(29):18092–18098) (Vanden Hoek T.L., Becker L.B., Shao Z., Li C., Schumacker P.T. Preconditioning in cardiomyocytes protects by attenuating oxidant stress at reperfusion. Circ. Res. (2000) 86:534–540).

Isolated cardiomyocytes demonstrate significant preconditioning protection with exposure to a 10-min ischemic preconditioning trigger just before 1 h of ischemia and reperfusion. In these studies, cell death (measured with PI exclusion dye) in non-preconditioned was cells was 47% versus 14% in preconditioned cells. Oxidant generation was observed to occur in during the brief 10 min of preconditioning ischemia that could be attenuated with **antioxidants (2-mercaptopriopionyl glycine**) and mitochondrial inhibitors (myxothiazol). When 2-mercaptopriopionyl glycine was added only during the preconditioning period in an effort to inhibit this oxidant generation only during the preconditioning stimulus, the protection of preconditioning prior to ischemia was lost. **Under these conditions, increased cell death is the result of adding an antioxidant—that has been protective under other conditions.** This observation has been confirmed in several other laboratories that have reported how preconditioning can be produced by ischemia induced oxidants or by direct infusion of the oxidant peroxynitrate and that **antioxidants (DMSO or MnTBAP)** when added during the preconditioning phase interfere with the induction of preconditioning. Likewise the "triggering" role for ROS in the induction of late precondition has been established in the whole animal. **The addition of 2-mercaptopropionyl glycine was able to abrogate late preconditioning while exogenous oxidants were able to induced late preconditioning in conscious rabbit infarction model, thus confirming the central and protective roles of ROS in protection pathways in animals** (Tang X.L., Takano H., Rizvi A., et al. Oxidant species trigger late preconditioning against myocardial stunning in conscious rabbits. Am. J. Physiol. Heart Circ. Physiol. (2002 (January)) 282(1):H281–H291).

The signaling pathways that connect the triggering ROS to induction of preconditioning protection have been the subject of much investigation. A central role in this protection pathway has been established for the mitochondrial ATP-sensitive K channel with opening of the channel cardioprotective during ischemia and reperfusion. Following mitochondrial K-channel opening, both ROS and NO appear to be generated in isolated cardiomyocytes which leads to the cardioprotected or adapted state. Thus, **we must appreciate the beneficial effects of ROS.** The clinical significance of this physiology and the protective effects of ROS are uncertain but likely to be important in designing human trials.

The continuous generation of ROS within our tissues is now recognized as a central signaling mechanism for a vast range of metabolic pathways and networks.

Living organisms have not only adapted to protect against ROS, they have developed mechanism for the beneficial uses of free radicals (Droge W. Free radicals in the physiological control of cell function. Physiol. Rev. (2002 (January)) 82(1):47–95).

ROS signaling is important in health as well as under conditions of ischemia. It is not surprising that **one must be careful when altering antioxidant defenses.** For example, Bai and Cederbaum created a stable transfection of HepG2 cells that over expressed mitochondrial catalase and **these cells were indeed more resistant to hydrogen peroxide and antimycin-induced oxidant stress (**Bai J., Cederbaum A.I. Mitochondrial catalase and oxidative injury. Biol. Signals Recept. (2001 (May–August)) 10(3–4):189–199**).**

However, these cells also developed increased sensitivity to tumor necrosis factor-induced apoptosis due to a redox change in the mitochondria. This highlights the careful balance and control mechanisms evolved within our tissues in our oxygen rich environment.

ROS are likely to play an important regulatory role in energy production, fertilization, survival kinases activation, ion channel regulation, apoptosis signaling, preconditioning, necrosis, oxygen sensing, inflammatory system, redox homeostasis, and regulation of vascular tone (Droge W. Free radicals in the physiological control of cell function. Physiol. Rev. (2002 (January)) 82(1):47–95).

Some of these important cellular functions are under the control of oxidant inducible genes that code for transcription factors like oxyR or soxR which have been reported to signal entire families of stress response proteins. These induced proteins include antioxidants like Mn-SOD, catalase, glutathione reductase, as well as other protective systems such as NFkB, insulin receptors, glutaredoxin, hydroperoxidase I, alkylhydoperoxide reductase, heat shock proteins, and others; more are currently being described. The emerging picture is that **cells maintain a delicate balance between the protective oxidant signaling versus detrimental effects and this balance seems a critical aspect of aerobic life.**

While the evidence is quite strong that significant reperfusion injury can be demonstrated in cellular systems of simulated ischemia and reperfusion, the evidence for reperfusion injury at the whole organ or whole animal level remain contradictory with both positive and negative studies.

3.0.5.0 Antioxidant failures

Despite many studies and a wide array of antioxidant agents, **there are as yet no clinical indications for the routine use of an antioxidant in the setting of ischemia and reperfusion**.

It is not for lack of trying as multiple clinical trials have attempted to use antioxidants in a wide variety of settings. Flaherty et al. studied the administration of human SOD in the setting of acute myocardial infarction patients who were undergoing percutaneous translumenal coronary angioplasty and **found no benefit** (Flaherty J.T., Pitt B., Gruber J.W., et al. Recombinant human superoxide dismutase (h-SOD) fails to improve recovery of ventricular function in patients undergoing coronary angioplasty for acute myocardial infarction. Circulation (1994 (May)) 89(5):1982–1991).

A large trial of Vitamin E and beta-carotene likewise failed to show any protective cardiovascular effects when smokers with acute myocardial infarction were treated long term with these agents (Rapola J.M., Virtamo J., Ripatti S., et al. Randomised trial of alpha-tocopherol and beta-carotene supplements on incidence of major coronary events in men with previous myocardial infarction. Lancet (1997 (June 14)) 349(9067):1715–1720).

In a 2003 recommendation paper on the need for antioxidants in diet an expert panel came to the non-specific conclusion that we should "eat more fruits and vegetables" (McKevith B., Kelly C., Stanner S., Hughes J., Buttriss J. The Food Standards Agency's antioxidants in food programme—a summary. J. Hum. Nutr. Diet. (2003 (August)) 16(4):257–263).

There have been positive studies using antioxidants, but the data is **not yet compelling**. If oxidants play such an important role in reperfusion injury and cardiovascular disease, why is the clinical data so weak at this time?

Several possible explanations may offer insight into the failure of clinical studies of antioxidants. Some experts have suggested that more than one antioxidant is required for clinical effectiveness. The rationale is that antioxidants exist as a "network" wherein both lipid soluble (like tocopherals) and water soluble (ascorbate, glutathione, dihydrolipoic acid) molecules work in a network for the removal of oxidant stress plus the regeneration of oxidant defenses. Work in the isolated rat heart revealed that both vitamin E and dihydrolipoic acid have synergistic functional effects during ischemia and reperfusion. To date clinical trials have generally not used synergistic combinations of agents despite the theoretical advantages and basic science demonstrations of effectiveness.

Another cited explanation for the failure of clinical antioxidant studies is that by inhibiting the normal production of ROS, another "toxic" condition may be produced if these agents or by-products lead to a reduced oxidative phosphorylation and ATP production (Siems W., Sommerburg O., Schild L., Augustin W., Langhans C.D., Wiswedel I. Beta-carotene cleavage products induce oxidative stress in vitro by impairing mitochondrial respiration. FASEB J. (2002 (August)) 16(10):1289–1291).

For example, **the beta-carotene cleavage products have been shown to strongly inhibit state 3 respiration in isolated liver mitochondria**. Persistent decreased ATP production has been reported and may be an important consideration following ischemia.

Therapies **and antioxidants** must become more specific for site of action, not have deleterious effects on other signaling pathways, be targeted to a specific ROS or cellular compartment, and the time sensitive challenge of delivering the correct therapy at precisely the correct time must be surmounted for us to predict reliable clinical success.

3.0.6.0 British Nutrition Foundation says eat more fruits and vegetables (2001)

In 2001, the British Nutrition Foundation (BNF) was contracted to evaluate projects from the *Antioxidants in Food* research programme, now funded by the Food Standards Agency and previously the Ministry of Agriculture, Fisheries and Food. The programme aimed at testing the 'antioxidant hypothesis'.

Methods The evaluation was conducted with support and guidance from a Steering Group of experts. The final report sets out BNF's recommendations for the future of the *Antioxidants in Food* research programme.

Results It was recommended that future research should consider a wider scope of potential mechanisms of action of substances within foods; more emphasis should be placed on studying bioavailability of a range of plant derived substances, and the impact of genotype, age and disease should be investigated.

Conclusions The research programme has been important as it has focused attention on disease prevention rather than on treatment, and has helped progress identification of biomarkers. From human observational and intervention studies there is evidence of an association between a diet rich in plant foods (particularly fruit and vegetables) and health benefits. However, as **there is no evidence that any particular nutrient or class of bioactive substances makes a special contribution, currently the most prudent public health advice is to increase vegetable and fruit consumption** (The Food Standards Agency's antioxidants in food programme – a summary. B. McKevith, C. Kelly, S. Stanner, J. Hughes and J. Buttriss. Journal of Human Nutrition and Dietetics.Volume 16 Issue 4, Pages 257 – 263).

3.0.7.0 Fruits, veggies slash breast cancer risk: U.S. study

12/15/08 **Certain breast cancer survivors who load up on fruits and vegetables, eating far more than current U.S. guidelines, can slash their risk the tumors will come back by nearly a third**, according to a U.S. study released on 12/15/08. **The finding only held for women who did not have hot flashes after their cancer therapy**, the researchers said -- a finding that suggests fruits and vegetables act on estrogen.

Their analysis suggests an explanation for why some studies have shown that eating more fruits and vegetables lowers the risk that breast cancer will come back, **while others do not.** It may depend on the individual patient, they report in the **Journal of Clinical Oncology.**

"Women with early stage breast cancer who have hot flashes have better survival and lower recurrence rates than women who don't," said Ellen Gold of the University of California Davis, who helped lead the study. Several studies have shown this. And this study showed that **women who had hot flashes after treatment for breast cancer had lower estrogen levels than women who did not.**

As estrogen drives the most common type of breast cancer, this suggests that eating extra servings of fruits and vegetables -- above and beyond the five servings a day recommended by the U.S. government -- may lower harmful estrogen levels in cancer survivors, the researchers said.

"**It appears that a dietary pattern high in fruits, vegetables and fiber, which has been shown to reduce circulating estrogen levels**, may only be important among women with circulating estrogen levels above a certain threshold," said John Pierce of the University of California San Diego.

The researchers took a second look at data from **3,000 breast cancer patients** in a study aimed at seeing whether a diet low in fat and high in fruits and vegetables might keep their cancer from coming back. Such a diet has been shown to lower overall risk of ever getting breast cancer in the first place.

The women were on average 53, and half were told to double their fruit and vegetable intake to 10 servings a day, eat more fiber and lower fat intake more than government recommendations. "We compared the dietary intervention group to a group that received '5-a-day' dietary guidelines," the researchers wrote.

About 30 percent of the original 3,000 breast cancer survivors said they did not have hot flashes -- a common side-effect of breast cancer treatment.

The researchers looked at the data on these women specifically and found that only 16 percent of those who doubled up on fruits and vegetables had their tumors come back after seven years, compared to 23 percent of those merely given advice on food guidelines.

Women who had been through menopause lowered their risk by 47 percent if they loaded up on salads, fruit and other plant food. **I believe that this is due to the fact that estrogen is an antioxidant, which creates an EMOD insufficiency state.**

3.0.8.0 Hypertension

3.0.8.1 Antioxidants fail to stop hypertension

Hypertension is associated with increased vascular oxidative stress; however, there is still **a debate whether oxidative stress is a cause or a result of hypertension.** Animal studies have generally supported the hypothesis that increased blood pressure is associated with increased oxidative stress; however, **human studies have been inconsistent**.

Oxidative stress promotes vascular smooth muscle cell proliferation and hypertrophy and collagen deposition, leading to thickening of the vascular media and narrowing of the vascular lumen. In addition, increased oxidative stress may damage the endothelium and impair endothelium-dependent vascular relaxation and increases vascular contractile activity. All these effects on the vasculature may explain how increased oxidative stress can cause hypertension. Treatment with antioxidants has been suggested to lower oxidative stress and therefore blood pressure. However, to date, **clinical studies investigating antioxidant supplements have failed to show any consistent benefit**.

It is noteworthy that **lowering blood pressure with antihypertensive medications is associated with reduced oxidative stress.** Therefore, **it seems that oxygen stress is not the cause, but rather a consequence, of hypertension** (Does Increased Oxidative Stress Cause Hypertension?

Ehud Grossman. Diabetes Care 31:S185-S189, 2008).

To identify oxidative stress as a cause of hypertension, several criteria should be fulfilled: *1*) Oxidative stress should be associated with hypertension. *2*) The mechanism by which oxidative stress causes hypertension should be known. *3*) Oxidative stress should cause hypertension in experimental animals. *4*) Antioxidation should lower blood pressure. **There is no evidence to support the concept that hypertension is caused by oxidative stress**.

Unlike the findings in animal models, **the association between oxidative stress and hypertension in humans is less consistent**, and results vary depending on the marker of oxidative damage being investigated (Ward NC, Croft KD: Hypertension and oxidative stress. *Clin Exp Pharmacol Physiol* 33:872–876, 2006).

Reductions in superoxide dismutase and glutathione peroxidase activity have been observed in newly diagnosed untreated hypertensive subjects compared with control subjects, with superoxide dismutase activity being inversely correlated with blood pressure within the hypertensive group, but not control subjects (Pedro-Botet J, Covas MI, Martin S, Rubies-Prat J: Decreased endogenous antioxidant enzymatic status in essential hypertension. *J Hum Hypertens* 14:343–345, 2000). **I believe that this is due to the increased peroxide production by SOD. Remember that peroxide is a vasodilator.**

Higher production of hydrogen peroxide has also been observed in treated and untreated hypertensive subjects compared with

normotensive subjects, with a significant correlation between hydrogen peroxide levels and systolic blood pressure (Lacy F, Kailasam MT, O'Connor DT, Schmid-Schonbein GW, Parmer RJ: Plasma hydrogen peroxide production in human essential hypertension: role of heredity, gender, and ethnicity. *Hypertension* 36:878–884, 2000).

Studies examining more specific markers of oxidative damage have not been as conclusive. **Concentrations of F2-isoprostane measured in spot urine were found to be the same in subjects with mild-to-moderate untreated hypertension and normotensive control subjects** (Cracowski JL, Baguet JP, Ormezzano O, Bessard J, Stanke-Labesque F, Bessard G, Mallion J: Lipid peroxidation is not increased in patients with untreated mild-to-moderate hypertension. *Hypertension* 41:286–288, 2003).

Ward et al.have recently demonstrated **no difference in either plasma or 24-h urinary F2-isoprostanes in treated or untreated hypertensive subjects compared with normotensive control subjects** (Ward NC, Hodgson JM, Puddey IB, Mori TA, Beilin LJ, Croft KD: Oxidative stress in human hypertension: association with antihypertensive treatment, gender, nutrition, and lifestyle. *Free Radic Biol Med* 36:226–232, 2004).

Tse et al.did not find differences in levels of some antioxidants between hypertensive patients and normal control subjects (Tse WY, Maxwell SR, Thomason H, Blann A, Thorpe GH, Waite M, Holder R: Antioxidant status in controlled and uncontrolled hypertension and its relationship to endothelial damage. *J Hum Hypertens* 8:843–849, 1994).

Different macronutrients induce a distinct pattern of increase in ROS generation (Aljada A, Mohanty P, Ghanim H, Abdo T, Tripathy D, Chaudhuri A, Dandona P: Increase in intranuclear nuclear factor kappaB and decrease in inhibitor kappaB in mononuclear cells after a mixed meal: evidence for a proinflammatory effect. *Am J Clin Nutr* 79:682–690, 2004).

Glucose induces a peak in ROS generation by both mononuclear cells and polymorphonuclear leukocytes at 2 h, whereas lipid produces a peak at 1 h. **The peak increase in ROS generation is the greatest with glucose and the least with protein**. Lipid intake causes a prolonged increase in lipid peroxidation. In obese subjects, caloric restriction and weight loss, over a short period of 4 weeks, lead to a decrease in ROS generation by leukocytes and oxidative damage to lipids, proteins, and amino acids (Dandona P, Mohanty P, Ghanim H, Aljada A, Browne R, Hamouda W, Prabhala A, Afzal A, Garg R: The suppressive effect of dietary restriction and weight loss in the obese on the generation of reactive oxygen species by leukocytes, lipid peroxidation, and protein carbonylation. *J Clin Endocrinol Metab* 86:355–362, 2001).

Moreover, **in normal subjects, a 48-h fast reduced ROS generation, total oxidative load, and oxidative damage to amino acids** (Dandona P, Mohanty P, Hamouda W, Ghanim H, Aljada A, Garg R, Kumar V: Inhibitory effect of a two day fast on reactive oxygen species (ROS) generation by leucocytes and plasma ortho-tyrosine and meta-tyrosine concentrations. *J Clin Endocrinol Metab* 86:2899–2902, 2001).

Indeed several studies showed that oxidative stress plays a role in the pathogenesis of hypertension in various animal models (Touyz RM: Reactive oxygen species, vascular oxidative stress, and redox signaling in hypertension: what is the clinical significance? *Hypertension* 44:248–252, 2004).

However, others failed to show that oxidative stress induces hypertension. Zhang et al. investigated the involvement of reactive oxygen species on changes in the hemodynamics of conscious normotensive rats. They studied blood pressure responses and cardiovascular mitogen-activated protein kinase (MAPK) activities induced by acutely administered Ang II, or phenylephrine, an α-adrenoceptor agonist, with or without treatment with the antioxidant tempol. They found that Ang II rapidly increased mean arterial blood pressure and phosphorylated MAPKs (ERK1/2, JNK, p38) and thiobarbital reactive substances in the aorta and cardiac left ventricle. Tempol suppressed the augmented phosphorylation of cardiovascular MAPKs and increased thiobarbital reactive substance levels induced by Ang II, but had no effect on arterial pressure elevation. Administration of phenylephrine also showed tempol-sensitive cardiovascular MAPK activation and tempol-insensitive blood pressure elevation. These data indicate that **Ang II or phenylephrine provoked an increase in oxidative stress in the cardiovascular tissues and that oxidative stress might not have a major contribution to the hypertensive responses elicited by the vasoconstrictors** (Zhang GX, Kimura S, Nishiyama A, Shokoji T, Rahman M, Abe Y: ROS during the acute phase of Ang II hypertension participates in cardiovascular MAPK activation but not vasoconstriction. *Hypertension* 43:117–124, 2004).

Similarly, Elmarakby et al. showed in Sprague-Dawley rats fed a high-salt diet that two antioxidants, tempol and apocynin, prevented an endothelin-1–mediated increase in plasma 8-isoprostane, an indicator of oxidative stress, and aortic superoxide production, but failed to attenuate blood pressure rise. These findings also **suggest that oxidative stress might not have a major contribution to**

the hypertensive responses elicited by endothelin (Elmarakby AA, Loomis ED, Pollock JS, Pollock DM: NADPH oxidase inhibition attenuates oxidative stress but not hypertension produced by chronic ET-1. *Hypertension* 45:283–287, 2005).

Some studies in animal models of hypertension, such as Ang II–induced hypertension and salt-sensitive hypertension, and in spontaneously hypertensive rats showed that **antioxidation may reduce blood pressure** (Laursen JB, Rajagopalan S, Galis Z, Tarpey M, Freeman BA, Harrison DG: Role of superoxide in angiotensin II-induced but not catecholamine-induced hypertension. *Circulation* 95:588–593, 1997) (Schnackenberg CG, Welch WJ, Wilcox CS: Normalization of blood pressure and renal vascular resistance in SHR with a membrane-permeable superoxide dismutase mimetic: role of nitric oxide. *Hypertension* 32:59–64, 1998) (Akpaffiong MJ, Taylor AA: Antihypertensive and vasodilator actions of antioxidants in spontaneously hypertensive rats. *Am J Hypertens* 11:1450–1460, 1998) (Virdis A, Neves MF, Amiri F, Touyz RM, Schiffrin EL: Role of NAD(P)H oxidase on vascular alterations in angiotensin II-infused mice. *J Hypertens* 22:535–542, 2004) (Fujii S, Zhang L, Igarashi J, Kosaka H: L-arginine reverses p47phox and gp91phox expression induced by high salt in Dahl rats. *Hypertension* 42:1014–1020, 2003).

However, **others failed to show that antioxidation reduces blood pressure** (Elmarakby AA, Loomis ED, Pollock JS, Pollock DM: NADPH oxidase inhibition attenuates oxidative stress but not hypertension produced by chronic ET-1. *Hypertension* 45:283–287, 2005) (Zhang GX, Kimura S, Nishiyama A, Shokoji T, Rahman M, Abe Y: ROS during the acute phase of Ang II hypertension participates in cardiovascular MAPK activation but not vasoconstriction. *Hypertension* 43:117–124, 2004).

The data from **clinical studies are less convincing.** A number of trials have investigated the use of antioxidant supplements; however, most of the studies did not focus on blood pressure as a primary end point. Galley et al. showed in a small group of normotensive and hypertensive subjects (n = 38) that short-term oral high-dose combination antioxidant therapy reduces blood pressure, possibly via increased availability of nitric oxide (Galley HF, Thornton J, Howdle PD, Walker BE, Webster NR: Combination oral antioxidant supplementation reduces blood pressure. *Clin Sci (Lond)* 92:361–365, 1997).

Several studies showed the efficacy of vitamin C in reducing blood pressure (Duffy SJ, Gokce N, Holbrook M, Huang A, Frei B, Keaney JF, Vita JA: Treatment of hypertension with ascorbic acid. *Lancet* 354:2048–2049, 1999) (Fotherby MD, Williams JC, Forster LA, Craner P, Ferns GA: Effect of vitamin C on ambulatory blood pressure and plasma lipids in older persons. *J Hypertens*

18:411–415, 2000) (Hajjar IM, George V, Sasse EA, Kochar MS: A randomized, double-blind, controlled trial of vitamin C in the management of hypertension and lipids. *Am J Ther* 9:289–293, 2002).

Unlike these studies, **many other studies failed to show blood pressure reduction with antioxidant supplementation.** One of the largest studies, undertaken by **the Heart Protection Collaborative Group, observed no improvement in blood pressure after treatment with an ascorbic acid, synthetic vitamin E, and β-carotene combination versus placebo after 5 years in subjects thought to be at high risk of cardiovascular disease** (Heart Protection Study Collaborative Group: MRC/BHF Heart Protection Study of antioxidant vitamin supplementation in 20,536 high-risk individuals: a randomised placebo-controlled trial. *Lancet* 360:23–33, 2002).

Kim et al. observed no reduction in blood pressure with long-term moderate doses (500 mg/day) of vitamin C supplementation (Kim MK, Sasaki S, Sasazuki S, Okubo S, Hayashi M, Tsugane S: Lack of long-term effect of vitamin C supplementation on blood pressure. *Hypertension* 40:797–803, 2002).

3.0.9.0 Antioxidants fail to reduce hypertension

Ward et al. recently showed **a significant increase in both ambulatory systolic and diastolic blood pressure in treated hypertensive subjects after 6 weeks of combination vitamin C and grape-seed polyphenols versus placebo or either treatment alone** (Ward NC, Hodgson JM, Croft KD, Burke V, Beilin LJ, Puddey IB: The combination of vitamin C and grape-seed polyphenols increases blood pressure: a randomized, double-blind, placebo-controlled trial. *J Hypertens* 23:427–434, 2005).

Palumbo et al. failed to show a blood pressure–lowering effect with vitamin E. They studied the effect of vitamin E supplementation (300 mg/day) on clinic and 24-h ambulatory blood pressure in 142 treated hypertensive patients. After 12 weeks, clinic blood pressure decreased whether or not patients were randomized to vitamin E. Ambulatory blood pressure showed no change in systolic blood pressure and only a small decrease in diastolic blood pressure (Palumbo G, Avanzini F, Alli C, Roncaglioni MC, Ronchi E, Cristofari M, Capra A, Rossi S, Nosotti L, Costantini C, Calvalera C: Effects of vitamin E on clinic and ambulatory blood pressure in treated hypertensive patients: Collaborative Group of the Primary Prevention Project (PPP)–Hypertension study. *Am J Hypertens* 13:564–567, 2000).

In another large study, **Rumbold et al. failed to show blood pressure reduction with antioxidant supplementation in nulliparous women between 14 and 22 weeks of gestation.** In this multicenter randomized trial, nulliparous women were assigned to daily supplementation with 1,000 mg vitamin C and 400 IU vitamin E or placebo until delivery. Of the 1,877 women enrolled in the study, 935 were randomly assigned to the vitamin group and 942 to the placebo group. There were no significant differences between the vitamin and placebo groups in the risk of preeclampsia, death, or serious outcomes in the infant or having an infant with a birth weight below the 10th percentile for gestational age. **Unexpectedly, women in the vitamin group had an increased risk of being admitted antenatally for hypertension and being prescribed antihypertensive drugs. This large study showed that supplementation with vitamins C and E during pregnancy does not reduce blood pressure** (Rumbold AR, Crowther CA, Haslam RR, Dekker GA, Robinson JS: Vitamins C and E and the risks of preeclampsia and perinatal complications. *N Engl J Med* 354:1796–1806, 2006).

In the large **Heart Outcomes Prevention Evaluation (HOPE) study, 9,541** subjects ≥55 years of age who were at high risk for cardiovascular events were randomly assigned to receive either 400 IU vitamin E daily from natural sources or matching placebo for a mean of 4.5 years. **There were no significant differences in the primary end points or in the number of deaths from cardiovascular causes, myocardial infarction, or stroke between the treatment groups.** Data on blood pressure levels were not published, which suggests that vitamin E in this study did not reduce blood pressure (Yusuf S, Dagenais G, Pogue J, Bosch J, Sleight P: Vitamin E supplementation and cardiovascular events in high-risk patients: the Heart Outcomes Prevention Evaluation Study Investigators. *N Engl J Med* 342:154–160, 2000).

Thus, **the evidence to support using antioxidants as a blood pressure–lowering agent is limited.** It is noteworthy that antihypertensive drug therapy, in addition to the blood pressure–lowering properties, also has beneficial effects on both oxidative stress and endothelial function. **Treatment with a β-blocker or Ang receptor blockers has been shown to reduce both blood pressure and markers of oxidative damage** (Saez GT, Tormos C, Giner V, Chaves J, Lozano JV, Iradi A, Redon J: Factors related to the impact of antihypertensive treatment in antioxidant activities and oxidative stress by-products in human hypertension. *Am J Hypertens* 17:809–816, 2004).

Similarly, **other studies have reported beneficial effects on blood pressure, oxidative stress, and endothelial function after treatment with**

ACE inhibitors (Ghiadoni L, Magagna A, Versari D, Kardasz I, Huang Y, Taddei S, Salvetti A: Different effect of antihypertensive drugs on conduit artery endothelial function. *Hypertension* 41:1281–1286, 2003) **or calcium antagonists** (Taddei S, Virdis A, Ghiadoni L, Versari D, Salvetti G, Magagna A, Salvetti A: Calcium antagonist treatment by lercanidipine prevents hyperpolarization in essential hypertension. *Hypertension* 41:950–955, 2003).

Because many blood pressures–lowering agents reduce oxidative stress, it seems logical that **lowering blood pressure per se rather than the agents used reduces oxidative stress.**

The potential value of antioxidant supplements to reduce blood pressure via reductions in oxidative stress is limited. In some cases, their use may even be detrimental. On the other hand, lowering blood pressure is associated with reduced oxidative stress. Therefore, it seems that **oxygen stress is not the cause, but rather a consequence, of hypertension.** (Does Increased Oxidative Stress Cause Hypertension? Ehud Grossman. Diabetes Care 31:S185-S189, 2008).

3.1.0.0 EMODs in veins vs arteries

Reactive oxygen species (ROS) are by-products of oxygen metabolism, normally present in low levels inside cells, where they participate in signaling processes. The delicate balance in the continuous cycle of ROS generation and inactivation is maintained by enzymatic and nonenzymatic endogenous systems. Overwhelming production of ROS (by such sources as the mitochondrial electron transport chain, NADPH oxidase, xanthine oxidase, or uncoupled nitric oxide synthase), when inadequately counteracted by destruction through antioxidant systems (such as superoxide dismutase or catalase), leads to a prooxidant state also known as oxidative stress. Increased levels of ROS and markers of oxidative stress have been consistently found in such cardiovascular diseases as atherosclerosis or hypertension, although controversy still exists over the pathophysiological role of oxidative stress in these conditions. ROS can modulate vascular function either by direct oxidative damage or by activating cellular signaling pathways that lead to abnormal contractile, inflammatory, proliferative, or remodeling properties of the blood vessel. Most current research focuses on these processes in arteries, leaving veins, "the other side" of vascular biology, in obscurity. Veins are different structurally and functionally from arteries. Equipped with a smaller smooth muscle layer compared to arteries, but being able to accommodate 70% of the circulating blood volume, veins can modulate cardiovascular homeostasis and contribute significantly to hypertension pathogenesis. Although the reports on the quantitative differences in ROS production in veins compared to arteries had conflicting results, **there is a clear qualitative difference in ROS metabolism and utilization between the two vessel types.** This review will compare and contrast the current knowledge of ROS metabolism in arteries *versus* veins in both physiological and pathophysiological conditions. Our understanding of the mechanisms underlying vascular diseases would greatly benefit from a more thorough exploration of the role of veins and venous oxidative stress (A Comparison of Arteries and Veins in Oxidative Stress: Producers, Destroyers, Function, and Disease. Theodora Szasz, Keshari Thakali, Gregory D. Fink and Stephanie W. Watts. *Experimental Biology and Medicine* 232:27-37 (2007).

3.1.1.0 Producers and Destroyers of Reactive Oxygen Species

ROS Producers:
Mitochondrial respiratory chain
Superoxide dismutase family **ROS destroyers**

NOX and DUOX families
Catalase **ROS destroyers**

Xanthine Oxidase
Glutathione system **ROS destroyers**

Superoxide dismutase family
Selenoproteins (glutathione peroxidase, thioredoxin reductase, etc.) **ROS destroyers**

Uncoupled nitric oxide synthase
Monamine oxidase
Peroxiredoxins **ROS destroyers**

Lipoxygenase
Antioxidant ROS scavengers (A, C, E vitamins, ceruloplasmin, ubiquinone, uric acid, bilirubin, etc.) **ROS destroyers**

Cyclooxygenase
Cytochrome P450
Nitric oxide **ROS destroyers**

Haber-Weiss and Fenton reactions
Uncoupling proteins (?)**ROS destroyers**

Environment (ionizing radiation, smoke, etc.)
Nitric oxide (reactive nitrogen species)

3.1.2.0 Mito-chondrial Respiratory Chain.

The mitochondrial respiratory chain is the main energy source for the cell. Situated in the inner mitochondrial membrane, it catalyzes electron transfer using more than 80 peptides organized in four complexes. The transfer of electrons, shuttled by coenzyme Q and cytochrome C, usually leads to the formation of ATP by the fifth complex. However, a certain amount (1–2% *in vitro*) of electrons leak, principally from complex III but also from complex I, generating superoxide.

The rate of mitochondrial ROS production, the levels of mitochondrial DNA oxidative damage, and the degree of membrane fatty acid unsaturation (potentially a target of lipid peroxidation by ROS) are all inversely linked to maximum longevity in animals (Barja G. Free radicals and aging. Trends Neurosci27(10):595–600, 2004).

These facts are among the evidence supporting the free radical theory of aging. Because **superoxide production is directly dependent on the proton motive force**, a feedback mechanism has been proposed for the uncoupling proteins (UCP 1, 2, and 3). Activated by superoxide and lipid peroxidation, these proteins seem to act by slightly reducing the proton motive force and hence energy production as a trade-off for a decreased ROS production from the mitochondrial complexes I and III.

The Nox family of NADPH oxidases is another major source of ROS. **Xanthine oxidoreductase (XOR) is an enzyme that catalyzes the last steps of purine metabolism: the transformation of hypoxanthine and xanthine to uric acid, with superoxide/H_2O_2 generated as by-products.**

I believe that this is reminiscent of the formation of peroxide with each molecule of ascorbic acid in animals possessing gulonolactate, i.e., for each molecule of antioxidant synthesized there is a prooxidant molecule created simultaneously. The body is producing redox pairs!

A central role in the regulation of ROS levels is attributed to superoxide dismutases (SODs), a family of enzymes responsible for superoxide breakdown, with the consecutive production of **hydrogen peroxide**.

There is a great body of evidence supporting the beneficial role of SOD. Knock-out experiments showed **neonatal lethality of mice lacking MnSOD and reduced lifespan and multiple function abnormalities in mice lacking CuZnSOD** (Huang TT, Yasunami M, Carlson EJ, Gillespie AM, Reaume AG, Hoffman EK, Chan PH, Scott RW, Epstein CJ. Superoxide-mediated cytotoxicity in superoxide dismutase-deficient fetal fibroblasts. Arch Biochem Biophys344(2):424–432, 1997) (Macmillan-Crow LA, Cruthirds DL. Invited review: manganese superoxide dismutase in disease. Free Radic Res34(4):325–336, 2001) (Faraci FM, Didion SP. Vascular protection: superoxide dismutase isoforms in the vessel wall. Arterioscler Thromb Vasc Biol24(8): 1367–1373, 2004) (Johnson F, Giulivi C. Superoxide dismutases and their impact upon human health. Mol Aspects Med26(4–5):340–352, 2005).

Furthermore, **overexpression studies of SODs strongly suggest a protective role of these enzymes in many diseases, as well as in aging** (Huang TT, Yasunami M, Carlson EJ, Gillespie AM, Reaume AG, Hoffman EK, Chan PH, Scott RW, Epstein CJ. Superoxide-mediated cytotoxicity in superoxide dismutase-deficient fetal fibroblasts. Arch Biochem Biophys344(2):424–432, 1997) (Macmillan-Crow LA, Cruthirds DL. Invited review: manganese superoxide dismutase in disease. Free Radic Res34(4):325–336, 2001) (Faraci FM, Didion SP. Vascular protection: superoxide dismutase isoforms in the vessel wall. Arterioscler Thromb Vasc Biol24(8): 1367–1373, 2004) (Johnson F, Giulivi C. Superoxide dismutases and their impact upon human health. Mol Aspects Med26(4–5):340–352, 2005).

Additionally, **mutations in the *SOD1* gene leading to the production of a changed, toxic variant of CuZnSOD are linked to 20%–25% of cases of familial amyotrophic lateral sclerosis (Lou Gehrig's disease),** a fatal neurologic condition (Potter SZ, Valentine JS. The perplexing role of copper-zinc super-oxide dismutase in amyotrophic lateral sclerosis (Lou Gehrig's disease). J Biol Inorg Chem8(4):373–380, 2003).

In addition to providing protection from superoxide, **SOD activity also results in production of hydrogen peroxide,** a diffusible molecule far more stable than the superoxide anion. **Hydrogen peroxide can act both by affecting gene expression as a signaling molecule** and by continuing the ROS cascade with the formation of the hydroxyl radical. The latter, generated through a reaction with transition metals, such as Fe^{2+} *via* the Fenton/Haber-Weiss chemistry, is a highly reactive radical that to our knowledge cannot be destroyed enzymatically. The only protection from its dangerous oxidative potential is therefore left to antioxidant scavengers and metal chelators.

Because of their widespread therapeutic use as antioxidants, endogenous ROS scavengers, such as vitamin C and E, should also be noted. However, when considering the antioxidant properties of such compounds, it should be appreciated that **they are not enzymes, and, thus, a new molecule is needed for each superoxide anion that is scavenged. These vitamins are therefore poor ROS scavengers**, and numerous other factors (such as the insufficient doses or their unknown intracellular concentration and activity) have been overlooked in some antioxidant clinical studies.

3.1.3.0 Arteries and Veins: A Comparison of Structure and Function

Arteries and veins, two separate components of the vascular system, are different structurally and functionally. Although arteries carry oxygenated blood from the heart to the peripheral tissues at a high pressure, therefore requiring a more elastic and muscular structure, veins carry blood from the tissues back to the heart at a low pressure, providing capacitance, therefore requiring more distensible, less muscular walls.

Both artery and vein are composed of similar layers: the innermost layer or the tunica intima containing endothelial cells; the tunica media, which is largely composed of smooth muscle, elastin, and collagen; and the outermost tunica adventitia containing mainly fibroblasts, collagen, and elastin. Small blood vessels called *vasa vasorum* integrate into the adventitia of larger vessels, providing nutrients to the vascular wall itself.

Several characteristics, in addition to a different distribution and relative abundance of these layers, distinguish arteries from veins. The delineation of the three layers is more obvious in an artery compared to a vein. This is particularly illustrated when viewing the thoracic vena cava *versus* the thoracic aorta from the same rat. The media of an artery, flanked by two elastic laminas, is typically thicker than that of a vein, whereas the elastic component of a vein is smaller compared to that of an artery. The greater relative contribution of the smooth muscle layer to the vascular wall thickness in arteries compared to veins can be appreciated. These differences are confirmed by immunohistochemical staining for α-actin, a smooth muscle marker. Larger veins possess venous valves on the luminal side of the wall, which help prevent backflow of blood. **The cardiovascular system should not be envisioned as being abruptly split into the two components but rather as a gradual transition from the heart to the large elastic arteries, then smaller muscular arteries/arterioles to, finally, the capillary section, having just one endothelial layer, and then back from the peripheral tissues, through less muscular venules, to large capacitance veins possessing all the components of the vessel wall and back to the heart.**

Due to these structural differences, there are also inherent differences in the contractility and synthetic properties of arteries and veins that can impact overall cardiovascular function. One can easily envision the mechanism by which arteries can affect blood pressure: by changing their tone through vasoconstriction or their structure through remodeling, they can increase total peripheral resistance, a major determinant of blood pressure. It is more difficult to picture a role for veins in the pathogenesis of hypertension. However, **by accommodating 70% of circulated blood, veins can influence blood volume distribution** and trigger adaptive remodeling from the arterial side that can drive a sustained increase in blood pressure.

The magnitude of the contractile force developed by a vein in response to receptor-dependent and -independent agonists is less compared with that developed by an artery. The time needed to reach half this maximal contraction, a measure of response speed, is shorter for a vein than for an artery. The capacity to relax in response to agonists that induce the production of endothelium-derived relaxant factors is decreased in veins compared to arteries. Similarly, specific differences exist in the contractile response of arteries and veins to a series of receptor-dependent agonists, the best studied of them being endothelin-1, a potent, though not selective, venoconstrictor.

Different properties of arterial and venous grafts used in bypass surgery, leading to different outcomes, have stimulated research on comparing these vessel types and the factors that influence their long-term patency. Venous smooth muscle cells appear to have a higher growth rate compared with their arterial counterparts, both in basal conditions and in response to various mitogenic stimuli. Endothelium function is also different in veins compared to arteries. Venous endothelium produces less prostacyclin and NO than arterial endothelium, and its overall response to atherogenic stimuli is different.

Because larger blood vessels of both kinds have different structural and functional properties compared with smaller ones, intuitively it makes sense that their potential contribution to vascular pathogenesis and dependence on ROS is also different.

3.1.4.0 Vascular EMOD production: veins have more EMODs

Few studies have compared basal ROS production in arteries and veins, and their **conclusions were contradictory. Basal superoxide production, measured through nitroblue tetrazolium reduction to formazan, was increased in porcine venous grafts compared to arterial grafts** (Shi Y, Patel S, Davenpeck KL, Niculescu R, Rodriguez E, Magno MG, Ormont ML, Mannion JD, Zalewski A. Oxidative stress and lipid retention in vascular grafts: comparison between venous and arterial conduits. Circulation 103(19):2408–2413, 2001). **I had predicted this. I believe that the increased peroxide levels in veins from SOD contributes to less atherosclerosis in veins than in arteries.**

Using lucigenin-enhanced chemiluminescence, **no difference in basal superoxide production was found in rings from human internal mammary artery (IMA) compared to human saphenous vein (HSV)** (Guzik TJ, Sadowski J, Kapelak B, Jopek A, Rudzinski P, Pillai R, Korbut R, Channon KM. Systemic regulation of vascular NAD(P)H oxidase activity and nox isoform expression in human arteries and veins. Arterioscler Thromb Vasc Biol 24(9):1614–1620, 2004).

Basal hydrogen peroxide production was higher in rat vena cava compared to aorta (Thakali K, Demel SL, Fink GD, Watts SW. Endothelin-1–induced contraction in veins is independent of hydrogen peroxide. Am J Physiol Heart Circ Physiol 289(3):H1115–H1122, 2005).

Unpublished data from our laboratory show increased superoxide production in rat veins compared to corresponding arteries as measured by lucigenin-enhanced chemiluminescence (inferior vena cava [VC] compared to thoracic aorta [Ao]:VC = 210 ± 42 % Ao; and mesenteric vein [MV] compared to mesenteric artery [MA]: MV = 267 ± 48 % MA). The increase in superoxide release, following the addition of the NOS inhibitor, L-NMMA, was greater in human arteries (IMA) compared to veins (HSV). This suggests a greater basal NO production in arteries that contributes to the quenching of superoxide in comparison to veins. Accordingly, basal peroxynitrite formation was higher in IMA compared to HSV.

Hydrogen peroxide modulates vascular tone, acting as a contraction-inducing agent in some vascular beds and as a relaxant in others (Thakali K, Davenport L, Fink GD, Watts SW. Pleiotropic effects of hydrogen peroxide in arteries and veins from normotensive and hypertensive rats. Hypertension 47(3):482–487, 2006) (Gao YJ, Lee RM. Hydrogen peroxide is an endothelium-dependent contracting factor in rat renal artery. Br J Pharmacol 146(8): 1061–1068, 2005).

There is a greater contraction to H_2O_2 in veins compared to arteries, possibly reflecting a difference in K^+ channel activity and Ca^{2+} influx (Thakali K, Davenport L, Fink GD, Watts SW. Pleiotropic effects of hydrogen peroxide in arteries and veins from normotensive and hypertensive rats. Hypertension47(3):482–487, 2006).

3.1.5.0 NADPH Oxidases: "the vascular oxidase"

NADPH oxidases are perhaps the best studied enzymes involved in ROS production in the blood vessels. Several features of Nox enzymes expressed in blood vessels, that distinguish them from the generic phagocyte NADPH oxidase, have made researchers in the field collectively term **them "the vascular oxidase." Compared with superoxide production from the phagocyte NADPH oxidase, vascular oxidase basal superoxide production is significantly lower (less than 1%).** Although phagocyte NADPH oxidase activity is primarily inducible, vascular oxidase has a constitutive activity that can be further increased by such agonists as angiotensin II. The cellular site of superoxide production by vascular oxidase also appears to be different: vascular oxidase–produced superoxide has been repeatedly detected intracellularly. Finally, **the physiological role of superoxide production by the blood vessel cells is distinct: instead of cytotoxic superoxide production as a defense mechanism against pathogens, ROS released by the vascular oxidase participate in cell signaling, consistent with their comparative low tissue levels.**

In atherosclerosis, increased arterial intracellular super-oxide production is observed.

3.1.6.0 Xanthine Oxidase

Xanthine oxidase expression in blood vessels has been difficult to prove.

Normal endothelial function, crucial in maintaining cardiovascular homeostasis, depends on normal NOS functioning, among other things.

3.1.7.0 SODs

The blood vessel wall of both arteries and veins expresses all three SODs. The cytosolic CuZnSOD has ubiquitous and high expression throughout the vascular layers. Mitochondrial MnSOD is relatively less expressed compared with CuZnSOD and EC-SOD but is also ubiquitous. **Extracellular SOD, produced largely by VSMC, is localized between arterial intima and media** and is thought to contribute substantially to the total SOD activity in the vasculature. No difference has been found between human arteries (IMA) and veins (HSV) in terms of their CuZnSOD and MnSOD protein expression and activity.

ROS involvement in cellular signaling has been reviewed extensively elsewhere (Finkel T, Holbrook NJ. Oxidants, oxidative stress and the biology of ageing. Nature 408(6809):239–247, 2000).

In summary, a series of major signaling pathways, such as MAPK, PI3K/Akt, NF-κB, ERK, JNK, p53, and the heat shock response, can potentially be activated in response to ROS or oxidative stress.

The presence of increased markers of oxidative stress (peroxidized lipids, oxidized proteins, increased GSSG, 8-oxoguanine, DNA breaks, etc.) has been identified in many pathophysiological situations. However, in most cases, **establishing whether oxidative stress plays a causal role or is a mere reflection of the effects of the disease process itself on cellular function has proved to be a difficult task.**

3.1.8.0 Atherosclerosis

ROS appear to be involved in the pathophysiological events leading to atherosclerosis, the underlying cause of most cardiovascular diseases. Common risk factors for atherosclerosis, such as hypertension, aging, smoking, diabetes, and hypercholesterolemia, as well as local oscillatory shear, all result in increased ROS.

Although atherosclerosis is essentially an arterial disease, when exposed to circulatory conditions similar to those of an artery, vein grafts can also undergo athero-sclerotic processes. These, together with thrombosis and intimal hyperplasia, are the main causes of the failure of venous grafts (vein graft disease).

3.1.9.0 Hypertension

A great body of evidence supports the idea that ROS are involved in the pathogenesis of hypertension. Increased markers of oxidative stress are found in human hypertensive subjects, as well as in various animal models of hypertension. Treatment of these models with ROS scavengers (Tempol), inhibitors of NADPH oxidase, inhibitors of xanthine oxidase, SOD mimetics, BH_4 or targeted gene delivery of SOD, or NADPH oxidase inhibitors, normalizes blood pressure or prevents the development of hypertension and in some cases improves vascular and renal function. Furthermore, genetic deficiency in ROS-generating enzymes protects some animals from experimental hypertension, whereas lack of antioxidant capacity causes increased hypertension in others. Increased NADPH oxidase and XO expression or activity is also observed in some experimental models of hypertension. **RMH Note: Large RCTs have failed to reverse or prevent hypertension in human trials.**

As much as we would like to be able to present a comprehensive diagram of all the differences in ROS metabolism between arteries and veins, as well as their implications on vascular function and disease, the knowledge today is simply insufficient to do so. (A Comparison of Arteries and Veins in Oxidative Stress: Producers, Destroyers, Function, and Disease. Theodora Szasz, Keshari Thakali, Gregory D. Fink and Stephanie W. Watts. *Experimental Biology and Medicine* 232:27-37 (2007).

3.2. 0.0 A comparison of EMODs in aorta vs vena cava

Reactive oxygen species (ROS) are important mediators in vascular biology. Venous function, although relevant to cardiovascular disease, is still understudied. We compared aspects of ROS metabolism between a major artery (the aorta) and a major vein (the vena cava, VC) of the rat, **with the hypothesis that venous ROS metabolism would be overall increased compared with its arterial counterpart.**

Superoxide and hydrogen peroxide (H2O2) release in basal conditions was higher in VC compared with aorta.

The antioxidant capacity for H2O2 was also higher in VC than in aorta.

Exogenous superoxide induced a higher contraction in VC compared with aorta.

Protein expression of three major ROS metabolizing enzymes, xanthine oxidase (XO), CuZn-SOD, and catalase, was higher in VC compared with aorta.

Because XO seemed a likely source of the higher VC ROS levels, we examined it further and **found higher mRNA expression and activity of XO in VC compared with aorta.** We also investigated the impact of XO inhibition by allopurinol on aorta and VC functional responses to norepinephrine, ANG II, ET-1, and ACh. Maximal ET-1-mediated contraction was decreased by allopurinol in VC but not in the aorta. Our results suggest that **there are overall differences in ROS metabolism between aorta and VC, with the latter operating normally at a higher set point**, releasing but also being able to handle, higher ROS levels. We propose XO to be an important source for these differences. The result of this particular comparison may be reflective of a general arteriovenous contrast (A comparison of reactive oxygen species metabolism in the rat aorta and vena cava: focus on xanthine oxidase. Theodora Szasz, Janice M. Thompson, and Stephanie W. Watts. Am J Physiol Heart Circ Physiol 295: H1341-H1350, 2008). **I have argued for years that the venous system must have a higher level of EMODs in order to oxidize microaggregates before they can form plaque. This paper verifies my predictions.**

3.2.1.0 Obese children risk thyroid damage

12/3/08 Obese children may be damaging their thyroids, creating a vicious cycle of metabolism and overweight, Italian researchers reported on 12/3/08.

Obesity may cause inflammation that damages the thyroid, which secretes hormones to regulate metabolism and other important functions, Dr. Giorgio Radetti of the Regional Hospital of Bolzano in Italy and colleagues said. They evaluated 186 overweight and obese children for about three years, testing thyroid hormone levels and thyroid antibodies and imaging the thyroid gland using ultrasound.

"Our study shows that alterations in thyroid function and structure are common in obese children and we may have uncovered the link," Radetti said in a statement. **"We found an association between body mass index and thyroid**

hormone levels which suggests that fat excess may have a role in thyroid tissue modification."

Writing in the **Journal of Clinical Endocrinology & Metabolism**, they said 73 of the children had inflamed-looking thyroids, but apparently not a condition called Hashimoto's thyroiditis, an autoimmune disease in which T-cells mistakenly attack the thyroid. But the children lacked antibodies that are also involved in the disease.

"The ultrasound findings are a bit mysterious," Radetti said. "However, the findings do suggest the existence of a low-grade inflammation state, which has been known to characterize obesity." More study is needed to show whether losing weight would normalize the thyroid and return the children to health, he said.

Low thyroid function can be linked to weight gain, although stimulating the thyroid does not automatically cause weight loss. Losing weight, however, has been shown to restore thyroid function in some cases.

I believe that this may be related to fats, acting as double bonded antioxidants, which are creating an EMOD insufficiency and thus, blocking iodination and T4 production. EMODs are vital to normal thyroid function, as peroxide serves as a substrate for thyroid peroxidase.

3.2.2.0 American Heart Association Says Antioxidants do not decrease CVD

Consumption of a diet rich in food sources of antioxidants and other cardioprotective agents--not supplementation with antioxidants-is a more likely pathway to prevention of cardiovascular disease (CVD), according to a new Science Advisory released by the American Heart Association (AHA) in the August 3 issue of *Circulation* (110, 5: 637-641, 2004).

While numerous meta-analyses and randomized clinical trials have been conducted on the relationship between various antioxidants and heart disease, they have typically failed to validate the hypothesis that antioxidant supplements have a beneficial effect on CVD morbidity and mortality. Further, the studies have differed with regard to subject populations studied, dose and type (e.g., synthetic or natural) of antioxidants or antioxidant cocktails, study length and study end points. In addition, the studies have historically been conducted on subjects who have had myocardial infarctions or subjects at high risk for CVD, rather than healthy subjects representative of the general population, and have been conducted over periods as varied as one year and 12 years.

To complicate matters, some studies have shown antioxidant supplements may have potentially adverse effects on CVD. For example, one study showed postmenopausal women with coronary disease receiving hormone replacement therapy given vitamin E plus vitamin C had an unexpected, significantly higher all-cause mortality rate and a trend for an increased cardiovascular mortality rate compared with vitamin placebo women (Waters DD et al. "Effects of hormone replacement therapy and antioxidant vitamin supplements on coronary atherosclerosis in postmenopausal women: a randomized controlled trial." *JAMA*. 288, 19: 2432-2440, 2002.) (http://jama.ama-assn.org). Similarly, in another study, subjects with angiographically demonstrated coronary artery disease taking simvastatin/niacin and an antioxidant cocktail including vitamin E, beta-carotene, vitamin C and selenium had a 0.7 percent progression in stenosis (narrowing or constriction of the diameter of a bodily passage or orifice) after three years, compared with a 0.4 percent regression in the group on simvastatin/niacin only (Brown BG et al. "Simvastatin and niacin, antioxidant vitamins, or the combination for the prevention of coronary disease." *New Engl J Med*. 345, 22:1583-92, 2001.) (www.nejm.org).

In general, the studies showing either positive or negative effects of antioxidant supplementation on CVD end points are much smaller studies than the larger clinical trials that have consistently failed to show any beneficial effects of antioxidant supplements on several CVD end points.

Moreover, the advisory said, CVD risk reduction should be pursued not through antioxidant supplementation but though long-term consumption of a diet consistent with AHA Dietary Guidelines (Krauss RM et al. "AHA Dietary Guidelines: revision 2000: a statement for healthcare professionals from the Nutrition Committee of the American Heart Association." *Circulation*. 102, 18:2284-99, 2000.) (www.circulation.org)--which include reduction of saturated and trans fats; increase in dietary fiber consumption; and increased consumption of fruits, vegetables, whole grains, low-fat or nonfat dairy products, fish, legumes, poultry and lean meats--the long-term maintenance of a healthy body weight by balancing energy intake with regular physical activity, and the attainment of desirable blood cholesterol and lipoprotein profiles and blood pressure levels; however, no consistent data suggest consuming micronutrients at levels exceeding those provided by a dietary pattern consistent with AHA Dietary Guidelines will confer additional benefit with regard to CVD risk reduction, the advisory said.

The advisory concluded that, although past clinical trials have not necessarily ruled out a role for oxidative mechanisms in the pathogenesis of human atherosclerosis, the existing scientific database of epidemiological evidence does not justify routine use of antioxidant supplements for prevention and treatment of CVD and called for further research to clarify the relationship between antioxidants and CVD.

"The Council on Responsible Nutrition [CRN] agrees that further research is needed," said Annette Dickinson, Ph.D., President of CRN, in a statement released by CRN. "In the meantime, people whose dietary patterns include the regular use of antioxidant supplements have no reason to change those habits. Antioxidants have been shown to enhance overall immune function, protect the eyes from cataracts and macular degeneration, slow the progression of Alzheimer's disease and reduce the risk of some cancers. In addition, while many of the studies on vitamin E and heart disease have been disappointing, some have been positive. The AHA seems to be trying to prematurely close the door on supplement use, even while more studies continue." http://www.naturalproductsinsider.com/articles/491online11.html. Accessed 2-3-09.

3.2.3.0 Vitamins C, E don't protect against cancer: studies

12/09/08 CHICAGO (AFP) —Vitamins C and E do not appear to reduce the risk of cancer, according to a pair of new studies which debunk earlier research suggesting supplements might provide some protection against the often deadly ailment.

Some 15,000 men aged 50 and older participated in the study, which included an eight-year follow-up period, but neither vitamin appeared to appreciably reduce their cancer risk, according to the studies appearing in the January 7, 2009 issue of the Journal of the American Medical Association (JAMA).

The findings are disappointing news for the more than half of American adults take vitamin supplements -- many in the hope of warding off illness.

They appear to refute earlier observational studies that linked use of vitamins E and C with reduced risk of certain forms of cancers, including cancer of the prostate.

One of the two studies -- the Selenium and Vitamin E Cancer Prevention Trial (SELECT) -- found that vitamin E or selenium supplements, whether taken alone or in combination, appear not to reduce the risk of prostate cancer, which is the second leading cause of cancer death in the United States.

"It may be time to give up the idea that the protective influence of diet on prostate cancer risk can be emulated by isolated dietary molecules given alone or in combination to middle-aged and older men," Peter Gann of the University of Illinois at Chicago reflected in a JAMA editorial.

SELECT researchers studied the supplements' effects over seven years on some 35,533 men, aged 50 years or older.

The researchers said that "large-scale, randomized trials" still must be conducted on the use of vitamin supplements and cancer.

Until that next generation of trials, **"physicians should not recommend selenium or vitamin E or any other antioxidant supplements to their patients for preventing prostate cancer,"** said Gann

3.2.4.0 Supplementation with vitamin E or selenium does not reduce risk of prostate cancer

In perhaps the largest cancer chemoprevention trial ever conducted, researchers have found that supplementation with vitamin E or selenium, alone or in combination, was not associated with a lower risk of prostate cancer or other cancers. This study, along with another cancer prevention study, will be published in the January 7 issue of *JAMA*, and both reports are being released early online because of public health implications.

The number of prostate cancer deaths in the United States has declined in recent years, but this cancer remains one of the most common malignancies in U.S. men, with approximately 186,000 new cases and 29,000 deaths (the second leading cause of cancer death) estimated for 2008. An effective prevention strategy for prostate cancer would have substantial public health benefits, according to background information. Previous studies have indicated the potential of selenium and vitamin E for preventing prostate cancer.

Scott M. Lippman, M.D., of the University of Texas M. D. Anderson Cancer Center, Houston, and Eric A. Klein, M.D., of the Cleveland Clinic Lerner College of Medicine, Cleveland, and colleagues conducted the Selenium and Vitamin E Cancer Prevention Trial (SELECT) to examine the effects of selenium and vitamin E, alone or in combination, on the risk of prostate cancer and other health outcomes in relatively healthy men. The trial included 35,533 men, age 50 years or older for African-American men and age 55 years or older for other men at the start of the study, from the U.S., Canada, and Puerto Rico. The participants were randomly assigned to receive one of four interventions between August 2001 and June 2004 for a planned minimum follow-up of 7 years: selenium (200 µg/day); vitamin E (400 IU/day), selenium + vitamin E, or placebo.

On September 15, 2008, the independent data and safety monitoring committee recommended the discontinuation of study supplements because the alternative hypothesis of no evidence of benefit from either study agent was convincingly demonstrated and there was no possibility of a benefit to the planned degree with additional follow-up. The notice to discontinue study supplements went out to all active study sites on October 23, 2008, when median (midpoint) overall follow-up was 5.46 years.

The researchers found that there were no statistically significant differences in the absolute numbers (or 5-year incidence rates) of prostate cancer diagnoses between the four groups: placebo, 416 cases (5-year rate of 4.43 percent); selenium, 432 cases (4.56 percent); vitamin E, 473 cases (4.93 percent); selenium + vitamin E, 437 cases (4.56 percent). There were nonsignificant increased risks of prostate cancer in the vitamin E group and type 2 diabetes mellitus in the selenium group, but not in the selenium + vitamin E group.

"In conclusion, SELECT has definitively demonstrated that selenium, vitamin E, or selenium + vitamin E (at the tested doses and formulations) did not prevent prostate cancer in the generally healthy, heterogeneous population of men in SELECT. These data underscore the prudence that is needed in considering recommendations to use agents for the prevention or control of disease in the absence of convincing clinical trial results. These findings also compel the medical research community to continue the search for new, effective agents for prostate cancer prevention," the authors write.

(JAMA. 2009;301[1]:doi:10.1001/jama.2008.864. Available pre-embargo to the media at www.jamamedia.org)

Editor's Note: Please see the article for additional information, including other authors, author contributions and affiliations, financial disclosures, funding and support, etc.

3.2.5.0 Editorial: Randomized Trials of Antioxidant Supplementation for Cancer Prevention-First Bias, Now Chance—Next, Cause

In a *JAMA* editorial, Peter H. Gann, M.D., Sc.D., of the University of Illinois at Chicago, comments on the "disappointing news" that two major trials (SELECT and Physicians' Health Study II, which were "conceived **during the wave of hope**" of earlier studies suggesting that cancer might be prevented by selenium or vitamin E) showed that neither selenium nor vitamin E produced any reduction in prostate cancer or other cancers.

"... single-agent interventions, even in combinations, may be an ineffective approach to primary prevention in average-risk populations. It may be time to give up the idea that the protective influence of diet on prostate cancer risk ... can be emulated by isolated dietary molecules given alone or in combination to middle-aged and older men. ... On the other hand, nonpharmacological dietary prevention of prostate cancer is probably more complex and may involve certain inconvenient truths. Fortunately, no dietary change this profound is likely to be beneficial for prostate cancer alone. If it requires whole foods, extracts, or dietary patterns, it may be necessary to give up the reductionist need to know which molecule is most responsible and perhaps give up the notion of placebo controls as well."

"Epidemiology teaches that every statistical association has only 3 possible explanations: bias, chance, and cause. However, I impugn this statement and would add to this 1) partial fabrication of data, 2) unscrupulous manipulation of data and 3) completely made up data, aka, lying.

Regarding nutritional prevention of prostate cancer, first-generation phase 3 trials were too reliant on biased interpretation of prior research, second-generation trials may have been too reliant on chance, yet there is every reason to believe that the next generation will have a firmer basis for causal hypotheses. Until then, **physicians should not recommend selenium or vitamin E—or any other antioxidant supplements—to their patients for preventing prostate cancer."**

(JAMA. 2009;301[1]:doi:10.1001/jama.2008.863. Available pre-embargo to the media at www.jamamedia.org)

3.2.6.0 Nutritional Chemoprevention for Prostate Cancer Strikes Out Twice

HOUSTON, Dec. 9 -- Vitamins E and C and selenium failed as prevention against prostate cancer in two large clinical trials. In the larger of the two studies, neither selenium nor vitamin E nor the combination of the two reduced the risk of prostate and other cancers in healthy men.

In fact, vitamin E was associated with a trend toward an increased risk of prostate cancer, and the selenium group had more new cases of type 2 diabetes, Scott Lippman, M.D., of the University of Texas M. D. Anderson Cancer Center, and colleagues reported online in the *Journal of the American Medical Association.*

Similarly, the second study, reported in the same issue, showed no protection from prostate cancer or total cancer among men taking vitamin E and C supplements.

"These data provide no support for the use of these supplements for the prevention of cancer in middle-aged and older men," reported J. Michael Gaziano, M.D., of Harvard, and colleagues.

In an accompanying editorial, Peter H. Gann, M.D., Sc.D., of the University of Illinois at Chicago, suggested **chemoprevention has run its course, which led to a dead end.**

"It may be time to give up the idea that the protective influence of diet on prostate cancer risk . . . can be emulated by isolated dietary molecules given alone or in combination to middle-aged and older men," said Dr. Gann.

Dr. Lippman and coauthors reported findings from the Selenium and Vitamin E Cancer Prevention Trial (SELECT), which involved 35,533 men enrolled at sites in the United States, Canada, and Puerto Rico.

The participants were healthy men with a serum PSA level less than 4 ng/mL, and a normal digital rectal exam. African-Americans were no younger than 50 and all other men were 55 or older.

The men were randomized to four daily supplement groups:

- Selenium plus vitamin E
- Vitamin E plus a selenium placebo
- Selenium plus a vitamin E placebo
- Placebos for both selenium and vitamin E

After a median follow-up of 5.46 years (range 4.17 to 7.33 years), the prostate cancer hazard ratio for vitamin E versus the double-placebo group was 1.13. The hazard ratio was 1.04 for selenium alone and 1.05 for selenium plus vitamin E.

The authors also found no significant differences among treatment groups for any other cancer-related end points.

Patients treated with vitamin E alone had a slightly elevated risk of prostate cancer (*P*=0.06), and the selenium group had a type 2 diabetes hazard ratio of 1.07 versus the double-placebo group.

Dr. Gaziano and colleagues reported findings from the Physicians' Health Study II, which evaluated the effect of supplementation with vitamins C and E on the risk of prostate cancer and total cancer.

The study involved 14,641 male physicians who were 50 or older at enrollment, including 1,307 men with a history of cancer.

The participants were randomized to vitamins E and C, vitamin E or matching placebo, vitamin C or matching placebo, or placebos for both vitamin E and C.

The primary outcome measures were the rates of prostate cancer and total cancer.

During a mean follow-up of eight years, investigators documented 1,008 cases of prostate cancer and 1,943 total cancers.

As compared with the double-placebo group, vitamin E was associated with hazard ratios of 0.97 for prostate cancer and 1.04 for total cancer.

In the vitamin C group, the hazard ratios versus placebo were 1.02 for prostate cancer and 1.01 for total cancer.

Analyses of other types of cancer revealed no significant differences.

In his editorial, Dr. Gann noted that a statistical association has only three possible explanations: bias, chance, and cause. With regard to nutritional cancer prevention, first-generation studies relied on biased interpretation of prior research, he said. Second-generation studies might have relied too much on chance.

"There is every reason to believe that the next generation will have firmer basis for causal hypotheses," said Dr. Gann. "Until then, physicians should not recommend selenium or vitamin E -- or any other antioxidant supplements -- to their patients for preventing prostate cancer."

The SELECT study was supported by the National Cancer Institute and the National Center for Complementary and Alternative Medicine. Study agents were provided by Perrigo Company, Sabinsa Corporation, Tishcon Corporation, and DSM Nutritional Products.

The Physicians' Health Study was supported by the National Institutes of Health and by BASF Corporation. Study agents were provided by BASF, Wyeth Pharmaceuticals, and DSM Nutritional Products.

Primary source: Journal of the American Medical Association

Source reference:

Lippman SM, et al "Effect of selenium and vitamin E on risk of prostate cancer and other cancers. The selenium and vitamin E cancer prevention trial (SELECT)." *JAMA*. 2009; 301: DOI:10.1001/jama.2008.864.

Additional source: Journal of the American Medical Association

Source reference:

Gaziano JM, et al. "Vitamins E and C in the prevention of prostate and total cancer in men. The physicians' health study II randomized controlled trial." *JAMA*. 2009; 301: DOI:10.1001/jama.2008.862.

Additional source: Journal of the American Medical Association

Source reference:

Gann PH. "Randomized trials of antioxidant suppleme ntation for cancer prevention. First bias, now chance-next, cause." *JAMA*. 2009;301:doi:10.1001/jama.2008.863.

3.2.7.0 Vitamins and antioxidants 'do not cut cancer risk'

12/09/08 Taking vitamins or antioxidants does not protect against developing cancer, according to two major new studies

Scientists found no evidence of any significant effect from the supplements in either study, involving a total of more than 50,000 men. Previous studies have suggested that vitamins and antioxidants like selenium, a mineral that naturally occurs in the body, could have anti-cancer properties, but the results were not definitive.

The studies looked at the effects of vitamins E and C and of selenium on the risk of prostate and any other form of cancer.

In the larger trial, 35,533 men from America, Canada and Puerto Rico were given either selenium, vitamin E, both or a placebo for between four and seven years.

The trial was stopped ahead of its original 12 year deadline because of a lack of any noticeable benefit.

Of the four groups, **those taking the placebo had the lowest levels of cancer**, although the difference was not statistically significant.

The authors of the study, led by Dr Scott Lippman, from the University of Texas, said that **their research "has definitively demonstrated that selenium, vitamin E or selenium plus vitamin E did not prevent prostate cancer in the generally healthy, heterogeneous population of men in** (the trial)."

Previous studies had suggested that men with low levels of selenium in their blood were twice as likely to go on to develop the disease as those with high levels of the mineral.

The other study, by scientists at Harvard university, followed **14,641 American doctors aged 50 or older who were given different combinations of vitamin C, vitamin E** and a placebo. **Neither vitamin reduced the risk of prostate or any other type of cancer**, the results, published in the Journal of the American Medical Association (Jama), show.

Writing in the same journal Dr Peter Gann, from the University of Illinois in Chicago, said that the findings were "disappointing news".

Dr Gann added: "It may be time to give up the idea that the protective influence of diet on prostate cancer risk... can be emulated by isolated dietary molecules given alone or in combination to middle-aged and older men."

Dr Jodie Moffat, from Cancer Research UK, said: "There are a lot of studies looking at whether vitamin and mineral supplements can reduce the risk of cancer but many of them, like this one, don't support a link.

"This new research means it is even less likely than we previously thought that supplements can protect against prostate cancer.

"Supplements don't substitute for a healthy diet and some studies have shown that they may actually increase the risk of cancer. "Eating a diet that is high in all types of fruit and vegetables is the best way to get the vitamins and minerals that we need."

4.0.0.0 Importance of oxygen levels

Earth is a spherical shaped solar collector, just like the moon. **(RMH Note: Our eyes are photon collectors to the brain.).** Both receive an almost constant income of solar photons. The main difference is not the income, but the outflow of energy. At the moon, photons from the sun that are not directly reflected to space, will convert to heat, and those converted joules will almost all emit to space within 24 hours. The photons that planet earth receives travelled from the sun in 8 minutes and 19 seconds. About one third continues its journey directly as reflected photons. The remaining two thirds become part of a unique labyrinth of activities on earth: an energy / matter interplay like a giant pinball game. **(RMH Note: the captured photons are then converted into oxygen via photosynthesis. We then eat the plants, utilize the oxygen for sustenance and regenerate carbon dioxide to feed the plants.)**

The enormous flow of solar income is not in itself sufficient to explain the growth that can be observed during the existence of earth. It is the ability to store and retrieve solar energy for various periods of time, that make-up the uniqueness of planet earth. The main physical enabler of this phenomenon is the earth's mass, and especially its mass of water. Its influence is extensively studied in the present-day climate models. In the model, mass as such is not discussed, since energy conversions do not change the amount of mass on earth in a significant way.

Some 2.5 billion years ago, the plant kingdom came against their limits to growth as a consequence of their waste product: oxygen. The result was the **Oxygen Catastrophe**: a crisis that would be noticed in dramatic changes of the amount of stored memory and stored joules.

The oxygen catastrophe is an example in the earth's history where the amount of memory, encapsulated in DNA, increased the probability of a carrying capacity crisis. Yet at the same time the memory volume raised the probability of a DNA pool that –eventually– could overcome the crisis. In this case, that memory pool enabled the creation of species that use oxygen (and hydrocarbons), and produce carbon dioxide as a waste product that can again be used by plants. So it seems that more memory means a greater probability of both a carrying capacity crisis *and* a solution of that crisis. Bridging the two is of course the difficult part.

After the oxygen crisis, the synthesis of plants and animals triggered a renewed growth in the stocks of memory on earth. Before human civilisation, the memory stock of planet earth mainly consisted of DNA in living organisms, plus whatever memory there was in the living brains of those organisms. The knowledge about DNA surfaced only recently. The first Nobel Prize in the field was awarded to Crick, Watson and Wilkins in 1962. With that knowledge, the stock of DNA information now becomes more and more retrievable by humans, even after the original organisms are long dead.

Human civilisation itself started more than ten thousand years ago with the storage of reproducible information via written symbols. **(Jeu-de-Joule: a conceptual earthly energy model. Anton W. Trijssenaar.).**

4.0.1.0 The importance of adequate oxygen levels: altitude sickness

12/10/08 **A brain swelling condition related to low oxygen levels in the air may have caused many of the deaths of people climbing Mount Everest**, researchers said on 12/10/08. An international team led by Paul Firth of Massachusetts General Hospital studied the 212 reported deaths from 1921 to 2006 on Mount Everest, the highest on Earth.

Hazards awaiting those who dare to climb the 29,000-foot (8,850 meter) Himalayan mountain include extreme cold, whipping winds, changing weather, treacherous climbs and avalanches. **Oxygen content in the air is only a third of that at sea level.**

"Nobody was attacked by any Yeti or anything else," Firth said, referring to the "abominable snowman" of legend. Firth said that while the cause of some deaths could not be determined with certainty, many appeared to have been the result of high-altitude cerebral edema. In this condition, **low oxygen levels cause cerebral blood vessels to leak fluid into surrounding brain tissue, triggering swelling. Confusion and loss of coordination follow.**

Many deaths occurred **above 26,000 feet in an area dubbed "the dead zone,"** particularly among people who already reached the summit and were climbing back down. "Of the guys who died up at 8,000 meters (26,000 feet), a large number of them were developing neurological symptoms. In other words, **they were getting confused, comatose or they were having a loss of coordination,"** said Firth, whose findings appear in the British Medical Journal.

This seemed consistent with high-altitude cerebral edema, he said in a telephone interview. "If you go too fast and you haven't adapted to the low oxygen levels, then you can get various types of high altitude illness." **He had expected to find more lung problems but in fact they were rare.**

The researchers speculated that many of the deaths attributed to falls or the person vanishing during the climb may have been due to high-altitude cerebral edema. The study showed that 1.3 percent of mountaineers who climbed above their Everest base camp died.

4.0.2.0 Low Brain Oxygen Ups Alzheimer's Risk

Lab mice living in low oxygen levels show worse memory and more brain plaque.

Nov. 20, 2006 -- **Low levels of brain oxygen may boost Alzheimer's risk**, a new study in mice shows. Researchers included Weihong Song, MD, PhD, of the psychiatry department and Brain Research Centre at Canada's University of British Columbia.

Song's team studied mice that had a gene tied to Alzheimer's disease. The researchers **kept some mice in cages with low-oxygen air for 16 hours a day for a month. They kept the other mice in cages with normal oxygen levels.**

In humans, conditions such as stroke that hamper blood flow in the brain can limit the brain's oxygen supply. After the month, the researchers tested both sets of mice on a memory test in which they were timed while swimming through a water maze to reach a hidden platform.

The mice that had lived in low oxygen performed worse. Those mice also had more amyloid beta plaque -- a hallmark of Alzheimer's disease -- in their brains, compared to the mice with normal brain oxygen levels.

Song and colleagues also studied the mice's genes. Under the influence of low brain oxygen levels, the BACE1 gene upped production of amyloid beta, the key protein in Alzheimer's brain plaque. Even a "slight" rise in BACE1 activity "could lead to a dramatic increase in [amyloid beta] production," the researchers write.

Low brain oxygen levels might also affect other genes and may spur brain cell death, worsening memory in Alzheimer's disease, Song's team notes. **Boosting brain oxygen levels may benefit Alzheimer's patients,** the researchers say. However, their study did not test that theory.

The report appears in *Proceedings of the National Academy of Sciences*' online early edition.

4.0.3.0 Anesthetic/Low Brain Oxygen Ups Alzheimer's Risk

April 28, 2008 (UPI) -- **An anesthetic and low oxygen during surgery have been linked to a build-up of amyloid-beta proteins associated with Alzheimer's disease**, a U.S. study found. Cell studies showed a common anesthetic -- desflurane -- did not cause a build up of amyloid-beta protein, however, when the anesthetic was combined with low oxygen it linked to more production of the proteins associated with Alzheimer's disease.

Bin Zhang, Yuanlin Dong, Rudolph Tanzi, Zhongcong Xie and colleagues at Massachusetts General Institute for Neurodegenerative Disease, Massachusetts General Hospital/Harvard Medical School in Boston said **hypoxia said low oxygen -- by itself -- did not have this effect.**

The findings, published in the **Journal of Biological Chemistry**, were produced from **human brain cell culture experiments** and should next be confirmed by animal models. The preliminary findings suggest it is important to ensure anesthetic patients maintain sufficient brain oxygen, the researchers said. The study exposed human brain cells to 12 percent desflurane for six hours -- mimicking surgical conditions -- and found no observable changes in either the production of amyloid-beta protein or the rate of cell death. However, **desflurane combined with low oxygen levels of 18 percent could stimulate both of these cellular change.**

4.0.4.0 Low Oxygen Accelerated the Great Dying (Permian-Triassic period)

April 19th, 2005. The biggest mass extinction in Earth history some **251 million years ago** was preceded by elevated extinction rates before the main event and was followed by a delayed recovery that lasted for millions of years. New research by two University of Washington scientists suggests that **a sharp decline in atmospheric oxygen levels was likely a major reason for both the elevated extinction rates and the very slow recovery**.

Earth's land at the time was still massed in a supercontinent called Pangea, and most of the land above sea level became uninhabitable because **low oxygen made breathing too difficult for most organisms to survive,** said Raymond Huey, a UW biology professor.

What's more, in many cases nearby populations of the same species were cut off from each other because even low-altitude passes had insufficient oxygen to allow animals to cross from one valley to the next. That population fragmentation likely increased the extinction rate and slowed recovery following the mass extinction, Huey said.

"Biologists have previously thought about the physiological consequences of low oxygen levels during the late Permian period, but not about these biogeographical ones," he said.

Atmospheric oxygen content, about 21 percent today, was a very rich 30 percent in the early Permian period.

However, previous carbon-cycle modeling by Robert Berner at Yale University has calculated that **atmospheric oxygen began plummeting soon after, reaching about 16 percent at the end of the Permian and bottoming out at less than 12 percent about 10 million years into the Triassic period.**

"Oxygen dropped from its highest level to its lowest level ever in only 20 million years, which is quite rapid, and animals that once were able to cross mountain passes quite easily suddenly had their movements severely restricted," Huey said.

He calculated that when the **oxygen level hit 16 percent, breathing at sea level would have been like trying to breathe at the summit of a 9,200-foot mountain today. By the early Triassic period, sea-level oxygen content of less than 12 percent would have been the same as it is today in the thin air at 17,400 feet, higher than any permanent human habitation.** That means even animals at sea level would have been oxygen challenged.

Huey and UW paleontologist Peter Ward are authors of a paper detailing the work, published in the April 15, 2005 edition of the journal **Science**. The work was supported by grants from the National Science Foundation and the National Aeronautics and Space Administration's Astrobiology Institute.

Not only was atmospheric oxygen content dropping at the end of the Permian, the scientists said, but carbon dioxide levels were rising, leading to global climate warming.

"Declining oxygen and warming temperatures would have been doubly stressful for late Permian animals," Huey said. **"As the climate warms, body temperatures and metabolic rates go up. That means oxygen demand is going up, so animals would face an increased oxygen demand and a reduced supply**. It would be like forcing athletes to exercise more but giving them less food. They'd be in trouble."

Ward was lead author of a paper published in Science earlier this year presenting evidence that extinction rates of land vertebrates were elevated throughout the late Permian, likely because of climate change, and culminated in a mass extinction at the end of the Permian. The event, often called **"the Great Dying,"** was **the greatest mass extinction in Earth's history, killing 90 percent of all marine life and nearly three-quarters of land plants and animals.**

Ward said paleontologists had previously assumed that Pangea was not just a supercontinent but also a "superhighway" on which species would have encountered few roadblocks while moving from one place to another. However, it appears **the greatly reduced oxygen actually created impassable barriers that affected the ability of animals to move and survive, he said.**

"If this is true, then I think we have to go back and look at oxygen and its role in evolution and how different species developed," Ward said. **"You can go without food for a couple of weeks. You can go without water for a few days. How long can you go without oxygen, a couple of minutes? There's nothing with a greater evolutionary effect than oxygen."**

An unimaginable number of synapses converge, combining their action potentials, sending the signal back to a central processor for analysis, sending it out for further clarification, and finally moving a new series of ions across membranes to terminate in the movement of fingers across a keyboard. Irradiatus.

Exponential numbers of oxygen molecules are hurriedly scurrying throughout my body and brain, shuffling through my electron transport chain, carrying on instantaneous corporeal and cellular cross talk, generating energy-rich ATP, thus, allowing me to utilize its combined prooxidant je ne sais quoi to present this lecture to you. RMH 1-29-10

4.0.5.0 Cell's Power Plants (mitochondria) Also Sense Low Oxygen

June 8, 2005. Researchers have produced the strongest evidence yet **that mitochondria—the organelles that generate energy to power the cell—also monitor oxygen concentration in the cell.** If oxygen slips below a critical threshold, the mitochondrial "sensor" triggers protective responses to promote survival.

Understanding how the cell senses and protects itself against hypoxia (low oxygen) has both important basic and clinical implications for biology and medicine, said one of the study's senior authors, M. Celeste Simon, a Howard Hughes Medical Institute investigator at the University of Pennsylvania.

"Oxygen is absolutely essential for life, so the biological mechanisms underlying response to low oxygen are central to the cell," she said. "For example, **during early development, the embryo exists in a naturally hypoxic environment until it is connected to the maternal cardiovascular system.**

"In the adult, **changes in oxygen levels occur during inflammation and atherosclerosis; and even transient oxygen starvation can have a profound impact on the brain**," said Simon. "For example, **the well-known case of the late Terry Schiavo, in which a cardiac episode reduced her to a vegetative state, was the result of only brief oxygen starvation."**

The new studies may suggest ways to enhance the body's natural protective response to low oxygen environments. These strategies might be employed to help the brain fend off the effects of **transient oxygen starvation that can quickly cause irreversible brain damage.**

The research team that included Simon and senior author Paul T. Schumacker of the University of Chicago, as well Ulrich Hammerling and colleagues from Memorial Sloan-Kettering Cancer Center, reported their findings in two articles published in the **June 2005 issue of the journal *Cell Metabolism*.** A third article in the same issue by Navdeep Chandel and his colleagues at Northwestern University presented additional evidence that **mitochondria function as oxygen sensors.**

According to Simon, the idea that mitochondria sense cellular oxygen concentrations has been controversial. "It has been a reasonable idea around for many decades, because **mitochondria are the primary consumers of oxygen in the cell,"** she said. "However, the idea was discarded, because it appears that the mitochondrion still functions perfectly well in a range of oxygen concentrations where it is known that limiting oxygen results in an accumulation of HIF." HIF, or hypoxia inducible factor, is the protein that triggers the cell's broad protective response to low oxygen conditions.

In previous studies, Simon and her colleagues had found evidence implicating mitochondria as oxygen sensors. They found that **in response to low oxygen, mitochondria produce chemicals called reactive oxygen species (ROS)—such as hydrogen peroxide—that trigger the activity of HIF**.

However, other researchers had performed experiments that argued against a mitochondrial role in oxygen sensing. They showed that **enzymes called prolyl hydroxylases (PHDs), which normally inhibit HIF activity, depend on oxygen**. Thus, low oxygen would reduce PHD activity, triggering HIF. "As a result of these findings, **in many people's minds, PHDs, became the long-sought-after oxygen sensor,"** said Simon.

In their latest experiments, which sought to demonstrate more conclusively that mitochondria were oxygen sensors, the researchers used new techniques to produce cells with defective mitochondrial machinery, or in which they could transiently switch off that machinery. They also used a new technique to precisely measure ROS levels in hypoxic cells.

"Our studies of cells with mitochondrial deficiencies showed that they do not accumulate HIF in response to moderate hypoxia," said Simon. **"Also, our highly sensitive probe for ROS showed that the cells do not produce these species, either.** Further, **we found that in these cells, we can supply the missing signal that triggers HIF accumulation by adding back ROS."**

One of the group's most important observations, according to Simon, was finding that **reducing oxygen levels to near zero, called anoxia, triggers an entirely different protective response that is independent of the mitochondria. This response involves the enzyme PHD as the oxygen sensor.**

"So, now we think we have something for everybody," said Simon. **"In oxygen ranges that are moderately low, the mitochondria control the protective response by releasing ROS. But when you get to a really low level**

of anoxia, the PHD becomes the oxygen sensor." Such a dual-mode mechanism makes evolutionary sense, said Simon, because it enables the cell to adjust to a wide range of low oxygen levels, even the "emergency" created by total oxygen starvation.

The group's findings might also have implications for cancer therapy since **tumors use this protective response to thrive in a low-oxygen environment.** If one could develop drugs to block that response, it could potentially take away one of the survival strategies exploited by tumors, said the researchers.

Simon said that **tumor growth seems to depend on the tumor's ability, via the HIF-triggered machinery, to adapt to low oxygen levels until it can develop its own blood supply.** Thus, she said, results from her laboratory are being used as a guide to develop drugs that inhibit HIF in tumors, to render them vulnerable to hypoxia and thwart their ability to grow blood vessels.

4.0.6.0 High altitude native Tibetans with high oxygen saturation survive better

High-altitude native populations are exposed to lifelong ambient hypoxia that stresses the oxygen delivery system and elicits adaptations. The genetic bases and thus the evolutionary interpretation of the adaptive traits of high-altitude populations are generally unknown, with the exception of oxygen saturation of hemoglobin among high-altitude native Tibetans. Tibetans at a given high altitude vary widely in percent oxygen saturation of hemoglobin despite uniform ambient hypoxic stress. A putative major gene (an inferred locus) with a recognizable quantitative effect having an autosomal dominant mode of inheritance that is associated with 6% higher oxygen saturation has been detected in two areas of the Tibet Autonomous Region. The high oxygen saturation genotypes may have greater Darwinian fitness because they are less physiologically stressed, in the sense of having higher arterial oxygen content and less departure from the internal milieu that evolved at sea level. Here, we test the hypotheses that Tibetan women with high oxygen saturation genotypes have higher fertility or lower offspring mortality than women with low oxygen saturation genotypes.

These findings suggest that high-altitude hypoxia is acting as an agent of natural selection on the locus for oxygen saturation of hemoglobin by the mechanism of higher infant survival of Tibetan women with high oxygen saturation genotypes. (Higher offspring survival among Tibetan women with high oxygen saturation genotypes residing at 4,000m. Cynthia M. Beall, Kijoung Song, Robert

C. Elston, and Melvyn C. Goldstein PNAS. September 28, 2004. vol.101, no. 39, 14300–14304).

4.0.7.0 High summits 'could harm brain'

10/20/08 **Top mountaineers may be suffering subtle brain damage each time they reach the upper slopes of the world's highest peaks**, say scientists. Italian researchers scanned ""world-class"" climbers before and after expeditions, publishing their results in the European Journal of Neurology.

They found changes in brain tissue even though, outwardly, the climbers had no obvious new neurological problems. **The most likely cause was a lack of oxygen at high altitudes,** they said. At the summit of Everest, the world's highest mountain, the concentration of oxygen in the air is reckoned to be only a third of that found at sea level, more than 8,000m lower.

All of the nine male climbers involved in the study, at the IRCCS Fondazione Santa Lucia in Rome, had reached their summit without the use of a supply of extra oxygen, a frequent practice among leading mountaineers. Before the trip, they underwent MRI scans, and were checked for any neurological illnesses, then matched against ""control subjects"" of the same age and sex, who had never climbed above 3,000m. Three of the climbers reached the top of at least one 8,000m peak, while the remainder reached altitudes of at least 7,500m, spending in excess of 15 days above 6,500m.

When they were scanned eight weeks after returning, compared with the ""controls"", there was a fall in the density and volume of brain tissue in two parts of the brain, the ""left pyramidal tract"" and the ""angular gyrus"".

However, Dr. Margherita Di Paola, who led the study, said that this reduction did not appear to have a direct impact on their neurological performance. ""The climbers in our study did not suffer any significant neuropsychological changes after the expedition,"" she said. However, some abnormal results on both the ""before"" and ""after"" tests, she said, might be the result of small, progressive brain damage caused by repeated trips to high-altitude.

These included tests on memory and brain functions such as the ability to anticipate outcomes and adapt to changing situations. Dr. Mike Grocott, from University College London, who has himself helped carry out research high on Everest into the effects of altitude, said that there was other evidence of the potential impact of high-altitude mountaineering on the brain. He said: ""Most climbers are aware that if you are going over 8,000m, there may be a small amount of damage to the brain associated with that.""Even a year later, people might not be as sharp as they were before.""

He said that the research did not show this type of climbing to be unacceptably dangerous, but should be viewed alongside other sports such as football, where studies suggests that even too much time spent heading the ball could cause subtle brain injuries.

4.0.8.0 'Earthly organisms developed in two sets' based on oxygen levels

12-23-08 **Life on Earth went from single microscopic cells to blue whales and giant sequoias in 3.5-billion years in two distinct bursts** tied to the planet's geological evolution, according to a study published on Monday. The study, published in the **Proceedings of the National Academy of Sciences**, goes against the common hypothesis that life slowly evolved from a single-celled organism to complex multi-celled organisms.

"We were surprised to observe that nearly all of the increase in size occurred in two distinct time-intervals," said Michal Kowalewski, a co-author of the study and professor of geosciences at Virginia Tech. "And what is more, **those intervals followed two major oxygenation events."**

In analysing fossil records, the study found that the two size jumps were from bacteria to eukaryotic cells, and from unicellular to multi-cellular organisms. **Only bacteria-like fossils were found in the first 1.5-billion years of recorded life on Earth, and they did not grow until more complex organisms developed around 2-billion years ago after the appearance of eukaryotic cells.**

About three billion years ago, **primitive bacteria "invented" photosynthesis**, nourishing themselves from the sun's energy and carbon dioxide. **They thrived in low-oxygen environments.**

But **the oxygen they released into the atmosphere allowed for more complex cellular structures to develop, and thus the eukaryotic cell was born**.

During about two hundred million years, organisms grew from cells invisible to the naked eye to organisms about the size of a thumbnail. "In a way, thus, an increase in size and complexity was a consequence of geobiological interactions between life and earth. **Life itself enabled life to become more complex**," Kowalewski said. **I believe that oxygen, itself, allowed "life to become more complex."**

It was not until another big increase in oxygen levels - reaching as much as 10 percent of current oxygen concentration - about 540-million years ago, that life developed into multi-cellular, tissue-forming organisms.

"What is really interesting is that each of these 'steps' correlate with a time in life's history where there is innovation in the complexity of life, **the first one being the eukaroytic cell and the second is the multicellularity of life,"** said Virginia Tech researcher Jennifer Stempien, another study co-author.

Through the 3.5-billion years of documented history of life on Earth, the scientists found that organisms' maximum body size increased by 16 times.

To date, marine animals like blue whales or vascular plants like the giant sequoia - the largest known form of life - can reach body sizes greater than the biggest dinosaurs.

4.0.9.0 High Tumor Oxygen Level essential for radiotherapy and chemotherapy

In a discovery that might help explain why widely used cancer therapies are less than optimal, Duke University Medical Center researchers have found that **a tumor's oxygen level and blood flow can fluctuate rapidly.** The Duke animal study, which contradicts previous assumptions about tumors, could be important because the two major cancer treatments, **radiation and chemotherapy, depend on a constant high oxygen level and steady blood flow within a tumor, scientists said.** "These fluctuations in oxygen level and blood flow are not predictable and might represent an impediment to radiation therapy and drug therapy," said Mark Dewhirst, co-director of the radiation oncology and hyperthermia program at Duke Comprehensive Cancer Center and associate professor of pathology. "Before this work, there was no way to reliably measure these values."

Dewhirst prepared the findings for presentation in 2004 at an American Association for Cancer Research meeting. His study, which was done in collaboration with Rod Braun, assistant professor in radiation oncology, was funded by the National Cancer Institute. A report based on the results of this study has been accepted for publication by the **American Journal of Physiology**. **High oxygen levels are crucial for effective radiation therapy, Dewhirst explained, because radiation kills tumor cells by forming oxygen radicals -- highly reactive oxygen atoms that damage DNA**.

Chemotherapy might be affected by the fluctuations, Dewhirst said, because if tumor blood flow drops, the drugs might not be delivered efficiently throughout the tumor.

While low oxygen levels, called hypoxia, are known to exist in certain tumors, researchers had not measured changes in oxygen levels over time. In the current study, Dewhirst and his colleagues measured oxygen levels in mammary tumors in **seven rats** using an electrochemical probe that produces an electrical current depending on the amount of oxygen present in the tissue.

The scientists found unexpectedly that no tumor had stable oxygen levels. According to Dewhirst, **60 percent of their measurements demonstrated acute hypoxia** -- in which oxygen levels dipped below the cutoff point for hypoxia of 10 mm of oxygen pressure. **A full 25 percent of measurements were chronically hypoxic -- never above 10 mm of oxygen -- a condition known to increase tumor radiation resistance.** The remainder, 15 percent, had oxygen levels that were always higher than 10 mm but still were not stable.

The clinical implications of such fluctuations could be serious, Dewhirst said. For example, fluctuations from low to high oxygen levels might reduce sensitivity to radiation, even for those tumors usually above hypoxic levels. In particular, the large fluctuations might be enough to simulate a condition called "hypoxia-reoxygenation injury" that can occur when oxygen levels increase in oxygen-starved tissues, Dewhirst said.

When oxygen is suddenly restored to an oxygen-deprived area, an enzyme called xanthine oxidase produces oxygen radicals from the newly supplied oxygen, leading to tissue damage. This hypoxia-reoxygenation injury can occur in conditions such as a stroke: a brain region already damaged by low-oxygen from the cutoff of blood flow can suffer additional damage when oxygen is restored, due to xanthine oxidase.

Cells that survive hypoxia-reoxygenation injury are likely to have developed defenses against damage from oxygen radicals, Dewhirst said. Likewise, tumor cells could develop protection against oxygen radicals if the oxygen level fluctuation is enough to mimic hypoxia reoxygenation. Thus, even if the tumor is irradiated at a time when the oxygen level is high and radiation should work, the tumor might not respond to therapy.

To understand whether such fluctuations also are present in other tissues, the researchers compared measurements in tumors to those in rat leg muscle. While they found similar frequencies of fluctuations in both tissues, the size of the fluctuations was much larger in tumor than in muscle, Dewhirst said.

He speculates that a phenomenon known as "vascular remodeling" -- in which blood vessels are formed and die quickly, quickly changing blood flow patterns within a tumor -- might underlie the mechanism responsible for the rapid, large fluctuations within tumors. Another hypothesis is that the low tumor oxygen levels might stimulate structural changes in red blood cells, causing the blood to thicken and thus reducing blood flow.

Dewhirst emphasized the importance of making measurements of tumor oxygenation and blood flow in human tumors as soon as the technology is available.

(http://www.scienceblog.com/community/older/1999/B/199901242.html. Accessed 12/10/08)

4.1.0.0 Breast cancer

4.1.1.0 Estrogen therapy increases breast cancer risk

Results from the **Women's Health Initiative trial** raise new questions regarding the effects of estrogen therapy (ET) and estrogen plus progestin therapy (EPT) on breast cancer risk.

We analyzed data from **126,638 females, ages 50 to 71 years at baseline, who completed two questionnaires (1995-1996 and 1996-1997) as** part of the NIH-AARP Diet and Health Cohort Study and in whom 3,657 incident breast cancers were identified through June 30, 2002. Hormone-associated relative risks (RR) and 95% confidence intervals (CI) of breast cancer were estimated via multivariable regression models.

Results: Among thin women (body mass index <25 kg/m^2), **ET use was associated with a significant 60% excess risk after 10 years of use. EPT was associated with a significantly increased risk among women with intact uteri, with the highest risk among current, long-term (≥10 years) users** (RR, 2.44; 95% CI, 2.13-2.79). These risks were slightly higher when progestins were prescribed continuously than sequentially (<15 days/mo; respective RRs of 2.76 versus 2.01). EPT associations were strongest in thin women, but elevated risks persisted among heavy women. EPT use was strongly related to estrogen receptor (ER)-positive tumors, requiring consideration of this variable when assessing relationships according to other clinical features. For instance, ER- ductal tumors were unaffected by EPT use, but all histologic subgroups of ER+ tumors were increased, especially low-grade and mixed ductal-lobular tumors.

Conclusions: **Both ET and EPT were associated with breast cancer risks with the magnitude of increase varying according to body mass and clinical characteristics of the tumors**. (Menopausal Hormone Therapy and Breast Cancer Risk in the NIH-AARP Diet and Health Study Cohort. Louise A. Brinton et al. Cancer Epidemiol Biomarkers Prev 2008;17(11):3150–60).

4.1.2 0 Hormone Therapy-Breast Cancer Tie Grows

12/13/08 **Taking menopause hormones for five years doubles the risk for breast cancer**, according to a new analysis of a big federal study that reveals the most dramatic evidence yet of the dangers of these still-popular pills.

Even women who took estrogen and progestin pills for as little as a couple of years had a greater chance of getting cancer. And when they stopped taking them, their odds quickly improved, returning to a normal risk level roughly two years after quitting.

Collectively, these new findings are likely to end any doubt that **the risks outweigh the benefits for most women.**

It is clear that breast cancer rates plunged in recent years mainly because millions of women quit hormone therapy and fewer newly menopausal women started on it, said the study's leader, Dr. Rowan Chlebowski of Harbor-UCLA Medical Center in Los Angeles.

"It's an excellent message for women: You can still diminish risk (by quitting), even if you've been on hormones for a long time," said Dr. Claudine Isaacs of Georgetown University's Lombardi Comprehensive Cancer Center. "It's not like smoking where you have to wait 10 or 15 years for the risk to come down."

Study results were given Saturday at the San Antonio Breast Cancer Symposium.

They are from the Women's Health Initiative, which tested estrogen and progestin pills that doctors long believed would prevent heart disease, bone loss and many other problems in women after menopause. The main part of the study was stopped in 2002 when researchers saw surprisingly higher risks of heart problems and breast cancer in hormone users.

Since then, experts have debated whether these risks apply to women who start on hormones when they enter menopause, usually in their 50s, and take them for shorter periods of time. Most of the women in the federal study were in their 60s and well past menopause.

So the advice has been to use hormones only if symptoms like hot flashes are severe, and at the lowest dose and shortest time possible. The new study sharpens that message, Chlebowski said.

"It does change the balance" on whether to start on treatment at all, he said.

Even so, **most women will not get breast cancer by taking the pills short-term. The increased cancer risk from a couple of years of hormone use translates to a few extra cases of breast cancer a year for every 1,000 women on hormones.** This risk accumulates with each year of use, though.

4.1.3.0 Hormone therapy may cut breast cancer risk in some

9/23/08 Hormone replacement therapy, which raises breast cancer risk for some women, appears to reduce the risk for those with a certain genetic mutation linked to the disease, researchers said on Tuesday.

Dr. Steven Narod of Women's College Hospital in Toronto and colleagues looked at hormone replacement therapy or HRT in post-menopausal **women with a BRCA1 gene mutation that greatly increases their chances of developing breast cancer.**

Among 472 women from nine countries, those who used HRT were 42 percent less likely to develop breast cancer than those who did not, Narod's team reported in the Journal of the National Cancer Institute.

Many women with a BRCA1 mutation choose to have their ovaries removed in order to reduce their risk of getting breast cancer, but the operation brings on menopause. HRT can relieve menopausal symptoms such as hot flashes and night sweats.

Earlier studies raised alarms about HRT because it raised the risk of breast cancer, stroke and other heart conditions.

But the impact on the risk of breast cancer in post-menopausal women with a BRCA1 gene mutation was unclear, Narod's team said.

Narod said the findings should reassure women with the mutation who want to have their ovaries removed before menopause to lower their risk of getting breast or ovarian cancer, but are worried about using HRT to relieve the symptoms that will follow.

"Certainly in my practice in Toronto at Women's College Hospital, I have no hesitance whatsoever in prescribing hormone replacement therapy to young women who have a BRCA1 mutation and surgical menopause," Narod said in a telephone interview.

"We want to be able to get the benefit of the ovariectomy in terms of preventing cancer but maintain the best quality of life. And we think that the best way to maintain the quality of life is to use hormone replacement therapy," Narod added.

Hormone replacement therapy can involve estrogen alone or estrogen along with progesterone or progestin, a synthetic hormone with effects like those of progesterone.

Narod found no difference in risk reduction between estrogen-only or estrogen-progesterone hormone therapies.

Not everyone was convinced. Two experts who wrote a commentary in the same journal accompanying the study said the findings "provide some evidence for safety but are insufficient to reliably inform routine clinical practice."

"As a result, continued caution in prescribing hormone therapy to women with BRCA1 mutations who are at high risk for breast cancers remains prudent," Dr. Rowan Chlebowski of University of California Los Angeles and Ross Prentice of the Fred Hutchinson Cancer Research Center in Seattle wrote.

Please remember that estrogen is an antioxidant.

4.2.0 0 Quercetin

4.2.1.0 Quercetin blocks EMOD induced apoptosis ==

The antioxidant, rather than prooxidant, activities of quercetin on normal cells: - quercetin protects mouse thymocytes from glucose oxidase-mediated apoptosis. (Lee J.-C.; Kim J.; Park J.-K.; Chung G.-H.; Jang Y.-S. Experimental Cell Research, Volume 291, Number 2, 10 December 2003 , pp. 386-397). **This indicates that the FRS drink advertised and promoted by Lance Armstrong is capable of blocking the oxidative killing of cancer cells.**

4.2.2.0 Quercetin acts as a prooxidant ==

The effects of **carnosine, rutin and quercetin on oxidative processes and metmyoglobin (MetMb)-reducing activity** in a beef model system were investigated. Ground beef was mixed with antioxidant solution at two concentrations. Storage period and antioxidant treatment negatively affected colour, colour stability and thiobarbituric acid-reactive substances values. Carnosine, rutin and to lesser extent quercetin accelerated discolouration, accumulation of MetMb and lipid peroxidation in the meat. The results suggest that **these antioxidants acted as a pro-oxidants under the specified experimental conditions.** The pro-oxidant activities were in the following order: carnosine>rutin>quercetin. The MetMb-reducing activity was not correlated with storage time, colour parameters, MetMb (%) or lipid oxidation. The MetMb-reducing activity was significantly reduced by 1 mM carnosine. However, there was no association between MetMb-reducing activity and colour stability during post-mortem storage (Pro-oxidant activities of carnosine, rutin and quercetin in a beef model system and their effects on the metmyoglobin-reducing activity. Bekhit, A.; Geesink, G.; Ilian, M.; Morton, J.; Sedcole, J.; Bickerstaffe, R. European Food Research and Technology A, Volume 218, Number 6, May 2004 , pp. 507-514).

4.2.3.0 Antioxidant and prooxidant effects of quercetin on GPDH

Anti- and prooxidant properties of quercetin under different conditions were investigated using glyceraldehyde-3-phosphate dehydrogenase, a glycolytic enzyme containing essential cysteine residues. **Quercetin was shown to produce hydrogen peroxide** in aqueous solutions at pH 7.5, this resulting in the oxidation of the cysteine residues of the enzyme. Quercetin significantly increased oxidation of GAPDH observed in the presence of ferrous ions, particularly when FeSO(4) was added to the solution containing GAPDH and quercetin. The results suggest **the formation of hydroxyl radical in the case of the addition of FeSO(4) to a quercetin solution.** At the same time, quercetin protects GAPDH from oxidation in the presence of ascorbate and Fe(3+). In the absence of metals, quercetin protects SH-groups of GAPDH from oxidation by the superoxide anion generated by the system containing xanthine/xanthine oxidase (Antioxidant and prooxidant effects of quercetin on glyceraldehyde-3-phosphate dehydrogenase. Food and chemical toxicology. 2007;45(10):1988-93)

4.3.0.0 Vitamin D

4.3.1.0 What you need to know about vitamin D

By SHARI ROAN. LOS ANGELES TIMES

December 11, 2008

The new star of the nutritional world is clearly vitamin D. Most people don't get enough of this wonder nutrient and increase their risk of several diseases by being deficient. In the past month, several major medical groups have called for a range of policy changes regarding vitamin D, including an increase in the current recommended daily allowance and new testing guidelines to look for deficiencies. Here's an update:

- **A group of 18 vitamin D researchers at the University of California has issued a "call to action," recommending that the daily intake of vitamin D for adults be revised by the government to 2,000 international units a day.** (The current recommendation is 200 IU for people up to age 50, 400 IU for people 51 to 70 and

600 IU for people 70 and older.) "While more research on this topic is highly desirable, it should not delay recommending a 2,000 IU daily intake of vitamin D for most people," a member of the consortium, Dr. Anthony Norman, said in a news release. An editorial on vitamin D by Norman, a University of California, Riverside biochemist, was published Monday in the American Journal of Clinical Nutrition.

- A review article published Tuesday in the Journal of the American College of Cardiology includes recommendations for screening for vitamin D deficiency and treatment in people with cardiovascular disease. The recommendations are needed, according to the authors of the paper, because of the growing body of evidence that links **vitamin D deficiency to cardiovascular problems.** They say that cardiovascular patients with a deficiency should receive 50,000 IU of vitamin D2 or D3 (forms of the vitamin) once a week for eight to 12 weeks followed by maintenance therapy.
- In October, the American Academy of Pediatrics published a recommendation that the amount of vitamin D for infants, children and adolescence should be doubled to 400 IU a day.

The American Academy of Pediatrics on Oct. 13, 2008, recommended a doubling of the amount of vitamin D children receive. The doctors, meeting this week in Boston, said infants, children and teenagers should get 400 international units of vitamin D each day, up from 200 IU that had been prescribed in the past.

The recommendation probably means that kids who don't already take a daily vitamin supplement will have to start. "Supplementation is important because most children will not get enough vitamin D through diet alone," said Dr. Frank Greer, chairman of the AAP Committee on Nutrition.

The new recommendation is aimed at preventing the bone-softening disease rickets in children. Adequate vitamin D intake, however, may also help prevent the future development of osteoporosis and other diseases. Research in adults shows vitamin D plays a key role in preventing infections, autoimmune diseases, cancer and diabetes.

The guidelines emphasize that infants who are breast-fed should begin receiving vitamin D supplements in the first few days of life because many women do not get enough vitamin D and their breast milk may be deficient. Non-breast-fed babies and older children who do not drink one quart per day of vitamin D fortified milk should also receive a supplement

Studies have linked vitamin D deficiency with an increased risk of hypertension, obesity, diabetes, heart attack, stroke and some types of cancer.

"Vitamin D deficiency is an unrecognized, emerging cardiovascular risk factor, which should be screened for and treated," Kansas City cardiologist James H. O'Keefe, a co-author of the JACC article, said in a news release. "Vitamin D is easy to assess, supplementation is simple, safe and inexpensive."

Optimal levels of vitamin D can be achieved by a combination of sunlight, supplements and foods such as fish, eggs and cod liver oil. Foods such as milk and some cereals are fortified with vitamin D but at levels that aim for 400 IU a day — which is now thought to be much too low. Vitamin D toxicity (taking too much) is rare but is possible if the intake is greater than 20,000 IU per day.

4.3.2.0 Please remember that vitamin D is a prooxidant.

Antioxidants are reducing agents, and limit oxidative damage to biological structures by passivating free radicals. **Passivation** is the process of making a material "passive" in relation to another material prior to using the materials together. **I do not believe that "passivation" is the basic process in redox reactions. Neither oxidizers nor reducers are rendered passive by their interaction.**

4.3.3.0 Vitamin D often low in mothers and newborns

More than one third of mothers and more than half of their infants have vitamin D deficiency at the time of birth, investigators report. What's more, prenatal vitamin D supplements do not fully protect against this deficiency, according to data released at Pediatric Academic Societies annual meeting 5-4-09.

Anne Merewood, Director of the Breastfeeding Center at Boston Medical Center, and her associates measured vitamin D levels in 433 women and 376 newborns using blood samples obtained within 72 hours of birth. They also collected data from questionnaires completed by the mothers and from the mothers' medical records. The results showed that **vitamin D deficiency was present in 36 percent of mothers and 58 percent of the babies. The deficiency was classified as severe in roughly two-thirds of the cases.**

Among women who took the vitamin D prenatally five or more times a week during the third trimester, more than 30 percent were still deficient at the time they gave birth.

Women who were vitamin D deficient at the time they gave birth were more than five times as likely to have an infant with vitamin D deficiency as women who were not vitamin D deficient.

Other risk factors for vitamin D deficiency in infants included winter birth versus summer birth, African American race, and severe maternal obesity.

Merewood called for measures to ensure that women of childbearing age maintain an adequate vitamin D intake. "The most obvious way to correct deficiency is sensible sun exposure," she said. "While a sunburn should be avoided, even a small amount of time spent outdoors was protective against deficiency." Other vitamin D sources include cod liver oil tablets, vitamin D fortified milk, and fatty fish, she said.

The Boston researcher emphasized that the results need to be interpreted cautiously given the ongoing debate among experts on the definition of vitamin D deficiency.

Few children who are technically classified as vitamin D deficient have any apparent physical signs of deficiency, she explained. "More research is needed to determine the exact definition of deficiency, especially in children."

4.3.4.0 Vitamin D prevents cancer

A review of 13 cancer registries found 416,134 cases of skin cancer and 3,776,501 cases of non-skin cancer as a first cancer. Rates from cancer registries in sunny countries (such as Australia and Spain) and less sunny countries (such as Canada and Iceland) were compared. The researchers concluded that **vitamin D production in the skin decreases the risk of several solid cancers, especially stomach, colorectal, liver and gallbladder, pancreas, lung, female breast, prostate, bladder, and kidney cancers.** The apparently protective effect of sun exposure against second primary cancer is more pronounced after non-melanoma skin cancers than melanoma.

Although some studies have reported an association between low blood levels of these antioxidant vitamins and a higher risk for cancer, supplements of vitamins A, C, and E appear to have few advantages in most cases. And there are some studies finding higher cancer risks with high intakes of antioxidants. For example, **a 2003 study reported a higher risk in melanoma in people with vitamin-C rich diets. Another study also reported a higher risk for cancer in male smokers who took multivitamins plus A, C, or E.**

Unfortunately, although it is clear that vitamins are required to prevent deficiency diseases, high doses of vitamin C, vitamin E, and beta carotene supplements may also have pro-oxidant effects, which can be harmful in patients with cancer. In these people, **high doses of antioxidant vitamins may actually protect cancer cells** just as they do healthy cells.

4.4.0.0 Antioxidants and the free radical myth

Both the reasons for the continued failure of antioxidant vitamins to demonstrate health benefits for degenerative diseases of aging in clinical trials, and for some studies to even suggest possible risks at doses above normal dietary levels, has to do with popularized misconceptions of the benefits of antioxidants and dangers of free radicals. Things aren't as black and white as that. **Free radicals actually play a role in normal, healthy physiological processes like our immune system and promote beneficial oxidation**; while in excess they can produce harmful oxidation that causes cell damage. Similarly, **many vitamins and supplements classified as antioxidants are actually *redox agents*, meaning they act as antioxidants in some instances and pro-oxidants in others** and can produce harmful levels of free radicals.

An editorial in the *Journal of the American Medical Association* accompanying the HOPE trials, written by researchers at the University of Washington School of Medicine in Seattle, said that the HOPE trials add **to a growing list of null clinical trials of vitamin E and effectively closes the door on the prospect of a major protective effect of this supplement for heart disease or cancer.** More importantly, the carefully done HOPE trial "reemphasizes the importance of controlled clinical trials for testing important hypotheses deriving from basic biological findings or from epidemiological observations. The latter can mislead; well designed clinical trials rarely do."

They added that this is a teaching opportunity:

> *HOPE-TOO allows physicians to educate their patients as with the following response to inquiries about vitamin E, "In nearly 68,000 patients studied to date,*

> *there is no compelling evidence that higher doses of vitamin E reduce cardiovascular risk or cancer; there are even some hints that vitamin E, in excess of normal daily intake, may slightly increase the risk of ischemic events or of heart failure. You may hear that vitamin E is a 'natural,' yet effective, way to prevent heart disease or cancer, but this has proven to be a false hope.*

The continued resistance to accepting the null findings of many of these clinical trials on vitamin and antioxidant supplements originates in another misconception of vitamins and supplements: that only natural sources of vitamins work and that they're different from synthetic versions. As explained in more depth here, **this is a marketing concept, but has no scientific basis or biological plausibility.** The molecular structure of a synthetic vitamin molecule is identical to one from natural sources and indistinguishable in all respects to our body.

Names can lead us to wrongly believe that one type of vitamin is less bioactive than another, such as vitamin E. The d-form (most often termed 'd-alpha tocopherol') comes form vegetable oils and other 'natural' sources. It's different from the dl-form (dl-tocopherol) commonly called the 'synthetic' type of vitamin E. But *biologically,* one isn't better than the other. That's because, to put it simply, the dl-form is a combination of d-form and l-form, but ***the body only uses the d-form.*** **The l-form is just excreted by the body.** So the *dosages will be different* on the labels of dl-form and d-forms (half) — but the bioeffective vitamin dose is the same.

'Natural' vitamins are said to have hundreds of other, unknown substances found in whole foods that aren't found in synthetic vitamins, but there are no credible clinical studies supporting such claims that these ingredients potentiate or improve the action or absorption of the vitamins or offer any special benefits. Vitamin pills extracted from foods undergo a process that changes their place in that food and it's implausible that the miniscule amount of some unknown factor that might survive that process in a tiny pill has any special vital essences or health promoting properties.

For men and their loved ones who may have had their lives shaken up this week by news of **the SELECT study being halted because of safety concerns**, hopefully, realizing that the risks weren't even statistically significant and seeing the bigger picture and the scientific evidence to date has helped. (http://junkfood-science.blogspot.com/2008/10/no-statistically-significant-risks-seen.html. Accessed 12-24-08.).

4.4.1.0 Oxidative aging theories lack support

The early observations on the rate-of-living theory by Max Rubner and the report by Gershman that oxygen free radicals exist in vivo culminated in the seminal proposal in the 1950s by Denham Harman that reactive oxygen species are a cause of aging (free radical theory of aging). The goal of this review was to analyze recent findings relevant in evaluating Harman's theory using experimental results as grouped by model organisms (i.e., invertebrate models and mice). In this regard, we have focused primarily on recent work involving genetic manipulations. Because the free radical theory of aging is not the only theorem proposed to explain the mechanism(s) involved in aging at the molecular level, we also discuss how this theory is related to other areas of research in biogerontology, specifically, telomere/cell senescence, genomic instability, and the mitochondrial hypothesis of aging. They also discuss where we think the free radical theory is headed.

It is now possible to give at least a partial answer to the question *whether oxidative stress determines life span* as Harman posed so long ago. Based on studies to date, we argue that **a tentative case for oxidative stress as a life-span determinant can be made in *Drosophila melanogaster*.** Studies in mice argue for a role of oxidative stress in age-related disease, especially cancer; however, **with regard to aging per se, the data either do not support or remain inconclusive on whether oxidative stress determines life span** (Trends in oxidative aging theories. Florian L. Muller, Michael S. Lustgarten, Youngmok Jang, Arlan Richardson and Holly Van Remmen. Free Radical Biology and Medicine. Volume 43, Issue 4, 15 August 2007, Pages 477-503).

4.4.2.0 The free radical theory and aging

(From Wikipedia) The free-radical theory of aging states that organisms age because cells accumulate free radical damage over time. A free radical is any atom or molecule that has a single unpaired electron in an outer shell. **While a few free radicals such as melanin are not chemically reactive,** most biologically-relevant free radicals are highly reactive. For most biological structures, free radical damage is closely associated with oxidative damage. **(RMH Note: this is not true.)** Antioxidants are reducing agents, and limit oxidative damage to biological structures by passivating free radicals.

Strictly speaking, the free radical theory is only concerned with free radicals, but it has since been expanded to encompass oxidative damage from reactive oxygen species such as O_2^-, H_2O_2, or OH_-. **Actually superoxide and the hydroxyl radicals are radicals but peroxide, singlet oxygen and hypochlorous acid are not radicals.**

Denham Harman first proposed the free radical theory of aging in the 1950s, and in the 1970s extended the idea to implicate mitochondrial production of reactive oxygen species (Harman, D (1956). "Aging: a theory based on free radical and radiation chemistry". *Journal of Gerontology* 11 (3): 298–300) (Harman, D (1972). "A biologic clock: the mitochondria?". *Journal of the American Geriatrics Society* 20 (4): 145–147).

In some model organisms, such as yeast and Drosophila, there is evidence that reducing oxidative damage does, as the theory would predict, extend lifespan. In mice, interventions that enhance oxidative damage generally shorten lifespan. **Whether reducing oxidative damage below normal levels is sufficient to extend lifespan remains an open and controversial question.**

The free radical theory of aging was conceived by Denham Harman in the 1950s, when prevailing scientific opinion held that free radicals were too unstable to exist in biological systems, and before anybody had invoked free radicals as a cause of degenerative diseases. Harman drew inspiration from two sources: 1) the rate of living theory, which holds that lifespan is an inverse function of metabolic rate, which is proportional to oxygen consumption; and 2) **Rebbeca Gershman's** observation that hyperbaric oxygen toxicity and radiation toxicity could be explained by the same underlying phenomenon: oxygen free radicals.

Noting that radiation causes "mutation, cancer and aging" **Harman argued that oxygen free radicals produced during normal respiration would cause cumulative damage which would eventually lead to organismal loss of functionality, and ultimately death. (RMH Note: But, he was wrong.).**

In later years, the free radical theory was expanded to include not only aging *per se*, but also age related diseases. **Free radical damage within cells has been linked to a range of disorders including cancer, arthritis, atherosclerosis, Alzheimer's disease, and diabetes.** Free radical chemistry is an important aspect of phagocytosis, inflammation, and apoptosis. Cell suicide, or apoptosis, is the body's way of controlling cell death and involves free radicals and redox signalling. Redox factors play an even greater part in other forms of cell death such as necrosis or autoschizis.

More recently, the relationship between disease and free radicals has led to the formulation of a greater generalization about the relationship between aging and free radicals. In its **"strong" form**, the hypothesis states that aging *per se* is a free radical process. The **"weak" hypothesis** holds that the degenerative diseases associated with aging generally involve free radical processes and that, cumulatively, these make you age. The latter is generally accepted, but the "strong" hypothesis is presently controversial pending further investigation. Both models trace back to Harman's work.

Evidence

- A large body of comparative biochemical evidence suggests that longer lived species exhibit decreased levels of oxidative damage, decreased susceptibility to oxidative stress, and decreased generation of reactive oxygen species.
- Results have demonstrated that **the overexpression of catalase, an enzyme involved in the decomposition of hydrogen peroxide, increased both the average lifespan and maximum lifespan of mice by 20%** (Schriner SE, Linford NJ, Martin GM, Treuting P, Ogburn CE, Emond M, Coskun PE, Ladiges W, Wolf N, Van Remmen H, Wallace DC, Rabinovitch PS (2005). "Extension of murine life span by overexpression of catalase targeted to mitochondria". *Science* 308 (5730): 1909–11). **However, the authors of that paper also indicated that the lifespan extension effect had apparently lessened in new generations of these mice.**
- Mutant strains of the roundworm *Caenorhabditis elegans* that are more susceptible to free radicals have shortened lifespans, and vice versa (Larsen P (1993). "Aging and resistance to oxidative damage in Caenorhabditis elegans". *Proc Natl Acad Sci U S A* 90 (19): 8905–9) (Ishii N (2000). "Oxidative stress and aging in Caenorhabditis elegans". *Free Radical Research* 33 (6): 857–64). **However, increasing atmospheric oxygen tension above the normal 21% O_2, does not meaningfully decrease lifespan of C. elegans.**
- **Drosophila that have mutations in enzymes relating to reactive oxygen species metabolism have also been shown to have dramatically reduced life-spans,** increased susceptibility to oxidative stress and ionizing radiation, partial female and complete male sterility, and a general "enfeebled" phenotype characterized by deformed wings and abdomen (Helfand S, Rogina B (2003). "Genetics of aging in the fruit fly, Drosophila melanogaster". *Annu Rev Genet* 37: 329–48) (T Parkes, K

Kirby, J Phillips, A Hilliker. 1998. "Transgenic analysis of the cSOD-null phenotypic syndrome in Drosophila". *Genome* 41: 642–651). **I believe that the shortened life span is related to a deficiency of SOD and consequently a deficiency in hydrogen peroxide.**

- While genetic manipulations that increase the levels of oxidative damage generally do shorten lifespan in mice, **there is at present very limited evidence that decreasing free radicals below their normal levels actually extends average or maximum lifespan.**
- **Consumption of high levels of antioxidants**, which should increase lifespan under the theory, **may extend average but not maximum lifespan in mice. The effect, if present, is weak and only inconsistently observed.**
- **Phenybutylnitrone (PBN) was shown to produce about a 10% extension of maximum lifespan in experimental animals** (Saito K, Yoshioka H, Cutler RG (1998). "A Spin Trap, N-*tert*-Butyl-α-phenylnitrone Extends the Life Span of Mice". *Bioscience, Biotechnology, and Biochemistry* 62 (4): 792–794) in one laboratory, **however, this finding has not been reproduced by other laboratories.**
- **Antioxidant supplementation has not been conclusively shown to produce an extension of lifespan in a mammal**

4.4.3.0 Mitohormesis: increased EMODs increased lifespan

Oxidative stress may promote life expectancy of *Caenorhabditis elegans* by inducing a secondary response to initially increased levels of reactive oxygen species (Schulz TJ, Zarse K, Voigt A, Urban N, Birringer M, Ristow M (2007). "Glucose restriction extends Caenorhabditis elegans life span by inducing mitochondrial respiration and increasing oxidative stress". *Cell Metabolism* 6 (4): 280–93).

This observation was initially named **mitohormesis, or mitochondrial hormesis** on a purely hypothetical basis (Tapia PC (2006/2005(epub)). **"Sublethal mitochondrial stress with an attendant stoichiometric augmentation of reactive oxygen species may precipitate many of the beneficial alterations in cellular physiology produced by caloric restriction, intermittent fasting, exercise and dietary phytonutrients**: "Mitohormesis" for health and vitality". *Medical Hypotheses* 66 (4): 832–43).

In mammals, the question of the net effect of reactive oxygen species on aging is even less clear (Sohal R, Mockett R, Orr W (2002). "Mechanisms of aging: an appraisal of the oxidative stress hypothesis". *Free Radic Biol Med* 33 (5): 575–86) (Sohal R (2002). "Role of oxidative stress and protein oxidation in the aging process". *Free Radic Biol Med* 33 (1): 37–44) (Rattan S (2006)."Theories of biological aging: genes, proteins, and free radicals". *Free Radic Res* 40 (12): 1230–8).

Recent epidemiological findings do not support the process of mitohormesis in humans, and even suggest that antioxidants may increase disease prevalence in humans (Bjelakovic G, Nikolova D, Gluud LL, Simonetti RG, Gluud C (2007)."Mortality in randomized trials of antioxidant supplements for primary and secondary prevention: systematic review and meta-analysis". *The Journal of the American Medical Association* 297 (8): 842–57).

4.4.4.0 Calorie restriction

Severe caloric restriction has been found to reduce reactive oxidative species and to increase the life-span of rodents, possibly by promoting mitohormesis. Studies have shown that both calorie restriction and reduced meal frequency or intermittent fasting can suppress the development of various diseases and can increase life span in rodents by 30-40% by mechanisms involving stress resistance and reduced oxidative damage. **Extreme calorie restriction, over 50%, resulted in increased mortality** (Mattson MP (2005)."Energy intake, meal frequency, and health: a neurobiological perspective". *Annual Review of Nutrition* 25 (25): 237–60) (Schulz TJ, Zarse K, Voigt A, Urban N, Birringer M, Ristow M (2007)."Glucose restriction extends Caenorhabditis elegans life span by inducing mitochondrial respiration and increasing oxidative stress". *Cell Metabolism* 6 (4): 280–93).

One of the most prominent proponents of calorie restriction as a way to longer life was the late Dr. Roy Walford (*1924-2004*), formerly Professor of Pathology at the University of California, Los Angeles School of Medicine. **Dr. Walford died of Amyotrophic Lateral Sclerosis (ALS).**

4.4.5.0 EMODs may add to longevity and antioxidants may be harmful

The precise mechanistic sequence producing the beneficial effects on health and lifespan seen with interventions as diverse as caloric restriction, intermittent fasting, exercise, and consumption of dietary phytonutrients is still under active characterization, with large swaths of the research community kept in relative isolation from one another. Among the explanatory models capable of assisting in the identification of precipitating elements responsible for beneficial influences on physiology seen in these states, the hormesis perspective on biological systems under stress has yielded considerable insight into likely evolutionarily consistent organizing principles functioning in all four conditions. Recent experimental findings provide the tantalizing initial lodestones for an entirely new research front examining molecular substrates of stress resistance. In this novel body of research, a surprising new twist has emerged: **Reactive oxygen species, derived from the mitochondrial electron transport system, may be necessary triggering elements for a sequence of events that result in benefits ranging from the transiently cytoprotective to organismal-level longevity.**

With the recent appreciation that reactive oxygen species and reactive nitrogen species function as signaling elements in a interconnected matrix of signal transduction, the entire basis of many widely accepted theories of aging that predominated in the past may need to be reconsidered to facilitate the formulation of **a new perspective more correctly informed by the most contemporaneous experimental findings.** This perspective, the mitohormesis theory, can be used in many disparate domains of inquiry to potentially explain previous findings, as well as point to new targets of research. The utility of this perspective for research on aging is significant, but beyond that this perspective emphasizes the pressing need to rigorously characterize the specific contribution of **the stoichiometry of reactive oxygen species and reactive nitrogen species in the various compartments of the cell to cytoprotection and vitality.** Previous findings regarding the influences of free radical chemistry on cellular physiology may have represented assessments examining the consequences of isolated elevation of signaling elements within a larger signal transductive apparatus, rather than definitive characterizations of the only modality of reactive oxygen species (and reactive nitrogen species) influence. In applying this perspective, it may be necessary for the research community, as well as the practicing clinician, to engender a more sanguine perspective on organelle level physiology, as **it is now plausible that such entities have an evolutionarily orchestrated capacity to self-regulate that may be pathologically disturbed by overzealous use of antioxidants, particularly in the healthy** (Tapia PC (2006/2005(epub)). **"Sublethal mitochondrial stress with an attendant stoichiometric augmentation of reactive oxygen species may precipitate many of the beneficial alterations in cellular physiology produced by caloric restriction, intermittent fasting, exercise and dietary phytonutrients**: "Mitohormesis" for health and vitality". *Medical Hypotheses* 66 (4): 832–43).

4.4.6.0 EMODs challenge dogma: EMODs are anti-inflammatory

For a long time, reactive oxygen species (ROS) produced by the phagocyte NADPH oxidase (NOX2) complex have been considered harmful mediators of inflammation owing to their highly reactive nature. However, **there are an increasing number of findings suggesting that ROS produced by the**

NOX2 complex are anti-inflammatory and prevent autoimmune responses, thus challenging existing dogma. ROS might not only be produced as a mechanism to eradicate invading pathogens, but rather as a means by which to fine-tune the inflammatory response, depending on when, where and at what amounts they are produced. In this review, we aim to describe the current findings highlighting ROS as regulators of autoimmune inflammation, focusing on autoimmune arthritis (Trends Immunol (2009) 0:The protective role of ROS in autoimmune disease. M Hultqvist, LM Olsson, KA Gelderman, R Holmdahl).

4.4.7.0 Inconsistencies of the free radical theory

The present state of the mitochondrial free radical theory of aging is reviewed. **Available studies do not support the hypothesis that antioxidants control the rate of aging because: (a) they correlate inversely with maximum longevity in vertebrates, and (b) increasing their concentration by different methods does not increase maximum lifespan.**

On the other hand, comparative studies consistently show that long-lived mammals and birds have low rates of mitochondrial reactive oxygen species (ROS) production and low levels of oxidative damage in their mitochondrial DNA. Furthermore, **caloric restriction, which extends longevity, also decreases mitochondrial ROS production at complex I and lowers mtDNA oxidative damage.**

Recent data show that these changes can also be obtained with protein restriction without strong caloric restriction. **Another trait of long-lived mammals and birds is the possession of low degrees of unsaturation in their cellular membranes. I believe that the lower levels of unsaturated lipids, which serve as EMOD traps, helps avoid an EMOD insufficiency state, which helps to maintain adequate EMOD levels and to decrease disease and helps prevent aging.**

This is mainly due to minimizing the presence of highly unsaturated fatty acids such as 22:6n-3 and emphasizing the presence of less unsaturated fatty acids such as 18:2n-6 in long-lived animals, without changing the total amount of polyunsaturated fatty acids. This leads to lower levels of lipid peroxidation and lipoxidation-derived protein modification in long-lived species. **Taken together, available information is consistent with the predictions of the mitochondrial free radical theory of aging, although definitive proof and many mechanistic details are still lacking** (Is the mitochondrial free radical theory of aging intact? Sanz A, Pamplona R, Barja G. Antioxid Redox Signal. 2006 Mar-Apr;8(3-4):582-99). Actually, any real proof is lacking.

4.5.0.0 Synta anticancer mechanism: STA-4783 causes EMOD apoptosis. NAC blocks apoptosis ==

By Mike Nagle, 01-Oct-2007

Although it is over forty years since scientists realised cancer cells don't have the anti-oxidant protective capabilities of normal cells, it seems that only one pharma company has developed a drug to exploit this fact. Synta Pharmaceuticals, based in Massachusetts, US, is preparing to test its lead drug, STA-4783, on skin cancer patients in the final stage of clinical development.

"We are all taught free radicals are really bad, but scientists have found that cancer cells have increased levels of ROS and their ability to keep that in check is severely compromised," explained Dr Tony Williams, vice president of clinical research at the company.

By increasing the number of reactive oxygen species (ROS) in cells, STA-4783 can tip tumors cells beyond the breaking point into a death pathway (apoptosis). While these cells die, normal cells have less ROS and can shield themselves against the drug's effects.

In fact, when the drug has been tested in normal cell lines, there is no measurable increase in ROS levels, according to Williams.

Although the interest in this mechanism has rocketed in recent years (in 2006, there were over 3500 papers in journals about it, almost doubling the total number ever), Synta claims to be the only pharmaceutical industry pursuing it.

Williams explained that although some anticancer drugs increase ROS levels indirectly to a lesser extent, none do it as or directly, like Synta's molecule. The drug is not potent enough to work as a monotherapy unless the dose is dangerously high, said Williams; instead the drug is seen as a method of increasing a cell's sensitivity to chemotherapy. In this setting, it has shown promising results in clinical studies so far. Dr Williams was speaking to DrugResearcher.com before presenting the Phase II trial results to delegates at the European Congress of Clinical Oncology (ECCO) in Barcelona, Spain.

"The median progression free survival was 1.8 months in the group who got chemotherapy alone, but 3.7 months in the group who got the combination," he said. "This doubling in progression free survival is impressive for this cancer, *and the result was achieved without substantial additional toxicity."*

He added: *"Progression-free survival was linked to improvements in overall survival. Patients on the experimental combination survived on average for 12 months after being diagnosed, while those getting only paclitaxel survived on average 7.8 months.* ***This is the first time an improvement in survival has been seen in a randomised, double-blind, multi-centre controlled trial for metastatic melanoma."***

While investigating the drug's mechanism, the team at Synta discovered that **once melanoma cells are exposed to the drug, levels of Heat Shock Protein 70 (Hsp70) shoot up over 300-fold in just one to three hours.** However, this is a "futile response," said Williams and over the next two to three hours, a switch inside the cell's mitochondria is triggered and the cells begin to die.

Although Hsp70 is not the target of the drug, as some have mistakenly thought, the increase in Hsp70 is, however, useful as a biomarker to prove the therapy is working. **For example, if the drug is given alongside antioxidants (such as NAC, N-AcetylCysteine), no extra Hsp70 is produced and the cells survive as normal.**

Williams said the company is unwilling to disclose the target as yet but hopes to soon once the programme is fully protected in terms of intellectual property (IP).

NAC is normally administered to people who have taken a paracetamol (acetaminophen) overdose, and Williams assured DrugResearcher.com that normal dietary levels of antioxidants shouldn't prevent STA-4783 from working, although he did say that **patients in the upcoming Phase III trial were told not to take any vitamin E supplements (an antioxidant).**

Melanoma is easily treated with surgery in its early stages and five-year survival rates are 99 per cent for localised disease, according to the American Cancer Society. However, once the cancer progresses to later stage, metastatic disease, survival rates plummet to just 15 per cent. STA-4783 is being tested in patients with advanced disease (stage IV metastatic melanoma), who desperately need more treatment options.

Most of the world's biggest pharma companies are developing drugs for melanoma. Pfizer's CP-675206 (tremelimumab/ticilimumab) and Bristol-Myers Squibb's (BMS) ipilimumab are both in Phase III clinical trials, the latter being developed in conjunction with Medarex. The drugs are antibodies against cytotoxic T-lymphocyte antigen-4 (CTLA-4), which is thought to suppress the immune system's T cell response to cancer.

AstraZeneca is testing a MEK inhibitor in Phase II trials. MEK is so called after the MAPK/ERK kinase pathway it belongs to. This cascade of extracellular signal-regulated kinases (ERK) or mitogen-activated protein kinases (MEPK) are thought to be involved in a number of processes that promote cancer, including cell growth and survival.

Novartis is utilising a different target in the same pathway, namely b-RAF kinase to design melanoma drugs. RAF265 is currently in Phase I clinical trials. Roche and Plexxikon's PLX4032/R7204 is at the same stage of development and targets the same protein.

Genzyme is looking at a transforming growth factor (TGF)-beta inhibitor, GC-1008, as a means of treating melanoma in Phase I/II clinical trials. Astellas Pharma's YM155, a survivin expression inhibitor is in Phase II trials.

With these and other melanoma drugs filling oncology pipelines globally, the outlook for patients with advanced melanoma might not be so bleak in the future.

This is not as good as my singlet oxygen generating system, which I could not get patented.

4.5.1.0 Brain plays key role in appetite by regulating free radicals: appetite controlled by EMODs

July 30, 2008 - 12:36 in Health & Medicine

Researchers at Yale School of Medicine have found **the brain's appetite center uses fat for fuel by involving oxygen free radicals**—molecules associated with aging and neurodegeneration. The findings, reported in the **journal *Nature***, suggest that antioxidants could play a role in weight control. The study's lead authors were Sabrina Diano and Tamas Horvath, who are an associate professor and professor, respectively, in the Departments of Obstetrics, Gynecology & Reproductive Sciences and Neurobiology. Horvath is also chair of the Section of Comparative Medicine.

"In contrast to the accepted view, the brain does use fat as fuel," said Horvath. "Our study shows that **the minute-by-minute control of appetite is regulated by free radicals, implying that if you interfere with free radicals, you may affect eating and satiety**."

The results also imply, added Horvath, "that each time a feeling of fullness or satiety is reached during a meal, you may be chipping away some time from your maximum lifespan as **the most free radicals are produced when satiety-promoting brain cells are active."**

Diano, Horvath and colleagues conducted the study in mice to better understand how the brain mediates neuronal activation in response to ghrelin, a hormone produced in the stomach and previously associated with growth hormone release, appetite, learning and memory.

They found that **ghrelin-induced increase in appetite is driven by burning fat in hypothalamic mitochondria, which produces free radicals that are scavenged by a mitochondrial protein called uncoupling protein 2 (UCP2).**

"The timing of taking antioxidants may be critical for the control of appetite," said Diano. **"If taken on an empty stomach antioxidants may further increase appetite**, however when taken with food, they may affect satiety. Further studies are needed to determine whether any regiment of orally taken antioxidants could be used to control appetite in animals and humans."

4.5.2.0 Exercise suppresses appetite by affecting appetite hormones

(Dec. 11, 2008) – A vigorous 60-minute workout on a treadmill affects the release of two key appetite hormones, ghrelin and peptide YY, while 90 minutes of weight lifting affects the level of only ghrelin, according to a new study. Taken together, the research shows that aerobic exercise is better at suppressing appetite than non-aerobic exercise and provides a possible explanation for how that happens. This line of research may eventually lead to more effective ways to use exercise to help control weight, according to the senior author, David J. Stensel of Loughborough University in the United Kingdom.

The study, "The influence of resistance and aerobic exercise on hunger, circulating levels of acylated ghrelin and peptide YY in healthy males," appears in the online edition of the *American Journal of Physiology-Regulatory, Integrative and Comparative Physiology*, published by The American Physiological Society. The authors are David R. Broom, James A. King and David J. Stensel of Loughborough University, and Rachel L. Batterham of University College, London. **I believe that exercise is increasing EMODs, which are limiting appetite, as in the above paper by** Sabrina Diano and Tamas Horvath.

4.5.3.0 Treadmill versus weight lifting

There are several hormones that help regulate appetite, but the researchers looked at two of the major ones, ghrelin and peptide YY. Ghrelin is the only hormone known to stimulate appetite. Peptide YY suppresses appetite.

Ghrelin was discovered by researchers in Japan only about 10 years ago and was originally identified for its role as a growth hormone. Only later did its role in stimulating appetite become known. Peptide YY was discovered less than 25 years ago.

In this experiment, 11 male university students did three eight-hour sessions. During one session they ran for 60 minutes on a treadmill, and then rested for seven hours. During another session they did 90 minutes of weight lifting, and then rested for six hours and 30 minutes. During another session, the participants did not exercise at all.

During each of the sessions, the participants filled out surveys in which they rated how hungry they felt at various points. They also received two meals during each session. The researchers measured ghrelin and peptide YY levels at multiple points along the way.

They found that the treadmill (aerobic) session caused ghrelin levels to drop and peptide YY levels to increase, indicating the hormones were suppressing appetite. However, a weight-lifting (non-aerobic) session produced a mixed result. Ghrelin levels dropped, indicating appetite suppression, but peptide YY levels did not change significantly.

Based on the hunger ratings the participants filled out, both aerobic and resistance exercise suppressed hunger, but aerobic exercise produced a greater suppression of hunger. The changes the researchers observed were short term for both types of exercise, lasting about two hours, including the time spent exercising, Stensel reported.

"The finding that hunger is suppressed during and immediately after vigorous treadmill running is consistent with previous studies indicating that strenuous aerobic exercise transiently suppresses appetite," Stensel said. "The findings suggest a similar, although slightly attenuated response, for weight lifting exercise."

4.5.4.0 Focus on active ghrelin

Previous studies have been inconclusive about whether exercise decreases ghrelin levels, but this study may help explain those mixed results, according to the researchers.

Ghrelin comes in two forms, acylated and non-acylated.The researchers measured acylated ghrelin, also called active ghrelin, because it can cross the blood-brain barrier and reach the appetite center in the brain. Stensel suggests that future research concentrate on active ghrelin.

While the study showed that exercise suppresses appetite hormones, the next step is to establish whether this change actually causes the suppression of eating.

4.6.0 0 Asbestos increases antioxidant enzymes

Despite numerous experiments, **the cytotoxicity of asbestos is still far from being well understood.** There is increasing evidence which supports the contribution of free oxy-radicals resulting from the phagocytosis of asbestos fibres concerning macrophages neutrophils, pulmonary epithelial and endothelial cells. **Both in vitro and in vivo studies revealed an asbestos-induced generation of hydrogen peroxide, hydroxyl radical and superoxide anion.** The intensity of the process varies with the physico-chemical properties of the asbestos fibres. Oxygen free radical activity accounts for the lipid peroxidation of cell membranes as well as for the damage of structural proteins and DNA. **However, the cells contain antioxidant enzymes such as catalase, superoxide dismutase, etc., which prevent the toxic effect of oxidants. Their activity increases when the cells are exposed to asbestos** (The role of oxygen free radicals in asbestos cytotoxicity. Lewczuk E, Owczarek H. Med Pr. 1992;43(4):335-42). **I believe that we may have again tricked mother nature. Asbestos is a synthetic chemical, which was not part of the evolutionary process. WBCs engulf it and generate EMODs trying to destroy it, but it is basically indestructible. Our cells have not yet learned how to successfully deal with this situation, just as it has not learned how to deal with ishcemia reperfusion.**

4.6.1.0 Free oxygen radicals and kidney diseases--part I

ADVERSE EFFECTS OF OXYGEN: **Adverse effect of oxygen on anaerobes implies oxidation of the basic cell constituents NAD(P)H, thiols,**

iron-sulphur proteins, pteridines and others) and inactivation of the essential components of the active site of enzymes. Oxygen can also adversely affect the aerobes, especially if long-term influence is taken into consideration, while exposition to high-pressure oxygen causes considerable damages. Direct influence of oxygen on aerobes due to slow and limited enzyme inactivation (for example glutamate decarboxylase) and small number of affected "targets" is not responsible for total adverse effects of oxygen. Even in 1954 it was supposed that oxygen free radicals are the most responsible for the adverse effects of oxygen.

ATMOSPHERIC (TRIPLET) OXYGEN: **Electron configuration of triplet oxygen explains its reactivity since it is a biradical.** The reactions of oxygen with non-radicals are possible with participation of transition metals **(except zinc),** while its reactivity is much more expressed in case of reactions with other radical species.

ACTIVE OXYGEN: More reactive forms of oxygen, known as singlet oxygen, can be generated by an input of energy to triplet oxygen. **Singlet-oxygen is obtained mainly by photoexcitation in the presence of initiators (methylene blue, chlorophyll etc.) and as a product of reactions of ozone with certain biomolecules.**

REDUCED FORMS OF OXYGEN: **If a single electron is added to the triplet oxygen, it must enter one of the antibonding molecular orbitals** and produce the superoxide radical--(O2.-). Addition of one more electron produces peroxide ion--O2(2-), which forms **hydro peroxide in presence of H+, the most common two-electron reduction product of oxygen in biological systems. The four-reduction product of oxygen in biological systems is water.**

SUPEROXIDE RADICAL: The in vivo production of superoxide radical is possible in many different ways mentioned in this paper. This radical species is unstable in water solutions because of dismutation reaction leading to non-enzymic generation of hydroperoxide. The most reactive radical species--hydroxyl radical is produced from hydro peroxide by Fenton or Haber-Weiss reactions in the presence of catalytic transition metals (iron or copper).

HYDROXYL RADICAL: Hydroxyl radicals are the most reactive radical species. The way of their generation has been shown in detail in this paper with special emphasis given to Fenton and Haber-Weiss reactions, that is, transition metals (iron and copper) as **catalizators** for these reactions. The reactivity of hydroxyl radical can be recognized by monitoring the second-order rate constants for reactions of the hydroxyl radical with some organic compounds in aqueous solution presented in this paper. Although the number of compounds that can be affected and damaged by hydroxyl radicals is great, until now, attention has been paid mostly to investigation of attacks of these radical species on lipids, proteins and DNA.

LIPID PEROXIDATION: Radicals react with lipids and cause oxidative destruction of unsaturated, that is, polyunsaturated fatty acids, known as lipid peroxidation. Both lipids in biological systems and lipids as food constituents are submitted to this process. Lipid peroxidation is a chain reaction and its mechanism has been shown in detail in this paper. Lipid peroxidation in cells leads to direct damage of cell membranes with indirect damages of other cell constituents, caused by reactivity of secondary products of this reaction, aldehydes. This complex reaction is responsible for damages of many tissues and progress of some diseases (atherosclerosis).

OXIDATIVE STRESS: Protection of an organism from oxygen free radicals implies activity of enzymatic (catalase, SOD, glutathione peroxidase, glutathione reductase etc.) and nonenzymatic (vitamin E. vitamin C. glutathione, uric acid etc.) systems of protection. Disturbance of the balance between production of oxygen free radicals (or some other radical species) and activity of antioxidative system of protection causes the **so called oxidative stress. An organism can tolerate a mild oxidative stress** but a higher disturbance between the production of free radicals and the activity of the antioxidative protection results in lipid, protein and DNA as well as numerous diseases (Free oxygen radicals and kidney diseases--part I. Sakac V, Sakac M. Med Pregl. 2000 Sep-Oct;53(9-10):463-74).

4.7.0.0 The eye

The cornea has no blood vessels and the lens sits behind it. Clouding of the lens is due to cataract formation. **Some are born with cataracts, which I believe discounts the theory that they are caused by EMODs, since there is no time for stochastic accumulation of ROS. Also, the lens has no blood vessels.**

Actually, EMODs are used with photodynamic therapy to repair macular degeneration.

4.7.1.0 Cataracts

Although older age is the primary risk factor for cataracts, experts are **still not certain about the exact biologic mechanisms that tie cataracts to aging.**

One of the functions of the human lens is filter light between 300–400 nm from reaching the retina. The lens is therefore continually under photooxidative stress. It can be concluded that light is most likely one of the causative factors in cataractogenesis.

A readily oxidized compound, such as the primate UV filter 3OHKyn. represents an oxidative stress within the lens and that **such oxidative processes can be exacerbated if the concentration of oxygen within the lens is increased**. This factor may account for the evolution of **unusually high levels of glutathione reductase in human lenses. I believe that this may be part of the problem, i.e., high antioxidant levels cause an EMOD insufficiency and does not allow for oxidation to breakdown the pre-cataractous aggregates.**

Some ot the following was taken from: The Photobiology of the Human Lens by Joan E. Roberts. http://www.photobiology.info/AdvModsVisionRoberts.asp.html. Accessed 12-23-08.

Oxygen Tension. **The oxygen tension in the lens is very low** (Roberts, McLaurn) **but is sufficient for photooxidation to occur**.

Defense Systems. The lens has a very efficient defense system. **The lens contains antioxidant enzymes, superoxide dismutase (SOD) and catalase, and antioxidants (e.g. Vitamin E, C, lutein, glutathione)** that serve to protect it against oxidative and photoinduced damage. Unfortunately, **most of these antioxidants and protective enzymes decrease beginning at forty years of age** and leaving the lens defenseless against light damage.

Repair. Although the retina and cornea repair light damage very efficiently, **the lens does not.** The peripheral lens epithelial cells are able to repair UV-B induced DNA cross-links (cyclobutane pyrimidine dimers and 6-4 pyrimidine-pyrimidone) (Andley et al, 1999), but any additional exposure to UV-A (Zigman et al 2000) or UV-B(Andley et al, 1999; Ayala et al, 2000) interferes with cell repair.

As there is little turnover of lens proteins, damage to lens proteins acumulates.

4.7.2.0 Mechanisms of Light Damage to the Lens

Ocular damage from light can occur through either an inflammatory response or a photooxidation reaction. In an inflammatory response, an initial insult to the tissue provokes a cascade of events that eventually results in wider damage to the tissue. This damage generally develops over at least twenty-four hours and in the lens is usually associated with the very short, high intensity wavelengths of UV-B.

The eye is immune privileged, which means that there is a very limited immune response when this organ is provoked. When this severe insult to the lens occurs, there is a release of interleukin I (IL-I) which summons macrophages to come into the damaged part of the eye. **These macrophages then release a cascade of reactive oxygen and reactive nitrogen species that then damage that portion of the eye.**

With less intense light, the eye is damaged through a phototoxidation reaction. In photooxidation reactions, a chromophore in the eye absorbs light and oxidizes certain amino acids and/or nucleic acids which results in damage to the whole lens. The chromophore may be endogenous (natural) or exogenous (a dye, cosmetic or drug that has accumulated in the eye). Absorption of light excites the chromophore to an excited singlet state, which then undergoes intersystem crossing and reaches the triplet state. In its triplet state, the chromophore then proceeds either via a Type I (free radical) or Type II **(singlet oxygen)** mechanism to cause the eventual damage. Photooxidation can occur in the lens can proceed by either a Type I or a Type II mechanism or both concurrently.

The chromophores is the adult human lens may be excited by light but they come down from this excited state (singlet) very quickly (nanoseconds) and so they don't have the chance of reaching a triplet state, making damaging active intermediates and therefore causing damage in the lens. However when the efficient photosensitizers, xanthurenic acid, it's glucoside and n-formyl kynurenine are present in the lens and the lens is exposed to UV radiation, they are capable are making triplets with sufficient efficiency (quantum yield) to **form reactive oxygen species** and free radicals which then in turn damage lens tissue.

4.7.3.0 Cataracts

The orderly arrangement of protein fibers in the lens normally causes the lens to be highly transparent. As the lens proteins (alpha, ß, gamma crystallins) become denatured or the lens epithelial cells can not longer repair damage from either chronic exposure to sunlight or short term exposure to sunlight in the presence of a photosensitizing medication, there is a resultant loss of transparency. The lens becomes finally becomes sufficiently cloudy to obstruct vision, and the individual is said to have a cataract. Cataracts reduce vision by scattering light and limiting the ability both to resolve and see contrast (Chylack, 1998).

Maintenance of structural integrity is particularly important for lens alpha -crystallin because of its role as a molecular chaperone. alpha -Crystallin is an aggregate of two polypeptides, alpha A and alpha B, which are small heat shock proteins that prevent ultraviolet (A and B) induced protein aggregation [93,94]. *Another study identified the specific amino acids that are modified in photooxidation of* alpha *-crystallin (Finley et al, 1997).*

By adding and removing alpha -crystallin production from lens epithelial cells, Andley has shown α-crystallin confers natural protection against UV light damage to these lens cells. [Andley, 1998, 2000]. alpha -Crystallin also protects against UVA inhibition of protective (catalase) enzyme activity (Horwitz and Zigman, 1997). The specific sites of damage to alpha -crystallin with both endogenous and exogenous chromophores have been detected using mass spectrometry.

Additional information on the mechanism of cataract induction has been possible now that human lens epithelial cells have been immortalized. It has been found that both UV-A and UV-B induce precataractous changes. Other specific targets for damage by UV-A radiation are lens cell membrane lipids, the **antioxidant enzyme catalase**, and the cytoskeletal elements of human and rabbit lens epithelial cells in culture.

4.7.4.0 Protection of the Lens Against Light Damage: antioxidants

The lens may be completely protected from light damage by removing UV A and B transmission with sunglass with appropriate filters. However these glasses must also be wrap around glasses (Sliney) to block reflective light or ***more*** rather than less damage may occur.

Another approach is to **supplement the age related decreased levels of antioxidants in the lens, with vitamins and antioxidants** present in fruits and vegetables. **But it must be the right combination of antioxidants** (Truscott et al.) for instance, Vitamin E, lutein, cysteine or N-acetyl cysteine (to replace glutathione) (Roberts et al.) **or the supplementation will not be effective in retarding age related cataracts [NIH study].** Green tea, which contains polyphenols (epigallocatechin gallate), has also been shown to retard light induced damage to the lens [Zigman, 100]. Other nutrients and botanicals, which may benefit cataract patients or help prevent cataracts, include pantethine, folic acid and bilberry. **I believe that there has been an overall failure of the antioxidants to either protect or reverse cataract formation.**

4.7.5.0 Conclusion

We have known for some time that exposure to intense sunlight either causes or exacerbates age-related cataracts diseases. Also, it is now clear that light damage can be enhanced by certain dyes and drugs, **and be enhanced or prevented by herbal supplements and vitamins. (RMH Note: That is not true.)**

In the future, earlier diagnosis, in conjunction with ocular protection against light (sunglasses) and prescribed specific supplementary antioxidants (lutein, zeaxanthin, vitamin E) may retard or eliminate this blinding disorder in the elderly. (**The Photobiology of the Human Lens** by Joan E. Roberts. http://www.photobiology.info/AdvModsVisionRoberts.asp.html).

4.8.0.0 Congenital cataracts

Congenital cataracts usually are diagnosed at birth. If a cataract goes undetected in an infant, permanent visual loss may ensue. Unilateral cataracts are usually isolated sporadic incidents. They can be associated with ocular abnormalities (eg, posterior lenticonus, persistent hyperplastic primary vitreous, anterior segment dysgenesis, posterior pole tumors), trauma, or intrauterine infection, particularly rubella.

Bilateral cataracts are often inherited and associated with other diseases. They require a full metabolic, infectious, systemic, and genetic workup. **The common causes are hypoglycemia, trisomy (eg, Down, Edward, and Patau syndromes), myotonic dystrophy, infectious diseases (eg, toxoplasmosis, rubella, cytomegalovirus, and herpes simplex [TORCH]), and prematurity.**

Incidence is unknown. Although the World Health Organization and other health organizations have made outstanding strides in vaccinations and disease prevention, the rate of congenital cataracts is probably much higher in underdeveloped countries.

- Metabolic and systemic diseases are found in as many as 60% of bilateral cataracts. Some cataracts are static, but some are progressive. This explains why not all congenital cataracts are identified at birth.

Leukocoria or white reflex can be the presenting sign of a cataract. In fact, in a 2008 study by Haider et al, 60% of patients who presented with leukocoria had congenital cataracts (18% unilateral and 42% bilateral). Other causes included **retinoblastoma** (11% unilateral and 7% bilateral), retinal detachment (2.8% unilateral and 1.4% bilateral), bilateral persistent hyperplastic primary vitreous (4.2%), and unilateral Coats disease (4.2%).

4.8.1.0 Causes

- The most common etiology includes intrauterine infections, metabolic disorders, and genetically transmitted syndromes. **One third of pediatric cataracts are sporadic;** they are not associated with any systemic or ocular diseases. However, they may be spontaneous mutations and may lead to cataract formation in the patient's offspring. As many as **23% of congenital cataracts are familial.** The most frequent mode of transmission is autosomal dominant with complete penetrance. This type of cataract may appear as a total cataract, polar cataract, lamellar cataract, or nuclear opacity. All close family members should be examined.
- Infectious causes of cataracts include **rubella (the most common), rubeola, chicken pox, cytomegalovirus, herpes simplex, herpes zoster, poliomyelitis, influenza, Epstein-Barr virus, syphilis, and toxoplasmosis.**

I believe that congenital cataracts negate the theory of oxidative stress as being causal of cataracts. Also, if cataracts are due to EMODs, adults should have primarily equally developed bilateral cataracts, but that is not the case. Also, the association of cataracts with infections indicates to me that these patients have low EMOD levels because they can not get rid of the infections and are also subject of allowance of cataract formation.

The lens of the eye is behind the iris, which is the colored part of the eye. The lens changes its shape to focus light onto the retina. **About 35% of the lens is**

made up of protein and the remaining 65% is water. As people age, the lens' proteins can naturally deteriorate, which can cause cataracts. Congenital cataracts in newborns are caused by genetic defects or an infection or disease in the mother during pregnancy. Traumatic cataracts are caused by a foreign body entering or trauma to the lens or eye. People with illnesses such as diabetes and eye diseases can have cataracts as complications, which is why these types are called complicated cataracts. Cataracts can also be caused from exposure to chemicals, such as **steroids**, and from exposure to the sun's ultraviolet (UV) rays. Lifestyle factors, such as smoking, alcohol consumption, and a diet high in saturated fats may also contribute to the formation of cataracts.

Congenital cataracts may be inherited. **The gene for such cataracts is dominant (autosomal dominant inheritance), which means that the defective gene will cause the condition even if only one parent passes it along.** In families where one parent carries the gene, there is a 50% chance in every pregnancy that the child will be affected.

Congenital cataracts can also be caused by infections affecting the mother during pregnancy, such as rubella. They are also associated with metabolic disorders such as galactosemia. Risk factors include inherited metabolic diseases, a family history of cataracts, and maternal viral infection during pregnancy.

4.9.0.0 Sugar Cataracts

There is strong evidence to show that diabetes is associated with increased oxidative stress. However, the source of this oxidative stress remains unclear. Using transgenic mice that **overexpress aldose reductase (AR)** in their lenses, we found that the flux of glucose through the polyol pathway is the major cause of hyperglycemic oxidative stress in this tissue. The substantial decrease in the level of reduced glutathione (GSH) with concomitant rise in the level of lipid peroxidation product malondialdehyde (MDA) in the lens of transgenic mice, but not in the nontransgenic mice, suggests **that glucose autoxidation and nonenzymatic glycation do not contribute significantly to oxidative stress in diabetic lenses.** AR reduction of glucose to sorbitol probably contributes to oxidative stress by depleting its cofactor NADPH, which is also required for the regeneration of GSH. Sorbitol dehydrogenase, the second enzyme in the polyol pathway that converts sorbitol to fructose, also contributes to oxidative stress, most likely because depletion of its cofactor NAD+ leads to more glucose being channeled through the polyol pathway. Despite a more than 100% increase of MDA, **oxidative stress plays only a minor role in the development of cataract in this acute diabetic cataract model. However,**

chronic oxidative stress generated by the polyol pathway is likely to be an important contributing factor in the slow-developing diabetic cataract as well as in the development of other diabetic complications (Lee, A.Y.W., Chung, S. S. M. Contributions of polyol pathway to oxidative stress in diabetic cataract. FASEB J. 13, 23-30 (1999).

4.9.1.0 Vitamin D deficiency cataracts

Although hypocalcemia from various causes has been associated with cataracts, only a few case reports have linked congenital cataracts with vitamin D deficiency. This case report from Marshfield, Wisconsin, describes a four-month-old infant with congenital cataracts who was the twelfth child born to an Old Order Amish woman. (None of his 11 siblings has cataracts.) Women in this religious group cover themselves completely when they are outdoors. Blood samples from both the child and the mother showed abnormally low vitamin D levels and elevated alkaline phosphatase. Physicians should be aware that women who wear clothing that completely conceals their skin are prone to vitamin D deficiency, especially if they live in northern latitudes and do not drink vitamin D-fortified milk. Women who have given birth to many children may be at especially high risk of deficiency, and children born to these women may become deficient in utero. The frequency with which fetal vitamin D deficiency leads to congenital cataracts has not been established (Edward B Blau, Congenital Cataracts and Maternal Vitamin D Deficiency, Lancet 34 7(9001):626 (2 Mar 1996). **Vitamin D is a strong prooxidant. Thus, a deficiency of vitamin D equates to an EMOD insufficiency.**

Cataracts are also seen with vitamin E deficiency, radiation exposure, steroid treatment, vitamin G deficiency, tryptophane deficiency, etc.

4.9.2.0 Vitamins C and E do not prevent cataract development or progression

Recently, **a 7-year controlled intervention trial of a daily antioxidant supplement containing 500 mg of vitamin C, 400 IU of vitamin E, and 15 mg of beta-carotene in 4,629 men and women found no difference between the antioxidant combination and a placebo on the development and progression of age-related cataracts** (A randomized, placebo-controlled, clinical trial of high-dose supplementation with vitamins C and E and beta carotene for age-related cataract and vision loss: AREDS report no. 9. Arch

Ophthalmol. 2001;119(10):1439-1452). **This reinforces my belief that cataracts are not caused by EMODs.**

Therefore, the relationship between vitamin C intake and the development of cataracts requires further clarification before specific recommendations can be made.

4.9.3.0 Vitamin E deficiency and long-term prednisolone treatment are subliminal cataractogenic risk factors

Investigators studied the relationship between vitamin E deficiency and prednisolone-induced cataract formation, long-term examination of lens changes was performed in rats under the condition of vitamin E deficiency or supplementation and administration of prednisolone. Rats were divided into six groups: normal chow (N), vitamin E–deficient chow (ED), normal chow with prednisolone instillation (NP), vitamin E–deficient chow with prednisolone instillation (EDP), NP treatment with vitamin E supplementation (NP+VE), and EDP treatment with vitamin E supplementation (EDP+VE). Prednisolone (1 mg/kg · d) and vitamin E (5%; 10 µL per administration per eye, 1 mg/kg · d) were applied in the cul-de-sac. Lens changes were documented and analyzed. Vitamin E status was confirmed by measuring peroxide-induced hemolysis.

After 15 months, 91.7% of the eyes in the EDP group showed development of anterior and posterior cortical cataracts. Supplementation with vitamin E significantly reduced cataract formation (to 38.9% of eyes). Neither a vitamin E–deficient diet nor prednisolone treatment alone significantly increased cataract formation. Hemolysis-susceptibility tests confirmed the expected vitamin E status of rats fed vitamin E–deficient chow and rats supplemented with eye drops containing vitamin E.

Vitamin E deficiency and long-term prednisolone treatment together cause cataracts. Singly, however, both conditions are subliminal cataractogenic risk factors (Low Vitamin E Level as a Subliminal Risk Factor in a Rat Model of Prednisolone-Induced Cataract. Masami Kojima et al. *Investigative Ophthalmology and Visual Science*. 2002;43:1116-1120).

5.0.0.0 Vitamin E does not prevent CVD

Vitamin E is thought to have a role in preventing atherosclerosis by inhibiting the oxidation of low-density lipoprotein (LDL) (Fuller CJ, Huet BA, Jialal I. Effects of increasing doses of alpha-tocopherol in providing protection of low-density lipoprotein from oxidation. *Am J Cardiol.* Jan 15 1998;81(2):231-3) (Hathcock JN. Vitamins and minerals: efficacy and safety. *Am J Clin Nutr.* Aug 1997;66(2):427-37).

Several epidemiologic studies have indicated that high dietary intake of vitamin E is associated with high serum concentrations of alpha tocopherol, as well as with lower rates of ischemic heart disease (Traber MG, Frei B, Beckman JS. Vitamin E revisited: do new data validate benefits for chronic disease prevention?. *Curr Opin Lipidol.* Feb 2008;19(1):30-8).

However, **although the Cambridge Heart Antioxidant Study supported this hypothesis, a subsequent report, the prospective Heart Outcomes Prevention Evaluation Study, did not** (Hathcock JN. Vitamins and minerals: efficacy and safety. *Am J Clin Nutr.* Aug 1997;66(2):427-37) (Stephens NG, Parsons A, Schofield PM, et al. Randomised controlled trial of vitamin E in patients with coronary disease: Cambridge Heart Antioxidant Study (CHAOS). *Lancet.* Mar 23 1996;347(9004):781-6) (Yusuf S, Dagenais G, Pogue J, et al. Vitamin E supplementation and cardiovascular events in high-risk patients. The Heart Outcomes Prevention Evaluation Study Investigators. *N Engl J Med.* Jan 20 2000;342(3):154-60).

5.0.1.0 Failures of antioxidants to prevent cataract formation

Age-related cataract (ARC) is the leading cause of blindness in the world, particularly in developing countries. In contrast, cataract surgery has become the most frequent surgical procedure in people aged 65 years or older in the Western world, causing a considerable financial burden to the health care system. The development of cataracts is mainly an age-related phenomenon, although socio-economic and lifestyle factors appear to influence their development, e.g. smoking has been found to directly influence ARC. A key role in the pathomechanism of the crystalline lens alteration is played by glucose metabolism and associated effected redox potential, which **may induce oxidative damages.** Aldose reductase blockers were able to prevent the development of diabetic cataracts in experimental studies, however clinical trials were interrupted due to unclear side effects. Other drugs with radical scavenging properties were effective in in vitro and in vivo experiments, but **could not be proven to be efficient and safe in preclinical human trials.** A number of epidemiological studies showed an increased risk of nuclear or cortical cataract in people with low blood levels of vitamin E. It is also known that the measured levels of ascorbic acid decline with increasing age in the lens. ß-Carotin and other non-polar carotenoids seem to be missing and may therefore only play a minor role. Polarized carotenoid lutein and zeaxanthin are available in low concentrations and may therefore have some direct effects.

The results of the present **interventional studies are still controversial**. While the Linxian studies indicated that the prevalence for nuclear cataract was reduced by the supplementation with retinol/zinc or vitamin C/molybdenum, the AREDS trial showed no effect of the antioxidant formulation on the development or progression of ARC. (A randomized, placebo-controlled, clinical trial of high-dose supplementation with vitamins C and E, beta carotene, and zinc for age-related macular degeneration and vision loss: AREDS report no. 8. Arch Ophthalmol. 2001; 119:1417-36).

Again, while the REACT study demonstrated a statistically significant positive treatment effect 2 years after treatment for the US patients and for both subgroups (US & UK) after 3 years, no effect was observed in UK patients alone. In another US study, the Physician Health Study, no positive or negative effect of ß -carotin was observed. **Taken together, these studies suggest that any effect of antioxidants on cataract development is likely to be very small and probably is of no clinical or public health significance,** thus removing a major rationale for anticataract antioxidants; vitamin supplementation among health-conscious individuals (Augustin A (ed): Nutrition and the Eye. Dev Ophthalmol. Basel, Karger, 2005, vol 38, pp 103-119).

Whether certain medications can reduce the risk of cataracts is controversial. **The results of trials of medications, such as aspirin or hormone replacement therapy, have been contradictory.** Some researchers have proposed that antioxidant vitamins from foods or vitamin supplements might help prevent cataracts by protecting against free radicals--unstable oxygen molecules that over time can damage various components of the lens. Population studies have found a link between high intakes of antioxidants and a reduced incidence of cataracts, but **results from the Age-Related Eye Disease Study, a large,**

randomized, placebo-controlled trial, found no such benefit from antioxidant supplements.

According to the website for **the Harvard School of Public Health, "The evidence accumulated thus far on antioxidant vitamins isn't promising. Randomized trials of vitamin C, vitamin E, and beta-carotene haven't revealed much in the way of protection from heart disease, cancer, or aging-related eye diseases** (website accessed 2/09/06).

The 2000 National Academy of Sciences report stated that there is not enough evidence to support claims that taking high doses of antioxidants (such as vitamins C and E, selenium, and beta carotene) can prevent chronic diseases. http://www.cancer.org/docroot/ETO/content/ETO_5_3X_Vitamin_E.asp. Accessed 12-24-08.

The most reliable studies on this issue are controlled clinical trials, such as the large study of antioxidant vitamins and cancer that was conducted in 1994 by the National Cancer Institute (NCI) in the United States and the National Public Health Institute of Finland. The study was designed to find out if antioxidant vitamins in higher doses than the RDA (eg, 50 mg) could reduce the incidence of lung cancer and other cancers and illnesses among **29,000 male smokers. The study found no beneficial effect of vitamin E supplements on lung cancer incidence and mixed results for other cancers. The study did find lower rates of prostate and colorectal cancer among those who received vitamin E, but higher rates of bladder, stomach, and other cancers. (American Cancer website: http://www.cancer.org/docroot/ETO/content/ETO_5_3X_Vitamin_E.asp. Accessed 12-24-08.)**

5.0.2.0 Antioxidants not recommended

Oxidative damage is involved in cardiovascular diseases. Intervention with alpha-tocopherol, ascorbic acid and beta-carotene does not appear to reduce pathogenesis. The purpose of this review is to describe alternative antioxidant mechanisms that may be involved. RECENT FINDINGS: Antioxidants with different chemical properties may recharge each other in an antioxidant network. The total antioxidant content of dietary plants may therefore be a useful tool for testing the "antioxidant network" hypothesis. Several berries, fruits, nuts, seeds, vegetables, drinks and spices have been found to be high in total antioxidants. Initial studies in animals and humans are supportive as to the beneficial effects of dietary plants rich in total antioxidants. Additionally, antioxidants and other plant compounds may also improve the endogenous antioxidant defence through induction of antioxidant and phase 2 enzymes. Dietary plants rich in such compounds include broccoli, Brussels sprouts, cabbage, kale, cauliflower, carrots, onions, tomatoes, spinach and garlic. SUMMARY: **Although initial studies have indicated that antioxidants may reduce oxidative stress, human intervention studies do not support a beneficial effect of antioxidant supplements.** Further research is needed to clarify whether other plant antioxidants, plants rich in a combination of antioxidants, or plant compounds that induce the endogenous antioxidant defence can reduce pathogenesis of cardiovascular disease and other oxidative stress-related diseases (Dietary antioxidants and cardiovascular disease. Blomhoff R. Curr Opin Lipidol. 2005 Feb;16(1):47-54).

5.0.3.0 ATBC study fails to prevent cataracts

Investigators studied if long-term supplementation with alpha-tocopherol or beta-carotene is associated with cataract prevalence and severity. METHODS: An end-of-trial random sample of **1828 participants** from the **randomized, double-blind, placebo-controlled clinical trial the alpha-tocopherol, beta-carotene cancer prevention study.** The alpha-tocopherol, beta-carotene cancer prevention study was originally designed to examine whether supplementation with alpha-tocopherol or beta-carotene would reduce the incidence of lung cancer in male smokers. The participants for this study lived in Helsinki City or Uusimaa province and were at entry to the alpha-tocopherol, beta-carotene cancer prevention study 50 to 69 years old and smoked at least 5 cigarettes per day. They received alpha-tocopherol 50 mg/day, beta-carotene 20 mg/day, a combination of the two, or placebo supplements for 5 to 8 years (median 6.6 years). Outcome measures were: cortical, nuclear, and posterior subcapsular cataract, differentiated and quantified with lens opacity classification system (LOCS II). Lens opacity meter provided a continuous measure of cataract density. RESULTS: Supplementation with alpha-tocopherol or beta-carotene was not associated with the end-of-trial prevalence of nuclear (odds ratio 1.1 and 1.2, respectively), cortical (odds ratio 1.0 and 1.3, respectively), or posterior subcapsular cataract (odds ratio 1.1 and 1.0, respectively) when adjusted for possible confounders in logistic model. Neither did the median lens opacity meter values differ between the supplementation groups, indicating no effect of alpha-tocopherol or beta-carotene on cataract severity. CONCLUSION: **Supplementation with alpha-tocopherol or beta-carotene for 5 to 8 years does not influence the cataract prevalence among middle-aged, smoking men** (Long-term supplementation with alpha-tocopherol and beta-carotene and age-related cataract. Teikari JM, et al. Acta Ophthalmol Scand. 1997 Dec;75(6):634-40).

5.0.4.0 Antioxidants not recommended for Adult Macular Degeneration

Investigtors evaluated the effectiveness of dietary antioxidants in the primary prevention of age related macular degeneration (AMD). Data sources Search of seven databases without limits on year or language of publication, and retrieval of references in pertinent reviews and articles.

Methods Two reviewers independently searched the databases and selected the studies, using standardised criteria. Randomised clinical trials and prospective cohort studies were included. Of the 4192 abstracts initially identified, 12 studies (nine prospective cohort studies and three randomised clinical trials) met the selection criteria and were included. Data extraction and study quality evaluation were independently reviewed, using standardised criteria. Results were pooled quantitatively using meta-analytic methods.

Results The nine prospective cohort studies included **149,203 people**, with 1878 incident cases of early AMD. The antioxidants investigated differed across studies, and not all studies contributed to the meta-analysis of each antioxidant. Pooled results from prospective cohort studies indicated that vitamin A, vitamin C, vitamin E, zinc, lutein, zeaxanthin, αcarotene, βcarotene, βcryptoxanthin, and lycopene have little or no effect in the primary prevention of early AMD. The three randomised clinical trials did not show that antioxidant supplements prevented early AMD.

Conclusions **There is insufficient evidence to support the role of dietary antioxidants, including the use of dietary antioxidant supplements, for the primary prevention of early AMD** (Dietary antioxidants and primary prevention of age related macular degeneration: systematic review and meta-analysis. Elaine W-T Chong, et al. *BMJ* 2007;335:755-755 (13 October).

5.0.5.0 Omega-3 Fatty Acids Appear To Impact AMD Progression

6-22-09 Omega-3 fatty acids found in fatty fish such as tuna and salmon may protect against progression of age-related macular degeneration (AMD), but the benefits appear to depend on the stage of disease and whether certain supplements are taken, report researchers at the Laboratory for Nutrition and Vision Research (LNVR), Jean Mayer USDA Human Nutrition Research Center on Aging (HNRCA) at Tufts University.

The researchers calculated intakes of **docosahexaenoic acid (DHA)** and eicosapentaenoic acid (EPA) from dietary questionnaires administered to 2,924 men and women, aged 55 to 80 years, participating in an eight-year supplement trial, the Age-Related Eye Disease Study (AREDS) of the National Eye Institute (NEI). The AREDS trial results suggest taking supplements of antioxidants plus zinc prevents progression of late-stage AMD. AREDS study participants were randomly allocated to receive either a placebo or supplements containing the antioxidants vitamins C and E and beta carotene, the minerals zinc and copper, or a combination of both.

"In our study, we observed participants with early stages of AMD in the placebo group benefited from higher intake of DHA, but it appears that the high-dose supplements of the antioxidants and/or the minerals somehow interfered with the benefits of DHA against early AMD progression," says senior author Allen Taylor, PhD, director of the LNVR at the USDA HNRCA. Taylor is also a professor at the Friedman School of Nutrition Science and Policy at Tufts and Tufts University School of Medicine (TUSM).

The antioxidant supplements did not seem to interfere with the protective effects of DHA and EPA against progression to advanced stages of AMD. Participants who consumed higher amounts of DHA and EPA appeared to have lower risk of progression to both wet and dry forms of advanced AMD. The results are published on-line ahead of print in the British Journal of Ophthalmology.

"Data from the present study also shows the supplements and omega-3 fatty acids collaborate with low-dietary glycemic index (dGI) diets against progression to advanced AMD," says corresponding author Chung-Jung Chiu, DDS, PhD, a scientist in the LNVR and an assistant professor at TUSM. "Our previous research suggests a low-GI diet may prevent AMD from progressing to the advanced stage. We hypothesize that the rapid rise of blood glucose initiated by high-GI foods results in cellular damage that retinal cells cannot handle, thus damaging eye tissues."

dGI is a scale used to determine how quickly carbohydrates are broken down into blood sugar, also known as blood glucose. Foods such as sweetened drinks, sodas and white bread are high-GI because they trigger a sharp rise and fall of blood sugar. Low-GI foods, such as whole grain versions of pasta and bread, have a milder effect on blood sugar response. Earlier data published by Taylor and Chiu suggests that daily substitution of five slices of whole grain bread for white bread out of a total intake of 250 g of carbohydrate might cut out almost 8% of advanced AMD over five years. This is readily achievable with little diet behavior modification.

Eating two to three servings of fatty fish such as salmon, tuna, mackerel, shellfish, and herring every week would achieve the recommended daily intake of DHA and EPA. However, the majority of AREDS participants and Americans eat a much lower level than recommended. "If changing dietary habits is not easy, supplementation is an option," says Chiu.

The authors stress it is still premature to conclude dietary recommendations for people with AMD and more studies are warranted. **"Taken together, these data indicate that consuming a diet with higher levels of omega-3 fatty acids, antioxidants and low-GI foods may delay compromised vision due to AMD**," says Taylor. "The present study adds the possibility that the timing of a dietary intervention as well as the combination of nutrients recommended may be important."

AMD is a progressive disease that attacks central vision, resulting in a gradual loss of eyesight and, in some cases, blindness. The NEI reports that AMD is the most common causes of non-remediable vision loss in Americans over 60.

5.1.0.0 Hyperbaric Oxygen Therapy (HBOT)

HBOT has a long history. The first chamber used to treat patients was constructed in 1662 by Henshaw. And yes, that date is correct, which makes **HBOT 350 years old**. HBOT treatments involve placing you in a chamber, and breathing pure oxygen. This saturates the tissues with oxygen and reverses any areas of hypoxia. As a comparisobn, **the average person breathes in about 6 pounds of oxygen a day, which is about the same amount by weight of food and water intake.**

During a single hour of HBOT, a person will take in about 2.4 pounds of oxygen. This increases the oxygen content of the tissues by a factor of 10-15. Some of the effects this has are to promote the growth of new blood vessels, decreases swelling and inflammation, deactivates toxins, increase the body's ability to fight infections, clears out toxins and metabolic waste products, and improve the rate of healing. **Patients with cataracts may experience accelerated maturation of the cataract, but the treatments do not cause cataract formation.**

5.1.1.0 Oxygen therapy benefit in autism

3-13-09 A decompression chamber may help children with autism, say researchers. After 40 hours of hyperbaric treatment autistic children showed significant improvements in social interaction and eye contact compared with controls. The BMC Pediatrics study could not show if the results were long-lasting but should prompt further investigation of the treatment, the US team said.

One theory is **that oxygen can help reduce inflammation and improve flow of oxygen to brain tissue**. Hyperbaric treatment has been shown to havee some fenefit in other neurological conditions such as fetal alcohol syndrome and ceerebral palsy.

Some studies have looked at the treatment in children with autism but they have not compared with a dummy procedure raising questions around a "placebo effect". In the latest study, carried out at six centres in the US, 62 children aged two to seven with autism were randomly assigned to receive 40 hours of treatment over a month with 24% oxygen at increased atmospheric pressure (1.3 atm) or normal air in a slightly pressurised room (1.03 atm).

Children who received the treatment showed significant improvements in overall functioning, receptive language, social interaction, eye contact, and sensory or cognitive awareness.

New research in *BMC Pediatrics* may give the therapy more credibility as a treatment for autism. The **randomized, double-blind controlled study of 62 children found that those who received 40 hours of treatment over a month were less irritable, more responsive when people spoke to them, made more eye contact and were more sociable than kids who didn't receive it.** They were also less sensitive to noise (some autistic children experience a kind of sensory overload from loud sounds and background noise). The most improvement was observed in kids older than five (the study included children ages two to seven) who had milder autism.

It's not clear why the treatment helped, says study co-author Dan Rossignol, a family physician at the International Child Development Resource Center in Melbourne, Fla., which treats children with developmental disorders. But the pressure may reduce inflammation believed to restrict blood flow to regions of autistic children's brains that control speech, or improve its ability to absorb oxygen, he tells *ScientificAmerican.com*.

"We're not saying it's a cure," Rossignol said, "but … if you can improve understanding so a kid doesn't run in front of a car, or improve sleep, that would be a benefit."

While the study only treated and tracked the children for four weeks, kids who receive the same number of sessions outside of research settings often remain better for longer, Rossignol says. Others get better after 80 sessions, according to Robert Hendren, executive director of the University of California Davis M.I.N.D. Institute, a large autism research center. He adds that some parents also buy chambers (approved by the Food and Drug Administration) and give their children periodic "tune-ups" at home, though those treatments haven't been studied.

While most children tolerate the treatment well, it can cause claustrophobia, bruising of the eardrums, sinus pain and, rarely, seizures, Rossignol says.

An estimated one in 150 children in the U.S. have autism in what some are calling an epidemic of the disorder, according to the Centers for Disease Control and Prevention (CDC).

Hendren, who wasn't involved in the study, says the research was "well done" but that the findings need to be confirmed by others before hyperbaric oxygen therapy is recommended as an autism treatment. He adds that the results will likely be used by doctors and parents petitioning insurers to pay for the treatment, which costs around $120 to $150 per session and isn't typically covered for autism. He speculates that 10 percent of autistic children are getting the therapy.

"It's going to cost a lot of money and yet if it works, it would be important to provide children with this kind of treatment," Hendren tells *ScientificAmerican.com*. "It may help reverse, theoretically, some of the process that's causing the autism.

I believe that the take-home-message is that oxygen therapy, which is known to generate increased EMOD levels, does not cause any harm and appears to only have positive effects. Further, the same oxygen effect may be able to be obtained by using peroxide in a nebulizer.

There are many indications for this therapy. In most diseases, blood flow to the diseased tissue is compromised which in turn decreases the amount of oxygen available for tissue healing. Hyperbaric therapy is able to increase tissue oxygen levels in diseased tissue which improves and speeds healing, improves the body's ability to fight infections, and reduces inflammation and swelling. Hyperbaric oxygen therapy is both a primary treatment and a complementary therapy. Consequently, hyperbaric oxygen therapy may be used alone or in conjunction with conventional therapies.

5.2.0.0 HBOT general information from emedicine

The use of increased atmosphere pressure for medical therapy has intrigued many physicians, scientists, and lay persons for hundreds of years. Vague accounts of increased atmosphere pressures used on humans date to the fifth century BC. Henshaw, a British clergyman, built the first sealed chamber, termed the *Domicilium,* in 1662. This chamber compressed air (21% oxygen) for numerous ailments such as inflammation, scurvy, arthritis, and rickets but likely had too little compression to do any physical good.

Following Priestley's discovery of oxygen in the late 1700s, Beddoes developed a pneumatic laboratory enriched with oxygen to treat chronic conditions such as leprosy. In the early 1930s, the *Junod* reported improvement in patients with cardiorespiratory disorders when treated in 2 atm of pressure in a copper compression chamber. These early reports spawned the creation of a number of "pneumatic institutes" in Europe. These chambers were able to treat up to 10 people at once and reached pressures of 2 or more atm. Compression therapy became the **"in vogue" spas of the day**. Pneumatic spas came to North America in 1860, with the first compression chamber built in Oshawa, Ontario, Canada.

The French surgeon Fontaine built a mobile compressorized operating suite in 1879. Patients reportedly had better outcomes because of improved oxygenation and decreased postoperative vomiting and cyanosis. Easier reduction of hernias was noted. Corning introduced the therapeutic compression chamber to the US in 1891 to treat nervous and mental afflictions. This chamber was the first operated by electric power.

Orville Cunningham noted 25 years later that patients with certain cardiovascular disorders improved when moved from high altitudes to sea-level altitudes. **He discovered this during the Spanish flu epidemic in 1918, which resulted in more than 500,000 deaths. Many of these victims died in a cyanotic state.** Under the care of Dr Cunningham, a rather sick resident physician was treated in the compression chamber and recovered completely. Cunningham subsequently built an 88-ft long and 10-ft wide chamber to treat numerous patients, with **remarkable success**. The credibility of the compression chamber was reinforced during treatment of flu patients. One night when the chamber's power accidentally was shut off, all patients died. At the time, the interpretation credited hyperbaric therapy with keeping the patients alive. When the compression stopped, these patients died. However, the deaths were likely the result of rapid ascent from the compression rather than the secondary effects of the Spanish flu.

In 1928, Mr Timkin, an appreciative patient whose uremic state was resolved after receiving hyperbaric therapies, constructed for Cunningham an enormous 60-ft tall, 6-story hyperbaric hospital that looked like a **steel sphere**. Conditions such as hypertension, diabetes, syphilis, and cancer were treated here until 1930, when the local medical society closed the hyperbaric hospital **for lack of scientific evidence or merit. After 1930, much of the medical or scientific community did not look favorably upon the use of hyperbaric medicine.**

A flurry of interest in therapeutic hyperbaric medicine was fostered by Dr I. Boerema, who, while in Amsterdam in 1956, reported hyperbaric oxygen (HBO) as an aid in cardiopulmonary surgery, particularly for congenital conditions such as tetralogy of Fallot, transposition of great vessels, and pulmonic stenosis. A colleague of Boerema's, W. H. Brummelkamp, also interested in hyperbaric medicine, discovered in 1959 (and subsequently published in 1961) that **anaerobic infections were inhibited by hyperbaric therapy. Anaerobes lack superoxide dismutase to control oxygen free radicals.** Meanwhile, Boerema had published an article, "Life without blood," a report of fatally anemic pigs treated successfully with volume expansion and pressurized hyperoxygenation. Boerema often is credited as the father of modern-day hyperbaric medicine.

Superoxide dismutase (SOD), SOD+catalase (CAT), desferrioxamine, verapamil and disulfiram are all free oxygen radical (FOR) scavengers.

5.2.1.0 The Oxygen Revolution: Hyperbaric Oxygen Therapy

The Oxygen Revolution: Hyperbaric Oxygen Therapy: The Groundbreaking New Treatment for Stroke, Alzheimer's, Parkinson's, Arthritis, Autism, Learning Disabilities and More. by Paul G. Harch (Author), Virginia Mccullough (Author)

"Hyperbaric oxygen has been the Cinderella of modern medicine for several decades given that **oxygen is not a patentable drug**. Finally, thanks to the pioneering efforts of Dr. Harch, the man-on-the-street is becoming aware of this non-invasive therapy." –Kenneth P. Stoller, M.D., FAAP, President of the International Hyperbaric Medical Association

HOPE FOR MANY "HOPELESS" DISEASES, FROM ONE OF THE FOREMOST RESEARCHERS IN THE FIELD

When Randy McCloy, Jr., the sole survivor of the Sago Mine disaster, finally walked out of the hospital to rejoin his family, it was in part due to the miracle of hyperbaric oxygen therapy. **Hyperbaric oxygen therapy (HBOT) is based on an almost laughably simple idea: Oxygen can be used therapeutically for a wide range of conditions where tissues have been damaged by oxygen deprivation.** Restore that oxygen, goes the logical thinking, and you can restore much of the lost function. It seems too good to be true, but Dr. Paul G. Harch's research and clinical practice has shown that this noninvasive and painless treatment can help the tens of millions of Americans who suffer from a brain injury or disease, such as:

• Stroke

• Autism and other learning disabilities

• Cerebral palsy and other birth injuries

• Alzheimer's, Parkinson's, multiple sclerosis, and other degenerative neurological diseases

• Emergency situations requiring resuscitation, such as cardiac arrest, carbon monoxide poisoning, or near drowning

It can also improve conditions in which inflammation is the culprit, such as arthritis and asthma; promote healing in infections, burns, and skin grafts, such as diabetic foot wounds; and slow the aging process.

For the millions of Americans suffering from these seemingly "hopeless" diseases, here finally is the handbook of hope. Inspiring and informative, *The Oxygen Revolution* is the definitive guide to the miracle of hyperbaric oxygen therapy, from a pioneer in the field. **Publisher:** Hatherleigh Press (April 24, 2007)

5.3.0.0 Exercise

5.4.0.0 Pills To Replace Exercising Could Soon Become Reality

What can be greater than taking a pill that would make your fat disappear and your muscle work as if you were doing aerobic but actually, you weren't? What can be greater than that? Two pills that can do that for you discovered by scientists at the Salk Institute for Biological Studies in California and the Howard Hughes Medical Institute in La Jolla, California led by Prof. Ronald Evans.

It's true that **the pills were tried only on lab mice**. Keeping the body in great shape and fat-free, it reduces the risk of various types of cancers and heart disease as well. The pills could also help reverse the muscle frailty associated with aging, or disease such as muscular dystrophy.

The two "breakthrough" pills, as they were called, are labeled **AICAR and GW1516.** AICAR licensed by Schering-Plough Corp. is currently studied in humans to help control bleeding during open-heart surgery. **GW1516 used to be developed by GlaxoSmithKline as a drug against dyslipidemia, a disorder affecting cholesterol. However, side effects of the drug, made the company give up producing it**.

Four years ago, Prof. Evans and colleagues reported that they boosted endurance in mice by tweaking a mouse gene to **boost the activity of a protein called PPAR-delta.** Then the researchers tried to get the same result but this time without genetic engineering. More exactly, they squirted GW1516 into mice's mouths every day for a month. GW1516 boosts PPAR-delta and the mice who were given the pill were exercising. At the end of the month, the researchers were surprised to find out that **the mice ran 68 percent longer and 70 percent farther compared to when the experiment began**. On the other hand, **mice that were given GW1516, but were not exercising saw no improvements,** the researchers found.

Then the researchers focused on another protein called **AMPK** and did the same experiment for a month this time giving the mice a daily injection of AICAR, which boosts AMPK. The mice involved in the experiment were not working. **At the end of the follow-up period, mice given AICAR ran 23 percent longer and 44 percent farther than those who weren't given anything.**

How exactly the pills worked to lead to such good results is not a mystery. The researchers noted that **the drug seemed to change the physical composition of muscle by burning the excessive fat**, the same thing that happens in distance runners or those with intensive training in different sports. The pills can be easily synthesized in any laboratory.

Especially for this reason, Prof. Evans has devised a test to detect whether an athlete has taken the drugs and has made it available to the World Anti-Doping Agency, which prepares a list of forbidden substances for the International Olympic Committee. Anti-doping officials confirmed the collaboration with Prof.

Prof. Evans' findings come at a short time after another experiment on mice showed that **those fed with a diet supplemented with resveratrol did not live longer than other mice but were far healthier in several important measures.** The compounds, usually found in red wine, but also in the crust of peanuts and walnuts, in grapes, blueberries, peanut butter, pistachios and other foods appeared to ward off the effects of aging on heart, bones, eyes and muscle of mice, improving conditions that make the elderly very frail like cataracts, osteoporosis and poor motor coordination.

5.5.0.0 A possible "exercise pill"

When ordinary mice were fed two experimental drugs, they turned into marathon mice, capable of running 44 percent longer on a treadmill than before they were medicated, according to an article published 8-1-08 in the journal Cell. People who are willing to use artificial means to enhance their performance keep abreast of scientific discoveries that could help them, said Ted Friedmann, director of the Center for Molecular Genetics at the University of California San Diego.

Friedmann is a leading authority on gene therapy – the evolving medical technology that inserts healthy or modified genes into the body to treat diseases such as cystic fibrosis, cancer and immune system deficiencies.

It is a dangerous process that uses viruses to transmit new genes into the body, or the injection of genetic material into certain tissue, Friedmann said. It requires expensive laboratory equipment and specific scientific know-how. And it permanently alters a person's genetics, Evans said.

Although there are dozens of promising gene therapies under way, the field has suffered serious setbacks. In 1999, Jesse Gelsinger, an 18- year-old with a rare, inherited liver disease, died from a massive immune response to the viral vector used to deliver genetic material to his cells.

"The bottom line is that interfering with normal genetic mechanisms in living organisms are not to be taken lightly and not to be undertaken except for the treatment of serious disease," Friedmann said.

With Evans' method of using drugs to enhance endurance, the genetic effect disappeared when the mice were taken off the drugs. He said he pursued the possibility of drugs because of the impracticality of using viruses and bits of genes for genetic engineering.

Four years ago, his team discovered the gene responsible for increasing endurance. In that work, Evans showed that by genetically engineering mice to permanently activate a genetic switch known as PPAR delta, their endurance was enhanced. The mice were also resistant to weight gain even when fed a high-fat diet that caused obesity in ordinary mice.

5.6.0.0 Disulfiram

5.6.1.0 General information from emedicine:

Disulfiram (tetraethylthiuram disulfide [TETD]) has been used for more than 50 years as a deterrent to ethanol abuse in the management of alcoholism. Approximately 200,000 alcoholics take disulfiram, or Antabuse, regularly in the United States.

The first suggestion that disulfiram might be used in the treatment of alcoholism came in 1937 when an American physician noted that workers in the rubber industry who were exposed to TETD developed a reaction after drinking ethanol. A decade later, two Danish researchers at the RoyalDanishSchool of Pharmacy in Copenhagen made the same discovery. Jens Hald and Eric Jacobsen were experimenting with disulfiram as a potential antihelminthic, and each took small doses to determine potential side effects in humans. Several days later, they attended a cocktail party and both became ill. They concluded that the facial flushing and tachycardia they experienced must be due to the disulfiram.

Soon thereafter, physicians began prescribing disulfiram as a deterrent to ethanol abuse. It has also been proposed as a deterrent to cocaine abuse, and several studies have suggested improved retention rates in treatment programs for cocaine-dependent individuals treated with disulfiram. A study found diminished "high" or "rush" after intravenous cocaine administration to healthy volunteers pretreated with disulfiram, with no change in cardiovascular parameters.

The disulfiram-ethanol reaction (DER) is due to increased serum acetaldehyde concentrations generated by the metabolism of ethanol by alcohol dehydrogenase in the liver. Normally, this acetaldehyde is cleared rapidly by its metabolism to acetate via aldehyde dehydrogenase. Disulfiram blocks this enzyme, irreversibly inhibiting the oxidation of acetaldehyde and causing a marked increase in acetaldehyde concentrations after ethanol consumption. The discomfort associated with this syndrome is intended to serve as a negative stimulus, but the reaction may be severe enough to cause hypotension and death.

In considering disulfiram toxicity, a distinction must be made between the clinical manifestations of a disulfiram-ethanol reaction (DER) and the toxic effects of disulfiram itself. Direct disulfiram toxicity may be further divided into acute poisoning versus chronic poisoning. The directly toxic effects of disulfiram include neurologic, cutaneous, and hepatotoxic sequelae in addition to the disulfiram-ethanol reaction.

Disulfiram received US Food and Drug Administration (FDA) approval for use in the treatment of alcoholism in 1951. At that time, it was commonly prescribed in very high doses, up to 3,000 mg a day in some cases. This resulted in a relatively high rate of extremely severe or fatal reactions. Today, much lower doses are used, and the incidence of disulfiram toxicity has waned.

Disulfiram also directly inhibits hepatic microsomal enzymes (cytochrome P450), in particular CYP2E1. This interferes with the metabolism of certain drugs, most notably that of warfarin, phenytoin, and theophylline. Disulfiram may also increase the clearance of some benzodiazepines (diazepam, oxazepam, and chlordiazepoxide), caffeine, and some tricyclic antidepressants (desipramine and imipramine). The resulting possible elevation of serum concentrations of these medications has the potential to cause a corresponding toxicity.

Disulfiram is highly lipid soluble (accumulates in adipose tissue, crosses blood-brain barrier), highly protein-bound, and has 80% bioavailability after an oral dose of 350 mg. Approximately 5-20% is not metabolized and is excreted unchanged in the feces; the remainder is metabolized to both toxic and nontoxic metabolites. The elimination of disulfiram and its numerous metabolites is a very slow process. **Approximately 20% of the drug remains in the body for 1-2 weeks postingestion.** Most of these metabolites are then eliminated through the gastrointestinal (GI), renal, and respiratory routes. The prolonged effects of disulfiram occur not only because the drug is slowly eliminated from the body but also because it irreversibly inhibits aldehyde dehydrogenase. In order to regain the ability to metabolize acetaldehyde, the individual must therefore synthesize new stores of the enzyme.

Disulfiram metabolites cause clinically important effects in the body. The most important toxic metabolites are diethyldithiocarbamate (DDC) and its metabolite carbon disulfide (CS2). DDC chelates copper, thus impairing the activity of dopamine beta-hydroxylase, an enzyme that catalyzes the metabolism of dopamine to norepinephrine. In this way, DDC causes depletion of presynaptic norepinephrine and accumulation of dopamine. Although hypotension from the disulfiram-ethanol reaction is mainly attributable to the effects of acetaldehyde, depletion of the potent vasoconstrictor norepinephrine may also be a contributing factor.

Dopamine agonism may be implicated in some of the altered behavior associated with disulfiram toxicity. **Although no studies have directly examined the effects of low doses of disulfiram on psychotic symptoms, hypomania and psychosis have been documented in many reports among alcoholics taking high-dose disulfiram (up to 2,000 mg/d).** It is possible that disulfiram, like L-dopa and amphetamine, unmasks or exacerbates preexisting psychotic symptoms in susceptible individuals by increasing central dopamine levels.

I believe that this ties in with the studies showing that CGD patients have mental disorders also caused by an EMOD insufficiency.

Neurotoxic effects associated with disulfiram include extrapyramidal symptoms, and lesions of the basal ganglia have been described in patients after therapy with disulfiram. **Potential mechanisms for disulfiram-associated neurotoxicity include abnormal CNS metal accumulation from the chelation of copper by DDC, leading to free radical formation and neuronal oxidative stress**. In addition, one study found that disulfiram and DDC increase the release of glutamate from striato-cortical synaptic vesicles, both in vitro and in rats, suggesting yet another possible mechanism for DDC-mediated neuronal damage.

Other mechanisms implicated in DDC's cytotoxic effects include its ability to chelate nickel, to interfere with sulfhydryl groups in cytochrome P-450 enzymes, and to inhibit ADH and ALDH enzymes. Furthermore, **DDC inhibits superoxide dismutase, thereby impairing the ability to eliminate free radicals. DDC-induced methemoglobinemia can also occur** secondary to impairment (consumption) of glutathione-dependent methemoglobin reduction. **I believe that the blockage of SOD also blocks its ability to produce peroxide and leads to an EMOD insufficiency.**

Carbon disulfide (CS_2), another disulfiram metabolite from DDC metabolism, has neurotoxic effects when administered directly. Acute exposure to CS_2 causes rapid onset of headache, confusion, nausea, hallucinations, delirium, seizures, coma, and potentially death. CS_2 may cause seizures by interacting with pyridoxal-5-phosphate, a cofactor in the production of GABA from glutamate, thereby depleting GABA levels in the brain and leading to benzodiazepine-resistant seizures; this forms the basis for an important experimental rat model of status epilepticus. In addition to its neurotoxic effects (neurobehavioral toxin), CS_2 is hepatotoxic, inhibits cytochrome P-450, and is cardiotoxic.

5.7.0.0 Disulfiram to treat cancer

United States Patent 6288110
Publication Date:
09/11/2001

Bis(diethylthiocarbamoyl) disulfide or tetraethylthiuram disulfide, hereinafter **disulfiram**, is an inhibitor of various enzymes and a chelator of heavy metals. Disulfiram is known as an alcohol deterrent and is the active ingredient of the drug **Antabuse** used in aversion therapy, an adjunctive treatment for chronic alcoholism (Haley, 1979). Disulfiram has an ampiphilic nature, is soluble in water but it solubilizes better in hydrophobic solutions such as methanol, acetone or chloroform.

Once ingested and absorbed through the intestinal tract or injected intraperitoneally as a colloidal suspension, disulfiram is extensively distributed throughout the body including the brain (Faiman, 1978). It is quickly converted into its main metabolite, diethyldithiocarbamate (DDC) (Eneanya, 1981), whereby the disulfide is reduced to a sulfhydryl group. The DDC produced is then further metabolized via different ways which include a non-enzymatic degradation to diethylamine (DEA) (Brien, 1983).

Both disulfiram and DDC are potent chelators of copper, iron and zinc. Chelation of the metal portion of an enzyme by disulfiram or DDC might lead to the inactivation of such enzyme. Thus disulfiram was shown to inhibit various zinc-containing dehydrogenases, such as aldehyde dehydrogenases as well as oxidases, dopamine-β-hydroxylases and aldolases (Eneanya, 1981). Inhibition of aldehyde dehydrogenases by disulfiram inhibits glycolysis, the tricarboxylic acid cycle and the pentose phosphate shunt.

Disulfiram was shown to interfere with induction of cancer by various carcinogens, often by inhibiting their metabolic activation, as shown for bladder cancer in rats exposed to N-butyl-N-(4-hydroxybutyl)nitrosamine (Irving, 1979) or to N-butyl-N-(3-carboxypropyl)nitrosamine (Irving, 1983), for liver tumors in rats induced by dimethyl- or diethylnitrosamine (Schmahl, 1976), for intestinal cancer induced by azoxymethane in rats (Nigro, 1978) (probably by blocking the metabolism of azoxymethane), for neoplasia of the large bowl induced by 1,2-dimethylhydrazine (Wattenberg, 1978), and in neoplasia of the forestomach induced by benzo(a)pyrene in mice (Borchert, 1976). Disulfiram inhibited the metabolism of the carcinogen azomethane thus offering protection from the oxymetabolite neoplasia (Fiala, 1977). Disulfiram was also shown to inhibit tumor progression--from papilloma to squamous cell carcinoma--in the murine skin multistage carcinogenesis model (Rotstein, 1988), to inhibit transmammary carcinogenesis induced in mice by 7,12-dimethylbenz(a)anthracene (Rao, 1989) and to reduce the incidence of mammary tumors induced in rats by N-2-fluorenylacetamide or N-hydroxy-N-2-fluorenylacetamide through inhibition of their metabolic activation (Malejka Giganti, 1980). Since a cytosolic aldehyde dehydrogenase is induced during rat hepatocarcinogenesis (Allen, 1982), the inhibitory effect of disulfiram on various carcinogens may be related to its inhibitory effect on aldehyde dehydrogenases.

Disulfiram was shown to protect mice against ifosfamide- and cyclophosphamide-induced urotoxicity when administered simultaneously with said drugs without compromising their anti-tumor activity against Sarcoma 180, EL-4 leukemia or L1210 murine leukemia (Hacker, 1982; Ishikawa, 1991; Ishikawa, 1994). On the other hand, disulfiram did not show any protection against cisplatin nephrotoxicity in humans (Verma, 1990). Disulfiram protected rats against the toxic side effects of 1-(2-hydroxyethyl)-3-(2-chloroethyl)-3-nitrosourea (HECNU), without inhibiting its anti-tumor potency (Habs, 1981). Disulfiram was also shown to potentiate the anti-cancer activity of some agents such as to nitrogen mustard (HN2) cytotoxicity against murine leukemia at 3 mg/mouse (Valeriote, 1989).

Disulfiram, together with ascorbic acid, augmented inhibition of Meth A tumor cell proliferation in vitro by increasing the intracellular oxygen free radicals (Augmented inhibition of tumor cell proliferation in the combined use of disulfiram with ascorbic acid and the involvement of oxygen free radicals. Mashiba H, Matsunaga K. Jpn J Exp Med. 1990 Aug;60(4):209-14).

In addition, **disulfiram inhibited superoxide dismutase in vivo** (Forman, 1980; Ohman, 1986). **All of these could result in an increase in oxygen species toxic to the cell thereby making the cell more sensitive to damage by a variety of chemotherapeutic agents or radiation that produce superoxide anions species** (Goodman, 1977). Resistance to cyclophosphamide and oxazaphosphorines is related to aldehyde dehydrogenase activity (Magni, 1996; Rekha, 1994), and inhibition of this enzyme by disulfiram thus increase sensitivity to these chemotherapies.

U.S. Pat. No. 4,870,101 (Ku and Doherty, 1989) discloses a method for inhibiting the release of interleukin-1 in animals which comprises administering to said animals an amount of disulfiram effective to inhibit the release of interleukin-1, thus proposing disulfiram for the treatment of IL-1 mediated inflammations such as psoriasis, rheumatoid arthritis, diabetes and atherosclerosis.

Disulfiram, given 0.05% in diet for 2 years, did not increase any tumor type in rats (Cheever, 1990). The toxic dose for disulfiram in normal mice is about 6-10 mg/mouse/day. The LD_{50} of disulfiram given orally in rats is 8.6 g/Kg.

None of the above publications describes or suggests the use of disulfiram as an inhibitor of angiogenesis.

5.7.1.0 Alcohol increases EMOD production

Investigators studied the hepatocellular site of reactive oxygen species generation during acute ethanol metabolism. Reactive oxygen species production was detected using the 2′,7′-dichlorofluorescein fluorescence assay and cell injury was determined by lactate dehydrogenase release. Incubation **with 1 and 10 mM ethanol increased the production of reactive oxygen species by 72% and 151%, respectively, which was associated with mild decreases in cell viability. Antimycin, a mitochondrial complex III inhibitor, elicited a 17-fold increase in the levels of reactive oxygen species and markedly decreased hepatocyte viability and ATP levels (RMH Note: due to increased apoptosis).** Ethanol increased reactive oxygen species production and the cytosolic $NADH/NAD^+$ ratio in antimycin-treated cells. **Rotenone**, a mitochondrial complex I inhibitor that allows electron flow through the flavin mononucleotide (FMN), but prevents electron flow to complex III, **significantly increased reactive oxygen species production in untreated cells, but decreased reactive oxygen species production in antimycin plus ethanol-treated cells.**

Diphenyliodonium, a mitochondrial complex I inhibitor that inhibits electron flow through FMN, attenuated reactive oxygen species generation in all groups. Fructose prevented cytotoxicity in all treatment groups. Though they do not eliminate the participation of other intracellular compartments, these results indicate that the **NADH dehydrogenase complex, as well as complex III of mitochondria, are involved in ethanol-related production of reactive oxygen species** (Ethanol stimulates the production of reactive oxygen species at mitochondrial complexes I and III. Shannon M. Bailey et al. Free Radical Biology and Medicine. Volume 27, Issues 7-8, October 1999, Pages 891-900). **I believe that this helps the French Paradox, in that higher EMOD levels aid prooxidant protection against diseases.**

5.8.0.0 EMODs high in reproductive organs

EMODs are high in reproductive tissues, due to steroidogenesis and normal metabolic demands and these organs are under constant oxidative stress. The maintanenceof a high redox potential is essential for keeping the reproductive system in a healthy state. (Fundamental roles of reactive oxygen species and protective mechanisms in the female reproductive system. Junichi Fujii et al. Reproductive biology and endocrinology. 2005. 3:43.). **I believe that this is very telling in that this most vulnerable tissue has high EMOD levels. It appears that they are a prerequisite for a normally functioning reproductive system.**

5.9.0.0 WBCs

5.9.1.0 WBCs have an EMOD defect

The precise molecular mechanisms by which phagocytic cells effect their microbicidal function is unknown. Potential mechanisms that have been identified include low intracellular pH, lysozyme, cationic proteins, lysosomal hydrolases, and oxygen metabolites.

Largely from the study of leukocytes of patients with rare genetic deficiency diseases--which include:

chronic granulomatous disease (CGD),

t glutathione peroxidase, and the reductase deficiencies,

glucose-6-phosphate dehydrogenase deficiency and myeloperoxidase deficiency--it has emerged that **there exists a close correlation between the respiratory burst in normal phagocytic cells and their cytocidal activity**, both of which are impaired in CGD.

It has long been established that one of the early sequelae of the phagocytic event in macrophages is a stimulation of the hexose monophosphate (HMP) shunt, and recent studies indicate that the ability of macrophages to kill parasites intracellularly and possibly tumor cells extracellularly is dependent upon the oxidative burst and production of oxygen radicals including superoxide anion (O2-), hydrogen peroxide (H202), hydroxyl radical, and, possibly, singlet oxygen; 102.

(MACROPHAGEVARIANTS IN OXYGEN METABOLISM. GUIDO DAMIANI, et al. J. Exp. Med.Volume 152 October 1980 808-822).

5.9.2.0 WBC EMOD production inhibited by endothelial cells

CIRCULATING POLYMORPHONUCLEAR neutrophils (PMN) normally exist in a quiescent state. **When neutrophils ingest particles or react to specific stimuli such as chemotactic peptides, they interact extensively with the endothelial layer lining the vessel walls.** These interactions include increased adherence to endothelial cells, migration through the endothelium and into extravascular space, disruption of the plasma membrane, and **generation of an array of reactive oxygen species, including superoxide anion ($O^{-}_{2}\cdot$) and hydrogen peroxide** (Babior, B. M. Oxygen-dependent microbial killing by phagocytes (Abstract). *N. Engl. J. Med.* 298: 659, 1978) (Varani, J., S. E. G. Fligiel, G. O. Till, R. G. Kunkel, U. S. Ryan, and P. A. Ward. Pulmonary endothelial cell killing by human neutrophils: possible involvement of hydroxyl radical. *Lab. Invest.* 53: 656-663, 1985) (Weiss, S. J., J. Yong, A. F. LoBuglio, A. Slivka, and N. F. Nimeh. Role of hydrogen peroxide in neutrophil-mediated destruction of cultured endothelial cells (Abstract). *J. Clin. Invest.* 68: 714, 1981).

Thus vascular endothelial cells can be injured indiscriminately by neutrophils proximal to the inflammatory site (Martin, W. J., II. Neutrophils kill pulmonary endothelial cells by **hydrogen peroxide** dependent pathway. An in vitro model of neutrophil-mediated lung injury. *Am. Rev. Respir. Dis.* 130: 209-213, 1984).

Endothelial cells contain various antioxidant mechanisms such as superoxide dismutase (SOD), catalase, and glutathione reductase. Hoover and co-workers reported that **coincubation of neutrophils with endothelial cells markedly inhibited the extracellular release of $O^{-}_{2}\cdot$ from the subsequently activated neutrophils** (Hoover, R. L., J. M. Robinson, and M. J. Karnovsky. Adhesion of polymorphonuclear leukocytes to endothelium enhances the efficiency of detoxification of oxygen-free radicals. *Am. J. Pathol.* 126: 258-268, 1987) (Hoover, R. L., J. M. Robinson, and M. J. Karnovsky. Superoxide production by polymorphonuclear leukocytes is inhibited by contact with endothelial cells (Abstract). *J. Cell Biol.* 95: L10A, 1982).

In summary, treatment of endothelial cells with staurosporine, like treatment of neutrophils, prevented neutrophil activation as well as neutrophil-mediated endothelial ACE dysfunction and endothelial cytotoxicity. Treatment of endothelial cells with staurosporine potentiated the H_2O_2- and X/XO-mediated endothelial cytotoxicity. Endothelial cells or conditioned medium from staurosporine-treated

BPAE inhibited $O^{-}_{2}\cdot$ generation by activated neutrophils and increased neutrophil adherence to endothelial cells. Endothelial cells treated with staurosporine do not inhibit $O^{-}_{2}\cdot$ generated by X/XO. The inhibitory effects of endothelial cells treated with staurosporine on $O^{-}_{2}\cdot$ generation were not affected by the SOD inhibitor DTCA. Thus these data suggest **that a soluble factor is released by endothelial cells treated with staurosporine, which can inhibit neutrophil activation and neutrophil-mediated endothelial injury** (Release of a leukocyte activation inhibitor by staurosporine-treated pulmonary artery endothelial cells. Xilin Chen and John D. Catravas. Am J Physiol Lung Cell Mol Physiol 275: L184-L192, 1998).

6.0.0.0 Staurosporine induces apoptosis via EMODs

Staurosporine (0.03–0.5 μ*M*) induced a dose-dependent, apoptotic degeneration in cultured rat hippocampal neurons that was sensitive to 24-h pretreatments with the protein synthesis inhibitor cycloheximide (1 μ*M*) or the cell cycle inhibitor mimosine (100 μ*M*). Cultures treated with the antioxidants U-74500A (1–10 μ*M*) and *N*-acetylcysteine (100 μ*M*) also demonstrated reduced staurosporine neurotoxicity. These results suggest a fundamental role for both Ca^{2+} and reactive oxygen species in staurosporine-induced neuronal apoptosis (Ca^{2+} and Reactive Oxygen Species in Staurosporine-Induced Neuronal Apoptosis. J. H. M. Prehn et al. Journal of Neurochemistry. Volume 68 Issue 4, Pages 1679 – 1685. **Published Online:** 18 Nov 2002).

6.0.1.0 Debunking The Detox Myth

A group of over 300 young UK scientists and engineers who investigated the evidence behind claims made for products and diets, have started a public awareness campaign by publishing a dossier that shows **the word "detox" has no meaning outside of the clinical treatment of drug addiction and poisoning**.

Called the "Detox Dossier", the report describes the findings of the investigation by the Voice of Young Science (VoYS) network of over 300 early career researchers. They reviewed about 15 products, ranging from bottled water to face scrub, and found that **many detox claims were "meaningless",** said a BBC report.

It follows an earlier report titled "There Goes The Science Bit..." published with the charity Sense About Science about a year ago, where the authors exposed "dodgy" science claims by phoning manufacturers and asking questions about their products. After the first report was published the authors received offers of help and lots of examples where the word "detox" was used, and this led to the latest investigation.

According to a BBC report, the advertising regulators said they would look at such issues on a case by case basis. The Advertising Standards Authority said:

"If a product is making claims not substantiated by the evidence submitted by the company we would challenge that."

The Detox Dossier investigators found that:

- No two companies had the same definition for "detox".
- The word "detox" was used to promote a range of things from foot patches to hair straighteners, without consistent explanations of what the word means.
- In most cases no evidence was presented to back up the "detox" claims on products.
- In most cases, producers and retailers who the young scientists got in touch with were forced to admit that they were using the word "detox" instead of mundane things like "cleaning" or "brushing".
- The prices ranged from about 2 pounds for a detox drink to over 36 pounds for detox bath products.

The scientists involved in the research include physiologists, biochemists, doctors and pharmacists and they will be launching their own leaflet titled "Debunking Detox" outside high street shops in central London.

The leaflet explains how the human body already has a fantastic detox system, called the liver and the kidneys, and that there is no need to spend money on expensive treatments and products. Eating healthily and getting plenty of sleep is a better investment.

Tom Wells, a chemist and one of the investigators, told the BBC that: "The minimum sellers of detox products should be able to offer is a clear understanding of what detox is and proof that their product actually works." "The people we contacted could do neither," he said.

Another researcher who investigated a Garnier face wash that claimed to remove toxins from the skin said that the "toxins" were no more than the normal dirt, make up and skin oils that one might expect any face cleansing product to remove, reported the BBC.

Garnier said that all their products underwent "rigorous testing and evaluation to ensure that our claims are accurate and noticeable by our consumers."

On the leaflet they will be handing out to shoppers in London, the detox investigators said that shampoos, cleansers and moisturizers "can't

help your body remove excess substances and are no better than any other other shampoos/cleansers/moisturizers" although they may be more expensive.

Putting a detox patch on your skin may make the area sweat more, and while very small amounts of chemicals may come out in the sweat, the effect is very small and makes little difference to the overall amount of chemicals in your body, they said.

The investigators also said that detox tonics can't improve your liver or kidney function, and if you have too high a dose of some of the detox supplements you could become very ill and even die. They could also interact with other drugs like the contraceptive pill and reduce their effectiveness.

And, said the investigators, although detox diets are often recommended after periods of excess, such as Christmas and New Year, the "best diet you can have at anytime is a normal, balanced diet".

One of the detox diet plans investigated was a five day plan from Boots, which according to the BBC claimed to detoxify the body and flush away toxins. One of the investigators, Evelyn Harvey, said that consumers would benefit just from following the healthy diet that was recommended with the product, they wouldn't need the product itself.

A spokeswoman from Boots told the BBC that their five day detox plan encouraged consumers to drink water and the product contained natural ingredients that fought against toxins and helped "protect from the dangers of free radicals".

Click here for more information about the Detox Dossier (Sense about Science).

Sources: Sense About Science, BBC News. Written by: Catharine Paddock, PhD

As a nation we spend millions on detox products, especially in the new year following post-Christmas guilt. But scientists are now saying detox remedies are a waste of money and a glass of water and an early night is far more beneficial.

Tracey Brown, director of the charity Sense About Science, said they were advising the public not to buy into the detox myth. "The body detoxifies itself. The body is rehydrated with ordinary tap water and is refreshed with a good night's sleep," she said.

Mrs Brown condemned products such as detox tablets and detox socks saying they sowed confusion about how nutrition and chemistry actually work. She said her groups advice followed a number of leading scientists into the role of detox solutions.

6.0.2.0 Detox nonsense

Dr John Emsley, chemical scientist and popular science writer, said: "Our bodies are very good at eliminating all the nasties that we might ingest over the festive season.

"There is a popular notion that we can speed up the elimination process by drinking fancy bottled water or sipping herbal teas, but this is just nonsense.

"In fact, **many of the detox diets and supplements really aren't that good for you**, nor have they been properly tested."

Professor Martin Wiseman, visiting professor of human nutrition, University of Southampton, added: **"The detox fad - is an example of the capacity of people to believe in and pay for magic despite the lack of any sound evidence.**

"This is a trend that should worry us all."

6.1.0.0 Mangafodipir trisodium

The trisodium salt of mangafodipir with potential antioxidant and chemoprotective activities. Consisting of manganese (II) ions chelated to fodipir (dipyridoxyl diphosphate or DPDP), **mangafodipir scavenges oxygen free radicals such as superoxide anion, hydrogen peroxide, and hydroxyl radical**, potentially preventing oxygen free radical damage to macromolecules such as DNA and minimizing oxygen free radical-related chemotoxicity in normal tissues. **However, this agent may potentiate the chemotherapy-induced generation of oxygen free radicals in tumor cells, resulting in the potentiation of chemotherapy-induced cytotoxicity; tumor cells, with higher levels of reactive oxygen species than normal cells, possess a lower threshold**

for oxygen free radical-mediated cytotoxicity. Mangafodipir is traditionally used as an imaging agent in magnetic resonance imaging (MRI). http://www.cancer.gov/templates/drugdictionary.aspx?expand=M

6.1.1.0 Motexafin gadolinium

A synthetic metallotexaphyrin with radiosensitizing and chemosensitizing properties. Motexafin gadolinium accumulates in tumor cells preferentially due to their increased rates of metabolism, **generating reactive oxygen species (ROS) intracellularly and lowering the tumor cell apoptotic threshold to ionizing radiation and chemotherapy**.

6.1.2.0 Metoxafin lutetium

A pentadentate aromatic metallotexaphyrin with photosensitizing properties. Motexafin lutetium preferentially accumulates in tumor cells due to their increased rates of metabolism and absorbs light, forming an extended high energy conformational state that **produces high quantum yields of singlet oxygen**, resulting in local cytotoxic effects.

6.2.0.0 Sonodynamic therapy

The sonodynamically induced antitumor effect of protoporphyrin IX (PPIX) disodium salt was studied in mice bearing sarcoma 180 solid tumors. *Methods:* In order to determine the optimum timing of ultrasound exposure after administration of PPIX, the PPIX concentrations in plasma, skin, muscle and tumor were estimated by measuring the fluorescence intensity of tissue extractions with a fluorescence photometer based on the standard curve. Antitumor effects were estimated by measuring tumor size and calculating the average survival time of tumor-bearing mice after sonodynamic therapy; additionally, the morphological changes of **sarcoma 180 cells** were evaluated by transmission electron microscope observation in vivo. *Results:* Our experiments suggested a time of 24 h after the administration of PPIX to be best for ultrasound exposure. At an ultrasound intensity ≥5 W/cm² and a PPIX dose ≥5 mg/kg, a significant synergistic effect of ultrasound combined with PPIX was observed, reducing tumor volume and increasing average animal survival time; this synergistic effect was obviously stronger than ultrasound treatment alone, while PPIX alone showed no significant effect. Transmission electron microscope observation indicated that changes in cell ultrastructure, such as cell membrane destruction, mitochondria swelling and chromatin condensation, were important factors that inhibited tumor growth and even induced cell death. *Conclusion:* The results implied that **the antitumor**

effect of ultrasound could be enhanced in the presence of PPIX which might be involved in a sonochemical mechanism (Sonodynamic Antitumor Effect of Protoporphyrin IX Disodium Salt on S180 Solid Tumor. Quanhong Liu, Xiaobing Wang, Pan Wang, Lina Xiao. *Chemotherapy* 2007;53:429-436).

6.3.0.0 High-Intensity Focused Ultrasound Therapy: an Overview for Radiologists

The following was excerpted from: **High-Intensity Focused Ultrasound Therapy: an Overview for Radiologists.** Young-sun Kim et al. Korean J Radiol. 2008 August; 9(4): 291–302

High-intensity focused ultrasound therapy is a novel, emerging, therapeutic modality that uses ultrasound waves, propagated through tissue media, as carriers of energy. This completely non-invasive technology has great potential for **tumor ablation** as well as hemostasis, thrombolysis and targeted drug/gene delivery. However, the application of this technology still has many drawbacks. It is expected that current obstacles to implementation will be resolved in the near future. In this review, we provide an overview of high-intensity focused ultrasound therapy from the basic physics to recent clinical studies with an interventional radiologist's perspective for the purpose of improving the general understanding of this cutting-edge technology as well as speculating on future developments.

Focusing the sunrays onto a small spot with a magnifying glass to start a fire is a childhood experiment that many of us tried. High-intensity focused ultrasound (HIFU) therapy is a technology with similar principles using ultrasound (US) instead of sunrays. HIFU therapy can transport energy in the form of US waves through a media of intervening tissues to specific target points of body organs, and hence, increase the temperature or bring about other biological interactions in an absolutely non-invasive manner. No significant negative biological effects on the intervening tissue occurs as long as that the ultrasonic energy is appropriately located and focused. **Because of its non-invasive nature, this technology has attracted the attention of clinicians, investigators and companies from around the world as an innovative, interventional tool that might provide virtually complication-free therapy.**

The use of US for therapy predates its application in diagnosis. The biological effects of HIFU were recognized in 1927. Since the 1930s, unfocused, usually low-intensity US has been adopted for physiotherapy. In 1942, Lynn et al. demonstrated that highly localized biological effects could be produced by focusing US. In the 1950s, focused US was employed for brain therapy through a soft tissue window by Drs.

Fry for the first time, and then, clinical application was attempted for Parkinson's disease. However, this clinical application was overshadowed by the development of L-dopa, which was considered very successful at the time. After a long period of relative inactivity, technological advances within the past 10 or more years have caused a resurgence of this technology in clinical medicine. **The first report on the clinical use of HIFU for prostate cancer was published in 1994,** which was followed by many additional clinical studies on its use on a variety of body organs.

Although most clinical studies on HIFU therapy have dealt only with thermal ablations (focused US surgery; FUS) (discussed later), the range of its potential applications in medical science appears to be much wider when numerous on-going investigations on hemostasis, thrombolysis and targeted drug/gene-delivery systems are considered.

In this review, we provide information encompassing the basic physics of sound required for understanding this therapy, biological interactions of US, the mechanisms of action of HIFU therapy, clinical HIFU devices, methods for guiding and monitoring therapy, and the results of clinical studies from the viewpoint of interventional radiologists. Our goal is to improve the general understanding of the status of technological development of HIFU therapy as well as speculate on the future direction of this novel technology.

6.3.1.0 Basic physics of sound and ultrasound

Sound is defined as a disturbance of mechanical energy that propagates through a medium in the form of waves. As this definition implies, sound can transport energy from its source to another area as long as a medium is present. US is a form of sound that has a higher frequency (> 20,000 Hz) than the human ear can detect (20-20,000 Hz; audible ranges).

While other minimally invasive therapies such as radiofrequency ablation or microwave ablation use an electrode or antenna to deliver electromagnetic waves, HIFU therapy makes use of US waves as carriers of energy, which is propagated through human tissues. US has been shown to have no detrimental effect on the human body within the diagnostic ranges used. However, it must be noted that US waves carry energy that causes biological reactions in various ways (discussed later) although these are usually minimal. The main challenge of this technique is to maximize energy-accumulation at the target area in order to induce significant biological reactions without causing harm to the intervening tissues such as the skin and the tissues surrounding the target area. HIFU therapy has adopted two strategies to resolve this problem. It uses high energy US waves generated from numerous sources and focuses them to a small spot.

The various methods of focusing US waves have been another important issue. The simplest and cheapest (often most accurate) method may be a shelf-focusing, for instance, a spherically curved US source (transducer). An US transducer constructed according to this method, has a beam focus fixed at the position determined from the geometrical specifications of the transducer. To compensate for its lack of versatility, a flat US transducer with an interchangeable acoustic lens system was devised. The acoustic lens enables variation of focusing properties such as focal length and focal geometry. However, a drawback of the lens system is that US waves undergo sonic attenuation due to absorption by the lens. Recently, a phased-array US transducer technique was adopted for HIFU therapy. By sending temporally different sets of electronic signals to each specific transducer component, this technique enables beam-steering and focusing, which can move a focal spot in virtually any direction within physically allowed ranges. This system is not only more versatile than other systems but also highly efficient without any sonic attenuation.

6.3.2.0 Biological interactions of US

US beyond the diagnostic ranges can bring about various kinds of reactions when insonated into biological tissue. The resulting effects include thermal, mechanical, chemical and optical reactions. Mechanical effects, more specifically, may consist of acoustic cavitation, radiation force, shear stress, and acoustic streaming/microstreaming. Among them, the thermal effect and acoustic cavitation are the most significant, and their mechanisms of action have been relatively well-understood.

Acoustic cavitation, defined as the formation and activity of a gas- or vapor-filled cavity (bubble) in a medium exposed to an US field, plays a major role in the mechanical effects and minor roles in the chemical and the optical effects of US technology. If an US wave, more intense than a specific threshold, is insonated into biological tissue, negative pressure representing the rarefaction of an US wave, may be large enough to draw gas out of the tissue solution to form a bubble. It is easy to understand the underlying mechanism if this is compared to the numerous bubbles formed by vigorous rotation of a motorboat screw. This bubble either repeats radial oscillations in a resonant size with the insonated frequency (stable cavitation; non-inertial cavitation) or oscillates in a similar manner expanding gradually above its resonant size due to net influxes of vapor into the bubble (rectified diffusion), and finally disintegrates by a violent and asymmetrical collapse (unstable cavitation; inertial cavitation). Acoustic cavitation, particularly inertial cavitation, can cause a significant degree of mechanical and thermal effects as well as chemical and optical effects. The thermal effect caused by acoustic cavitation is larger than that caused by US absorption alone. Mechanical and thermal effects by acoustic cavitation are generally known to be complex, unpredictable, and, sometimes, detrimental. The threshold of acoustic cavitation depends on (negative) pressure amplitude and frequency of the sound and the tissue where cavitation occurs.

6.3.3.0 Clinical Devices in use

Since the 1990s, several commercial companies have developed different forms of clinical HIFU devices, which are now in the initial stages of their clinical applications. Generally, the devices are divided into transrectal and extracorporeal types according to their energy-delivery routes, and are also classified into US- and MR (magnetic resonance)-assisted devices according to their guiding and monitoring methods. Transrectal devices are exclusively used for the treatment of prostate pathology. There are two widely used clinical devices manufactured by companies in France (Ablatherm® HIFU system; EDAP, Vaulx-en-Velin) and the United States (Sonablate® 500 system; Focus Surgery, Inc., Indianapolis, IN). Both systems are guided and monitored by US imaging modalities.

Extracorporeal devices are relatively more versatile in application than transrectal. They can be used for benign or malignant pathology of the uterus, breast, liver, kidney, pancreas, thyroid, testis, extremities, and other organs where US can be delivered through an external surface of the human body. Clinically available extracorporeal HIFU devices have been developed by several companies in China (HAIFU System; Chongqing HIFU Technology, Co., Ltd., Chongqing, HIFU Tumor Therapy System; China Medical Technologies, Inc., Beijing, CZ901 HIFU System; Mianyang Sonic Electronic, Sichuan) and Israel (Exablate® 2000; InSightec, Haifa). Devices from China are US-assisted and those from Israel are MR-assisted. All Chinese devices utilize one or two single-element therapeutic transducers with an imaging transducer incorporated in their center. The transducers are spherically-curved so as to focus US waves to their geometrical focus and the area is mechanically manipulated in order to aim the US waves to the target spot. It has to be noted that the geometrical focus does not always coincide with the real beam focus at which the US intensity has its maximum. On the other hand, the MR-assisted device from Israel uses a phased-array transducer with approximately 200 elements that enables electronic manipulation of a focal zone within specific ranges. This range of focusing is complemented by the piezoelectric servo-motor system that also enables mechanical manipulation of the transducer.

6.3.4.0 Results of clinical studies

The clinical uses of HIFU therapy have been increasingly concentrated on treating tumors. The accessibility of US beams to the target organ is the most important determinant of whether or not HIFU therapy can be applied.

Prostate cancer has the longest history of clinical use of HIFU, therefore, many clinical studies have been performed on it. All of the clinical studies have been carried out with transrectal US-assisted equipment. FUS for early-stage, localized prostate cancer has been comparable to surgery in terms of local control, disease-free survival, and complication rates. The cumulative 5-year disease-free survival rates range from 68-78%. However, prospective randomized controlled trials have not been performed to date. FUS has also proven to be effective in the control of recurrent prostate cancer after an external beam radiation therapy.

The uterus provides a good target for FUS treatment because it is static and located close to the abdominal wall. Most clinical studies on uterine leiomyoma have been done with MR-assisted HIFU devices. It is the only disease entity that is approved by the FDA for treatment using this device at the time of writing this manuscript. FUS has been shown to be effective in controlling symptomatic uterine leiomyomas. Targeted symptom reduction rates have been reported to be 71% at six months and 51% at 12 months. However, the volume reduction rate of the tumors was not satisfactory (13.5% at 6 months). Neoadjuvant use of GnRH (gonadotropin releasing hormone) turned out to improve both the symptom control rate (83% at 6 months, 89% at 12 months) and the volume reduction rate (21% at 6 months, 37% at 12 months).

The breast is also a superficial and static organ. However, because of the difficulties in treating the axillary lymph nodes, the clinical application of HIFU therapy for breast cancer has been limited. The feasibility as a first line therapy has not been studied to date; only its local control rate has been evaluated (the local tumor progression rate 9.1%).

The liver, especially the right lobe, is not a suitable organ for the application of FUS because of the large respiratory excursions and the sonic shadowing caused by the ribs. Therefore, most clinical studies have been carried out on palliative applications rather than for curative purposes. FUS has proven to be effective in lengthening the survival of patients with advanced hepatocellular carcinomas in combination with transcatheter arterial chemoembolization. Liver cancer is a great prey of interventional oncologists. In order to overcome these problems, techniques utilizing FUS, which forms an excellent noninvasive weapon, are being investigated by researchers and manufacturers.

Pancreatic cancer is also a promising field for the palliative application of FUS. In one study, 100% of the patients experienced resolution of back-pain after the treatment. The effects of FUS on primary and metastatic renal cancers, malignant bone tumors, soft tissue sarcomas, testicular tumors, and brain tumors also have been evaluated and most have found application for palliative purposes useful.

6.3.5.0 Limitations and Future Works

Major differences of HIFU therapy from other interventional therapeutic modalities are its complete non-invasiveness and sharp, tailorable treatment margins, which may lead to treatments with very low complication rates. However, several complications have been known to occur after HIFU therapy. These are mostly due to high-energy US waves reflected on gas or bony structures. Skin-burn can be caused by poor acoustic coupling between the skin and the therapeutic window (e.g. poor shaving) or a previous operation scar. In cases of liver treatment, reflected US waves on ribs can induce overlying soft tissue damage including the skin. Gas-containing bowel loops act in the same manner and can cause thermal injury of the bowel wall. Sciatic nerve injury was also reported after HIFU therapy for uterine leimyoma. This complication is deemed to be caused either directly by high-energy US waves that pass the focal therapeutic zone or indirectly by elevated temperatures of the pelvic bone. If the focal zone is located superficially as in case of breast cancer, direct thermal injury of overlying skin can occur. Likewise, internal organs just anterior or posterior to the focal zone could be injured.

In addition to these complications, HIFU therapy at the time of writing this manuscript, has displayed several other limitations, which are hampering the effective use of this modality in clinical practice. These include a long procedure time, difficulty in targeting and monitoring moving organs, sonic shadowing by bones or gas in bowels, and the relatively high cost of this technique in relation to its effectiveness and limitations. However, recent technological advances are expected to resolve these problems. One example is the new MR-assisted HIFU device under development, which adopts the technique of an automatic on-line, spatiotemporal temperature control using a multispiral trajectory of the focal point and proportional, integral and derivative principles. This system claims to be able to make a thermal lesion faster and more stably under real-time thermal monitoring even in moving organs than the existing devices.

6.4.0.0 What is SPDT, PDT?

The following was taken from: http://www.prostate90.com/prostate_cancer/Metastasis.htm Accessed 6-15-09.

Whats onc, Photo Dynamic Therapy, SPDT?

Sonic Photo Dyanamic Therapy (SPDT) has evolved in 2005, from years of improving PhotoDynamic Therapy (PDT) which has been around since the 1900s, very successful, but limited by agents that were not very selective for cancer cells, very toxic, essentially Chemo.

Recently, about 1996, non-toxic agents have been developed of mainly algae/chlorophyll moving PDT into a whole new realm of healing. PDT involves getting an agent into the body, (originally by injection, **now orally**), which adheres to cancer cells, so that when light of the correct frequency is applied, **the agent "explodes" into free radical oxygen, instantly killing the cancer cells which cannot survive in oxygen**. "Rather than using a scalpel, you're using light and a molecule that then reacts with the cells," *Wired Magazine 4-07,* An older, very detailed explanation of Photodynamic Therapy, it's history and successes, is in Scientific American, January, 2003, New Light on Medicine, by N. Lane.

For total and permanent recovery, it is still necessary to address the causes and even more important to do complete cleansings of toxins from the body, especially including all the dead cancer cells. PDT is recently approved in the U.S., UK, and has been adopted by the Chinese Government. Experimental projects have recently been published in Toronto, Canada and other countries.

PDT in Australia, under Doctor Tom Cleary, MD, made great strides, during 2005, including extending the treatment period to 2 weeks (from 1 week), improved agents and not discharging any patient until the cancer is gone by every medical measurement. In early 2005, ultrasound treatment and agent were added to reach deeper tumors. Also, it has become clear that **some cancer cells die faster with sonic vibrations than light**, so patients have responded even more quickly. The result for patients, is more complete recovery, faster, with no pain or discomfort, save a "tiredness" as the cancer cells die off. So it is a very successful non drug, non invasive treatment for prostate, breast and other cancers, without any unpleasant or harmful side effects.

This from, Dr. Douglas Mitchell, Chairman, of the Opal Clinic, Melbourne, a Scientist of Distinction, PhD Chemistry, University Chancellor, and formerly a research director in the New York State Department of Health, for 15 years:

"Since 2002, Dr Tom Cleary, MD, now Chief Medical Officer at the Opal Clinic in Melbourne, Australia, has been treating cancer patients using photodynamic therapy (PDT). His PDT technology is to administer orally, a highly selective photosensitizer, a chlorophyll like substance which is selectively taken up by cancer cells. The patient is then treated with red and infra-red light to activate the photosensitizer and produce **free radical oxygen. This attacks and kills cancer cells.** This is a systemic (whole body) therapy which attacks cancer wherever it is in the body. Beginning early this year, (2006), he used a much more aggressive treatment protocol than before, and this dramatically improved results. Equally good results are reported by two clinics in China using the same technology.

His latest improvement incorporates ultra sound to activate a sensitizer, a technique called **sonodynamic therapy (SDT).** The **sonic sensitizer, another chlorophyll derivative**, has impeccable safety credentials, and is also designed to be selectively taken up by cancer cells. **It responds to ultra sound, producing free radical oxygen** and hence attacking cancer cells. The body is much more transparent to ultra sound than to light, so this improves performance with deep tumors. **Research shows that the two techniques together are better than either alone. The combined therapy is particularly effective in killing metastases,** something which is very difficult to do with conventional cancer therapies. Both treatments are painless, with minimal side effects. The most common side effect is tiredness, which is understandable as the treatment is killing tumors.

We are seeing fantastic results. Of our last ten patients, one had a grade I cancer, one grade III, and eight grade IV. Four are now clear of cancer, and five others report major health improvements (they are still being treated). One patient has mesothelioma, lung cancer and lymphoma. He reports that his night coughing has stopped and he sleeps better, breathing is not as painful and he can now inhale deeply. He has had "an amazing increase in energy ". Patients with mesothelioma, let alone mesothelioma and lung cancer, rarely get any benefits at all from any treatment.

Failures? Only one. A patient with a grade IV breast cancer with liver metastases failed to respond to the PDT, but she chose not to have the sonodynamic therapy."

Five of six recent prostate cancer patients, have had complete recovery, no symptoms, normal markers. The failed one was moribund, in very poor general health, PSA 9000, died of other causes, in retrospect, should not have been treated.

Working with the Chineese clinics, due to their 1000s of patients and complete latitude to experiment, **the intensity of the Ultrasound was increased In December 2005, by a magnitude of 12, and another 12 in 2006**, which has dramatically improved overall results, especially on deeper tumors. This is true of all the above clinics, all of which work with Dr D J Burke, MD, of Harvard Medical School.

Dr. Cleary, now heads the Xytos clinic as Medical Director. I have worked personally with Dr Cleary, for several years, first in his native Ireland and know him to be a very caring, conservative, wonderfully creative physician. Even more important are the major successful results I see him achieve with patients. I personally did the treatment in its then evolution, in Ireland in 2001 and again in 2006, at Xytos, to very successfully repair sun damage from 35 years of daily exposure in the Hawaiian Sun. I can recommend this treatment, now SPDT, without any reservation to those in need. **It is not a panacea,** however, you will need to be coached in eliminating the cancer causes and necessary detoxing in preparation for and follow-up of the treatment. Successful detoxing determines the success of long range healing.

The Dove Clinic, under Dr Julian Kenyon MD MB ChB, has now been approved in the UK, attesting to its many successes, in recent years.

The Rapha Clinic, under Dr. Anthony Jimenez, MD, Dr. Larry Clapp, PhD, and 6 other MDs, has a very comprhensive residential and take home SPDT protocol, complemented with Daily Songrams, Massage (including prostate), Biological Dental work, 3 major detox protocols, daily conferences with physicians and staff, all in a very homey oceanfront clinic, **in Playas**, a small Beach town. **Patients are met at San Diego airport and driven to the clinic, about a 20 minute drive.**

SPDT has reached a level of maturity and wide acceptance around the World, as a safe, very effective, cancer treatment, **void of harmful side effects.** When combined with addressing the causes and thorough detoxing we have seen patients have miraculous, complete recovery from cancers, including, "fatal" metastases.

When patients come to us wanting a high success rate, Non-Invasive treatment for prostate and other cancers, including metastases we are able to refer them to an increasing number of successful clinics, around the World, performing very advanced SPDT therapies:

1) Xytos.Clinic, located in Indianapolis, IN, FDA Approved,. 2 week stay, $100,000 + travel and lodging in local hotels. (Currently, not taking patients.)

2) Opal Clinic, located in Melbourne, Australia, 2 week stay, $50,000 + travel and lodging in local hotels.

3) Dove Clinic, located in England, UK Approved, 2 week stay, $40,000 + travel and lodging in local hotels.

4) Rapha Clinic, located in Playas, Mexico, 8 day stay, $30,000 including food & lodging, in the Ocean Front clinic, with optional take home treatment package for up to 6 months continued treatments at home.

A recent SPDT patient, Ben Sharp, was re-biopsied with a verdict of "no cancer" by Dr. Duke Bahn, MD, a very thorough Radiologist-Urologist, after a 10 year struggle with prostate cancer.

Dr. Thomas Cleary, MD will be working with patients in the clinic, May 7 to May 21, 2007. Dr. Cleary has the most experience treating cancer patients, with SPDT, since 2000, having been Medical Director in Ireland, Melbourne, and Xytos, in Indianapolis, (not currently taking patients). Dr. Cleary also has worked with Dr/ General Wong, treating 1000s of cancer patients, in China.

Limited appointments are available by email to info@hope4cancer.com or info@prostate90.com or calling 619-572-4060.

6.5.0.0 Light Therapy Spares the Scalpel and the Chemo

Cyrus Farivar. (*Wired Magazine*, 04.02.07)

Imagine you could treat cancer by taking a pill, then directing a laser light toward the location of the tumor. The growth would dissolve with no chemotherapy, and no harm to healthy tissue.

It might sound futuristic, but a **select number of cancer patients already benefit from the method, called photodynamic therapy**. An upgrade for the procedure could save thousands more cancer patients from the horrors of chemotherapy.

"It's an approach that I really like," said Karen Brewer, a professor of chemistry at Virginia Tech and lead author of the research on **04.02.07** at the American Chemical Society annual conference in Chicago. "We stand to make a really major improvement, instead of trying to treat one new kind of tumor or make the patient a little less sick."

Although chemotherapy has improved over the past decade, the treatment still damages healthy tissue and causes other unpleasant side effects like nausea and a weakened immune system. The researchers hope their work will spare patients from chemo's ravages and even the surgery usually necessary to remove a tumor.

"Rather than using a scalpel, you're using light and a molecule that then reacts with the cells," said William Phelps, scientific program director at the American Cancer Society.

The new treatment, however, still needs to be tested head to head with the current version of photodynamic therapy, Phelps said.

The technique starts with a compound called a photosensitizer, a type of molecule that latches itself onto a tumor and when exposed to focused light **excites oxygen, destroying the tumor cells. The treatment's reliance on oxygen, however, has been a limitation because smaller, newer tumors don't contain any**.

The new technology gets around the problem by killing the tumor with "supramolecules" -- large molecular assemblies that act as anti-cancer fighting forces. The supramolecules deliver the drug directly to the tumor's DNA -- a process known as **DNA cleavage**.

Once the drug (the set of supramolecules) is ingested (or in the case of skin cancer, applied as a cream), a light (usually from fiber optics or a laser) focused on the site of the tumor activates the DNA cleavage.

"This has a distinct virtue of being able to get the tumor before it's generated its own blood supply," said Brian Storrie, a professor of physiology and biophysics at the University of Arkansas for Medical Sciences.

But what if a tumor is inside the body, such as on the liver or other internal organs? As anyone who has played with a red laser pointer knows, **red light can permeate human tissue.** So **red or infrared light can reach some, but not all, tumors.** "Research is certainly underway to work on better light delivery methods," Brewers said. **I believe that this illustrates the advances of the Howes Singlet Oxygen Cancer system, in which hypochlorite and peroxide are used to generate singlet oxygen by injection.**

Brewer has performed tests using her technique on raw DNA, cell cultures and E-coli. She and her associates will begin tests on horses "any day now," because **horse skin cancer is remarkably similar to human skin cancer. I need to contact LSU vet. School and try to get permission to do some studies with my system.**

6.6.0.0 New light on medicine

The following was excerpted from: Scientific American. New light on medicine. Nick Lane. Pg. 38-45. Jan. 2003.

Chlorophyll, the plant pigment that absorbs the energy of sunlight in photosynthesis, is a porphyrin, as is heme, which is at the heart of the oxygen-transporter protein hemoglobin and of many enzymes vital for life, including cytochrome oxidase (which generates energy by transferring electrons to oxygen in a critical step of cellular respiration).

Porphyrins orchestrate the two most critical energy-generating processes of life: photosynthesis and oxygen respiration.

Porphyria arises because of a flaw in the body's heme-making machinery. The body produces heme and other porphyrins in a series of eight coordinated stages, each catalyzed by a separate enzyme. **Iron is added at the end to make heme**. In porphyria, one of the steps does not occur, leading to a backlog of the intermediate compounds produced earlier in the sequence. The body has not evolved to dispose of these intermediates efficiently, so it dumps them, often in the skin. The intermediates do not damage the skin directly, but many of them cause trouble indirectly. Metal-free porphyrins (as well as metalloporphyrins containing metals that do not interact with the porphyrin ring) can become excited when they absorb light at certain wavelengths; their electrons jump into higher-energy orbitals. The molecules can then transmit their excitation to other molecules having the right kind of bonds, especially oxygen, to produce reactive singlet oxygen and other highly reactive and destructive molecules known as free radicals. Metal-free porphyrins, in other words, are not the agents, but rather the brokers, of destruction. They catalyze the production of toxic forms of oxygen.

Photosensitive reactions are not necessarily harmful. Their beneficial effects have been known since ancient times. In particular, some seeds and fruits contain photosensitive chemicals (photosensitizers) called psoralens, which indirectly led scientists to experiment with porphyrins. Psoralens have been used to treat skin conditions in Egypt and India for several thousand years. They were first incorporated into modern medicine by Egyptian dermatologist Abdel Monem El Mofty of Cairo University, just over 50 years ago, when he began treating patients with vitiligo (a disease that leaves irregular patches of skin without pigment) and, later, those with psoriasis using purified psoralens and sunlight. When activated by light, psoralens react with DNA in proliferating cells to kill them.

Two American dermatologists, Aaron B. Lerner of Yale University and Thomas B. Fitzpatrick of Harvard University, were struck by the potential of psoralens. In the 1960s they showed that psoralens are activated by ultraviolet (UVA) rays, and the researchers later refined psoralen therapy using an ultraviolet lamp similar to those used in solariums today. Their method became known as **PUVA (short for psoralen with UVA) and is now one of the most effective treatments for psoriasis and other skin conditions.**

Thomas Dougherty's idea was the beginning of true photodynamic therapy, in which photosensitizers catalyze the production of oxygen free radicals. It was built on earlier work, which revealed two medically useful properties of the porphyrins: they accumulate selectively in cancer cells and are activated by red light, which penetrates more deeply into biological tissues than do shorter wavelengths, such as blue light or UVA.

The ideal drug to treat cancer would be not only potent and highly selective for tumors but also broken down quickly into harmless compounds and excreted from the body. This is exactly what my singlet oxygen delivery system does!

The first photosensitizing drug to fulfill most of the stringent criteria for potency and efficacy without causing photosensitivity, verteporfin (Visudyne), was approved in April 2000 by the FDA not to treat of cancer at all but to prevent blindness. As the theories converged with reality, researchers came to realize that **PDT can do far more than destroy tumors, such as treat adult macular degeneration and arterial plaques**.

Red light penetrates no more than a few centimeters into biological tissues

6.6.1.0 Down's syndrome

Trisomy 21, or Down Syndrome, is the most common genetic cause of learning disability in the UK, affecting 1 in 1000 live births. Neuronal depletion and structural abnormalities of the brain are seen even in infants with Down syndrome. Why the changes occur isn't fully understood, but **it has been suspected that the damage to the neural cells is caused by an increased activity of superoxide dismutase** that occurs in children with Down syndrome, **which increases concentrations of hydrogen peroxide**.

The presence of damaging superoxide dismutase led to a belief that high levels of antioxidants may reduce the effects of Down syndrome, improving language and psychomotor development. **Previous studies have investigated the effects of folate and antioxidants, with no significant effect being found.** However, due to commercial marketing claiming substantial benefits, many parents of children with Down syndrome give their children specialized vitamin and mineral supplements.

A study published by the British Journal of Medicine, finds that such supplements do not help. UK researchers studied the effect of specialized supplements on 156 babies under 7 months old with Down syndrome. The children were assessed for development after an 18 month period, and the researchers found that **the supplements made no difference.** This is important information for parents to consider before giving such supplements to their child, as there are potentially adverse effects from high doses of vitamins and minerals (February 2008. British Medical Journal).

6.6.2.0 Down's have lower risk of tumors, atherosclerosis and diabetic retinopathy

Health benefits of Down syndrome include greatly reduced incidence of many common malignancies except leukemia and testicular cancer — although it is, as yet, unclear whether the reduced incidence of various fatal cancers among people with Down syndrome is as a direct result of tumor-suppressor genes on chromosome 21 (such as Ets2), because of reduced exposure to environmental factors that contribute to cancer risk, or some other as-yet unspecified factor. In addition to **a reduced risk of most kinds of cancer, people with Down syndrome also have a much lower risk of hardening of the arteries and diabetic retinopathy**. (Yang

Q, Rasmussen SA, Friedman JM. Mortality associated with Down's syndrome in the USA from 1983 to 1997: a population-based study. *Lancet* 2002 23 March;359(9311):1019–25).

(http://www.answers.com/topic/down-syndrome.Accessed 7-21-09.) **(RMH Note: I believe that Down's patients have lower rates of cancer, diabetes and atherosclerosis is due to the increased activity of SOD on chromosome 21 and the subsequent production of hydrogen peroxide, an EMOD.This is a very important observation).**

6.6.3.0 Free Radicals and Kundalini

The following was taken from: http://biologyofkundalini.com/article.php?story=FreeRadicalsandKundalini

Longevity = *maximum ATP (energy) with a minimum of free radical production*

Free radicals are reactive oxygen molecules that have lost an electron in interactions with other molecules.As a result, these molecules are extremely unstable and they race around stealing electrons from other molecules creating more free radicals in the process, damaging cell components. Free radicals are produced by normal cellular processes, and the majority are produced during the production of ATP in the mitochondria. Other normal cellular enzymatic processes create free radicals include phagocytosis, inflammation, in prostaglandin synthesis, in the cytochrome P450 system and in reactions involving iron and other transition metals. Free radicals are also created from: exercise, sunlight, cigarette smoke, alcohol, pesticides, air pollution, stress, electromagnetic radiation.

The body produces several free radical quenching enzymes as its first line of defense.They are superoxide dismutase (SOD), catalase, and glutathione peroxidase. Additionally the body uses antioxidant vitamins, minerals and substances found in food to counteract free radicals. **Half the protein produced in the body every day is enzymes and our endogenous antioxidant Superoxide dismutase is the fifth most abundant protein in the body.**

Bacteria produce SOD and other vitamins like biotin and B12. Chlorine in drinking water, birth control pills, other steroids, antibiotics and even negative thinking will reduce intestinal bacteria and promote candida yeast growth.Thus the hormonal swings that are inevitable with kundalini awakenings could promote intestinal conditions that interfere with the body's free radical defense system.

There is an increase of free radical production in the body during metamorphosis because of increased hormone and neurotransmitter use and breakdown, increased metabolism and nerve energy flow, increased oxygen and glucose consumption, increased immune function, the increase breakdown and growth of cells, increase in stress hormone production and the impairment of normal digestion due to sympathetic-nervous-system hyperactivation. All these factors raise the free radical load on the bodymind during active kundalini. Free radicals overtax the immune system and keep it so busy fighting the breakdown of the body's own cells that it cannot fight off viruses, microbes, and infections that attack it from without. **(RMH Note: This is incorrect. It is the EMODs which protect us from pathogens and neoplasia.)**

It is likely that we will be stressed during an awakening in experiencing the extreme chemistry and expanded levels of perception. Having a spiritual practice would reduce this secondary stress by making us more adapted to changes in the autonomic nervous system and state. This stress would further over-excite the body and produce a flow of free radicals. High levels of cortisol cause cells to shift from maintenance to energy creation. Even muscle tissue is broken down for use as fuel during fight or flight chemistry. Also the breakdown of cortisol and adrenaline produces free radicals. Stress therefore is synonymous with oxidative damage.

How well we weather a kundalini crisis is partly determined by our antioxidant reserves, our blood-sugar/glycation history and our mineral and enzyme reserves. If our protein structures are strong and we have strong free radical defenses, then extra energy can pass through our system without excess friction or damage. Glucose is burned in the powerhouses of the cells, known as mitochondria to generate 90% of the energy used in the cell. Free radicals and ROS are created as toxic waste in this process. Consider also that since greater energy is generated and used during an awakening the numbers of mitochondria must correspondingly increase. The faster oxygen is used to burn glucose, the faster free radicals are produced as toxic waste.

The brain is susceptible to free radical damage due to the high content of polyunsaturated fats and high mitochondrial content. Levels of vitamin C in the brain are 50 times higher than elsewhere in the body to protect brain tissue and neurotransmitters from oxidation. (RMH Note: the high concentration of vitamin C may be for the production of hydrogen peroxide, just as seen with IV megadoses of ascorbate in

the treatment of cancer). The free radical damage to proteins in neurons reduces their efficiency. Raising antioxidant levels not only allows damaged proteins to repair, but increases neurotransmitter levels as well. Preventing morbid down swings or permanent neurological damage from kundalini awakening is a matter of increasing our ability to cope with these higher levels of free radicals.

To protect the brain from free radical damage during the heightened nerve flow we need to take hydrophobic (water repelling) antioxidants like pine bark, vitamin C-Ester and alpha lipoic acid, as the blood brain barrier is impervious to hydrophilic (water loving) substances. We must aim to get more antioxidant protection into the cerebrospinal fluid.

One way of interpreting the die-off being that it is a temporary collapse in which our ability to cope with the free radical oxidation load, specifically in the mitochondria of the nerves and the tissue in general. This overload often forces complete bed rest until the body's free radical defenses win out and the bodymind can begin to reinstate normal functioning. The average die-off therefore takes 3-5 days for this recuperation to occur. The shock and die-off phase of awakening constitutes a free radical oxidation crisis that we can attempt to adapt to by increasing antioxidant intake and upping our stress reduction techniques at this time.

Die-offs however should not be prevented because they are needed to dissolve the present structure and make way for the new. Thus die-off is an "essential" part of the process, however we do not have to be set back and regress if we know how to successfully weather these changes. If we have adequate mineral, enzyme and antioxidant reserves we will be able to weather the catabolic stages without complete collapse and damage, to achieve a higher level of resurrection. Once we intimately know the process of biological transmutation we can achieve a greater adaptation and higher-homeostasis.

Free radical interference with the ability of mitochondria to produce energy is no doubt implicated in various periods of intense **fatigue** that often accompany kundalini awakening. This must be one of the many processes occurring during the die-off period, when free radical overload is at max. The fatigue periods could also be brought on by free radical interference with nerve transmission. For serious fatigue situations try B-complex vitamins, alpha-lipoic acid, Co Q10 or Idebenone and magnesium along with NADH.

When there is inadequate exogenous and indigenous antioxidants cellular decay and ageing occurs. In fact the decline in faculty that occurs with age is largely because free radicals interfere with the messages transmitted by neurotransmitters, thus affecting reflexes, organ regulation, muscle contractions, blood flow, memory and learning ability. This is why the concentration of vitamin C in the central nervous system, the brain and spinal cord, is 50 times greater than in other tissues of the body.

Despite their destructive power, free radicals are in fact used by the body for useful purposes. Their killing power is used by the white blood cells to destroy invading organisms. Ironically it is the free radicals that the macrophages use in their fight against arterial cholesterol which kills them and turns them to foam cells thus producing arteriosclerosis. Free radicals also play a role in the synthesis of major biomolecules--proteins, carbohydrates, lipids and nucleic acids and in the detoxification of chemicals inside organelles in the interior of cells. Free radical reactions play a part in the generation of cellular energy in the mitochondria. So you see that **free radicals are indispensable to life,** but they need to be managed so that their usefulness outweighs their destruction.

Billions of free radicals are being produced in the body at any time. Our attitude and state of mind can actually contribute to our level of oxidative damage. For example each molecule of adrenaline produces two oxygen radicals as it metabolizes in the body, therefore too much stress can increase our oxidation damage and overwork our immune system. Stress also increases our endorphin production which in turn suppresses our nervous, immune and hormonal systems.

One of the best ways we can counter and overcome the stress in our lives is through regular exercise. However not all exercise is good for fighting the free radical war. In fact excessive exercise for which the body is not prepared for can actually cause extensive oxidative damage. Free radical production goes up during exhausting, high intensity workouts and such free radical activity is associated with oxidative damage in the muscles, liver, blood and other tissues. Hence at the heaviest training levels there is increased susceptibility to cancer, heart attacks, cataracts, premature aging and decreased immunity. **Some of the reasons why there is increased free radical damage during exercise are: the consumption of oxygen goes up 10-20 times, there is an increased output of Superoxide radicals by mitochondria**, there is oxygen deprivation from the increased demand by tissues and the bodies antioxidant defenses are over burdened. There is an increase in free radical production in both excess oxygen and lack of oxygen conditions.

Regular lower intensity exercise minimizes the production of free radicals while strengthening the indigenous antioxidants and enzymes. Without regular exercise the body's internal defenses against free radicals (SOD, GSH, Catalase) may become too fragile for the antioxidants in our food and supplements to have their full affect. Sedentary people are twice as likely to get cancer and heart disease as active individuals. Trained muscles are resistant to oxidative damage because of the increased supply of the bodies own antioxidants. Regular training prepares the bodymind to better handle unexpected physical and emotional stresses and strains. That is exercise builds up our resistance to free radical damage from all stressors. Fast walking at the pace of 12-15 minutes per mile is ideal for returning optimum endurance benefits, without creating excess free radicals and damaging tissues. Fast walking can be as effective as jogging without the risk of injury. To strengthen our endogenous free radical defenses we need to do at least 30 continuous minutes of brisk walking three times a week. Besides this we also need to do some weight bearing strengthening exercise and some stretching as well. By maintaining strength and subtly we prevent the aches, pains and free radicals that come from physical stress to an unconditioned body.

Free radicals do most of their damage to the outer layer of the cell because free radicals are drawn to areas that have the greatest density of molecules, hence the richest source of electrons. And since the *cell membrane* has the greatest concentration of molecules, it would be the primary target of the free radical. Since the outer portion of the cell is mostly fat, we need fat-soluble antioxidants to protect our cell membranes. So along with stable (non-reactive) fat intake you will also need to have a good supply of **fat soluble antioxidants** to protect the cell membranes such as Vitamin C ÔEster,' Alpha Lipoic Acid, DMAE, Vitamin E Tocotrienol, CoQ10, Acetyl L-Carnitine, Glutathione, NADH, Pycnogenol, Propolis.

Free radical damage to the cell membranes causes dehydration of the interior of the cells and edema or fluid collecting outside of the cells. Once the cell membrane becomes damaged by free radicals, it becomes unable to let nutrients in and wastes out. Wastes and salts, such as potassium, begin to take up increasing amounts of space within the cell. As a result the cell's water supply is pushed out, and the cell becomes dehydrated.

The sleep hormone **Melatonin is a major physiological antioxidant (and hormone) by directly reacting with hydroxyl and peroxyl radicals, or by stimulating the expression of superoxide dismutase, glutathione peroxidase, or glutathione reductase**. Melatonin has also been reported to inhibit nitric oxide synthetase.

There is an upcoming cancer cure that uses Vitamin C + Vitamin K in a specific ratio to create an oxidation environment that essentially blows up cancer cells. It can get rid of cancerous growths within one month. Vitamin C on the micro-level acts as an antioxidant, but combined with Vit K on the macro-level it oxidizes the cancer cell membranes and destroys their DNA.

6.6.4.0 TOP ANTIOXIDANT FOODS

- **Oxygen radical Absorbency Capacity or ORAC's:**
    - *Fruit:* Prunes 5770, Raisins 2830, Wolf berries 3472, Vitamin E oil 3309, Pomegranates 3037, Blueberries 2400, Blackberries 2036, Strawberries 1540.
    - *Vegetables:* Kale 1770, Spinach 1260, Brussel Sprouts 980, Alfalfa Sprouts 930, Broccoli 890.
- ***Other antioxidant substances are:*** Fresh raw fruit and vegetables are loaded with antioxidants. The fruits highest in antioxidants are blueberries and other berries and kiwifruit. Brewers yeast, bioflavonoids, pycnogenol, Co enzyme 10, hydergine,
    - PABA, RNA, BNT, BHA, Choline, Inositol, B_1, B_5, B_6, B_{15}, L-Dopa, Amino acids: NAC (N-acetyl-cysteine), L-methionine, L-glutathione.
- ***Antioxidant herbs include:*** Gingko, Rosemary, Chaparral, Astragalus, Ligustrum, Garlic, Shiitake mushrooms, Echinacea, Schizandra, Bilberry and Green Tea. In fact Green tea contains an antioxidant EGCG which is believed to be 200 times more powerful at inhibiting lipid peroxidation than Vitamin E.
- **NADH** -- NADH is an activated form of the B vitamin niacin and is the body's most powerful antioxidant. NADH increases overall energy, boosts the immune system, protects cells from damage and improves memory. NADH is the reduced (electron- energy rich) coenzyme form of vitamin B3, while NAD is the oxidized (burned) coenzyme form of B3. The molecular structure of NADH is a vitamin B3 (niacinamide) combined with a ribose (5-carbon sugar), a phosphate group and an adenine nucleotide (a DNA component).

Mitochondria produce the NADH necessary for the Oxidative Phosphorylation of food stuffs into ATP. **It is NADH, which captures the electrons thrown off during Krebs' cycle oxidation and shuttles them to the electron transport side chain energy production cycle.** Whether it is produced internally within the cell or enters the body from a dietary supplement, NADH will trigger increased cellular energy production. Energy is stored in the NADH molecule, and when it reacts with oxygen, energy is produced in the form of ATP. One NADH molecule leads to the formation of three ATP molecules. In addition NADH creates more energy when it reacts with oxygen and water forming nicotinamide (also known as vitamin B3) and ADP.

Free radicals interfere with cellular energy production by destroying enzymes and mitochondria. NADH is a high-energy hydrogen that occurs naturally in all our cells. NADH transfers the Hydrogen to oxidized (or damaged) glutathione to restore normal glutathione, and it can regenerate other important antioxidants as well. In the nucleus of the cell there is only one compound that can activate the nucleus DNA repair system: that compound is NADH. The better the DNA repair system functions the better our protection from chronic diseases such as cancer, arthritis, arteriosclerosis and immunodeficiencies.

The brain must produce and use 20% of the body's total ATP production in order to maintain normal function; depression reflects a lowering of the brain's energy status. Through its multiple roles in producing ATP energy, NADH energizes the brain thereby reducing depression, seizure and psychosis. Besides increasing brain energy NADH also increases the neurotransmitters dopamine and noradrenaline, which along with serotonin are frequently diminished during depression (brain cells use dopamine to make noradrenaline). And since NADH's spares tryptophan, more tryptophan is available for conversion to serotonin. For depression take NADH along with DL Phenylalinine, tyrosine and tryptophan or 5-HTP

NADH can be made in the liver and other cells from vitamin B3, so rather than the expensive activated form you could just take 50-100mg of vitamin B3 per day. NADH can also be made from the amino acid L-Tryptophan using 60mg tryptophan for 1mg B3. Tryptophan being the precursor to serotonin.

This book is a companion andcompliment to my other books on this subject. Please check out all of them at www.amazon.com.

www.ingramcontent.com/pod-product-compliance
Lightning Source LLC
Chambersburg PA
CBHW080226180526
45167CB00006B/2230

* 9 7 8 1 4 9 7 4 5 0 4 1 7 *